GLUTE LAB

The Art and Science of Strength and Physique Training

BRET CONTRERAS, PhD
and **GLEN CORDOZA**

Victory Belt Publishing Inc.

Victory Belt Publishing Inc.

ISBN-13: 978-1628603-46-0

This book is for educational purposes. The publisher and authors of this instructional book are not responsible in any manner whatsoever for any adverse effects arising directly or indirectly as a result of the information provided in this book. If not practiced safely and with caution, working out can be dangerous to you and others. It is important to consult with a professional fitness instructor before beginning training. It is also important to consult with a physician prior to training due to the intense and strenuous nature of the techniques outlined in this book.

Cover and Interior design by Charisse Reyes

Illustrations by Elita San Juan, Crizalie Olimpo, and Charisse Reyes

Photography by Glen Cordoza

Models: Katie Cordoza, Jamie De Revere, and Alex Sterner

Printed in Canada
TC 0622

Table of Contents

Foreword

It's always an honor being asked to write the foreword for a book by someone you respect and admire. It's particularly gratifying for me when that individual is Bret Contreras. There is no one I respect and admire more, both personally and professionally.

Those of you who are fairly new to fitness may not truly appreciate the magnitude of influence that Bret's had on the industry. In fact, it's no exaggeration to state that Bret has changed the way fitness enthusiasts and pros alike approach glute training.

All that's needed to fully comprehend Bret's contribution to the field is a perusal of the exercise literature in the years prior to his arrival on the fitness scene. You'll see that until the late 2000s, virtually every article on glute training advised people to go heavy and hard on squats and deadlifts. The occasional paper might have included a few sets of lunges or stiff-leg deadlifts, but many so-called authority figures were all too quick to dismiss lunges as a "sissy" exercise. To that end, cable kickbacks and the seated hip abduction machine were also for wimps. Bodyweight exercises, banded exercises, single-leg exercises, and high reps in general were regarded as ineffective for enhancing glute development. Back extensions were performed with the intention of targeting the lower back musculature, and the entire category of glute bridges and hip thrusts didn't even exist.

Bret spends the bulk of his days figuring out ways to further evidence-based glute training. No one devotes more time and energy to scouring the relevant literature and then testing out his applied theories in the trenches. Indeed, Bret invented barbell glute bridges, barbell hip thrusts, frog pumps, and nearly every other loaded bridge and thrust variation you can think of. Moreover, he invented glute-dominant back extensions (rounded back and feet turned out), side-lying hip raises, extra-range side-lying hip abductions, and many other popular glute exercises. He popularized turning the foot inward for frontal plane hip abduction exercises, greatly influenced the rise in popularity of mini bands and elastic loops for glute training, and helped make it acceptable to utilize machines, cables, and higher rep ranges for glute growth. Bret also created force vector terminology to differentiate glute exercise categories and aid in program design. The list goes on and on…

Bret's tireless research in the lab and in the gym has revolutionized the way we train glutes today; his reach on the topic spans the globe. While training strategies for the pecs, delts, lats, arms, quads, and hammies haven't changed much over the past few decades, the science and practice of glute training has progressed exponentially thanks to Bret. In the case of the hip thrust, nobody else in the world can be credited for inventing and popularizing an exercise that is now universally performed in fitness facilities on a daily basis. I still get a kick out of the fact that pretty much every time I hit the gym, I see someone performing an exercise that Bret devised. Suffice it to say, you'll never meet anyone as passionate about glutes as Bret Contreras, and I'm proud to have collaborated with him on dozens of published research studies, lay articles, and podcasts.

I know that Bret and Glen worked relentlessly on *Glute Lab* for two years, making sure that it communicates Bret's complete system of glute training in a manner that is easy for the masses to comprehend. Whether you are a personal trainer, strength coach, athlete, physical therapist, or just somebody looking to improve the strength and appearance of your glutes, do yourself a favor and read *Glute Lab;* I guarantee you won't be disappointed.

Yours in Fitness, Brad Schoenfeld, PhD

INTRODUCTION

If you could improve any part of your body, what would it be? For me, it's always been the gluteus maximus, or glutes.* Not because it's the largest muscle in the body or one of the most important. No, I first became fascinated with glutes because I didn't have any.

Long before I was known as the "Glute Guy," I was a skinny, lanky teenager. My flat backside in particular was a constant source of embarrassment. Some guys are shy to talk about it, but we all know that having nice glutes is both attractive and desirable; it's a symbol of health, strength, athleticism, and beauty. But I had nothing.

In high school, I would often overhear girls talking about my friends' butts. They'd say things like, "So-and-so has a nice butt," or, "His butt looks great in those jeans." I often wondered what they said about me. Then one incident, which I'll never forget, made it clear.

I was out golfing with my sister's boyfriend, and at one point I went to swing the club when he said, "You know, Bret, you have no butt." He was drawing a straight, vertical line in the air with his hand: "Your back just goes right into your legs!" I was devastated. He had just called attention to my biggest insecurity. Even worse, I now knew what the girls at school were saying about me. I thought, if this is what my sister's boyfriend thinks, imagine what all of the girls at school are thinking.

This was a turning point for me. Something needed to change. I needed to get glutes.

From then on, I was obsessed with glute training. My underdeveloped backside put me on a quest to find the best training methods and techniques for strengthening and developing the glutes. Now, after 28 years of training, coaching, and experimenting—and getting my PhD and publishing numerous research papers—I've developed the world's first comprehensive glute training system. This book is that system. You will learn why glute training is important, how your glutes function, the critical role they play in your body, and, most importantly, how to design a program and perform techniques that maximize glute development and performance.

But before I delve into the system, I want to share my journey because it explains why and how the system and techniques were developed.

*See page 6

When I use the word *glutes* in this book (and I use this word a lot), I'm actually referring to three gluteal muscles that make up your buttocks: the gluteus maximus, gluteus medius, and gluteus minimus. The names of the gluteals are derived from the Greek word *glutos,* meaning buttocks, and the Latin words *maximus* (great), *medius* (middle), and *minimus* (least). The gluteus maximus is the main muscle. It is the largest of the three and gives the shape and appearance of what we informally call the butt. For this reason, *glutes* refers primarily to the gluteus maximus, but also captures the other two smaller gluteal muscles. In Chapter 5, I describe all three muscles in more detail.

THE QUEST TO ATTAIN GLUTES

When I decided to get glutes, the first thing I did was read all of the bodybuilding magazines and books I could get my hands on. I wanted to learn everything I could about training the glutes. There was just one problem: nobody talked about glute training back then. Bodybuilders had a leg day, and it was assumed that the glutes would develop just fine as long as you included squats and deadlifts in your leg routine. So that is exactly what I did.

For years, I obsessively trained my glutes by squatting, deadlifting, and then eventually performing other leg exercises that worked the glutes, like step-ups and split squats. And it worked for a while. I got stronger, my physique improved, and I felt great. But at a certain point, my glutes stopped developing.

Looking back, there were two reasons for this.

First, my genetics were working against me. It turns out that genetics play a huge role in gluteal development; you will learn more about the role of genetics in Part 2. Some people have never worked out a day in their life and have a perfect butt, while others have to work tirelessly for years to get glutes. I was in the latter category. (If you're like me, don't let your glute genetics get you down. You can still improve your physique, health, and performance with the glute training techniques and programs outlined in this book.)

Second, the squat and the deadlift patterns—though great for building strength and muscle in the lower body—do not work the glutes to the same degree as the quadriceps (quads) and hamstrings (hams): the squat primarily works the quads, while the deadlift primarily works the hamstrings (especially the way I tend to deadlift, with high hips). Sure, multiple muscles are working simultaneously, but there is a dominant muscle powering the movement, one that is contracting to a higher degree than the other muscles.

So my poor glute development was due in part to genetics and the fact that I wasn't performing glute-specific exercises (or, as I refer to them later in this book, *glute-dominant exercises*). At the time, I was ignorant to the role of genetics, but I had learned enough about squatting and deadlifting to know that the glutes were not the primary muscle being worked.

Realizing that I needed to perform more glute-dominant exercises, I looked to the Internet to see what other coaches were doing. This is when I came across the work of Mark Verstegen, Joe DeFranco, Eric Cressey, Mike Robertson, Mike Boyle, and Martin Rooney. They were teaching a ton of glute exercises like glute bridges, bird dogs, and side-lying clams.

Although these were great glute exercises, they were bodyweight and banded movements. To get a good workout, you had to perform a ton of repetitions. In fact, these coaches weren't even using them to build glutes. They were considered low-load activation exercises, meaning that they were used to stimulate the muscles, not strengthen and grow them. For example, these exercises might be used as a warm-up for a workout or as corrective exercises to treat muscular imbalances (one glute that is larger than the other), postural issues (lower back pain), or poor movement patterns (squatting with bad form). They were certainly not being prescribed to build muscle.

It's important to realize that back in those days, everyone thought you had to lift heavy in order to put on muscle. (We now know you can build muscle with high repetitions, which you will learn about in Part 2.) So, when I came across these exercises, I loved them, but I didn't think they would give me the results I was looking for. I wanted bigger and stronger glutes, and to achieve that, I needed to perform a movement that not only targeted the glutes but could also be performed while lifting heavy. From what I could find, such a movement didn't exist.

Then it happened.

It was October 10, 2006. I was watching UFC fights with Jeanne, my girlfriend at the time. Ken Shamrock was facing Tito Ortiz, and I was hoping for a stellar fight. Ortiz had Shamrock pinned, and it looked like it was all but over. Not wanting the match to end just yet, I yelled, "Buck him off, buck him off!"

I suppose I was drawing on childhood memories of wrestling matches with my twin brother, Joel, when I would extend my hips violently in order to gain some wiggle room and get out from under him. (It turns out that this movement, referred to as *bridging,* is a fundamental technique in grappling arts like wrestling and jiu-jitsu.)

Obviously, in professional mixed martial arts, it's not that easy. But I knew bridging was easy from the floor. Then came the light bulb moment. I thought that if I could just add load or weight to the motion along with more range of motion, it would be a great way to strengthen and build muscle in the glutes.

After the match was over, I hurried out to the garage and called for Jeanne to come help me move some equipment around.

"It's 9:30 at night," she said. "I don't feel like doing this right now."

"Fine! I'll do it myself," I replied, as I shimmied the glute ham raise over to the reverse hyper.

After I got the equipment lined up, I draped a bunch of 45-pound plates around my waist with a dip belt and carefully positioned my back on the glute ham developer and my feet on the reverse hyper. Clearly, this is not the proper way to use the equipment. It was sketchy, to say the least.

I slowly bridged my hips up and down for 15 reps. I'd never felt such an intense glute burn in my life. By the fifteenth rep, my glutes were screaming for mercy. For the first time, I felt like my glutes were actually the limiting factor in a glute exercise; the set ended when they were too fatigued to carry out another rep.

When I look back on that moment, I realize that this experiment was as dangerous as it was effective. If those two machines had slipped apart, I easily could have broken my tailbone. But at the time, I wasn't thinking about safety. I knew that I had found a missing link to glute training: a full-range movement that targets the glutes the same way the squat targets the quads and the deadlift targets the hamstrings. What's more, it could be performed with load (weight).

As cheesy as this may sound, after I finished the set, I went out into the front yard, looked up into the sky, and said, "My life is going to change forever. I am going to make it my life's mission to make this exercise popular."

And so the hip thrust was born.

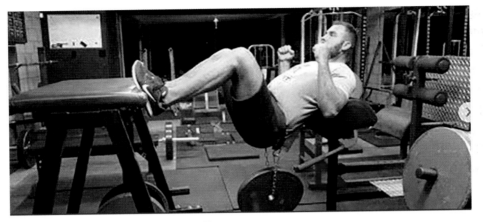

ORIGINAL HIP THRUST CONCEPT

WHAT TO NAME THE EXERCISE?

Upon inventing the hip thrust, I realized that I needed to name the movement. Several options came to mind. I could go the scientific route and call it the "supine bent-leg hip extension," but that seemed too wordy. I could have named it the "American hip extension" to give us an exercise to compete with exercises like the Bulgarian split squat, Nordic ham curl, and Romanian deadlift, but this didn't seem like a good strategy if I was striving for maximum popularity. I could have named it after myself and called it the "Contreras glute lift," but I didn't want the exercise associated with an individual. After contemplating the various options, I decided to go with "hip thrust" simply because that's what the exercise mostly mimicked to me: you're thrusting your hips.

THE THRUST IS A MUST

At this point in my life, I had been lifting weights for 15 years. I had graduated from college, received a master's degree, become a Certified Strength and Conditioning Specialist (CSCS), and worked briefly as a high school math teacher. I loved teaching, but my real passion was personal training. It's all I ever thought about. So, after six years of teaching school, I quit my job and devoted myself full-time to being a personal trainer.

Most of my clients loved glute training, and I was eager to share the hip thrust with them. So the day after that fateful night in the garage, I told my aunt, whom I was training at the time, about the new exercise I had devised. The downfall, I explained, was that getting the weight into place and worming your back up the pad was a huge chore. Moreover, not many people had access to a reverse hyper and a glute ham developer, and even if they did, the gym wouldn't allow them to maneuver them around and monopolize both pieces for a different purpose. It was a great exercise, but the logistics were so complicated that I feared no one would actually do it.

"So invent something," she told me.

To be certain no one had thought of it before me, I spent five days painstakingly searching the web for evidence of the exercise. I tried every pairing of "hip," "glute," "pelvic," "supine," and "floor" with "bridge," "thrust," "lift," and "raise." I also looked through all of the old classic strength training texts.

The only thing I found was an old picture in Mel Siff's and Yuri Verkoshansky's famous 1977 book, *Supertraining,* which depicts elevated bridging variations, but only with manual resistance or a kettlebell dangling from the non-working leg, which I didn't find very practical (or gym appropriate). It looked like I was good to go.

As a former high school math teacher turned personal trainer—and now inventor—I wasn't exactly the world's savviest designer. The earliest model of my machine, which I called the Skorcher, was pretty clunky. It was nearly impossible to adjust, and the padding on it was far from optimal. The subsequent model was a step in the right direction, but it still had drawbacks. To perform the movement with load (weight), for example, two spotters had to load a barbell in place. Nevertheless, it got the job done.

Using the Skorcher, I began incorporating the hip thrust into my clients' programs at my training studio, Lifts, in Scottsdale, Arizona. The results were nothing short of astounding. My clients would tell me things like, "Bret, I'm running faster and my butt is growing, and it's due to the hip thrust. I love it!"

Among all of the glute exercises we did—Bulgarian split squats, step-ups, lunges, squats, deadlifts, RDLs, back extensions, reverse hypers, glute ham raises, and hip thrusts (all of which are featured later in the book)—how could they possibly have known it was the hip thrust?

"When I'm running, I just feel my glutes like I do in the hip thrust. I can tell it's that," they would say.

It was clear that the hip thrust was the real deal. But I needed more than just anecdotal evidence. To earn the respect of fellow coaches and practitioners, I needed science to back it up.

At this time, the most comprehensive experiment on glute training I knew of was an unpublished study by the American Council on Exercise (ACE) from 2006 called "Glutes to the Max." In the experiment, the researchers used electromyography (EMG), which is an instrument that measures muscle activation, to compare the glute activation of several popular lower-body exercises.

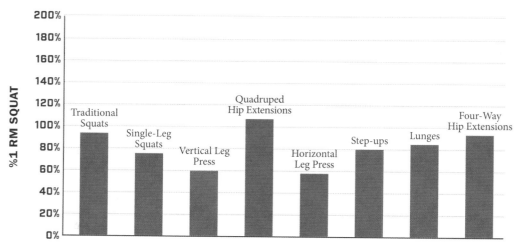

MEAN PEAK MUSCLE ACTIVATION FOR THE GLUTEUS MAXIMUS

ACE Glutes to the Max Experiment

I remembered reading that the biggest manufacturer of EMG equipment was located right in Scottsdale. So, without giving it a second thought, I called them up and ordered my own machine. Fortunately, they were gracious enough to teach me how to use it.

With my new EMG unit, I began testing the glute exercises we did at Lifts on my clients and myself. The initial results were promising. The hip thrust yielded higher levels of gluteal activation than the squat, deadlift, and other common glute training exercises. This is the kind of evidence-based science that I needed to validate the hip thrust as a legit glute-building movement. But then disaster struck.

The economy collapsed, the plaza in which Lifts was located went out of business, and I was forced to close the studio. At the same time, my efforts with investors to mass-produce the Skorcher went south.

My dreams of popularizing and validating the hip thrust as a legitimate strength training exercise and spreading the benefits of glute training would have to wait.

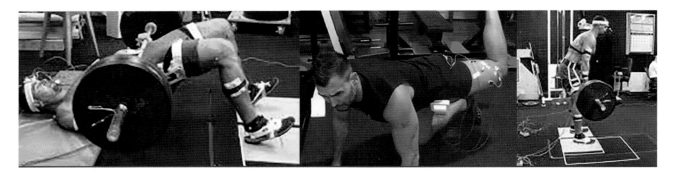

EMG RESEARCH

ENTER THE GLUTE LAB

With Lifts shut down, I needed a new platform to teach my methods. I started BretContreras.com and published everything I had learned about glute training through blog posts and articles. And I never stopped training and coaching. Although I was now training people out of my garage, my client base grew and the system continued to evolve. I experimented with different programs and found new, better ways to perform the hip thrust.

At Lifts, we used the Skorcher for hip thrusts. As I experimented with different ways to perform the hip thrust, it dawned on me that you could perform the exercise with your back braced against a bench. This turned out to be a much more practical approach to the hip thrust, and it is how many people do it today.

Glute training was still in its infancy, however. The strength and conditioning community still considered squats and deadlifts to be the best movements for strengthening and developing the glutes. But I suspected otherwise and set out to prove it.

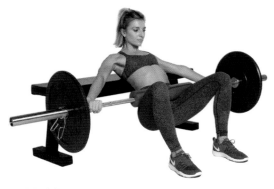

HIP THRUST WITH A BENCH

To spread my ideas, I started writing for popular strength training and bodybuilding websites and magazines. One article in particular, titled "Dispelling the Glute Myth," got some traction. It was written for T-Nation, one of the most well-respected websites for strength coaches, bodybuilders, and powerlifters. The article proposed that the squat and deadlift, though important exercises, were not the best movements for building bigger, stronger glutes.

Those who had been squatting and deadlifting as a primary strategy for developing their glutes had plenty of negative things to say in response. "What do you mean, the squat and deadlift aren't the best exercises for the glutes?! This is how it's been done for years!"

Needless to say, the article and my approach to glute training got people's attention. And while there were those who challenged my ideas, many were intrigued. The evidence was impossible to ignore. People were posting videos of themselves hip thrusting and commenting about how much they felt their glutes working during the exercise. It's worth noting here that you don't always feel your glutes contracting hard when you perform squats and deadlifts. When you hip thrust, on the other hand, you typically feel your glutes contracting to a high degree on every rep, which I will explain in the pages to come.

I believe that this was the turning point for the hip thrust. The movement was now out there, and it was up to the people to decide whether they wanted to include it in their programs and recommend it to others.

Although there was some negative pushback, I understood why some people were upset and closed off. When you devote yourself completely to a subject or idea and then someone comes along and tells you that there is a better way, there tends to be resistance.

I've always done my best to approach training with an open mind. I was lucky to learn this early on in my journey. Moreover, I wasn't discouraged by what people had to say about the hip thrust, because I knew it was not only safe but also effective. And I knew from EMG experiments that the hip thrust activated the glutes to a higher degree than both the squat and the deadlift. This was proof enough for me at the time, but if I wanted to popularize the hip thrust and my glute training methods, I needed even more science to back it up.

The problem was, I had no formal education in strength and conditioning. Sure, I had logged thousands of hours training, coaching, and reading, but that would not be enough. After all, who's going to a listen to a former high school math teacher turned personal trainer?

In order for my ideas to get accepted, I needed more credibility. What's more, I needed a place where I could innovate, test, experiment, and practice.

So, in 2011, I enrolled in the PhD program at the Auckland University of Technology (AUT) under Dr. John Cronin, specializing in biomechanics. As a doctoral student, I learned that quite a bit of research had been done on the glutes, and I devoured all of it. I was a kid in a candy store, totally obsessed. My study habits bordered on insane, reading anything and everything related to glute and strength training, day and night. Over time, I amassed a collection of more than 1,200 studies related to the glutes. It's worth noting here that when I started hunting for articles related to glute training, I didn't exactly know how to conduct research, nor did I have access to a database of studies. But all of that changed in the first year of my PhD program. I read, studied, and organized everything I could get my hands on.

The best part about studying at AUT was that I could do it from afar. I spent the first year in Auckland, but after that, I came home to Arizona to resume my studies. While working on my PhD remotely, I not only stayed current with the latest research but also blogged, trained, updated my sports science equipment, and, most importantly, coached clients.

As a personal trainer at Lifts, I had tested glute training methods on my clients and myself. Now I was doing it out of my four-car garage turned strength training gym. I called it the Glute Lab because, in addition to being a gym, it was also a place where I tested my ideas, theories, and techniques. I already had an EMG unit to test muscle activation, but I wanted to investigate more variables of interest, so I purchased a force plate to examine ground reaction forces during different movements and an ultrasound unit to look at changes in muscle thickness over time. The clients working with me at the time, "The Glute Squad," provided tons of feedback and helped me take a compilation of training methods and turn them into a system.

What's more, the experiments using EMG, ultrasound, and a force plate, along with the two training studies I conducted for my PhD, further validated the efficacy of what we were doing in the Glute Lab. The benefits of the hip thrust were no longer theoretical. I had science to prove it.

In addition to experimenting and testing new ideas, I continued innovating equipment. Just as the Skorcher was not practical, neither was performing the hip thrust against a bench. I needed something better—a piece of equipment specifically designed for hip thrusting.

So I went back to the drawing board.

WHAT IS THE GLUTE LAB?

The "Glute Lab" is what I called my four-car garage gym at my house in Phoenix, Arizona. It is where I trained my clients and myself and where I conducted most of the research for my PhD thesis. I used an awesome collection of glute-building equipment along with sports science technology, including an EMG unit, a force plate, and an ultrasound machine. In addition to publishing several original, peer-reviewed journal articles pertaining to the glutes, I used this gym and equipment to conduct dozens of smaller experiments and case studies.

Nowadays, the Glute Lab is more than just a gym; it is my system for strength and physique training. This is the book version of that system. And if you want to see me present the ideas contained in this book, you can attend one of my Glute Lab seminars or visit my gym in San Diego, California. In addition to training the Glute Squad, I continue to conduct research to enhance my understanding and application of glute training.

THE HIP THRUSTER

When you perform the hip thrust using a bench, the key is to jam the bench against something stable, like a wall or squat rack, to prevent it from sliding or tipping backward. Even though I was receiving a lot of positive feedback, it wasn't practical for large groups, and if you set it up incorrectly, it could be dangerous. It also was difficult to perform banded hip thrusts because you have to anchor the bands to something (such as heavy dumbbells or the feet of a power rack) that is just the right distance from the bench.

I realized that in order to perform the hip thrust exercise, I needed to attach the bench to a platform. Moving on from the Skorcher model, I developed something new—the Hip Thruster. With this new design, I could safely perform the movement using a barbell and I could perform hip thrusts with band resistance, and it was much more cost-effective.

My team and I loved the Hip Thruster, but it was met with some pretty staunch criticism.

I was reminded of the famous quote from German philosopher Arthur Schopenhauer, "All truth passes through three stages. First, it is ridiculed. Second, it is violently opposed. Third, it is accepted as being self-evident."

This progression has been especially true for the hip thrust and Hip Thruster. At first, people were outraged. Some of the biggest names in the industry called it stupid and dangerous. Then the detractors started writing it off as nonfunctional. With the hip thrust, you're lying on your back—referred to as the *supine position*—and you have three points of contact—your back is on the bench and both feet are on the ground. People view this position as nonfunctional because performing the movement doesn't require a lot of balance (which actually makes it safer) and because you're lying down, which doesn't mimic the actions of sport and life. I'll discuss how glute training can improve function and performance in Chapter 4.

Finally, to my surprise, people started saying that I hadn't invented the hip thrust. People would say that they'd been doing it for the past 20 years. Of course, no one had photo or video evidence to back up their assertions.

There will always be dissenters. But the before-and-after pictures—see "Transformations" on the next two pages—speak for themselves. And the research and articles I've published (which I cover in Part 2) validate the functional benefits for strength, health, and performance.

*

It's important to mention that you can still perform the hip thrust using a bench as described above. And if you don't feel comfortable doing it against a bench, there are other options, which I outline on page 310. My primary concern is this: I don't want you to think you need to spend money on a Hip Thruster in order to perform the movement. Later in the book, I demonstrate how to safely and effectively perform the hip thrust using a bench as well as using other variations. Put simply, you have options. Other, more expensive glute-building equipment is becoming more commonplace in commercial gyms.

GLUTE TRAINING IS HERE TO STAY

In the coming years, I expect more data from around the world to corroborate what my clients have been feeling all along: that the hip thrust is one of the most functional exercises there is. In addition to being an incredible glute builder, it is great for improving sprinting, jumping, horizontal pushing force, mid-thigh pulling force, and squat and deadlift strength.

In the meantime, I have learned that you don't simply publish one article, book, study, or thesis and expect everything to change all at once. People need time to adjust their views without feeling pressured. The wheels are definitely in motion, though. Thousands of coaches and athletes are incorporating the hip thrust and embracing my glute training methods. Thanks to social media, hip thrusts are now seen all over the world. The Rock, Kate Upton, and James Harrison have all posted videos of themselves performing hip thrusts.

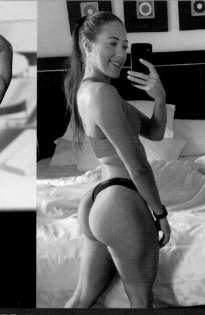
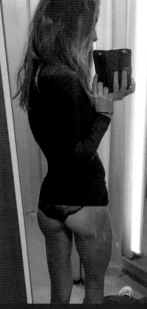

BETH CLARE (@bethclarefitness)

BETH SANDERS (@bethsanders98)

BRITTANY PERILLE (@brittanyperilleee)

KIANA LOOMIS (@nirvanafit)

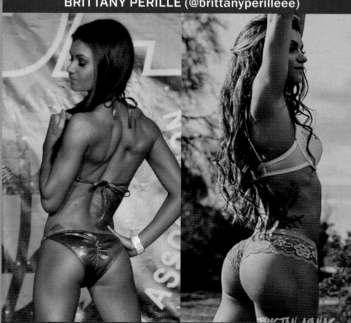

KRISTA ANTONIOU (@krista_mindtomuscle)

KRISTINA JENNESSEE (@kristinajennessee)

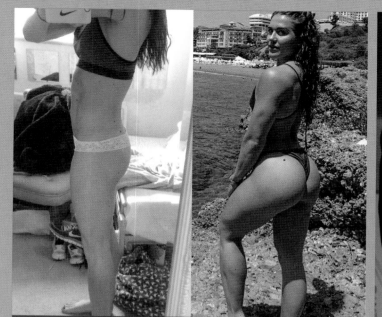
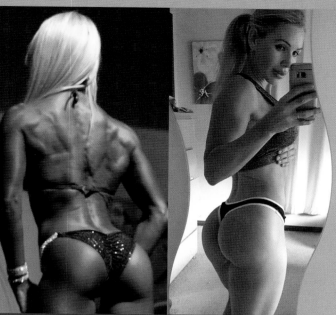

LUCY DAVIS (@lucydavis_fit)

MELISSA CROWTHER (@enduringfitness)

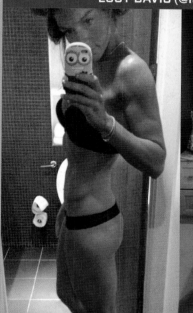
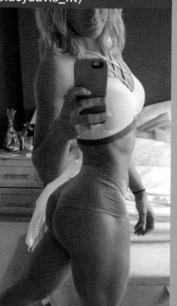
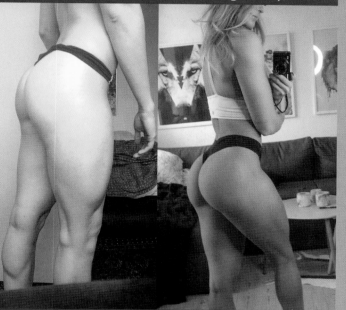

ROXY WINSTANLEY (@roxy_winstanley)

SARAH BARLOSE (@sarahbarlose)

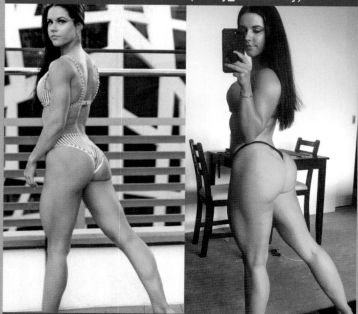
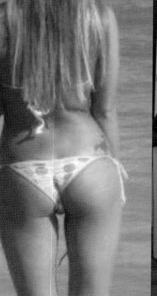
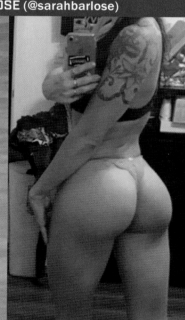

SHARELLE GRANT (@sharellegrant)

TINA (@liftwithtina)

So, while the opposition is busy getting inferior results, I'll stick to what can easily be demonstrated through scientific methods. Sure, science isn't perfect, but at least it allows us to continue to learn, experiment, refine ideas, and push the field forward—whether it's to build a better physique or to improve health, strength, and performance. The nice part is that people don't have to follow the science, or even believe in it, as long as they get results. As the saying goes, the proof is in the pudding.

I don't pretend to have all of the answers. I remain curious, and I do my best to think outside the box. And I will never stop searching for more effective training methods and techniques. If someone comes up with something better, I will embrace it. My goal is not to prove people wrong, but to help them achieve their goals. And I hope this book will help you achieve yours.

ORGANIZATION AND STRUCTURE

The lessons I've learned as a personal trainer, lifter, and student are numerous. And my knowledge of strength and physique training goes far beyond the specificity of glute training. For this reason, I've included strength and physique training principles, methods, and techniques that apply to all body parts. Put another way, this is not just a book about glute training; it's a book about strength and physique training with a glute training emphasis. For example, you will learn how to perform full-body movements—such as the squat and deadlift—but I keep it within the context of glute training. You will also learn about dietary strategies, training around and recovering from injury and discomfort, the science of muscle growth and progressive overload, and the principles of program design and periodization, which you can apply to all strength and physique training systems.

To make this book easier to navigate, I've organized it into five parts.

PART 1

THE IMPORTANCE OF GLUTE TRAINING

Part 1 explains how training your glutes can improve aesthetics, health, strength, and performance. In short, you will learn about the many benefits of glute training and why it is crucial to train your glutes—regardless of your goals, experience level, and body type.

PART 2

THE SCIENCE OF STRENGTH AND PHYSIQUE TRAINING

This part of the book outlines the anatomy and function of the glutes, the role of genetics, how muscle grows (hypertrophy), how to gain strength, and how to categorize glute training exercises. If you're new to science, don't worry; I've boiled it down to the essentials. In other words, don't let the word *science* turn you away from this section. After learning how your glutes work, the role of genetics, the mechanisms for muscle growth, how to implement progressive overload, and the best way to categorize exercises, you will be better equipped to perform and teach the exercise and programming principles covered in the subsequent parts.

Now, I'm not going to lie; some of this material is a bit dense. But if you can take the time to read and understand the chapters in this section, your knowledge of glute training (and strength and physique training as a whole) will exceed that of 90 percent of personal trainers and coaches.

SCIENCE SPEAK

If you're familiar with my work, or if you follow me on Instagram (@bretcontreras1) or frequent my blog, you know that I am a scientist at heart. I have my PhD in sports science with an emphasis in biomechanics, which applies math and physics to human movement, and—as I explained earlier—I'm constantly reading studies to further my understanding of strength training.

My intention with this book is to make the information accessible to everyone, regardless of experience and background. For this reason, I decided to keep the main body text as basic as possible and (for the most part) devoid of research studies, which can sometimes convolute the main theme. However, I didn't want to leave out important studies or the biomechanical explanations related to the topics being discussed. This would be a major disservice to my fellow academics or anyone interested in exploring the science behind glute training.

So, for those interested in delving deeper into research and the application of biomechanics, I have included sidebars titled "Science Speak" in Parts 1 and 2. You'll find the works cited in these sidebars in the references section at the back of the book.

Although this information is important (the science validates the techniques and concepts covered in the book) and I believe that everyone can benefit from reading these sidebars, it's not mandatory.

To put it another way, you don't need to understand all of the complicated terms and studies to effectively employ my system. If all you do is read the main text, you will learn everything you need to know about glute training. So feel free to skip these sidebars if the science and biomechanics do not interest you.

Another option—and this is a great approach for those who are new to glute training—is to read through the main text in each chapter first. This will give you a basic yet comprehensive overview of my system, as well as introduce some of the terms and definitions covered in the "Science Speak" sections. With this foundational knowledge under your belt, you will be better equipped to understand and digest the information when you revisit these academically dense sidebars.

THE ART OF STRENGTH AND PHYSIQUE TRAINING

Part 3 provides the fundamentals for optimal strength and physique training, from training frequency (how often you work out) and set and repetition or rep schemes (how many times your perform the exercise) to creating realistic goals and expectations, as well as dietary guidelines. You will learn both basic and advanced training methods that will help you maximize your time in the gym, as well as troubleshooting solutions for the most common problems relating to physique, exercise, and programming. You will also learn the program design variables, which include exercise selection, training frequency, tempo, rest periods, volume, load, effort, and exercise order. If the exercises are the ingredients, this part shows you how to make the recipe.

PART 4

PERIODIZATION AND PROGRAMS

The fourth part includes sample full-body programs with a glute training emphasis that cater to all fitness levels and templates that you can use for yourself or your clients. I provide beginner, intermediate, and advanced 12-week programs that incorporate most of the techniques and strategies outlined in this book. In addition to providing sample programs, I outline how I approach periodization or a long-term training plan, provide training splits (programming templates), and include sample glute training programs for bodybuilders, powerlifters, and CrossFitters.

I want to emphasize that the sample programs are exactly that—samples. Although you can follow these programs exactly as they are prescribed, they can and should be modified to cater to your or your clients' individual needs, which you will learn how to do in Part 3 and in the FAQ portion of Chapter 18. Think of the programs in this part as templates that you can change based on your goals, training frequency, experience level, and background.

PART 5

EXERCISES

This final part of the book contains all of the most important glute training exercises, from which there are a lot to choose. As I repeat throughout the book, performing a variety of exercises is crucial for strengthening and building your best glutes, legs, and body. To make the exercises easy to navigate, this part is divided into three chapters with sections for each movement pattern: Glute-Dominant Exercises, Quad-Dominant Exercises, and Hamstring-Dominant Exercises.

For short videos demonstrating the exercises included in this book, visit glutelabbook.com

Although each of these chapters focuses on exercises that emphasize a specific muscle group, they all work your glutes and body in slightly different ways. This is important because everyone is unique. The majority of people get the best results from prioritizing glute-dominant exercises, but everyone can benefit from performing a variety of lower-body movements. Throughout the book, I discuss specific strategies for exercise selection based on variables like goals, anatomy, anthropometry (torso, arm, and leg lengths), and experience. The important thing to note here is that variety is vital for building the best glutes possible.

WHAT ABOUT UPPER-BODY EXERCISES?

It's accurate to say that glute training is a system for developing your lower body. But it's important to realize that a lot of the glute training movements work your entire body. Squats, deadlifts, swings, sled pushes, and certain other glute exercises work the lower and upper body. So, even if you follow a glutes-only training program, you can still receive a little bit of upper-body stimulus.

Having said that, I still recommend upper-body-specific exercises. In Part 4, I offer training splits that include upper-body exercises as well as full-body programs with a glute training emphasis.

HOW TO NAVIGATE THIS BOOK

Although this book is supposed to be read in its entirety, it is also designed for browsing. For example, you can start following one of the programs in Part 4 while referencing the techniques in Part 5. However, I highly recommend you take the time to read and understand the science in Part 2 because it validates the methods presented in Part 3 and the techniques covered in Part 5.

Stated differently, if you're primarily interested in shaping a nicer butt or you're looking for a great glute workout, then you can skip to Part 4 and start following one of the many programs or templates that I offer. If you do, just be sure to reference the technique descriptions in Part 5 to ensure you're performing the movements correctly. But if you want to understand how your glutes work, why you should train them, and how to do it effectively, then you need to read the book straight through to the exercises in Part 5.

I believe in the principles, methods, and techniques broken down in this book because I have seen them work time and time again, both in the gym and in life. Whether you're male or female, and whether you're a bodybuilder, powerlifter, CrossFitter, personal trainer, strength coach, physical therapist, or someone who just wants a better butt and body—this book contains everything you need to know to build bigger, stronger, shapelier glutes.

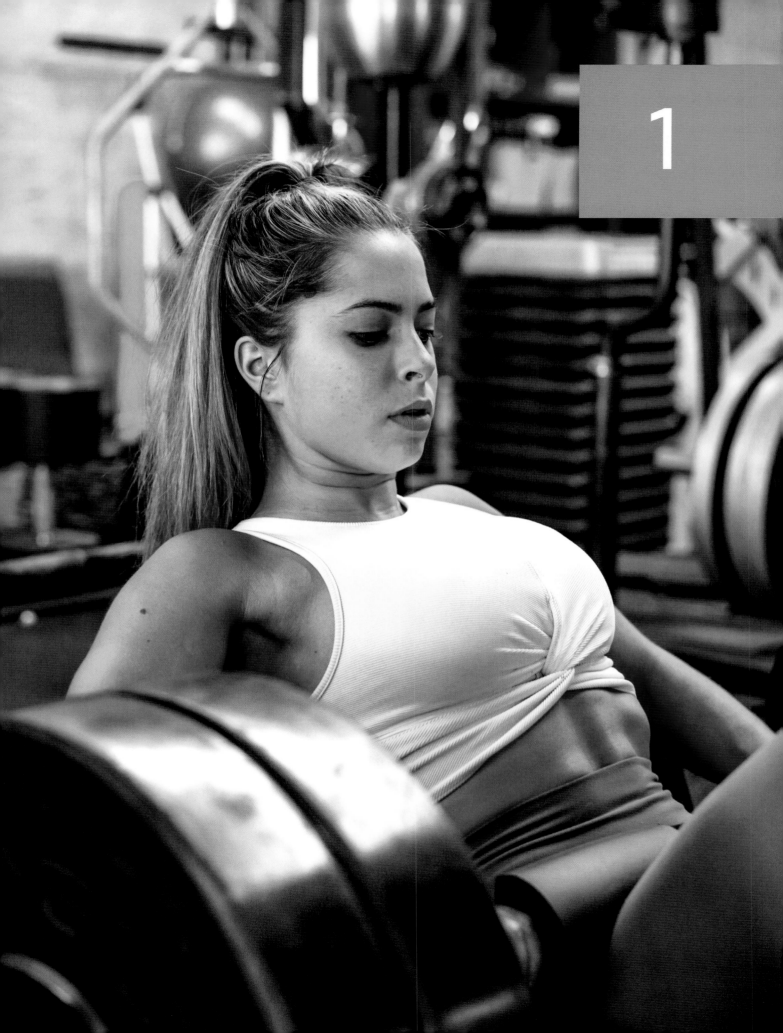

1

THE IMPORTANCE OF GLUTE TRAINING

You might be wondering why glute training is important. Sure, a big, strong butt looks great in a tight pair of jeans, and this is a good enough reason for most of you to start training your glutes. But what are the other benefits? And why should you prioritize your glutes in training?

To answer these questions, you first need to understand what makes the glutes special.

For starters, the glutes are the biggest and most powerful muscle group in the human body. In addition to being aesthetically appealing, the glutes control a wide range of functional movements. Walking uphill, getting out of a chair, picking something up off the ground—these actions would be very difficult to carry out without your glutes. What's more, having big, strong glutes sets you up to lift heavier, jump higher, sprint faster, and swing harder and can even play a role in preventing knee, hip, and lower back injuries. The glutes, in a nutshell, influence every aspect of your physical life: from the way you look and how you feel to your ability to run, jump, cut, lift, and twist. It's pretty safe to say that the glutes are the most important and versatile skeletal muscle in the body.

Does this mean you should neglect other areas of your body and focus primarily on your glutes? Well, it depends on your goals.

As you will learn in Part 3, programming is highly individualized, meaning that it is different for everyone. The exercises you like and need to program in order to reach your goals might look very different from the exercises and programs I follow or the ones that I write for my clients. This is why it's important to understand how to design your own programs. I do offer sample program templates in Part 4, and one of them might suit your needs just fine. But only you or your coach can determine which muscles you need to exercise, which movements you should perform, and how often you should train.

I don't want to leave you with the opinion that glute training is the be-all, end-all system for training. So let me be clear, because I don't want you to avoid training other muscles in your body. All muscles are important, and you should train your entire body.

But when it comes to function and aesthetics, the glutes reign supreme, and for most people, they should be prioritized in training. This might mean training your glutes twice a week as a supplement to your current strength training program, or it might mean training them five days a week. Whatever your commitment, it doesn't mean you're neglecting other areas of your body. Depending on your goals, you still need to train your upper body and perform a wide range of movements.

I also want you to realize that glute training is not muscle specificity training in the sense that you're working and isolating only one muscle group. This is actually impossible when it comes to training your glutes. Obviously, there are some exercises that specifically target your glutes, but the majority of movements target multiple muscle groups simultaneously. Hip thrusts, lunges, squats, deadlifts, back extensions—these exercises not only target your glutes, but also work your legs, your core, and (to a lesser degree) your upper body. So, when I say "glute training," I mean prioritizing your glutes by selecting exercises that target the gluteal muscles and by extension, your legs and trunk.

When I started my glute training journey, I was interested only in getting big, powerful glutes. I now realize that there is much more to glute training than building a better butt and body. This is important because we all have different reasons for training. Some people care mostly about aesthetics, or how they look: they want to lose fat, gain muscle, and improve body composition. Others train primarily to improve performance: they want to get stronger, faster, and better at their sport. And still others train simply because they enjoy it and want to lead healthier lives.

If you're like me, you train for all of these reasons. Strong, shapely glutes are my goal—and I will show you how to get exactly that in the pages to come—but I also want to get stronger overall, look younger, and feel better. And I want to have fun doing it. The value of a training program can be measured by its comprehensiveness and adaptability. It should cater to a broad range of goals and suit the needs of the individual. This is the basis of my glute training system. It sets the stage for looking and feeling your best and has the potential to improve your health, strength, and performance.

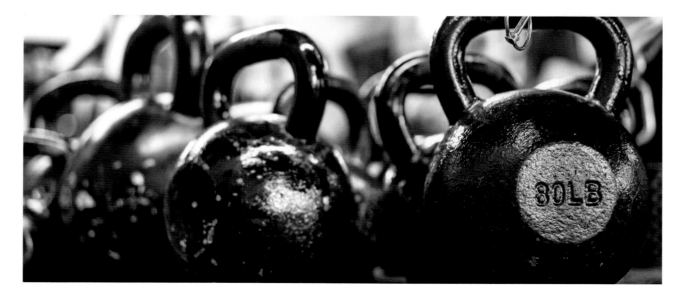

WHAT IS THE NUMBER ONE REASON YOU PERFORM HIP THRUSTS?

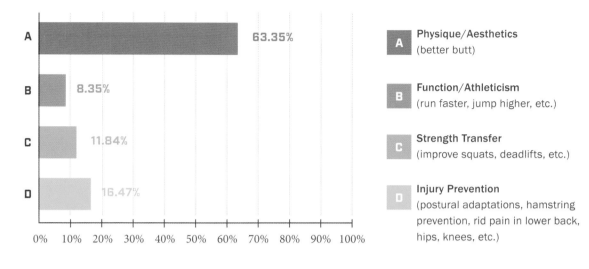

A	63.35%
B	8.35%
C	11.84%
D	16.47%

0% 10% 20% 30% 40% 50% 60% 70% 80% 90% 100%

A Physique/Aesthetics
(better butt)

B Function/Athleticism
(run faster, jump higher, etc.)

C Strength Transfer
(improve squats, deadlifts, etc.)

D Injury Prevention
(postural adaptations, hamstring
prevention, rid pain in lower back,
hips, knees, etc.)

A poll undertaken in July 2017 with 7,628 respondents indicates that the majority of exercisers (63 percent) hip thrusted for physique and aesthetic purposes (to get a better butt). The remaining respondents hip thrusted for injury/pain prevention (16 percent), strength transfer to squats and deadlifts (12 percent), and functional performance outcomes (8 percent). We need more polls to determine why people train their glutes. However, it's safe to say that the majority of people train hip thrusts primarily for aesthetics.

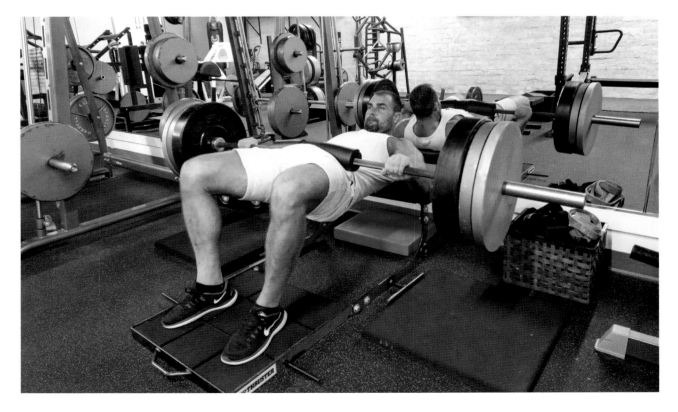

Glute Training for Aesthetics

The majority of people who come to me for coaching are primarily interested in one thing—improving their physique. They want to develop their bodies to suit their aesthetic goals, which usually means sculpting a bigger, leaner, stronger physique. Glute training is, in this context, a form of bodybuilding.

The term *bodybuilding* means exactly what it implies: you're building your body through weight training. Some think of it not as bodybuilding but as body *sculpting* because you're trying to change your appearance by lifting weights. Just as an artist creates sculptures using shaping techniques, a bodybuilder lifts weights to sculpt certain areas of the body.

While I love the idea of sculpting physiques, bodybuilding encompasses more than just physique training. It's a form of strength training and physical exercise. But, at its core, bodybuilding represents an important aspect of how we see each other as humans. For better or worse, we judge one another based on appearance. If someone is lean and muscular, you might see that person as athletic, healthy, and strong. Conversely, you might view someone who is morbidly obese as sedentary and unhealthy.

Whether these judgments are right or wrong, the fact remains: research shows that how you look impacts not only how others see you but also how you think of yourself. This is a complex and nebulous subject because everyone has different tastes and opinions, which are affected by genetics, culture, and environment. What I consider sexy, you might consider ugly. As the saying goes, "Beauty is in the eye of the beholder."

The questions you need to ask yourself are: What do you consider beautiful? How do you want your body to look? What makes you happy when you look in the mirror? Are there areas of your body that you want to change? If you think big, powerful butts are beautiful and you want stronger, shapelier glutes, then you can use the methods and techniques in this book to help sculpt your ideal physique. But it's important not to focus solely on the desired results because there are some things you can't change, like your genetics. If you're like me and you inherited horrible glute genetics, then trying to build a big butt may not be in your cards (at least not in the short term). So, when it comes to creating physique goals, it's imperative that you focus on the process (training) rather than the results (aesthetics).

Stated differently, you need to create realistic goals based on your genetics and body type and focus on things that you can control (more on this in Chapter 11). What you eat, the types of exercise you do, your activity level, how you manage stress, your quality of sleep—these things can have a massive effect on how you look, how you feel, and how you think of yourself. My job as a personal trainer is to help clients achieve their goals, whether the goal is to lose weight, enlarge muscles, or improve strength. Glute training can do all of these things while sculpting a physique that many people desire.

I suspect that most of you reading this book are interested in glute training because you want (for yourself or someone else) a better butt and body. As long as your goals are realistic and the training is safe and healthy, working to attain your ideal physique is perfectly acceptable. But there is a fine line between caring about how you look and wanting to look better, and obsessing about how you look and needing to look better. There's a spectrum. On one end, there's the overweight sedentary person who never exercises, and on the other, there's the obsessive lifter who spends all of their time in the gym and can't walk past a mirror without checking themselves out. Neither extreme is healthy, and it's up to you to find a balance.

You can, however, have a goal of getting a better butt and body without feeling guilty or self-absorbed. Wanting to improve your physique doesn't mean you're vain. It just means that you want to improve your body, which is something most people want, whether they're willing to admit it or not. This begs the question: what is it about the glutes specifically that makes them so aesthetically appealing? There are a few explanations.

THE ATTRACTION TO GLUTES

Research indicates a strong association between having big, strong glutes and being attractive and athletic. The instinct to check out a nice butt seems to be hard-wired into our genes. From an evolutionary perspective, it makes sense.

Imagine living in a hunter-gatherer society where activities like throwing, sprinting, and punching were as important as checking your email or driving a car. We know the glutes power functional movements, so it's not a stretch to think that those with powerful glutes were more proficient and capable of performing important actions necessary for survival. This is natural selection at work. The males and females with the bigger, stronger glutes were more likely to survive and triumph in their environment due to increased function and power.

This might be a bit of a stretch and is not proven fact, but it's an interesting idea. In warrior and hunter societies where people were fighting predators and other humans in hand-to-hand combat and sprinting to chase down food, there can be no doubt that the glutes would have played a small yet crucial role.

More likely, though, the glutes played a more prominent role in sexual selection—that is, the selection of traits (strong glutes) that enhanced mating success. It stands to reason that both males and females were attracted to nice glutes, instinctively making the connection between big, strong glutes and survival, reproduction, hunting, and protection. A woman might select a male based on his ability to hunt, fight, and protect. And such abilities might very well have been tied to his powerful glutes. A man might select a female for the same reasons, but with the added perception that bigger glutes meant better childbearing hips. It's the idea that the peacock with the most brilliant feathers gets to mate—but instead of feathers, we have muscles, with the glutes being among the most important and noticeable.

Today, these traits don't serve the same function, but our DNA doesn't know the difference. If you see someone with strong glutes on a balanced, lean, muscular frame, you automatically assume that person is fast, powerful, athletic, and probably attractive. It's the attraction part that typically draws people to my system. They want nice glutes not because it makes them stronger, faster, or more athletic, but because they want to look good from behind.

GETTING GLUTES

If you are glute training for aesthetic purposes, it's important to understand that it is difficult to get and maintain glutes. As you age, your glutes—like all muscles—start to decline. When neglected, they start to atrophy, meaning they weaken and sag. Some people have nice glutes in high school because they're young and active; they're walking around all day, playing sports, and so on. But as time goes on, they start to sit more and more, they're less active, and eventually their hard, round butts become weak and flat. You might look back on your youth and think, "Dang, I used have a nice butt and legs. I used to look really good. I want that back."

These are the people who tend to find me—people who went through the same process I went through. They're not getting the results they are looking for or they aren't satisfied with their physique, so they start following my training methods. They still train other areas of their bodies but perform a wide variety of glute exercises and train their glutes more frequently. Not surprisingly, they start getting the results they're looking for.

As I mentioned in the Introduction, the squat and deadlift develop the glutes but primarily target the quads and hamstrings. A lot of women I work with don't like their physique from just squatting and deadlifting. They tell me about their overdeveloped quads and hamstrings, which take away from their glutes. This is what typically happens when you don't perform glute-dominant exercises like the hip thrust—the quads and hamstrings grow disproportionately to the glutes, which makes the butt look smaller in comparison. But these are clients who are going for a specific look.

At the end of the day, you are your own physique artist. Training your glutes is just one way you can alter your appearance through exercise. If you want your butt to stand out and you're not satisfied with your shape, then following a specialized glute program might get you closer to your ideal physique based on your goals and body type. For example, if you have big quads and hamstrings and you want your butt to pop, then you need to focus on glute-dominant exercises over squats and deadlifts. Conversely, if you want to build your glutes and your legs, then employing all of the exercises in this book will get you closer to your goals.

For physique and aesthetics, women are going to value glutes more than men, but both need to prioritize them in training. The aesthetics has to be geared toward the individual, but I've developed the best system for helping both men and women develop their physique goals just by identifying which exercises activate the different regions of the glutes best and figuring out how to biomechanically tailor a program to the individual.

I can speak from experience, having always prioritized my glutes. Women I have dated have made comments like, "Oh man, you have a nice butt. My last boyfriend only trained his upper body." Women tend to appreciate nice butts on men just like men appreciate nice butts on women. But a lot of men don't realize this fact. Their egos hold them back. Men are looking in the mirror at their beach muscles while women are making fun of their chicken legs. They don't realize that women like nice glutes, too. When you have a nice set of glutes, you just look better. It gives you a powerful, athletic look that is mesmerizing and attractive.

If getting big, powerful glutes is your goal, then you will love following these programs and implementing these techniques into your exercise routine. But there's more to glute training than looking good from behind. A lot of people mistakenly assume that you sacrifice health, function, and performance when training for aesthetics. While that might be the case with some bodybuilding systems, it's not the case with my glute training system. It's all about selecting the right exercises and following a well-designed program.

Even if you're training only for aesthetics, as long as your programming and mechanics are good, you will get stronger and healthier and perform better as part of the package. Put simply, you don't need to sacrifice performance, strength, or—most importantly—your health when sculpting your physique.

SCIENCE SPEAK: IMPROVED AESTHETICS

SHAPE AND SIZE

Although your ability to change your appearance is partially determined by your genetics, you can significantly improve the shape of your buttocks through glute training (exercise selection and program design). The improvements in shape happen mostly through changes in muscle cross-sectional area (perpendicular to the muscle fibers). These increases tend to be greatest in the middle region when measuring from end to end,[1, 2] which is often the point of maximum diameter.[3, 4] Targeted glute training, in a nutshell, makes your glutes look rounder, creating a fitter, more athletic appearance.

BODY COMPOSITION

Training your glutes will also improve your overall body composition (increasing the percentage of muscle while decreasing the percentage of fat). In order to train your glutes, you need to perform exercises that emphasize powerful hip extension joint actions, such as hip thrusts, squats, and deadlifts. Performing these exercises ties in a lot of muscle groups, including the prime movers (gluteus maximus, three of the four hamstring muscles, and adductor magnus) and the trunk stabilizers (erector spinae and other core muscles). What's more, the key hip extension exercises involve many other muscle groups in both the upper and the lower body.

Glute training, in other words, works a lot of muscle groups, which leads to high metabolic cost (burning calories during and after a training session). This "afterburn" effect is called *excess post-exercise oxygen consumption,* or EPOC for short.[5] Although the number of calories burned during the EPOC period is relatively small in comparison with the calories burned during the workout, it can reach around 100 kcal per day and last for up to 72 hours![6] The EPOC effect is greater after strength training than after any type of aerobic exercise, including high-intensity interval training (HIIT). You can maximize the number of calories burned in the EPOC period by keeping volume fairly high. Shorter rest periods and heavier loads help,[7] and certain advanced training techniques, like rest pause (page 203), might be beneficial, too.[8]

Glute Training for Health

Although the majority of people train their glutes for aesthetic purposes, glute training conveys numerous health benefits that can have a profound impact on your quality of life.

First, training your glutes is a great way to shed unwanted weight. With the glutes being the largest muscle in the body and controlling a wide range of functional movements (see page 40), training your glutes burns more calories than training other body parts, especially when you perform glute exercises in a progressive manner. This causes you to "recomp," which means that you build muscle while simultaneously losing fat, assuming your diet doesn't change much. And this helps you lose fat all over, including the regions of your body that tend to store a lot of fat, like your hips, legs, and trunk. In addition to improving your physique, maintaining a healthy weight through exercise can reduce the risk of developing certain diseases, like type 2 diabetes and high blood pressure, which can cause a plethora of problems ranging from blood clots and kidney disease to heart attacks and strokes.

Second, training your glutes works your muscular, skeletal, and cardiovascular systems. As Part 2 explains, in order to get the best results based on what we currently know about training for muscular growth, you need to take a shotgun approach, meaning that you need to implement a variety of movements and perform a variety of set and rep schemes. For example, one day you might hip thrust for high reps and perform heavy bench presses, and the next day you might go heavy with deadlifts and perform higher-rep pull-ups.

Performing a variety of movements and hitting your body from different angles with different loads and speeds not only stresses and strengthens the bones and muscles involved in the movement but also gets your heart rate up and your blood pumping. This builds stamina and endurance by strengthening your cardiovascular system, which transports blood, oxygen, and nutrients throughout your body.

Just as training your glutes helps you lose weight and works your cardiovascular system, it also develops and strengthens your bones and muscles, which is very important to your health. As we age, we lose bone density and muscle, and as our bone density diminishes and our muscles weaken, we become more susceptible to injury and pain. So how do we develop and maintain strong bones and muscles? It's simple: by doing resistance training, or weight-bearing activities. This is how you set yourself up to better handle the wear and tear of daily life. To put it another way, you're setting yourself up to have solid, well-equipped knees, hips, and lower back.

But it's not enough to simply lift weights. In order to maintain strength and avoid pain and injury, you also have to perform full-range movements—that is, exercising through the full motion of a joint. For example, lowering the hips below the knees during a squat, as shown opposite, moves the hips through a full range of motion for most individuals.

In general, people who perform a variety of full-range movements—both in their daily lives and during exercise—have an easier time staying injury- and pain-free, as long as they don't overdo it in the gym. Glute training encompasses these full-range movements, and I have included plenty of options in Part 5 for variety.

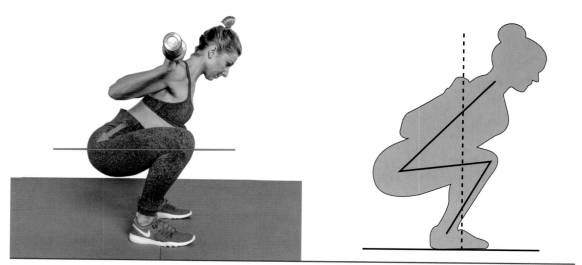

SQUATTING TO PARALLEL

To squat to parallel, you must bend your knees and lower your body until the tops of your legs at your hip joints are lower than the tops of your knees (that is, your hip joints are lower than your knee joints).

STRONG GLUTES, AN ANTIDOTE TO PAIN AND INJURY

Another important variable in managing and preventing pain and injury is having a strong, well-balanced frame. If one muscle is weak or underdeveloped, other muscles have to compensate by working harder. So, if you have deconditioned glutes, your back and leg muscles have to work extra hard to keep you moving. This means that any muscle or muscle group working in concert with the glutes during functional movements—like the hamstrings in sprinting, the quads and calves in jumping, the adductors in squatting, or the erectors in lifting—are at risk when the glutes are undeveloped or weak.

For example, let's say you rely heavily on your quads to lift and jump. This increases your chances of developing patellofemoral pain syndrome (generic knee pain) because you're loading your knees instead of the big engines of your hips. Stronger hips and glutes can change your mechanics and effectively take some of the loading off your knees, potentially safeguarding you from developing knee pain.

Another common example is an imbalance between the strength of the hamstrings and the strength of the glutes. In this case, you must rely more on your hamstrings to extend your hips. The hamstrings' leverage on the femur (thigh bone) can cause the ball (in the hip joint) to jut forward in the socket, which can lead to anterior hip pain. Strong glutes will pull rearward on the femur, causing it to center itself in the socket and reducing the likelihood of anterior hip pain.

In addition to creating a movement pattern that overworks synergistic muscles, weak glutes change the mechanics of how you move, putting even more wear and tear on the compensating muscles. Having big, strong glutes, on the other hand, can prevent poor mechanics by giving your body balance and stability. Here are a couple of examples:

- Knees: When your glutes are strong, it's easier to keep your knees in a stable position while running and landing from a jump. By *stable,* I mean that the knees don't cave inward. If the knees do collapse inward (referred to as *knee valgus*), which can happen in people with deconditioned glutes (other factors that can cause knee valgus, too), it can lead to pain or, even worse, knee injuries such as ACL tears.

- Hips and lower back: Your glutes help carry out hip extension. If your glutes are weak, you will end up using your back more when lifting, and your erector muscles will work extra hard to perform the task, and will do so dynamically rather than isometrically. The added stress on your spinal discs, ligaments, and muscles when lifting in this manner can lead to lower back pain, strains, and injury (such as a herniated disc).

Strong, well-developed glutes can prevent these kinds of injuries and help you avoid lower back pain. The exercises that target the glutes, specifically the glute-dominant hip thrust movements, train your body to rely on your glutes during hip extension—think standing up from a squat—and not your lower back or hamstrings. Moving from your hips and using your glutes make it easier to keep your back flat, which in turn reduces stress on your spine. In fact, training your glutes might even improve your posture by reducing anterior pelvic tilt (hyperextending in your lower back) and decreasing thoracic kyphosis (rounding in your upper back). Many lifters notice that after starting to deadlift, squat, and hip thrust, they begin standing taller and appear more athletic.

I'll take a closer look at how glute training can prevent pain and injury in the Science Speak sidebar that follows. For now, it's important to understand that pain is multifaceted and related to a variety of psychological and social factors, and it's not well correlated with tissue damage. That said, you're dealing with greater forces and stresses in the weight room and in sports than in everyday life, so the more glute strength and stamina you have, the easier it is to maintain a good position while standing, walking, and moving. And being in a good position while bearing heavy loads or moving rapidly decreases stress on the surrounding tissues, which can prevent pain and injury.

Now, when you look good (according to your own standards), you tend to stand taller and strut your stuff a bit more. In essence, you exude confidence. This confidence can play a role in how you interpret pain, how people view you, and how you feel about yourself. I'm not saying that glute training will automatically give you perfect movement mechanics and more confidence, but it can influence how you stand and how you carry yourself, which can have a broader impact on your health and outlook.

Activity in the form of movement and exercise is bedrock to a healthy life. Pain is a natural part of living, and we shouldn't think we can go through life without ever experiencing pain. Have you ever heard of an elite athlete who never suffered here and there? Me neither. If you stand with poor posture, experience lower back pain, or suffer from knee or leg injuries, training your glutes might help you. When you feel healthy and fit, other aspects of your training improve. You not only look and feel better, but your performance and strength also improve.

JOINT STABILITY

When it comes to training—whether for sport or for leisure—there is always an inherent risk of injury. Although chance plays a huge role and can make the underlying causes of injury hard to discern, there are things you can do to lower your chances of getting hurt, such as practicing good form, strengthening your body, and working on your weaknesses. Training your glutes might also help reduce your risk of injury to some extent.

Although high-quality research showing that glute training reduces injury risk is not available at this time, we can see from certain biomechanical studies (not to mention anecdotal evidence and common sense) that the gluteus maximus provides stability at several joints—the knee, hip, spine, and sacroiliac joint— which may reduce the risk of knee, hip, and spinal injuries. For example, the glutes prevent anterior tibial translation during lunges,[1] which is a mechanism for anterior cruciate ligament (ACL) tears and ruptures, probably through its insertion point on the iliotibial tract.[2]

You'll learn more about where the insertion and attachment points are in Chapter 5. Here's what's important to know now: the glutes help provide stability for your lower limbs and trunk, and the more stable the joint, the less likely you are to injure it. In this case, the additional knee stability provided by your glutes may help prevent ACL injuries. Though the lunge doesn't perfectly translate to all sporting movements, it is a loaded unilateral (single-leg) staggered-stance movement, which is common in most sports and activities.

And there's more: a recent modeling study concluded that excessive hamstring co-contraction (simultaneous contraction of the hamstring around the knee) during squats and other similar hip extension movements might increase the quadriceps muscle force and therefore raise patellofemoral joint pressure to damaging levels.[3]

For example, let's say you're performing a barbell back squat. If your glutes are weak and underdeveloped, you will rely more heavily on your hamstrings for hip extension power, which will require more output from your quads because hamstring activation works against them at the knee joint, thereby increasing the pressure on your knees. This pressure can cause a variety of issues in the various structures of your knees.

This underscores the importance of strengthening and developing your glutes for heavily loaded lower-body exercises, like barbell back squats, and for high-impact lower-body sports, such as volleyball, basketball, and other activities that involve drop landings (landing from a jump).

MUSCLE STRAIN

As I mentioned in the main text, the glutes work synergistically with other muscles during lower-body movements.[4] When you squat, for example, your glutes help distribute and share the load placed on your lower body with other muscles, like your quads and hamstrings. If your glutes are weak, in other words, other muscles have to compensate—that is, work harder to carry out the task. This places more stress on those other muscles (quads and hamstrings) during exercise and activity, which can increase your risk of experiencing a muscle strain.

Keeping with the squat, modeling studies show that the glutes work together with the quadriceps, hamstrings, and adductor magnus (the muscle on the inside of your thigh) to perform combined hip and knee extension (standing up from a squat).[5, 6] These same studies suggest that a lack of force produced by the gluteus maximus can result in excessive hamstring co-contraction during squats and other similar movements. So, in addition to increasing the risk of knee injury, weak glutes can increase the risk of hamstring muscle strain, which is common.[7] This might also apply to the quadriceps, which are often strained in soccer,[8] and the adductors, which are highly susceptible to muscle strains.[9] And there are good reasons to assume that the glutes work synergistically with the adductors in sprinting.[10]

KNEE VALGUS

As you will learn in Chapter 6, the gluteus maximus is an important hip external rotator (rotating your leg outward) and hip abductor (moving your leg away from your body). Hip external rotation and hip abduction muscle strength are key predictors of ACL injury.[11] In addition, gluteus maximus EMG amplitude (a measure of muscle activation) is reported to be moderately and negatively correlated with knee valgus (inward caving of the knee, which is a mechanism for ACL injuries) during step-down[12] and jump landings.[13]

It's important to point out that not all studies report a close relationship between glute strength and the degree of knee valgus. But this is probably due to the many other factors that affect knee valgus, such as ankle dorsiflexion range of motion (the ability to bring your toes toward your shin)[14] and motor control (coordination and form).[15]

Here's what we do know: the gluteus maximus is a key muscle for controlling knee valgus. It follows that the stronger and more functional your glutes, the more you can control or prevent your knee from twisting inward. And the more you can prevent the valgus knee fault, the less likely you are to injure your ACL.

PATELLOFEMORAL PAIN

Pain is a complex issue, and it is certainly not determined solely by postural or biomechanical factors. Even so, there are good indications that hip exercises, particularly those that focus on the gluteus maximus in its multiple roles as a hip extensor, hip external rotator, and hip abductor, are very effective for use in physical therapy programs designed to rehabilitate patellofemoral pain.[16]

HIP STABILITY

In addition to helping stabilize the knee, the glutes are vital for hip stability. Aspects of hip anatomy (including transverse and sagittal plane—see page 112 for more on planes of motion—neck angles, hip socket alignment, and hip socket shape) vary between individuals,[17, 18] meaning that some people are at greater risk of experiencing anterior hip pain. These individuals often find that their hip pain flares up during squatting.

What's more, the glutes exert a rearward pull on the hip during hip extension movements, which creates more space for the anterior femoral head to move inside the hip socket. This reduces the force exerted by the bone on the socket in the forward direction,[19] thereby helping it avoid contact with the sides.[20]

SPINAL STABILITY

When it comes to spinal stability, we know that the pelvis is balanced by a pair of force couples (muscles or muscle groups working in concert to move a joint), where one side of each couple (muscle) comprises the gluteus maximus (at the rear) and the abdominals (at the front).[21] The other muscles that produce movement around the hip and help stabilize the spine are the erector spinae (at the rear) and the hip flexors (at the front).

The gluteals, in a nutshell, are well placed to maintain a stable spine. Therefore, glute exercises can be helpful for people with poor spinal stability.[22] In particular, the role of the glutes in performing posterior pelvic tilt can help prevent excessive lumbar extension (hyperextension), which is associated with lower back pain.

PELVIC TILT

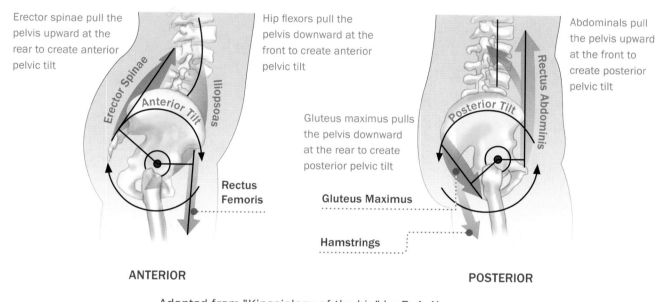

Erector spinae pull the pelvis upward at the rear to create anterior pelvic tilt

Hip flexors pull the pelvis downward at the front to create anterior pelvic tilt

Abdominals pull the pelvis upward at the front to create posterior pelvic tilt

Gluteus maximus pulls the pelvis downward at the rear to create posterior pelvic tilt

Erector Spinae
Anterior Tilt
Iliopsoas
Rectus Femoris

Rectus Abdominis
Posterior Tilt
Gluteus Maximus
Hamstrings

ANTERIOR

POSTERIOR

Adapted from "Kinesiology of the hip" by D. A. Neumann

SACROILIAC JOINT STABILITY

In addition to their role in stabilizing the pelvis, the glutes may play a specific role in preventing unnecessary movement of the sacroiliac (SI) joint. Anatomical investigations have found a deep region of the glutes with short fibers crossing over the SI joint.[23, 24] In addition, biomechanical models have shown that applying load through the gluteus maximus produces force closure of the joint (the muscles clamp down and pull the joint together, which reduces motion),[25, 26] and one experimental study has confirmed that contracting the hip extensors reduces SI joint mobility.[27]

Based on the research, it's safe to say that the glutes help stabilize the SI joint. Because a large number of lower back pain cases are thought to be SI related,[28] the glutes may help prevent certain types of mechanical lower back pain that arise from instability of the SI joint.

Glute Training for Strength

Getting strong is a common goal for most athletes and weightlifters, not just because lifting a lot of weight is cool, but also because, as most weightlifters can attest, it gives you something to train for. Put simply, training for strength is a great way to measure your progress. There's something special about setting new personal records (PRs) in the gym and lifting more weight than you've ever lifted before.

Although a lot of variables contribute to lifting more weight, such as technique, diet, rest, and programming, strength is one of the most concrete ways to measure progress. It's definitive. If you can lift more weight today than you did last month with the same form and same range of motion, you're a stronger version of yourself, and you can accurately conclude that your training is paying off.

In my experience as a personal trainer, the people who train to improve their strength are more likely to stay consistent. Unlike physique training, which is a lot harder to measure, training for strength is a powerful tool for building confidence and consistency. For this reason, I recommend that everyone—even those training for a better physique—train for strength. Most of the fitness models and bikini competitors I coach love working toward strength goals. They already look good, but they associate getting stronger with looking better, and rightly so. There's a direct (but imperfect) correlation between getting stronger and growing muscle (hypertrophy) and vice versa. As your muscles grow, so too does your strength. This is why a lot of bodybuilders use weights as another way of measuring progress in the gym.

Not everyone cares about aesthetics, and sometimes it's difficult to see physical changes. Your mind will play tricks on you when you use the scale or a mirror, but weights don't lie. And not everyone can put on muscle like the guys and gals in bodybuilding shows. For these people, training for strength becomes an important goal.

THE FOUR PRIMARY BENEFITS OF GLUTEAL STRENGTHENING

1. POSTURAL IMPROVEMENTS

2. INJURY AND PAIN PREVENTION

3. INCREASED ATHLETICISM, STRENGTH, AND POWER

4. PHYSIQUE IMPROVEMENTS

TINY BUT MIGHTY

A small percentage of people simply don't have the genetics to build muscle. They can train hard for as long as they want, but it's not in their genes to get naturally jacked. If you fall into this category, make training for strength your primary goal. Instead of trying to put on muscle, focus on lifting more weight. Make it your reason for training. It's a reward for your effort. You may not get buff, but you will get stronger and reap the health and performance benefits. And most people—even those who don't have the best muscle-building genes—will get a leaner, more defined physique by simply training for strength. I call this the "tiny but mighty" concept. You can feel confident in your body, even if it's not what you originally sought to achieve, because you know how hard you've worked and are proud of how strong you've become. Ever seen the athletes who proudly strut their stuff in *ESPN The Magazine*'s annual Body Issue? They don't all have what society deems ideal physiques, but they couldn't care less. They're world-class athletes, and they love their bodies because of what they're capable of doing on the field, regardless of how lean they are or how developed certain muscles are.

How do you improve strength? It's simple. To get stronger, you have to continually work toward lifting heavier weights. You do this by gradually increasing the resistance on your muscles over a given period. In strength training programs, this is accomplished using the progressive overload principle. If you're new to lifting, *progressive overload* simply means doing more over time. For example, adding more weight to a lift, performing more reps, and/or having more productive training sessions all fall into the category of progressive overload.

I'll dive deeper into progressive overload in Chapter 9. What I want you to understand here is that in order to improve your strength, you should be working toward lifting more weight. Although you want to improve strength in all of the lifts and movements that you perform, a few lifts are considered to be the ultimate tests in strength. This is where powerlifting enters the picture.

STRONGER GLUTES = HEAVIER LIFTS

Just as bodybuilders use weights to sculpt their bodies and the mirror to gauge their growth, powerlifters use three barbell lifts—the squat, deadlift, and bench press—and total weight lifted to measure their strength and progress. The good news is that you don't need to be a powerlifter to reap the benefits from these movements. In fact, these three lifts are bedrock to almost all strength training programs. Whether you're bodybuilding, CrossFitting, or just focusing on glute training, you can benefit from the big three power lifts.

For instance, the squat and deadlift are excellent ways to measure full-body strength, which includes your glutes. In fact, squatting and deadlifting are critical to glute development and function. Sure, the hip thrust variations and other glute-dominant exercises target the glutes more effectively, but it's still important to squat and deadlift. And because the glutes are involved in these movements, having stronger glutes can improve your strength when performing these movements. So, just as glute training is great for bodybuilders, it's also great for powerlifters, Olympic lifters, strongmen, or anybody who is performing heavy lifts.

Think about it like this. The hip thrust is a hip extension movement, meaning that you're adding load to your hips and then extending your hips into the weight to reach full extension.

Well, what do you think happens when you get stronger in this movement pattern? That's right; you increase your hip extension strength. If you're a powerlifter or someone who wants to increase your strength in the squat and deadlift, working the hip thrust or other glute-specific movements into your routine is a great way to make improvements.

Here's an all-too-common scenario that will help illustrate my point. Imagine someone trying to deadlift an enormous amount of weight. They've lifted it off the ground and pulled the bar past their knees, and then they start shaking and hitching in an attempt to lock out their hips. In other words, they've managed to get the weight off the ground, but they can't extend their hips and stand upright to complete the lift. You've probably seen this happen to someone you know, or you may have experienced it yourself. I know I have.

How do you prevent this from happening? A lot of variables could be at play here, such as grip failure or poor technique, but weak glutes might be one of them. If your glutes are weak, especially at end range (lockout), extending your hips to complete the lift might be a challenge. And this is the exact motion you're training when you perform glute-dominant exercises like the hip thrust. My point is this: by training your glutes and the hip extension motion (via the hip thrust, glute bridge, and so on), you can improve your mechanics and strength for movements that are most commonly used to measure strength, like the squat and the deadlift.

Although the power lifts are great ways to measure strength, you don't have to limit yourself to the squat and the deadlift. This is one of the main benefits of the hip thrust: it enables you to directly challenge your glutes with load. When it comes to measuring strength, everyone gravitates toward certain lifts. What's important to understand is that all of the popular lower-body exercises involve the glutes. This is true for variations of the squat, deadlift, lunge, good morning, hip thrust, leg press, and split squat. That means you will never be a great squatter or deadlifter if you have ultra-weak glutes. And you certainly can't hip thrust a ton of weight with weak glutes.

INCREASING GLUTE STRENGTH CAN INCREASE AND IMPROVE:

- Acceleration and top speed in forward sprinting
- Power in bilateral and unilateral vertical and horizontal jumping
- Agility and quickness in changing direction from side to side
- Acceleration and top speed in lateral sprinting
- Rotational power in swinging, striking, and throwing
- Running, jumping, and throwing performance in track and field events
- Squat and deadlift strength

- Snatch and clean and jerk power in weightlifting
- Strength and conditioning in strongman events
- Bridging and abduction strength for escapes, submissions, and defense in mixed martial arts (MMA)
- Incline sprinting and climbing strength and endurance
- Deceleration in backpedaling, lateral running, and rotational movements
- Ground-based horizontal pushing force

TESTING GLUTE STRENGTH

The squat, deadlift, and hip thrust are great ways to measure lower-body strength, but is there a way to test glute strength specifically? I get this question all the time. Unfortunately, there is no simple answer. For some people, simply testing the glutes with the squat, deadlift, and hip thrust is a great starting point. But even though all of these movements heavily involve the glutes, they're not an exact measure of glute strength. All hip extension exercises utilize the glutes, adductors, and hamstrings. When the knees are bent, the hamstrings contribute less and the glutes slightly more, but all three muscle groups are involved. If simultaneous knee extension occurs (think standing from a squat), then the quads are called into play, and if the spine and pelvis must be stabilized, then various core muscles need to work in concert with one another. It's accurate to say that the three aforementioned lifts are a great way to measure overall lower-body strength, but not strength for a specific muscle. Even hip abduction and external rotation glute exercises call other muscles into play, such as the gluteus medius and minimus, tensor fasciae latae, and deep external hip rotators.

Another way to test glute strength is simply to feel if the muscle is contracting during a movement. This requires a bit of mind-body connection. In a perfect world, we would all own EMG units and could measure the electromyographic output of the glutes while we performed different movements. However, this isn't realistic, and simply paying close attention can suffice. Do you feel your glutes activate maximally during the squat and the deadlift? Do you feel them more when performing a hip thrust? What about other movements, like the single-leg Romanian deadlift or the Bulgarian split squat? If your glutes are rock-solid and you feel them contracting very hard during a movement, you can say for certain that you're working the muscle, but this wouldn't be a test of glute strength.

In short, there is no single test or exercise that will accurately test glute strength because of the shared responsibilities of the muscles working synergistically to carry out hip extension, hip abduction, and hip external rotation. The closest you can get to measure indicators of glute strength is probably the one-rep max (1RM) hip thrust, but even then you'd want to gauge the density of the glute contraction and make sure the technique and range of motion are solid.

Remember when I said that there is a correlation between growing muscle and getting stronger in a variety of glute exercises and rep ranges? Well, if you're training your glutes and building muscle, you can bet that you're getting stronger with all of the movements that involve the glutes, assuming you're practicing them regularly. This encompasses jumping, sprinting, squatting, pulling, powerlifting, Olympic lifting, and strongman. Put another way, the glutes are involved in just about every feat of strength, whether it's for sport or for everyday activities. So, if your goal is to get stronger, you need to train your glutes.

I've been speculating for years as to whether the hip thrust (and glute training in general) improves strength in other lifts, such as the squat and deadlift. I always assumed that glute training—specifically hip thrusting—would improve hip extension strength and therefore improve strength in lifts that involve the hip extension motion. But until recently, I never had the science to back it up.

Four pieces of evidence definitively conclude that the hip thrust alone will improve squat and deadlift strength as well as overall hip extension strength.

TWIN EXPERIMENT

For this study, I trained a pair of identical twin sisters three times per week for six weeks using a daily undulated (DUP) approach—meaning that they performed the exercise three times per week in varying set and rep schemes.[1] One twin performed only squats for her lower body, and the other performed only hip thrusts. Here's what they did.

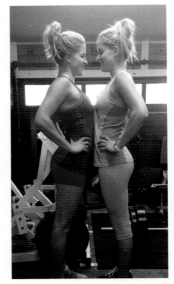

Three times per week, each twin performed 3 to 5 sets of 6 to 15 reps of her individual lift (hip thrusts or parallel back squats). Day one was 4 x 10 with around 75 percent of 1RM, day two was 5 x 6 with around 85 percent of 1RM, and day three was 3 x 15 with around 65 percent of 1RM. However, if the subject could perform more reps on the last set, she did, so the last set was an AMRAP set (which stands for "as many reps as possible").

After the lower-body lift, each twin performed 2 sets of incline presses, bench presses, or close-grip bench presses; then 2 sets of inverted rows, lat pull-downs, or negative chin-ups; and then 2 sets of ab mat crunches, straight-leg sit-ups, or hanging leg raises. The loads were increased each week.

I should point out that the twins were instructed to follow identical caloric and macronutrient plans throughout the study, and their weight didn't change much during the six-week period.

Squatting or hip thrusting 18 times over a six-week period in a DUP fashion elicited the following results:

	1RM SQUAT	1RM HIP THRUST	MAXIMUM HORIZONTAL PUSHING FORCE	UPPER GLUTEUS MAXIMUS THICKNESS	LOWER GLUTEUS MAXIMUS THICKNESS
Squat Twin	↑63%	↑16%	↑20%	↑20%	↑21%
Hip Thrust Twin	↑42%	↑54%	↑32%	↑28%	↑28%

As you can see, the twin who performed the hip thrust improved her squat strength by 42 percent without ever squatting. This clearly indicates that the hip thrust transfers very well to the squat and can improve squat strength without having to perform the squat movement itself. Conversely, the twin who performed the squat improved her hip thrust by only 16 percent, suggesting that the hip thrust transfers more to the squat than the squat transfers to the hip thrust.

RUGBY STUDY

The next piece of evidence is a study that I published as part of my PhD thesis. It was carried out on adolescent rugby players and—like the twin study—showed that the hip thrust improved front squat strength by 7 percent.[2] It wasn't a huge improvement, but it did show that the hip thrust improved squat strength without ever having to squat.

BASEBALL STUDY

This eight-week study investigated the effects of hip thrust training on the strength of 20 male college baseball players.[3] The players were divided into two groups: one group added hip thrusts to their baseball training regimen, while the other group followed only their regular baseball training routine. The results showed a 28 percent increase in squat strength in the hip thrust group (their squat strength increased from around 185 pounds to around 235 pounds)—again, without ever squatting.

LUMBAR EXTENSION STRENGTH STUDY

In this study, researchers tried to determine the effects that squatting and hip thrusting had on lumbar extension strength.[4] To carry out the study, trained males were divided into two groups: twice a week for four weeks, one group performed only squats, and the other group performed only hip thrusts. Interestingly, neither the squat nor hip thrust improved lumbar extension strength. But the group that performed only hip thrusts increased their squat strength by 7 percent, providing more evidence of strength transfer from one hip extension exercise to another.

HIP THRUST TRANSFER TO THE SQUAT

	POPULATION	DESIGN	PRE	POST	% CHANGE
Twin Study	2 female identical twins	3x/week for 6 weeks DUP back squats	95 lbs	135 lbs	42%
Rugby Study	28 adolescent male rugby players	2x/week for 6 weeks Periodized front squats	171 lbs	183 lbs	7%
Baseball Study	20 male college baseball players	3x/week for 8 weeks Periodized back squats	185 lbs	237 lbs	28%
Back Strength Study	14 trained male subjects	2x/week for 4 weeks	242 lbs	259 lbs	7%

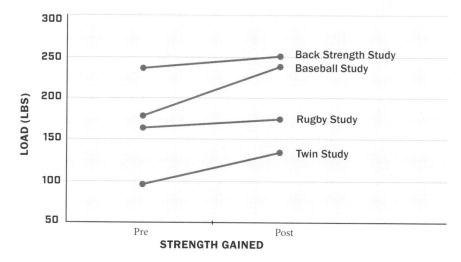

Glute Training for Performance

When I first started lifting weights over 20 years ago, bodybuilding was the most prevalent and widely accepted form of strength training. If you wanted to get strong, improve performance, and build muscle, you lifted weights and trained like a bodybuilder—meaning you performed a wide range of lifts that included both functional and isolated movements.

To clarify, functional movements work multiple joints and muscles simultaneously, and they are considered functional because they mimic the actions of sport and life. Squats, deadlifts, push-ups, and pull-ups are examples of functional movements. Isolated movements are exercises that work only one joint and typically target a specific muscle group. For example, the biceps curl works your elbow joint and primarily targets your biceps.

Why is this important, and how does it relate to glute training, you might ask? It's important because a lot of people consider glute training a form of bodybuilding, which it is. And this is a problem because many people view bodybuilding as being nonfunctional, for two reasons: 1) it incorporates isolated movements; and 2) the majority of bodybuilding is centered on aesthetics or physique training. But this doesn't make bodybuilding nonfunctional.

How did this happen? I'm sure there are a lot of reasons, but here's my observation: As functional fitness grew in popularity, people went through a transition whereby any movement that was not functional was criticized and then tossed out. Isolated movements were exercises for looking good and served no purpose. Though compound movements are important (they are bedrock to my system and to most bodybuilding programs), saying that isolated movements are not functional is simply wrong. Research has shown that lying leg curls, for example, increase sprinting speed, and the lumbar extension machine has been shown to increase Romanian deadlift strength.

And what happens if you get injured? What if you hurt your shoulder and can't do pull-ups, but you can do biceps curls? Should you avoid curls because they're not functional? You're still strengthening your elbow joints, wrists, biceps, and forearms. Just as a carpenter has specific tools for certain jobs, personal trainers and athletes need a set of exercises that not only work the entire body, but also hone specific areas. For example, let's say you're a personal trainer working with an athlete with underdeveloped glutes, and squats and deadlifts are not getting the job done. What are you going to do? Whether your intention is rooted in aesthetics or performance, you need both compound and single-joint movements to target the underdeveloped and weak areas.

In this book, you will learn how to perform both functional and isolated movements that target your glutes. You can lump glute training into the bodybuilding or physique training category, but saying that it is not functional is a false claim. I can confidently say that glute training is one of the most functional forms of strength training out there. How do I know this? Because your glutes—as I've established and will elaborate on in the next part—are one of the most important muscle groups in your body, and the best way to develop your glutes is by implementing the techniques outlined in this book.

Let's not forget that your glutes are responsible for extending your hips, pushing laterally, and rotating your body. This basically covers the entire range of functional movements. It stands to reason that if you train your glutes, you will improve function for movements that involve your glutes, which include sprinting, jumping, squatting, cutting, carrying, throwing, pushing, pulling, punching—the list goes on and on. Everyone can agree that the hips are important for function. Well, your glutes move your hips. And strong, powerful hips are often what separate elite athletes from average ones.

STRONGER GLUTES = BETTER ATHLETE

As athletes progress, they learn to incorporate their hip (glute) and leg muscles into their movements. This is common in boxing and martial arts. A fighter who is just starting out might throw a punch using the power of their shoulder. But as their technique advances, they begin to incorporate their hips and lower body into the movement, adding power and speed.

Another example is comparing a beginner shotputter who uses their upper body when throwing to an advanced shotputter who uses their entire body. Put simply, in order to advance, athletes must learn how to derive maximum power from their hips and legs. And in order for this advancement to take place, a foundation of adequate glute strength (to mention one example) is an absolute prerequisite.

Glute strength and size are important for sports for another reason: well-developed glutes have more potential for force development—that is, the ability to increase the strength or action of a movement. And this is generally true for all muscles. The bigger and stronger the muscle, the more force it can produce, assuming you dedicate ample time to practicing the actions you're trying to improve upon.

Glute-dominant movements also strengthen end-range hip extension, which is the zone involved in ground contact while sprinting—the most important zone for producing force and propelling the body forward. Everyone can agree that speed and acceleration are critical in most sports. So, by training your glutes, you're strengthening a critical motion involved in sporting action.

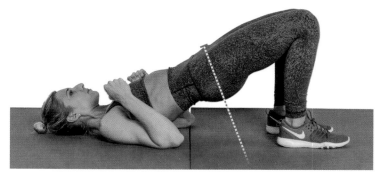

End-Range Hip Extension

FULL HIP EXTENSION

In addition to improving your ability to run, jump, lift, and twist, training your glutes can improve your balance. Whether you're standing on one leg or two, your glutes provide stability for your hips and legs.

Given these facts, it would be silly to make the argument that glute training is not functional. I would argue the opposite and say that you're actually *less* functional if you don't train your glutes.

The bottom line is that strong, healthy glutes make you look and feel better, help prevent injuries and pain, maximize strength, and improve performance.

For all of the reasons outlined in this chapter, I believe that everyone can benefit from glute training. It doesn't matter who you are or what your goals are; the information in this book will help you tremendously.

I have covered a lot of ground and touched on a lot of topics ranging from glute genetics and aesthetics to glute strength and function. In the next part, you will learn the anatomy of the glutes, the roles of the glutes, the mechanisms for growing muscle (hypertrophy), and a classification system for categorizing exercises.

SCIENCE SPEAK: FUNCTION AND PERFORMANCE

As we age, we often experience a reduction in our ability to perform basic activities of daily living, which include walking, climbing stairs, stoop and squat lifting, sit-to-stand movements, carrying objects, and maintaining a single-leg stance. As you can imagine, this can have a big negative impact on our quality of life. The good news is that you can avoid a lot of the negative ramifications of aging by strengthening and developing your glutes, as the studies outlined below help demonstrate.

Walking: The glutes are involved in walking, and activation increases with faster walking speed.[1, 2]

Stair Climbing: The glutes are involved in stair climbing, and activation increases with faster climbing speed.[3]

Sit-to-Stand Movement: The glutes are highly active in the sit-to-stand movement, and activation increases to a greater extent than other muscles with heavier loads.[4]

Carrying: The glutes are very active in carrying loads, and activation is greater with heavier loads held with two hands than with lighter loads held with one hand.[5, 6]

The fact that glute muscle activation increases with increasing walking and stair-climbing speeds and with greater sit-to-stand and carrying loads indicates that the glute muscles play an important role in these movements. Simply stated, strengthening your glutes will improve function in these foundational movement patterns.

IMPROVED HIP EXTENSION

When you extend your hips, you're using your glutes, hamstrings, and adductors (known as the hip extensors) to carry out the action. The hip extension action is central to a wide range of athletic movements, including sprinting, jumping, drop landing, climbing, decelerating and changing direction, cutting from side to side, throwing, swinging, striking, and even strongman events like the truck pull.[7, 8]

The importance of the glutes (and hamstrings and adductors) is underscored by the fact that their role increases with increasing load and speed. This is called the "increasing role of the hips" theory of sports performance. As loads get heavier (in the squat, lunge, conventional deadlift, and hex bar deadlift exercises) and running speeds and vertical jumps increase, the turning force requirements at the hips (hip extension torque) increase proportionally more to the movement, while turning force requirements at the knees (knee extension torque) increase proportionally less.[9]

Although the theory has been criticized on the basis that net joint moments are hard to interpret,[10] other methods of investigation (such as electromyography and musculoskeletal modeling) produce similar results.[11]

SPRINTING

The hip extensors, specifically the glutes, are responsible for increasing speed through increases in stride frequency at high speed.[12] They are also the most active muscle group in the final part of the swing phase and in the stance phase,[13, 14, 15] where they are critical for absorbing braking forces upon ground contact, as illustrated in the chart below.

Bear in mind that the glutes are also hip external rotators and abductors. While they extend the hips and help swing the legs downward, they also stabilize the pelvis in the frontal and transverse planes by preventing excessive hip adduction and internal rotation during the single-leg stance phase.[16]

CHANGING DIRECTION

The glutes play a crucial role in cutting from side to side or changing direction while running. The role of the glutes in producing force in multiple planes simultaneously is likely a feature of cutting from side to side or other lateral movements. In these scenarios, the different regions of the glutes must contract in a coordinated fashion to produce hip abduction, hip external rotation, and hip extension at the same time. It is commonly thought that hip abduction strength is more important for lateral movements than hip extension strength, but this is not the case—hip extension strength better predicts lateral movement ability than hip abduction strength.[17, 18]

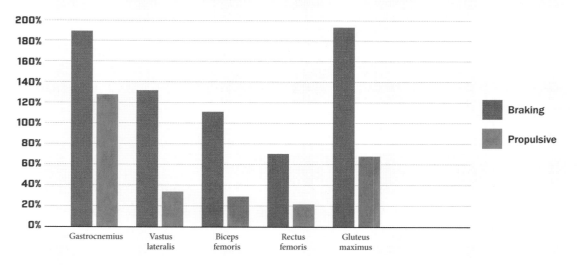

EMG AMPLITUDES (PERCENTAGE OF MAXIMUM ISOMETRIC VOLUNTARY CONTRACTION) IN THE STANCE PHASE OF SPRINT RUNNING

THROWING AND STRIKING

The glute of the rear leg works to perform both hip extension and hip external rotation when throwing[19] or swinging a club, bat, or racket. This explains why the glutes are so active during baseball pitching.[20, 21] The glutes, in summary, play a crucial role in sports that involve striking and throwing.

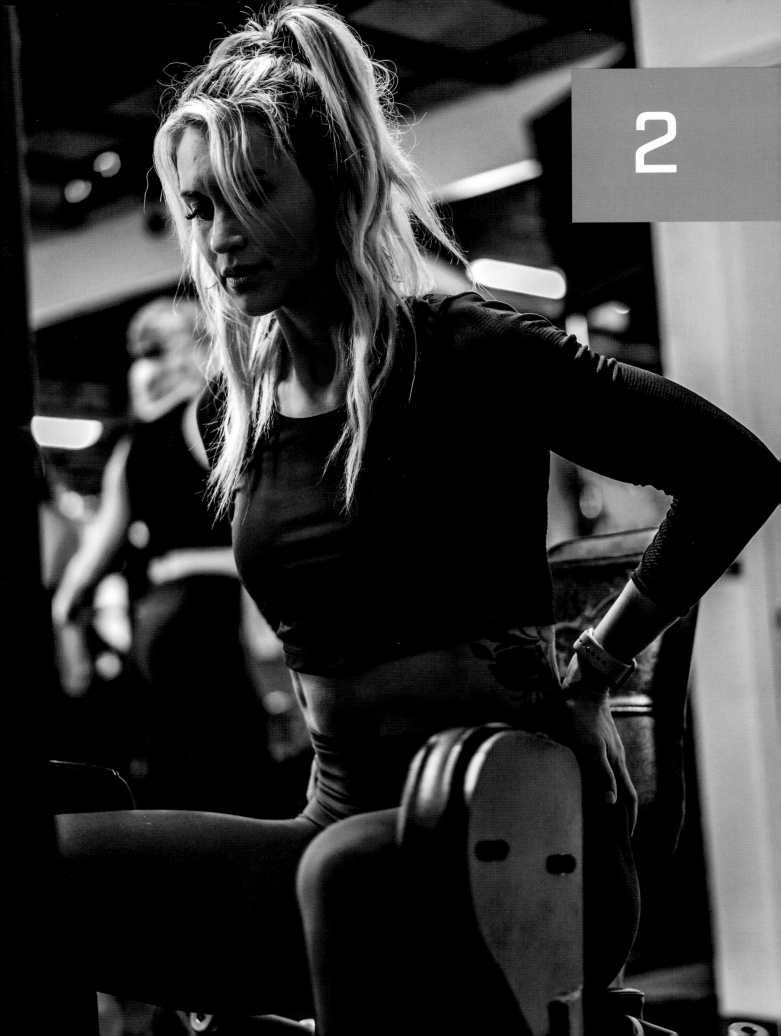

THE SCIENCE OF STRENGTH AND PHYSIQUE TRAINING

If you were to go back in time and tell my younger self that one day I would be known as the Glute Guy and would be the world's foremost expert on glute training, I never would have believed you. I would have given you a puzzled look and said, "Me, a Glute Guy?! You're crazy."

But it happened, not because I developed the most amazing glutes that anyone has ever seen (though that would've been awesome), but because I was the first person to start looking into the science of glute training. I wanted to understand why and how the glutes grow, how anatomy and the roles of the glutes affect movement and aesthetics, and the best exercises for targeting the glutes.

And I found the answers. Although there is still much to learn about the glutes and how best to train them, we do know a lot based on research, experiments, and observations. In this part of the book, I distill the most important glute training science into four chapters. You will learn the anatomy and function of the glutes and how they influence your appearance and movement. You will learn the science of muscle growth and the best methods for strengthening and building bigger glutes. Lastly, you will learn an exercise categorization system that explains why certain exercises are well suited for specific goals and why certain exercises work your glutes better than others.

While many people have skipped learning this information and gotten great results simply by performing the exercises and following the programs in the back of the book, you will never be the best physique competitor, athlete, or trainer or reach your true potential if you don't understand the fundamental science behind what you are doing. Why? Because when you understand how your glutes work and why they work the way they do (the science of glute training), you can attach meaning to the exercises you perform and the program you design (the art of glute training). You know what you are doing works, not because you've tested it on yourself or because it worked for someone else, but because you understand the science.

Anatomy of the Glutes

I'm going to assume that most of you reading this book are more interested in growing bigger, stronger glutes than learning about anatomy. This is not a bad thing. In fact, filling out my jeans in the hopes of looking more athletic and attractive is what put me on the path to becoming the Glute Guy. So I realize that learning the anatomy of the glutes might not be your chief objective. But here's the deal: whether or not you're interested in anatomy, it is crucial to understand—at least on a basic level—for several important reasons.

For starters, everyone can benefit from knowing how the body works. After all, I make a lot of recommendations and propose a ton of ideas that will help you grow and strengthen your glutes, but those recommendations aren't valid unless I discuss the muscles you're working so hard to develop. When you understand what the glutes look like, where they are located (I'm referring to the three gluteal muscles, which I will get to shortly), what structures they attach to, and why they are shaped the way they are, you will gain a whole new appreciation for their role and function, as well as for the glute training techniques and programs I offer later in the book. Equally important, understanding the anatomy will help you realize how magnificent and versatile your glutes are and why prioritizing them in training is so important.

Second, the anatomy of the glutes explains a lot about the aesthetic differences between individuals and highlights what you can and can't change. For example, if you're wondering why you can't get a wider butt no matter how hard you train, or why you have pronounced hip divots or hip dips (inward curves on the sides of your hips), knowing about anatomy will provide a clear and concrete answer. Put simply, anatomy partly explains your glute aesthetics and appearance.

Third, in order to appreciate the important role the glutes play in our daily lives—from posture and injury prevention to performance and overall health—you need to understand what is going on underneath the skin. As you work your way through this chapter, you will learn how hip anatomy determines how you move, and what adjustments you need to make based on your anthropometry (limb and torso proportions) to achieve your desired results, whether you're training your glutes for aesthetics, performance, or general health.

In addition to guiding your movement mechanics, understanding the anatomy of your glutes will help you relate what you are feeling when you perform an exercise. As I discuss in Chapter 8, picturing in your mind the muscle you are working during an exercise (referred to as the *mind-muscle connection*—see page 93) has been shown to enhance muscle growth. And understanding your gluteal anatomy will help you communicate where you are feeling an exercise—whether it is in your upper glutes, lower glutes, or somewhere else—which will allow you to make the necessary adjustments. In short, a basic knowledge of anatomy will help you refine your technique and choose exercises that are in line with your aesthetic and performance goals.

And if you happen to be a trainer, it's even more important to have a working knowledge of anatomy, especially if you intend on teaching my Glute Lab system. You have a duty to educate your clients. They will have questions, and it's up to you to provide answers backed by evidence-based science. For instance, clients might want to know why a particular exercise feels better than others, why their glutes are shaped the way they are, and why they need to perform certain exercises based on their anatomy and training goals. If you don't understand where the muscles are located and what they are designed to do, you won't have good answers. Not only will you fail to satisfy their curiosity, but you might lose their confidence, which is a primary driver for getting results. However, if you can explain the nuances of skeletal and muscle anatomy and how those determine the shape and function of their glutes, you can resolve their concerns, attach meaning to the programs you're putting them through, and keep them focused on the most important elements of training, which are having fun and staying consistent.

HIP AND PELVIS SKELETAL ANATOMY

The appearance and function of a muscle can be partly figured out by looking at its anatomy—what the muscle looks like and what it attaches to. Although your gluteal muscles give your hips shape, the skeletal anatomy of your pelvis and hips determines that shape. What's more, your hip and pelvis anatomy is an important variable for determining which exercises you should prioritize and how, based on your anatomy, you should approach those exercises. I discuss all of this in more detail in the pages to come, and I reference anatomy as it pertains to exercise mechanics and program design throughout this book.

So, before you glaze over the illustrations, understand that hip and pelvic skeletal anatomy is crucial not only for determining the appearance of your glutes, but also for determining the best exercises for your unique anatomical shape. But before I delve into these particulars in this chapter, you need to know what the main bones of the hip and pelvis are.

Don't feel like you need to memorize the name and location of each bone. This is just a primer to familiarize you with basic skeletal hip and pelvis anatomy. As you progress through this chapter, I will reference these bones and help you connect the dots between skeletal and anatomical differences (sizes and shapes) and how those differences create unique aesthetic characteristics and movement patterns.

Let's begin by looking at the anatomy of the pelvic region. As you can see, your pelvis and hips are made up of five main bones: the ilium, pubis, ischium, sacrum, and coccyx.

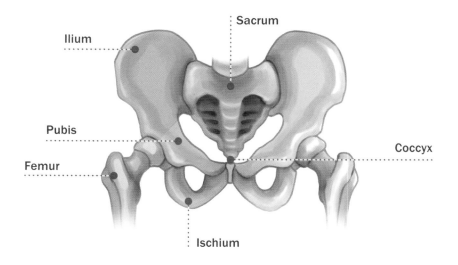

On the side of the pelvis are the acetabulum (hip socket) and the femur, which encompass the femoral head (ball), femoral neck, greater trochanter, and thigh bone.

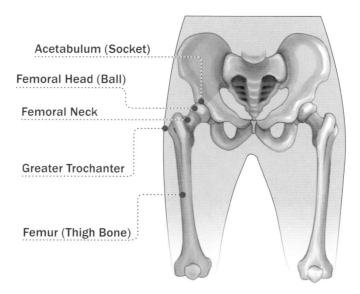

Acetabulum (Socket)

Femoral Head (Ball)

Femoral Neck

Greater Trochanter

Femur (Thigh Bone)

Here's how these bony structures fit together to make up your hip and pelvis anatomy.

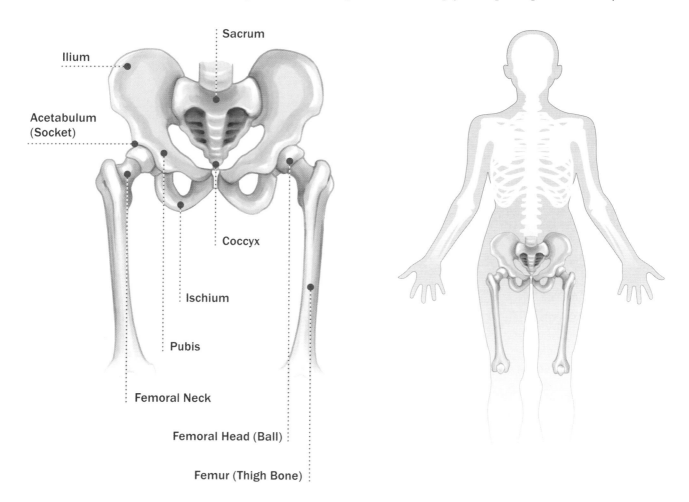

Sacrum

Ilium

Acetabulum (Socket)

Coccyx

Ischium

Pubis

Femoral Neck

Femoral Head (Ball)

Femur (Thigh Bone)

Whether I'm working with a man or a woman, I base the training strategy around their goals and select exercises based on their unique anatomy. Because everyone has different anatomical shapes, mobility, and injury histories, I treat every person as a unique case.

However, there are some general differences between male and female hip anatomy that are worth noting and that, in some circumstances, help explain certain aesthetic and movement characteristics. For example, the male pelvis is generally taller and narrower than the female pelvis, and the acetabulum is oriented more laterally in males than in females, which is more forward-facing.[1, 2] This means men tend to have relatively narrower and longer glutes compared to females, who tend to have wider and shorter glutes. Interestingly, relative overall glute size is nearly identical between men and women; male glutes are proportionately larger, though.[3]

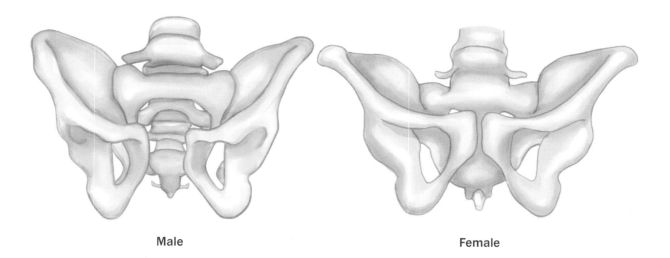

Male   Female

What's more, females on average have significantly greater acetabular depth and smaller femoral head diameters compared to males,[1, 4] which might make the hip joint more or less stable in certain positions and movements. We can't say for certain what these positions and movements are because it depends on so many variables. All we can do is make assumptions based on the average characteristics.

For instance, women tend to have relatively wider hips than males. For this reason, it is commonly thought that women have larger Q angles (line representing the resultant line of force of the quadriceps made by connecting a point near the ASIS to the midpoint of the patella) compared to males; however, this is not the case.[5] Nevertheless, women tend to possess more hip range of motion, allowing them to move through more range of motion during various glute exercises than males.[6, 7] Women also tend to portray greater knee valgus (inward movement of the knee) than men during various landing and squatting movements (eighth study) due to anatomical and neuromuscular factors.[8] Wider hips can make it appear that women are caving in more than men during various single-leg squatting movements, but sometimes this is just an illusion, and the knee isn't actually caving inward.

Women also tend to have greater standing sacral slope and lumbar lordosis angles (there is a 7- to 13-degree difference between females and males according to various studies).[9, 10] This explains why female glutes often appear to protrude more than male glutes and suggests that women have more range of motion in the lumbar spine. I've experienced this in my own practice. In fact, most of the women I train are more prone to hyperextension through the lumbar spine when squatting and deadlifting than men, and this might be due to a greater lumbar range of motion. For example, when I use the "chest up" cue, which reminds lifters not to round their backs when they squat or deadlift, some women tend to anterior pelvic tilt and overarch their backs, putting unnecessary increased stress on the lumbar spine. So the "chest up" cue is great for most men, but not for some women.

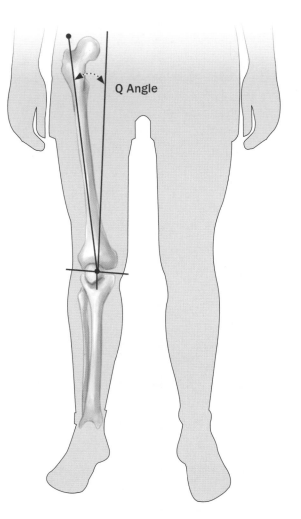

Although these examples are common, they're not universal. Some guys I train can squat to rock bottom, whereas some women I train can't get to parallel without butt winking (posterior pelvic tilting in the bottom of the squat). Some women I train have narrow pelvises, and some men I train have wide ones. Some women I work with never struggle with knee valgus or lumbar hyperextension, whereas some men I work with do. The point is, these averages don't take into account individual variability, which ultimately determines how each person looks and moves. So you can use these averages to help explain certain aesthetic and movement differences, but you also need to take into account the individual's injury history, mobility, experience level, and goals, as well as their skeletal anatomy.

Now that you're familiar with basic skeletal hip and pelvis anatomy, let's see how the different sizes and shapes of these bones create certain gluteal shapes. Then we'll look at how those differences create unique movement patterns.

HOW SKELETAL ANATOMY INFLUENCES GLUTEAL APPEARANCE

As you probably know, you cannot change your skeletal anatomy. It's completely dependent on your genetics. You can manipulate the appearance of your glutes by adding muscle and losing fat, but you can't modify your skeletal anatomy. For this reason—and I can't stress this enough—I implore you not to get hung up on the things you cannot change. Instead, focus on the things you *can* control, like your body composition (proportion of fat to muscle), muscle development, and exercise selection and, equally important, your diet, mindset, and lifestyle (sleep and stress management). Genetics matter, it's true, but other variables influence how you look, feel, and perform, and those are the ones you should focus on.

Later in the book, you will learn how to maximize muscle growth and alter the appearance of your glutes by targeting certain regions (upper and lower) with specific exercises. But for now, I want to focus on the different anatomical shapes and how these anatomical differences partially determine the shape of your glutes.

For instance, the size and width of the ilium (A), the length and angle of the femoral neck (B), the vertical distance between the ilium and greater trochanter (C), and the size of the greater trochanter (D) partially determine the shape of your hips, waist, and glutes when viewed from the front and back.

FACTORS THAT INFLUENCE GLUTE SHAPE

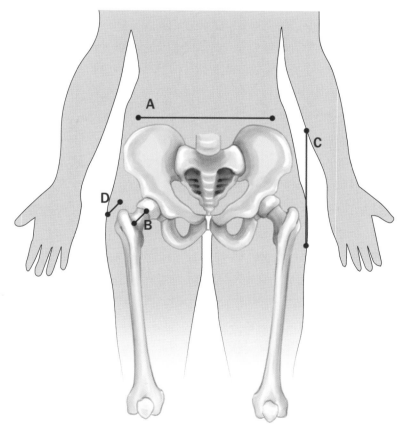

If you have wide ilium bones, long femoral necks, and pronounced greater trochanters, you might have a square or round butt. If you have medium or narrow ilium bones, long femoral necks, and pronounced greater trochanters, you might have a heart- or pear-shaped butt. And if you have wide ilium bones, short femoral necks, and small greater trochanters, you might have a V-shaped butt.

DIFFERENT TYPES OF GLUTE SHAPES

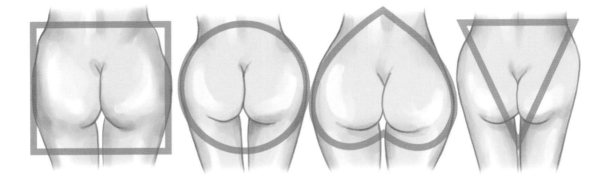

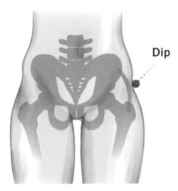

Dip

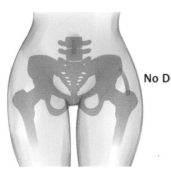

No Dip

And there's more: some people have outward curves, giving the bubble butt look, while others have inward indentations along the insides of their hipbones, which are often referred to as *hip dips* or *hip divots*. Just as hip and femur size partially determines gluteal shapes, it also partially determines how pronounced the inward depressions are. If you're lean and have wide hips (ilium bones), long femoral necks, and big greater trochanters, you might have more pronounced hip dips than someone who has narrow hips, small greater trochanters, and more body fat. What's more, the vertical distance between the ilium and hip socket also matters. If that distance is short, you may not have any hip dips, but if that distance is long, you may have more pronounced hip dips.

Other aspects of the skeleton that affect the appearance and shape of your glutes are the angle of the sacrum and the distance between the sacrum and femurs. Picture someone standing in front of you so that you're viewing them from the side. If the individual has a more horizontal sacrum and a greater horizontal distance from the sacrum to the femurs, their glutes will look rounder and larger. If the individual has a more vertical sacrum and a smaller horizontal distance from the sacrum to the femurs, their glutes will appear flatter and smaller. This is true regardless of the amount of gluteal muscle mass the person has. Some ethnicities are known for having more aesthetically pleasing glutes than others, and the angle of the sacrum plays a large role in this appearance.

Of course, all of the examples I have offered are gross generalizations; there are a lot more variables that determine these shapes, such as body composition and muscle size. My intention here is merely to highlight how the size and structure of the hip bones influence the shape and appearance of the glutes. In other words, they are far from concrete. Just because you identify with a certain shape doesn't mean your anatomy matches that shape. I've trained women who

THE DEGREE OF SACRAL SLOPE INFLUENCES GLUTEAL APPEARANCE

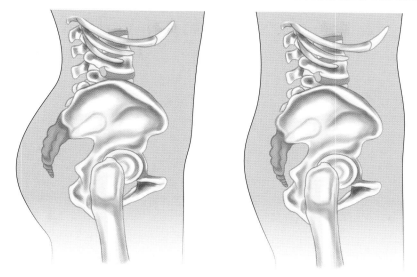

These two pelvises are the same except that the one on the left has a larger sacral slope, which creates a greater gluteal prominence.

have wide hips, long femoral necks, and pronounced greater trochanters who have no hip divots. My point is this: anatomy matters, but it's not everything. I can't emphasize this enough: you can alter your appearance by increasing the size of your glutes (adding muscle) or by adjusting your percentage of body fat (losing or gaining weight). And you will learn how to do exactly that in the following chapters.

Having covered the role that skeletal anatomy plays in appearance, let's look at how it affects movement.

HOW SKELETAL ANATOMY INFLUENCES MOVEMENT PATTERNS

Just as there is no all-encompassing approach to nutrition and program design, there is no universal way to perform a movement. The shape, orientation, and depth of the hip socket; the length of the femur; and the angle of the femoral head and neck, for example, vary from person to person and therefore influence the setup, execution, and exercises people should perform.

For instance, if someone has shallow hip sockets and long femoral necks, they might have access to more hip range of motion—say, squatting to full depth (hips below knee crease)—because their femurs are unobstructed by their hip sockets (acetabulum). If they have deep hip sockets and short femoral necks, on the other hand, they might not be able to squat as deep or lift their knees as high because their femur collides with the ridge of their acetabulum. And these are just two examples, which factor in only a couple of variables.

As I describe in Part 5, your stance, your technique, and the variation you choose to perform should be based on your experience, body type, and anatomy. And this is where the art of training and coaching comes into play. It takes some tinkering and experimenting to figure out which setup, execution, and exercise variation is best for you. But understanding anatomy will shed light on how you should move and may steer you in the right direction.

**DIFFERENCES IN FEMORAL NECK
LENGTHS AND ANGLES**

**DIFFERENCES IN HIP SOCKET
ORIENTATION AND DEPTH**

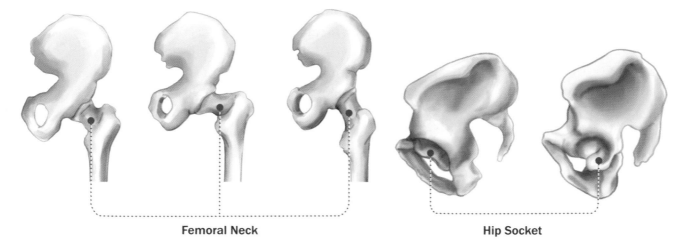

Femoral Neck

Hip Socket

For example, perhaps squatting deep from a narrow stance hurts your hips, while squatting to parallel from a wide stance is just fine. Some trainers will tell you that you need to squat deep to get the best results and that your poor mobility is the limiting factor when in fact it is your bony anatomy. Rather than spend time performing stretches that won't actually improve your mobility due to anatomy, you can focus on performing the variations that cater to your unique build.

Another example of how anatomy affects movement is femur and torso proportions (anthropometry). Take the deadlift and squat, for example. To maintain balance and perform the movement correctly, you must keep the barbell centered over the middle of your feet. Someone with a longer torso and short legs will necessarily have a more upright squat and deadlift, while someone with a shorter torso and longer legs will need to lean their torso forward.

**SHORT TORSO/LONG LEGS:
FORWARD LEAN**

**LONG TORSO/SHORT LEGS:
UPRIGHT**

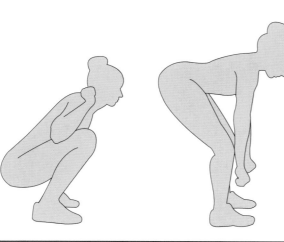

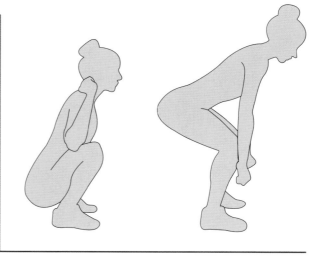

FORWARD LEAN
SQUAT

FORWARD LEAN
DEADLIFT

UPRIGHT SQUAT

UPRIGHT DEADLIFT

But this is not always the case. There are always exceptions and anomalies. There are people who have short torsos and long femurs who squat upright, which might be due to the orientation, shape, and depth of their hip sockets and the length, size, and angle of their femoral necks, along with other factors such as ankle dorsiflexion mobility and technique.

The point is, no two individuals move exactly the same, and they shouldn't. There is a wide range of skeletal shapes and sizes that affect how we move. So, if you ever hear a coach telling everyone to squat or perform a movement the same way, you should immediately question that coach's motives and experience.

It's also important to point out that these examples are simple generalizations. Like I said, there are exceptions to every rule, and I'm leaving out a lot of variables, such as mobility and motor control (coordination), which also highly influence how you move and the exercise variations you should perform. I'll dive deeper into these variables and look at all of this in more detail in Parts 3 and 4.

The key takeaway here is that skeletal anatomy varies from person to person, and these variations dictate not just how you look, but also your range of motion and movement mechanics.

GLUTEAL MUSCLE ANATOMY

Now that you have a basic understanding of skeletal anatomy, let's take a look at the gluteal muscles. As you know, the three muscles in each buttock—the gluteus maximus, gluteus medius, and gluteus minimus—are collectively referred to as the glutes.

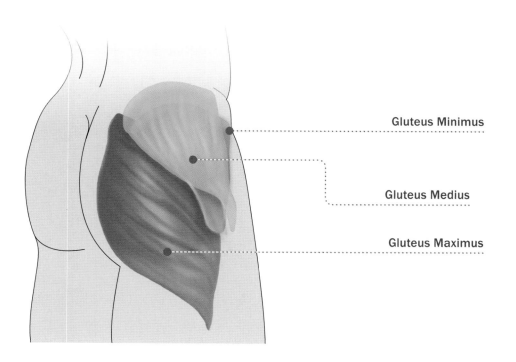

Gluteus Minimus

Gluteus Medius

Gluteus Maximus

GLUTEUS MAXIMUS

The gluteus maximus (or glute max) is the largest of the three gluteal muscles and gives your hips and butt shape. It is typically broken into two subdivisions—the upper and lower glute max. As you can see, the gluteus maximus builds the most superficial layer (the top layer closest to the skin), covering a portion of the gluteus medius (and the gluteus medius covers the gluteus minimus).

It's worth repeating that when I say "glutes," I'm referring mainly to the gluteus maximus because it makes up two-thirds of the glutes and is twice the size of the gluteus medius and gluteus minimus combined. When it comes to aesthetics as well as function and performance, it's easier to think of all three muscles as one. (This will make more sense after you read Chapter 6.)

With regard to exercise selection and glute sculpting—that is, targeting a specific region of the glutes with an exercise—I'll simply refer to the upper and lower subdivision of the gluteus maximus. For example, if you want to target your upper glutes to build what is commonly referred to as a *shelf,* it's best to perform hip abduction exercises. If you want to target your lower glutes, you might prioritize more squats and deadlifts. And if you want to target the upper and lower subdivisions simultaneously, performing hip thrusts and glute bridges will give you the best results.

UPPER AND LOWER SUBDIVISIONS OF THE GLUTE MAX

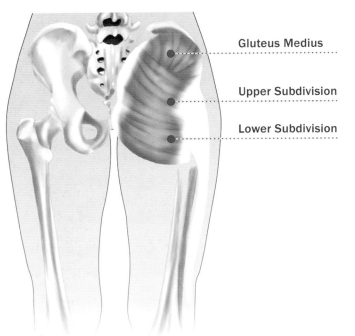

Gluteus Medius

Upper Subdivision

Lower Subdivision

BUTTERFLY SHAPE

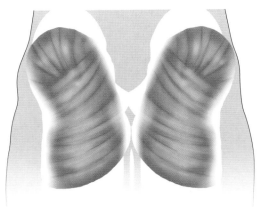

Well-developed, lean glutes take on a butterfly-shaped appearance.

Due to the anatomy and structure of the glute max, we don't think in terms of inner versus outer subdivisions because it's impossible to target the muscle in that way. When you look at the glute max, for example, you will notice that the muscle fibers are oriented diagonally and tend to run the entire length from the origins to the insertions. This helps explain the shape of the muscle and why it's difficult to target the inner versus outer regions.

As I will make clear in the forthcoming chapters, I recommend performing a variety of exercises to ensure maximal development. But what is important to understand here is that you can target the upper, lower, and both the upper and lower with specific exercises.

Untrained humans range from around 200 to 1,000 cm³ in gluteus maximus volume, a five-fold difference—and that's without training! With training, research shows that there are large discrepancies in the ways individuals respond physiologically. Much of this has to do with the way people's satellite cells behave. Satellite cells are muscle stem cells that surround the muscles' cells and lend their nuclei when it senses the muscles need it, which are the three primary mechanisms of hypertrophy. Think of satellite cells as a backup system signaling that the muscle needs to grow. Furthermore, skeletal anatomy and body fat levels profoundly impact the look of the glutes, both of which are highly influenced by genetics.

There are several ways to measure the size of a muscle, including anatomical cross-sectional area (CSA), muscle thickness, volume, and even weight. By any measure, the glutes are the largest muscle in the body.

The charts below show that the glutes are the heaviest[11] and largest[12] muscles in the lower body. Indeed, the gluteus maximus is certainly the largest muscle in the body when measured by anatomical CSA, with values in cadavers reaching 48.4 cm² [13] and many values recorded in living subjects using magnetic resonance imaging (MRI) or computed tomography (CT) scans reaching as high as 58.3 cm².[14, 15, 16, 17, 18, 19, 20]

When comparing gluteus maximus muscle volume between males and females, it's interesting to note that the relative measures are similar (as a proportion of total hip muscle volume), but the absolute measures are very different, with the whole muscle being 27 percent larger in males than in females.[21]

Across different sports, female athletes show different levels of gluteal development.[22] Those taking part in high-impact sports (volleyball players and high-jumpers), odd impact sports (soccer and squash players), and high-force sports (powerlifters) all tend to show much larger glute size than those taking part in repetitive impact sports (endurance runners) and repetitive non-impact sports (swimmers). Overall, those pursing odd impact sports had the greatest glute size, which may suggest that variety of loading types is one key to successful gluteus maximus development.

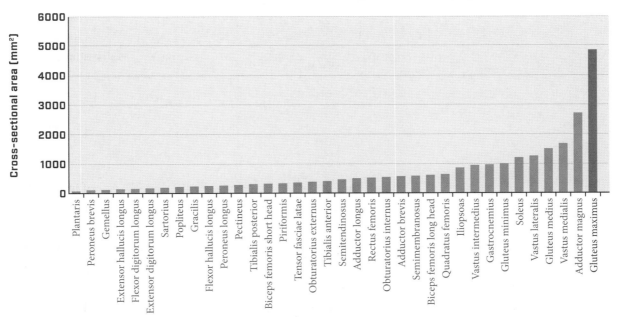

CROSS-SECTIONAL AREA OF THE LEG MUSCLES AS MEASURED IN A SINGLE MALE CADAVER (AGED 58 YEARS)

RELATIVE WEIGHTS OF THE LEG MUSCLES AS MEASURED IN A SINGLE MALE CADAVER (AGED 58 YEARS)

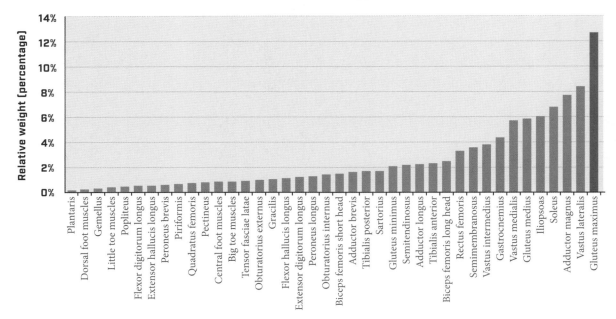

Gluteus Maximus Origin and Insertions

The function of a muscle can be partly figured out by looking at the attachment points, which are called the origins and insertions. The origins and insertions are where the muscle and its associated tendons attach to the bones of the skeleton. The origin is closer to the center of the body, while the insertion is more distant from the center of the body. When the muscle contracts, it pulls the origin and the insertion points closer together.

As the image on page 56 illustrates, the gluteus maximus runs diagonally downward from the rear of the pelvis to meet the femur and the iliotibial band (ITB). This diagonal direction of the muscle fibers—as you will learn more about in the next chapter—has important implications for exactly how the glutes function.

Interestingly, only around 20 percent of the gluteal fibers attach to bone; the remaining 80 percent attach to fascia (connective tissue). The gluteus maximus connects to the coccyx, sacrum, pelvis, femur, iliotibial band, pelvic floor muscles, thoracolumbar fascia, erector spinae, gluteus medius, and sacrotuberous ligament.

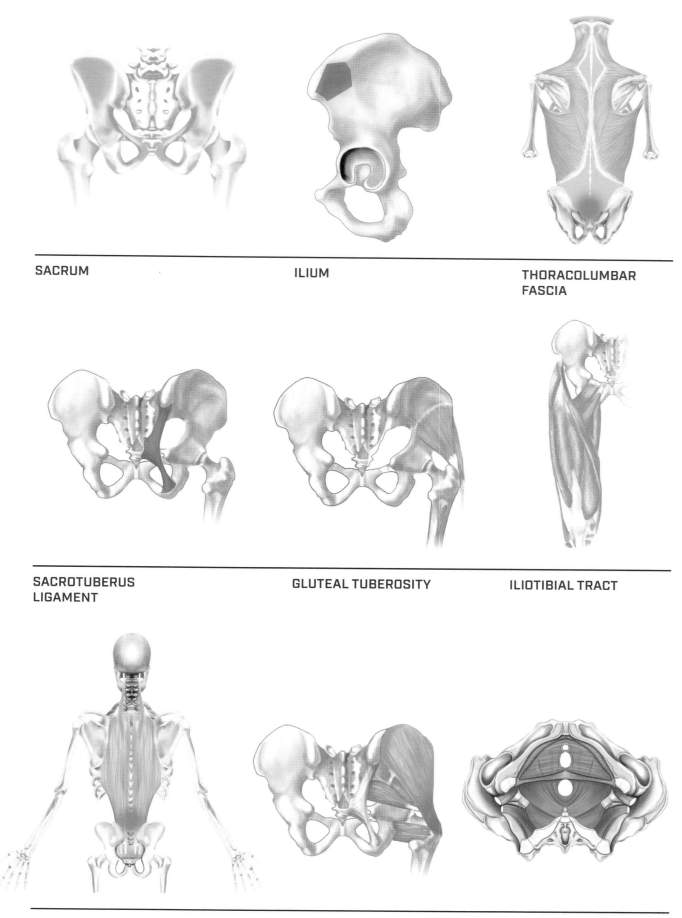

SACRUM

ILIUM

THORACOLUMBAR FASCIA

SACROTUBERUS LIGAMENT

GLUTEAL TUBEROSITY

ILIOTIBIAL TRACT

ERECTOR SPINAE

GLUTEUS MEDIUS

PELVIC FLOOR

From this list, it becomes apparent that the gluteus maximus is one of the most important muscles in the human body due to its vast attachments. For example, it connects to the humerus (the long bone in the upper arm) via the latissimus dorsi (lat) muscle through the thoracolumbar fascia, and it connects to the tibia (shin bone) via the iliotibial band, thereby influencing movement and transferring force throughout the entire body. What's more, these attachment points allow for hip extension, hip abduction, and hip external rotation, all of which are expressed in the movements of daily life.

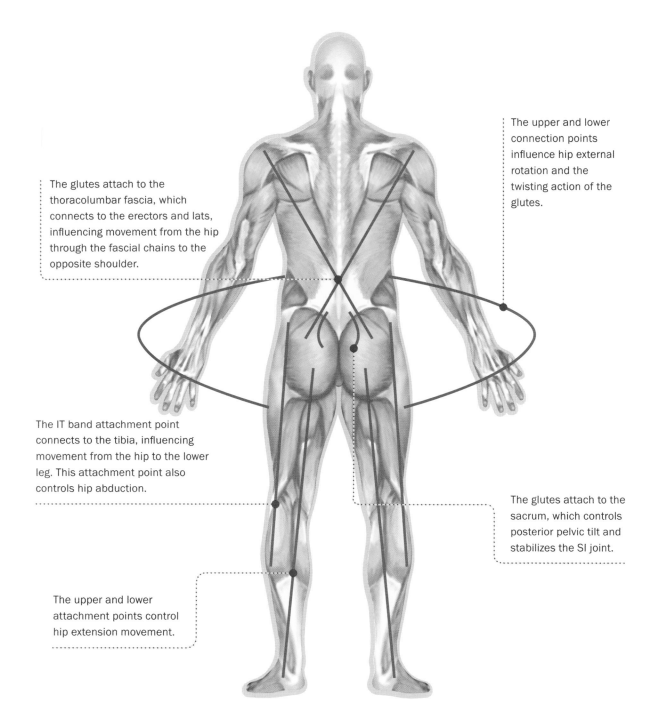

The glutes attach to the thoracolumbar fascia, which connects to the erectors and lats, influencing movement from the hip through the fascial chains to the opposite shoulder.

The upper and lower connection points influence hip external rotation and the twisting action of the glutes.

The IT band attachment point connects to the tibia, influencing movement from the hip to the lower leg. This attachment point also controls hip abduction.

The glutes attach to the sacrum, which controls posterior pelvic tilt and stabilizes the SI joint.

The upper and lower attachment points control hip extension movement.

Again, you will learn more about the function of the glutes in the next chapter—more specifically, the role of hip extension, hip abduction, and hip external rotation. For now, it's important to understand that these attachment points allow for a wide range of movements, from daily actions like squatting, bending over, standing upright, and walking to explosive movements like sprinting, jumping, and rotating.

GLUTEUS MEDIUS

The gluteus medius (or glute med) and gluteus minimus (or glute min) are commonly referred to as the *small gluteal muscles* and often are lumped into the same category when describing anatomy and function. The gluteus medius is located near or slightly above the hip joint, forms the middle layer of the glutes, and completely covers the gluteus minimus muscle. The glute med provides some shape to the upper butt region, but it's hard to isolate the muscle with specific exercises because it shares responsibilities with the upper subdivision of the glute max as well as the glute min.

Nonetheless, you'll hear a lot of trainers say, "You should do lateral band training to target your gluteus medius." The problem with this statement is that it's nearly impossible to know which subdivisions of which gluteal muscles you're working during a movement, especially when the hips move away from neutral in terms of flexion (bending your hips or lifting your leg), abduction (moving your leg away from your body), and rotation. In all likelihood, you're working all of them to a certain degree.

There are three subdivisions of the gluteus medius: the anterior, middle, and posterior regions. Each plays slightly different roles during functional movement. When you perform lateral band walks, you're working the gluteus medius, but you're also targeting the upper subdivision of the gluteus maximus and the gluteus minimus. Again, this is why I refer to the gluteal muscles collectively as the glutes and often distinguish only the upper and lower regions of the glute max.

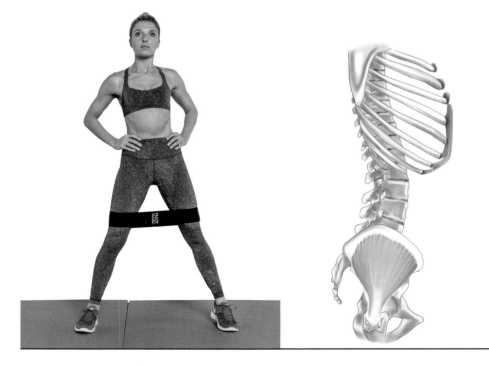

LATERAL BAND WALK   GLUTEUS MEDIUS

Gluteus Medius Origin and Insertion

The glute med originates on the ilium and inserts (with the gluteus minimus) at the greater trochanter of the femur. This connection serves as a primary stabilizer for your hip when you're balancing on one leg or walking and running. If your gluteus medius is deconditioned or weak, then your pelvis won't be as stable, and you will have more knee valgus—more specifically, one side of your pelvis will drop, and your knee will cave inward. Physical therapists home in on this muscle because when the pelvis drops to one side or another, it can create knee, hip, and lower back issues.

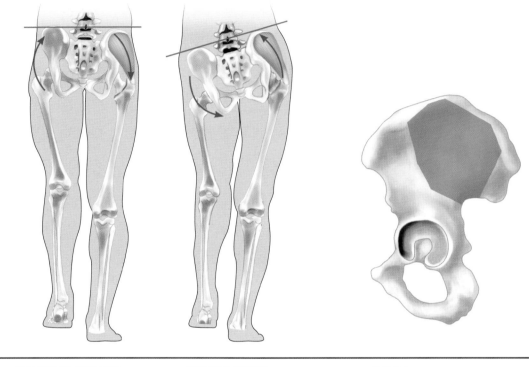

NEUTRAL PELVIS   PELVIC DROP   ILIUM

GLUTEUS MINIMUS

The gluteus minimus, the smallest of the gluteal muscles, is located under the gluteus medius. As I just mentioned, the glute min often is lumped into the same category as the gluteus medius because it shares the same origin and insertion points and performs similar movements. However, they are different muscles with slightly different functions. As is the case with the gluteus medius, there are three subdivisions of the gluteus minimus— the anterior, middle, and posterior regions—and each plays a unique role during functional movement. As you can see, the gluteus minimus originates on the ilium below the gluteus medius and inserts at the greater trochanter of the femur. Like the gluteus medius, this connection provides stability for your hips.

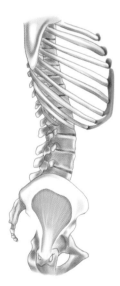

MUSCLE ARCHITECTURE

Just as your skeletal anatomy influences your appearance, form, and exercise selection, your unique muscle architecture or the physical organization of your muscles can play a huge role.

It should come as no surprise that we all have unique muscle architecture. Unlike your skeletal anatomy, you can change your muscle architecture through training, but those changes may or may not be visually noticeable. For example, increasing fascicle length or pennation angle (the length of the muscle itself) won't make your glutes look much different, but it will improve how the muscle functions, because when you increase the fascicle length, you essentially have a longer muscle, which translates to more rapid force production (more on this in the sidebar below), and when you increase the pennation angle, you have greater force production capabilities.

I think it goes without saying, though I'm going to say it anyway, that there is much more to your gluteal anatomy than what is covered in this chapter. My intention is to include only the essential information pertaining to glute anatomy and appearance.

In subsequent chapters, I tie in more anatomy, such as muscle fiber composition, the roles of the glutes, the mechanisms for increasing muscle size, and why performing a variety of exercises is essential to maximizing glute gains.

SCIENCE SPEAK: MUSCLE ARCHITECTURE

Muscle architecture refers to the way in which the muscle fibers are arranged within the overall muscle.[23] It is made up of three main factors: the length of the muscle fascicles (groups of muscle fibers), the fascicle angle (also called the pennation angle), and the cross-sectional area (CSA) relative to the direction of the muscle fascicles (called the physiological CSA).

Most muscles in the body are either long and thin, with long muscle fascicles (bundle of skeletal muscle fibers), low fascicle angles, and small physiological CSA; or short and fat, with short muscle fascicles, high fascicle angles, and large physiological CSA. Long and thin muscles are well suited for producing low levels of force at high speeds through large ranges of motion (ROM). Short and fat muscles are better suited for exerting high levels of force at low speed through small ranges of motion.

The gluteus maximus has unusual muscle architecture, displaying aspects of both broad types of muscle. It has a large fascicle angle, a large physiological CSA, and long muscle fascicles. So it seems to function both to produce high levels of force at low speed through small ranges of motion, as well as to produce lower levels of force at high speeds through large ranges of motion.[24, 25, 26, 27]

Scientists analyze various aspects of muscles that determine their size, shape, and characteristics. These unique architectural characteristics help explain why some people are well suited for a particular sport or activity. For example, muscles with longer fibers shorten faster and lend themselves well to explosive actions such as sprinting or jumping, whereas muscles with high levels of physiological CSA produce high levels of force, which lends itself well to high-force actions such as strongman or powerlifting. Again, this points to a variety of loading types as one key to successful glute development.

Function of the Glutes

The glutes are a true Swiss Army knife of a muscle equipped to handle a wide range of actions—from daily movements like walking, standing up from a chair, picking something up off the ground, and carrying groceries to sporting motions like running, cutting, lifting, jumping, throwing, and striking. And whether you're balancing on one foot, lifting heavy, moving explosively, or carrying out an endurance effort, your glutes are well suited to handle every task.

When you examine the anatomy of the glutes—the attachment points and the fact that they link the upper and lower body together—you can start connecting the dots between the muscle structure and the wide range of movements the glutes control. Just as understanding the anatomy of your glutes helps explain their appearance and can inform your exercise selection and program design, knowing the roles of your glutes—that is, the movements they produce—can help you develop a training strategy that caters to your goals.

But what exactly do the glutes do? We know that they control a wide range of actions, but how do we know these things, and what specific motions are we talking about?

This chapter contains the answers to those questions. But before I get into the specific joint actions, which refers to the motions of the joint, I want to clarify a commonly misunderstood idea.

You might be thinking that each gluteal muscle has a specific role when it comes to moving your body, and you're most certainly right, but we don't know exactly what those roles are. For example, you will hear people say that the gluteus maximus is responsible for hip extension (standing up from a squat) and the gluteus medius and minimus are responsible for hip abduction (moving your leg laterally away from your body) and some hip external rotation (rotating your thigh outward). While this might be partly true, we don't know the exact role of each muscle from every joint angle. I'm the Glute Guy, and I don't even know.

There are a couple of reasons for this. For one, there are subdivisions for each muscle. The gluteus maximus, as you learned in the previous chapter, can be broken into two subdivisions: upper and lower. You can also subdivide or characterize them as surface and deep muscle fibers, which have different functions. With the gluteus medius and minimus, you have three subdivisions—the anterior, middle, and posterior—which, again, do different things, meaning that the anterior fibers are performing different actions than the posterior fibers.

Two, the gluteal muscles perform different actions depending on your hip and foot position. For example, from an upright standing position, your gluteus medius is responsible for moving your leg outward, but when you squat (flex your hips), the role of the muscle changes. Instead of producing outward movement (driving your knees out), it creates inward movement (pulling your knees in). Stated differently, your gluteus medius controls external rotation when your hips are in extension and internal rotation when your hips are in flexion. It's hard to determine the exact role of each muscle because the role changes depending on the movement, range of motion, and joint angle.

I can confidently say that from an upright anatomical position, the gluteus maximus is responsible for hip abduction, hip external rotation, and hip extension and the gluteus medius and gluteus minimus are responsible for hip abduction. But we're rarely in an upright standing (anatomical) position when we're in motion. For this reason, I don't program exercises to target each specific gluteal muscle, but rather select exercises that target either the upper or lower subdivision of the glute max.

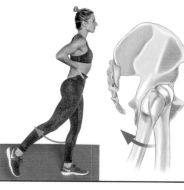 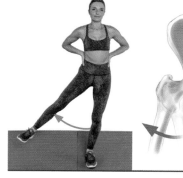 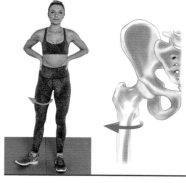

HIP EXTENSION **HIP ABDUCTION** **HIP EXTERNAL ROTATION**

JOINT ACTIONS

Although we have more to learn about the exact function of each gluteal muscle, we can confidently say that the glutes perform three primary joint actions: hip extension, hip external rotation, and hip abduction.

Even though most of the movements we perform involve a combination of these joint actions, understanding the role your glutes play in facilitating these actions will improve your comprehension of how your glutes function and why it's so important to train them using the methods and techniques provided in this book. Let's start with one of the most important joint actions of the human body: hip extension.

In many of the fundamental hip joint actions (including hip extension and hip external rotation),[1,2] the glutes are the prime movers, meaning that they are responsible for creating movement. This shows that the gluteus maximus muscle is not merely a conveniently placed synergist (helps with movement), but rather an essential player.

HIP EXTENSION

Hip extension is when you extend or open your hip joint, as in hip thrusting, standing out of a squat, or raising your torso from a deadlift.

HIP THRUST

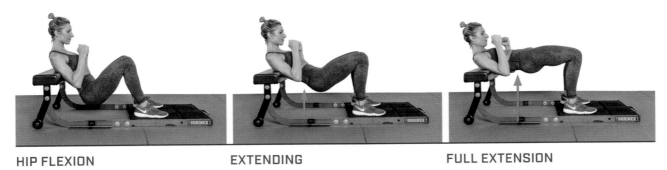

HIP FLEXION   EXTENDING   FULL EXTENSION

SQUAT

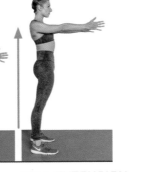
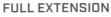
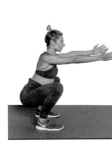

HIP FLEXION   EXTENDING   FULL EXTENSION

DEADLIFT

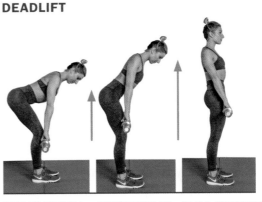

HIP FLEXION   EXTENDING   FULL EXTENSION

You can also extend your hip by moving your leg behind your body, such as in a kickback or quadruped hip extension.

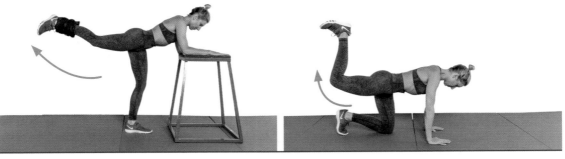

KICKBACK   QUADRUPED HIP EXTENSION

As you can see from the examples, you can perform hip extension movements while standing, while horizontal with your body facing downward (prone or quadruped position), or while horizontal with your body facing upward (supine position).

Maximum glute activation occurs at end-range hip extension. This implies that exercises that emphasize end-range hip extension in our programs, specifically hip thrusts and glute bridges, should always be included. (But depending on your position and the movement you're performing, your glutes will activate and develop to varying degrees. For example, when you perform a cable kickback or quadruped hip extension, you get a short but high spike in glute activation. When you squat, peak glute activation is reached when the glutes lengthen and stretch, which works the muscle differently compared to hip thrusts and other glute-dominant exercises. I'll talk more about glute activation and how each movement pattern influences glute strength and growth in the coming chapters. For now, you just need to understand that position, vector (line of resistance), and movement patterns influence the degree of glute activation even though they all involve the hip extension joint action.

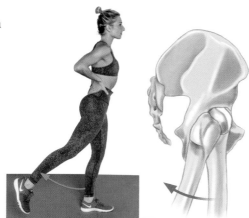

HIP EXTENSION

There's one more thing worth noting about hip extension: it is the same as tilting your pelvis backward, known as *posterior pelvic tilt.* This may seem confusing because hip extension and posterior pelvic tilt appear different when you look at the physical motion of the hips. But when you look at what's happening inside the hip joints, it's the same motion in that the femurs move rearward, or away from the fronts of the hip sockets.

In short, your glutes also control posterior pelvic tilting, and you can use this knowledge to achieve higher levels of glute activation. In other words, the majority of people feel their glutes more when they posterior pelvic tilt while hip thrusting.

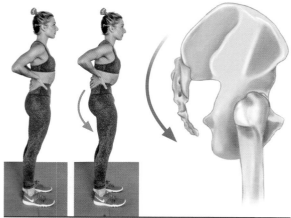

POSTERIOR PELVIC TILT

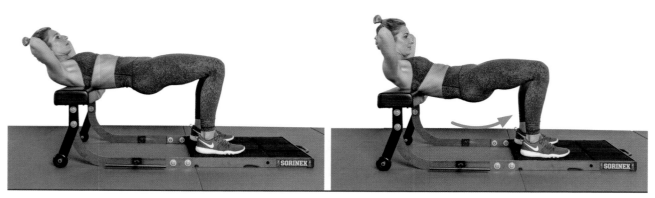

NEUTRAL SPINAL POSITION   **POSTERIOR PELVIC TILT**

We know that the glutes are a primary hip extensor from gross anatomy, muscle moment arms, and EMG. Gross anatomy is only broadly reliable as a way of assessing muscle function, as it is hard to identify the exact positions of the muscle in different joint positions when looking at a cadaver. Muscle moment arms (perpendicular distance between the line of force and axis of rotation) are a better way of determining muscle function, but only EMG can tell us how involved a muscle is in a joint action involving multiple muscles and supportive tension from passive structures.

Nevertheless, the origins of the gluteus maximus fibers on the rear of the spine and pelvis and its insertions on the femur[3] show us that this muscle is well placed to perform hip extension. Also, looking at the muscle moment arm lengths tells us that the glutes are effective hip extensors, just like the hamstrings and adductor magnus.[4, 5, 6]

Finally, EMG confirms what we can deduce from basic anatomy and from calculating muscle moment arm lengths, as maximum activation of the gluteus maximus can be achieved during isometric hip extension contractions. Hip flexion angle, though, is likely the biggest factor, with very high activation of the upper and lower regions of the glutes occurring in a position of full hip extension, irrespective of whether prone isometric hip extension or simple squeezing of the muscle in a standing position is performed.[7]

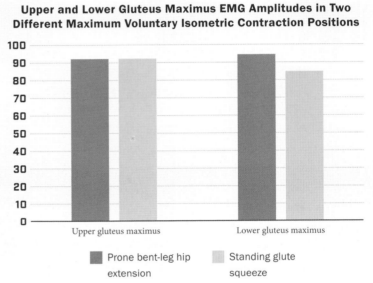

Upper and Lower Gluteus Maximus EMG Amplitudes in Two Different Maximum Voluntary Isometric Contraction Positions

Legend: Prone bent-leg hip extension | Standing glute squeeze

This may be why some research has found that the glutes are more active during a bodyweight quadruped hip extension (which has a peak contraction in full hip extension) than during a loaded barbell squat (which has a peak contraction in hip flexion).[8] Alternatively, this may be because combining hip and knee extension seems to emphasize the knee muscles more and the hip muscles less.[9]

This important finding about gluteal activation in hip extension movements was made nearly 50 years ago. It was discovered that gluteus maximus activation was substantially higher in full hip extension (the anatomical position) compared to in greater degrees of hip flexion, when exerting force to produce hip extension.[10] This was confirmed 30 years later in a more detailed experiment in which a number of joint angles were tested.[11]

These findings show us that the glutes are more active in producing hip extension when contracted (at short lengths) than when stretched (at long lengths). This can also be observed when producing forceful hip extension in positions of greater hip abduction,[12, 13] posterior pelvic tilt,[14] and hip external rotation.[15]

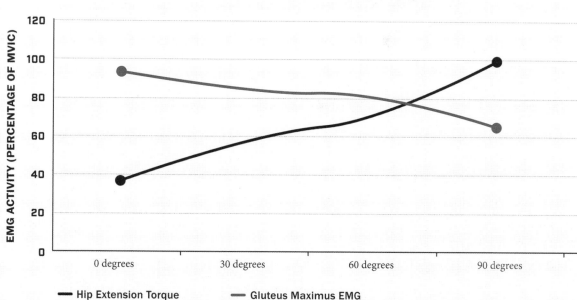

MEAN EMG AMPLITUDES OF THE HIP EXTENSORS AND MEAN HIP EXTENSION TORQUE

Y-axis: EMG ACTIVITY (PERCENTAGE OF MVIC) — 0, 20, 40, 60, 80, 100, 120

X-axis: 0 degrees, 30 degrees, 60 degrees, 90 degrees

━ Hip Extension Torque   ━ Gluteus Maximus EMG

This study showed that gluteus maximus activation actually increased from 64 percent of maximum voluntary isometric contraction (MVIC) levels at 90 degrees of hip flexion to 94 percent of MVIC levels when measured in full hip extension. It also showed that the hips are stronger in extension when in a flexed position compared to neutral.

From a training perspective, we can use this information wisely during many different exercises. Performing glute bridges and hip thrusts with a wider stance, or while resisting an elastic resistance band placed around the knees, can enhance gluteal activation.

Finally, we know that making it harder for the hamstrings to produce force by flexing the knees and contracting them below their optimal length also increases gluteus maximus activation.[16] This is called creating "active insufficiency" of the hamstrings.

Again, we can use this information to help us predict which exercises are likely to be best for the glutes. Exercises that involve straight legs are almost certainly going to have more hamstring and slightly less glute involvement than exercises performed with bent legs. In other words, bent-leg hip extension movements like the hip thrust and glute bridge variations involve more glutes because hamstring activation is decreased. (You will learn more about this in Chapter 10.)

So, even though back extensions are a great exercise for the glutes,[17] they do not involve quite as much glute activation as hip extension exercises with the knee flexed, which is such an effective position that it is used for the MVIC position during EMG testing.[18]

POSTERIOR PELVIC TILT

We know that the glutes can produce posterior pelvic tilt from gross anatomy and EMG. Gross anatomy is only broadly reliable as a way of assessing muscle function, as it is difficult to identify the exact positions of the muscle when in different joint positions from a cadaver. Even so, the clear origins of the gluteus maximus fibers on the rear of the spine and pelvis, and its insertions on the femur[138] show us that this muscle can easily posteriorly rotate the pelvis. Indeed, this should also be obvious because of the role that the glutes play as a key element of the pair of force couples that cross the pelvis, connecting the trunk and legs.[139]

EMG studies have confirmed what these basic anatomical investigations suggest. Performing posterior pelvic tilt when doing a hip extension action in a quadruped position increases gluteus maximus activation above the same hip extension action in anterior pelvic tilt.[140] Similarly, simply standing on a vibrating platform in posterior pelvic tilt leads to greater gluteus maximus activation than standing on the same platform in the same position but in either neutral or anterior pelvic tilt.[141]

HIP EXTERNAL ROTATION

Hip external rotation occurs when you turn your knee outward or rotate your thigh away from your midline. Hip external rotation also creates hip and full-body rotation. For example, if you rotate your hips with your feet planted as you would when performing a hip external rotation exercise or when throwing a punch or swinging a baseball bat, your glutes work in concert with other muscles to produce that motion.

BAND HIP EXTERNAL ROTATION

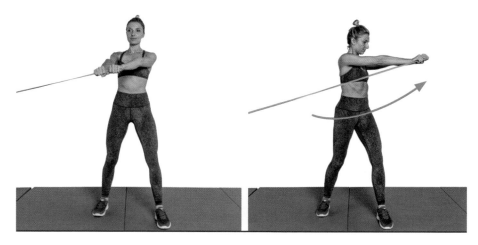

Hip external rotation helps stabilize your pelvis, knees, and ankles during a myriad of movements, especially double- and single-leg squat patterns and glute bridge and hip thrust patterns. To feel how your glutes control external rotation, simply stand in an upright position with your feet oriented straight and then squeeze your glutes. You'll notice that your pelvis rotates and spins your legs outward, causing you to feel outward pressure in your planted feet.

STANDING GLUTE SQUEEZE

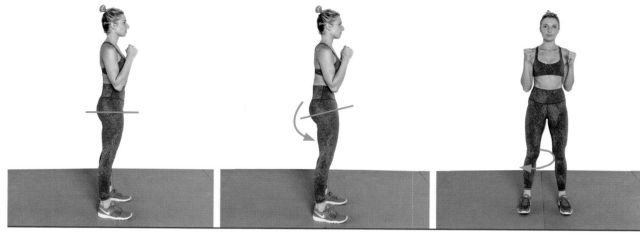

But external rotation often happens in conjunction with abduction. I'll use squatting to illustrate how this works. The three most common faults when squatting, which I cover in more detail in the Squat section beginning on page 410, are excessively hyperextending your back in the top position, allowing your knees to collapse inward (knee valgus), and excessively posterior pelvic tilting in the bottom position (butt wink).

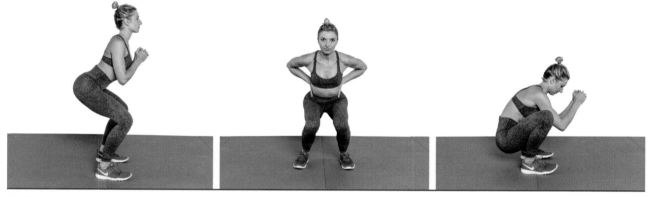

HYPEREXTENSION FAULT   **KNEE VALGUS FAULT**   **BUTT WINK FAULT**

By rotating your thighs outward (hip external rotation) and pushing your knees out (hip abduction), you stabilize the joints of your lower body, thereby preventing knee caving and even reducing posterior pelvic tilt.

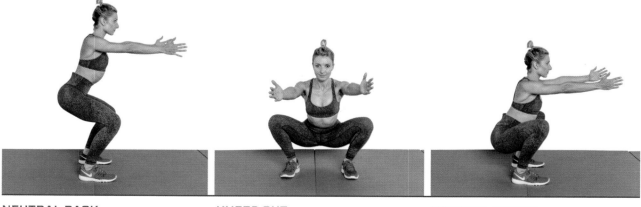

NEUTRAL BACK   **KNEES OUT**   **NEUTRAL PELVIS**

Some coaches cue athletes to screw their feet into the ground to create external rotation stability, but I don't think this is necessary. It might help you activate your glutes, so if it works for you, then by all means do it. But in my experience, simply turning the legs outward as soon as the descent begins and pushing the knees out when they are bent does the trick.

SCIENCE SPEAK: HIP EXTERNAL ROTATION

We know that the glutes are the most important hip external rotator[19] from gross anatomy, muscle moment arms, and EMG. Since the insertion point of the gluteus maximus is on the lateral surface of the greater trochanter of the femur,[20, 21] as the fibers of the muscle shorten, they naturally rotate the femur laterally in the hip socket. Indeed, this role as an external rotator may be as important as the role in performing hip extension. Based on logical assumptions about the anatomical line of pull of the gluteus maximus muscle, the authors of the study calculated that 71 percent of the maximum muscle force could be employed to perform external rotation.

Furthermore, careful assessment of muscle moment arm lengths reveals that the hip external rotation arm length of the gluteus maximus is substantial and is probably only shorter than that of the posterior fibers of the gluteus medius (which is quite a small region with little ability to produce force) and of the deep external rotators (also small and weak muscles).[22, 23] Finally, EMG confirms these findings, as several common hip external rotation exercises produce levels of muscle activation that are moderate or high, albeit not in excess of MVIC levels.[24] I have tested the band hip external rotation exercise and found that it generates extremely high levels of gluteus maximus EMG activity in the rear glute, indicating that the glute max is well suited for rotating the hip outward.

HIP ABDUCTION

Hip abduction occurs when you move your leg laterally away from your body, as in a fire hydrant or lateral band walk.

FIRE HYDRANT

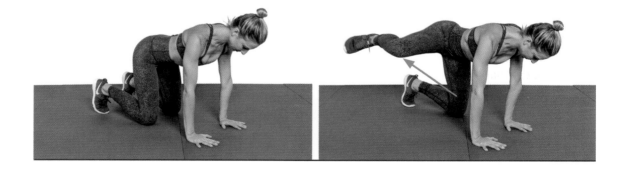

The majority of hip abduction exercises predominantly target the upper glute region. But your position determines the degree of upper to lower glute activation. For example, lateral band walks and standing cable hip abduction, which are considered "frontal plane" hip abduction exercises and are performed with a neutral hip position, highly activate your upper glutes, whereas seated hip abduction and fire hydrant exercises, which also involve hip external rotation and are considered "transverse plane" hip abduction exercises because they are performed with a flexed hip position, activate both the upper and lower glute regions.

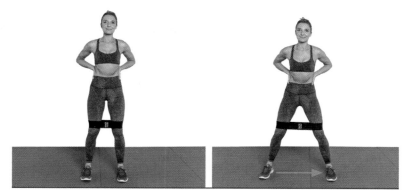

Abduction—as I just covered—also helps stabilize your back, hips, knees, and ankles in a myriad of movements. The most common examples are preventing pelvic lateral drop when walking (during gait) and driving your knees out when you squat or sumo deadlift. In addition to increasing glute activation, you're creating tension in the system, which prevents potentially harmful positions. Again, I cover these faults and corrections in more detail in the Squat section.

VARIETY IS ESSENTIAL

Your glutes are unique in that you can challenge the muscle in all three joint actions simultaneously. For example, when you perform a knee-banded barbell hip thrust, you're performing a combination of hip extension, hip external rotation, and hip abduction. This not only maximizes glute activation but also targets the upper and lower gluteal subdivisions.

TRIPLE-BANDED BARBELL HIP THRUST

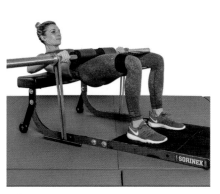

While the upper and lower glutes highly activate in most movements that involve hip extension, hip external rotation, and hip abduction, only the upper glutes activate during certain movements and positions, and the lower glutes activate much more than the upper glutes during certain movements and positions. This is due to the incredible number of attachment points on the skeleton, unique muscle architecture, and multiple subregions within the muscle. When you consider these facts, it becomes clear that optimal glute training requires a great deal of exercise and training variety.

In Chapter 10 and Part 5, you will learn how to choose exercises based on the area and muscle you want to target. The point I want to hammer here—and a point that I reiterate throughout the book—is that performing a variety of movements is crucial for fully developing the glutes. The next chapter looks at the role of genetics as it pertains to glute development, and then I'll home in on specific strategies for building bigger, leaner, stronger glutes.

The Role of Genetics

One of my greatest joys in life is helping people achieve their strength and physique goals. Nothing makes me happier than receiving testimonials showcasing the incredible physique changes credited to glute training, or helping a client lose weight and watching their confidence soar as they hit new personal records in the gym. Not only is it a testament to sound training strategies, but it also shows that hard work and consistency pay off.

In the following chapters, you will learn evidence-based principles for growing muscle and improving strength so that you can achieve similar results to my clients and the hardworking people following my training system. Of course, your rate of progress—like everything in fitness—depends on many factors (most of which are covered in this book). And the one factor that is rarely discussed is genetics.

There's no getting around it: genetics is one of the most important variables when it comes to improving strength and building muscle. We've already seen how your skeletal anatomy affects how your glutes look as well as how you move. It turns out that how you respond to resistance training is also partially determined by what your parents passed on to you. I wish I could lie and tell you that genetics don't matter, but the reality is, the way your glutes look before and after glute training will depend largely on your individual genetics.

GENETIC DIFFERENCES

You've heard it before, and certainly it's true: everyone is different, and genetics help explain those differences. As I've said, glutes come in all shapes and sizes. Some people are naturally stronger and more muscular than others. Consider the following outliers, for example. World record–setting powerlifter Andy Bolton squatted 500 pounds and deadlifted 600 pounds the first time he tried those exercises. Professional bodybuilder and six-time Mr. Olympia Dorian Yates bench-pressed 315 pounds on his first attempt as a teen. Arnold Schwarzenegger looked more muscular after a single year of lifting than most people do after ten.

The same certainly holds true for the glutes. One study found that in a sample of the general population, muscle volume varied from 198 to 958 ccm in men and from 238 to 638 ccm in women! So one man had glutes that were 384 percent larger than another man's glutes.

In addition to large differences in baseline levels of strength and size, there are big differences in how people respond to training. One study assessed how 585 untrained subjects responded to 12 weeks of strength training. The exact same program resulted in a shockingly wide range of responses. Those who responded the worst actually *lost* 2 percent of their muscle size and didn't gain any strength. In contrast, those who responded the best increased their muscle size by 59 percent and their strength by 250 percent. Another trial found that 26 percent of subjects failed to achieve any increase in muscle size after 16 weeks of strength training.

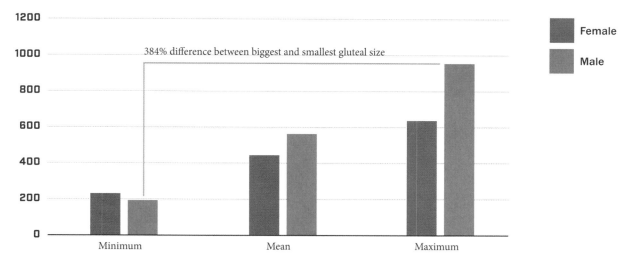

MINIMUM, MEAN, AND MAXIMUM GLUTEUS MAXIMUS VOLUMES (CCM) IN A RANGE OF MALES AND FEMALES AGES 19 TO 83

384% difference between biggest and smallest gluteal size

Female
Male

Minimum · Mean · Maximum

Although these findings highlight the unquestionable role of genetics and the differences among individuals, it's important to realize that the training programs used in the research studies didn't allow for individual variation. Everyone used the same program, with the same sets, reps, frequency, and exercises. They didn't involve any experimentation, tweaking, or autoregulatory training (adjusting your training based on how you feel, also referred to as *biofeedback*). So, before you label yourself as someone who has poor glute-building genetics, consider the fact that the program you are following might not be well suited to your individual needs.

For instance, a lot of people follow a coach's program because they want to look like the coach does. Social media has turned women with nice butts into glute trainers overnight because they know people will buy their programs in hopes of building a similar physique by working out the same way. While it may work for a select few, it's not a comprehensive strategy. And the last thing I want is for you to follow a program and then give up on training because you're not getting the results you were promised.

What's more, it is nearly impossible to determine whether someone has the genetics for building muscle and strength without a ton of time and experimentation. Of course, there are outliers, like the aforementioned examples who make any normal person look like a weakling their first day in the gym, and some people can practically glance at a barbell and put on muscle. But most of us respond well; you just need to find the programs and exercises that cater to your goals and unique physical traits.

CONTINUED EDUCATION: INDIVIDUAL DIFFERENCES

Research reports averages, which is not exactly accurate because many of us don't fall into the average category. In short, we all react differently to various training stimuli, and there are huge individual differences from one person to the next, which you can learn more about in this article: bretcontreras.com/individual-differences-important-consideration-fitness-results-science-doesnt-tell/

Although we haven't identified all of the muscle-building genes, we do know that some people have the genetics for building muscle all over their bodies, some have the genetics for building muscle in specific areas, and some have genetics that don't allow them to do either. I have great chest-building genetics, but I can't grow my quads to save my life. You can have great genetics for one muscle and poor genetics for another.

It's also important to acknowledge the genetics of how you look without training and the genetics of how you look after training. For example, just because someone starts with no glutes doesn't mean that they don't have the genetics to develop strong, shapely glutes. You might be a skinny twig without training, but once you start lifting weights, you will put on muscle and look jacked. The point is that your starting point is not reflective of your end point. You can't just train for three months and say, "I don't have the genetics to put on muscle." Sure, your rate of progress is partially determined by your genetics, but smart training, patience, and consistency will always produce results over a long enough period.

And there's more: some individuals respond very well to strength training, some barely respond, and some don't respond at all. It took me years of hard training and experimentation to figure out how to grow my glutes. If you're someone who, like me, has poor glute-building genetics, don't get discouraged. It's not all doom and gloom. You might not have the biggest glutes, but if you respond well to resistance training, you will build glutes fast. Conversely, you might have small glutes and have a hard time building muscle, but you'll be lean and strong as hell.

YOU CAN'T CONTROL YOUR GENETICS, BUT YOU CAN CONTROL YOUR MINDSET

Although you can't control your genetics, a lot of variables dictate your ability to improve strength and build muscle that *are* within your control. Regardless of where you fall on the muscle-building genetic spectrum, it's important to focus your attention on the variables you can regulate, such as sleep, eating habits, exercise selection, and training frequency. Some people respond best to variety, some to certain exercises, some to volume, some to effort, and some to frequency. You have to discover the best stimulus for your body, and that takes not only constant experimentation but also rationally considering your genetics and how that might affect your training strategies.

I wish I could provide a specific training protocol based on your unique genetic profile, but we're not there yet. There will come a day when you can get a genetic test that will tell you exactly what you should eat, how long you should sleep, and how you should train based on your genetic makeup. If you knew, for example, that you respond better to one of the three muscle-growing mechanisms covered in the next chapter, then you could more accurately determine the best exercises to perform. But we're still pretty far from that. Until we know more, it will remain more of an art than an exact science.

The fact is, everyone has genetics that they have to work around. Some people carry excess fat all over, while others are lean but have stubborn areas of fat (think stomach and hips). Some people have a hard time building muscle but are strong, while others can build muscle but have weak body parts. And then some of us have a combination of issues.

My list of genetic curses is a mile long, but I've managed to train my way to some decent glutes. Are they the biggest and strongest glutes? No. In fact, most people who see me would say, "That's the Glute Guy? He has mediocre glutes!" But if you looked at my starting point, you would see a big difference, and you might be impressed. Granted, it took me many years of hard work, but I've come a long way. And you can, too.

CONTINUED EDUCATION: BODYBUILDING GENETICS

Some people experience far greater results than others. Although training and diet have a huge impact on people's ability to put on muscle, the rate at which they progress is largely determined by their genetics, which I cover in more detail in this article: www.t-nation.com/training/truth-about-bodybuilding-genetics

In fact, I've yet to see a lifter who trains intelligently—meaning that they train consistently and experiment to find what works best for them—fail to see results. Of course, the rate and extent of the overall growth are highly influenced by genetics, but sound training methods will always produce good results. That is, you will probably lose fat, gain some muscular shape and density, and improve your strength. Even if you don't notice results right out of the gate, you can and will see results as long as you adopt the right mindset and remain consistent.

Remember, you can choose to train smart and work hard. You can choose to grow your knowledge to maximize your training results. You can choose to experiment to find out what works best for you. You can choose to sleep, eat, and live better. Embrace your genetics and fall in love with the training process. And praise your efforts and reward yourself for training consistently. We all have strengths and weaknesses. The key to sustained progress and overall happiness is to be proud of your strengths and work tirelessly to round out your weaknesses.

With this understanding in mind, you will have a better idea of how you need to approach the training strategies, exercise selection, and program design variables covered later in the book. Equally important, you will be able to create goals that will improve your self-image, confidence, and resolve toward training. People don't say knowledge is power for nothing. Use the knowledge you're gaining in this book not only to empower your training, but also to improve how you think about yourself.

The results you see in the gym are highly dependent on the extent to which the satellite cells—muscle stem cells that play a role in muscle hypertrophy—surrounding your muscle fibers can fuse their nuclei into your muscle fibers. Put simply, the satellite cells produce more genetic material that signals the muscle cells to grow.

We know this because one study found that the difference between excellent responders and average/ nonresponders in strength training boiled down mostly to differences in the degree of satellite cell activation.[1] Excellent responders have more satellite cells surrounding their muscle fibers as well as a greater ability to expand their satellite cell pool during periods of training, meaning it's easier for them to put on muscle.

In that study, excellent responders averaged 21 satellite cells per 100 fibers at baseline, which rose to 30 satellite cells per 100 fibers by the end of the program. This was accompanied by a 54 percent increase in mean fiber area. The nonresponders averaged just 10 satellite cells per 100 fibers at baseline. This level did not change post-training, and they didn't experience any muscle growth. In addition to changes in satellite cells, the key hypertrophy-signaling molecules' mechanogrowth factor (MGF), myogenin, and IGF-IEa were all upregulated to a much greater extent in responders than in nonresponders.[2]

Some people just win the genetic lottery, and the prize money is not insignificant. Some reviewers have suggested that genetic factors are responsible for 50 to 80 percent of the individual variability in muscle size[3] based on an analysis of twin studies.[4, 5, 6] That is not to say we have a perfect map of which genes are responsible for a person being an excellent responder to strength training. Rather, because methods for identifying the genes responsible for hypertrophic responsiveness are relatively new, research is still quite limited.[7] And while some researchers have already found a small number of different genetic traits and single nucleotide polymorphisms (SNPs) that may be related to a superior increase in muscle mass, the extent to which these can explain the inter-individual variability in responsiveness to training is small.[8]

While some folks hit the genetic jackpot, others get the genetic shaft. Genetically speaking, anything that negatively impacts the ability of the muscle fibers to increase the number of myonuclei in response to any type of mechanical loading (lifting weights) reduces the potential for increasing muscle size and strength. This ranges from the number of signaling molecules that are produced to the sensitivity of the muscle fibers to those signals to satellite cell availability to satellite cell pool expansion to miRNA regulation.

LAST WORD ON GENETICS

As I said, it is rare for anyone who trains consistently and intelligently and experiments to find out what works for them to not look much better after a couple of months of training. From a standing start, everyone loses fat and gains some muscular shape. So never use your genetics as a crutch not to train. Be patient and stay the course. Some of my most incredible transformations took place over the course of several years. If you need inspiration, check out the transformation photos on pages 14 and 15 or on my Instagram (@bretcontreras1).

How Muscle Grows

When I first started bodybuilding, my goal was simple: to build bigger, stronger glutes. It took me a couple of years to realize that I needed to train my glutes in a unique way, but like most beginners, I had no idea what I was doing. Although I was listening to the advice given to me by more experienced bodybuilders, following training programs in bodybuilder magazines, and copying other people in the gym who looked jacked, my form was horrendous, and my programming was lackluster because I omitted any exercise that felt off or was difficult to learn.

Now, you would think that I never would have gained any strength or size. After all, my training was far from systematic. But the truth is, I got results.

This is the biggest advantage of being a beginner: the vast majority of people will gain strength and size very quickly, as long as they're consistently training hard. The good times last only so long, though. Over a long enough period, your body adapts to the training, after which point you will struggle to meet your physique and strength goals. What's more, there's an inherent risk of getting hurt when you lift with improper form or train too hard, too fast.

This is exactly what happened to me. I was getting bigger and stronger, but I was picking up bad habits. Instead of mapping out a direct path to my goals, I trained hard and then waited to correct issues until something went wrong or my progress stalled, which makes no sense. It's like waiting to get lost before checking the GPS. If you want to get to your destination faster, you need to know where you are going and pick a clear path to get there. If your goal is to develop bigger, stronger glutes, certain knowledge will help you avoid mistakes that beginners (and advanced practitioners) commonly make.

Most of us know this intuitively. The more knowledge and experience we gain, the faster we reach our goals. Yet I see so many people making the same mistakes that I made when first starting out. It's not until their progress stalls or something goes wrong that they start looking for a map and seeking higher forms of knowledge.

My hope is that this book will serve as that map. Take it from me: training smart (that is, using science to guide your programs and workouts) is more important than training hard, though both are critical. By studying the principles and ideas outlined in this chapter, you can avoid a lot of the mistakes that I made and the majority of lifters make when they begin training. In other words, understanding how your muscles grow and the variables that contribute to muscle growth is essential if you want to reach your physique goals, and it will prevent you from getting derailed in your pursuit of muscular development.

HOW YOUR GLUTES INCREASE IN SIZE: THREE MECHANISMS OF HYPERTROPHY

The science of growing muscle is a complex and emerging field of research. When it comes to how muscles increase in size, we refer to it as *hypertrophy* (pronounced "hy-PER-tro-fee"), which is muscle growth or the enlargement of muscle fibers (muscle cells). Another way to think of hypertrophy is as the opposite of atrophy, which is losing muscle, or the degeneration of muscle cells.

Based on what we currently know, three mechanisms are thought to cause muscle growth: mechanical tension, metabolic stress, and muscle damage. While many experts contest muscle damage and metabolic stress, everyone agrees that mechanical tension is paramount for hypertrophy and is the most important factor by a long shot. The good news is, scientists are working to unravel the precise signals and sensors involved in muscle growth, which will allow us to focus on the exact mechanisms at play. But right now, we really don't know much about what causes muscle growth from a physiological perspective, so we take a shotgun approach—that is, we form training strategies that target all three mechanisms.

MECHANICAL TENSION

When you're lifting heavy weights, it sometimes feels like the muscle is about to rip off the bone due to the insane level of contraction and tension in the muscle. This is mechanical tension.

To better understand how this works, I need to briefly describe what I mean by tension. There are two ways to place tension on a muscle:

1. **The first is passive tension, in which you place tension on a muscle by stretching it passively. Think of bending over and performing a hamstring stretch. Your hamstrings get very taut and you feel tension mounting, even though the muscle isn't activated.**
2. **The second is active tension, in which you place tension on a muscle by flexing or contracting it. Think about flexing your biceps as hard as you can to show off your guns. This is an example of active tension.**

When you lift weights through a full range of motion, however, the muscles are placed under a combination of passive and active tension. In other words, they lengthen (eccentric phase) and shorten (concentric phase) while being activated through a full range of motion. And by "full range of motion," I'm referring to the full movement potential of your joint.

For example, say you're performing a heavy barbell back squat. Lowering your hips below your knee crease is considered a full range of motion because you're expressing a fairly complete degree of the movement potential of your hips, knees, and ankles—meaning you're fully opening (extension) and closing (flexion) the joints. And because you're performing a heavy barbell back squat, you have to contract your muscles sufficiently to raise and lower the weight, which creates a lot of tension in your muscles.

To maximize muscle growth by using the mechanical tension pathway, you must:

- Choose exercises that include both eccentric and concentric phases (see the Muscle actions sidebar on pages 83 and 84 for more on eccentric and concentric muscle actions)
- Move through a decent range of motion
- Create maximal activation and contraction in the muscle by lifting a lot of weight, lifting a moderate weight as many times as possible until you fail, or conscientiously contracting the muscle as hard as you can

Time under high tension is another important factor to consider. Your muscles need ample, regular signaling to grow larger, and they need enough stimulating reps to be enticed to grow. A stimulating rep is carried out slowly enough to achieve maximum tension by way of crossbridge formation at the sarcomere level. Put simply, ample time is required for the muscles to generate maximum tension. If the contraction is too fast, you won't achieve high enough levels of tension to stimulate growth at the molecular level. Even with full motor unit recruitment (motor units are groups of muscle cells that coordinate contractions of a single muscle), you can display lower levels of tension because of the rapid detachment of crossbridges that occur during activities such as jumping and sprinting. Only reps that are heavy enough—say, above 85 to 90 percent of your one-rep max (1RM)—or reps done with lighter weight but placed at the end of a set and performed to muscle failure will meet these two criteria. In fact, a 1RM and the last rep of a set to failure (say, rep 10 of a 10RM) are carried out at the same speed.

In truth, all reps build muscle, but their muscle-building potential exists on a continuum with heavy reps and reps close to failure packing by far the most muscle-building potential. If you perform only one full-range squat with light weight, you will not stress the muscle enough to adapt and increase in size. But if you focus on the three criteria above and regularly perform ample volume to expose your muscles to enough stimulating reps, you will put enough tension on the muscles to stimulate growth.

It's also worth mentioning that lifting heavy doesn't automatically confer high levels of mechanical tension on the muscles. For example, it's possible to move a large amount of weight without generating high levels of muscle tension using leverage, the contribution of other muscles, and more. For this reason, you need to carefully select exercises that target the muscle you're trying to grow—say, hip thrusts for your glutes—and strive to maximize muscle contraction by focusing intently on the area you're trying to develop. This is known as the mind-muscle connection, and I cover it in more detail later in this chapter.

Exercise Strategies for Creating Mechanical Tension

There are many ways to create mechanical tension. The most straightforward strategy is to lift heavy weight using the principles of progressive overload and the mind-muscle connection with low to medium reps (1 to 12 reps) and long rest periods between sets to allow for maximal recovery. You can also utilize advanced training methods such as the following, which I cover in Part 3:

- Mind-muscle connection (page 93)
- Progressive overload (page 102)
- Cluster/rest-pause reps (page 203)
- Heavy partial reps
- Enhanced eccentrics (page 206)
- Pause reps (page 210)
- Forced reps

Here are three exercise examples of achieving high levels of mechanical tension:

 Warm up thoroughly and perform heavy squats for 4 sets of 3 reps with 85 percent of your 1RM.

 Perform pause half-squats for 3 sets of 5 reps with a 3-second pause at the bottom of each rep with 60 percent of your 1RM.

 Say you're performing barbell hip thrusts with 275 pounds. This is your 6-rep max. Perform rest-pause hip thrusts and do a set of 6 reps to failure. Then rest for 10 seconds and perform 2 more reps. Then rest for 10 more seconds and perform 1 more rep, then rest for 10 more seconds and perform a final rep. By the end of the set, you will have gotten 10 reps with your 6-rep max.

MUSCLE ACTIONS (TYPES OF CONTRACTION)

Muscle action refers to the movement of a muscle relative to the joint. For the purposes of this book, I define three main muscle actions (there are more if you want to get geeky): isometric, eccentric, and concentric.

Isometric muscle actions occur when the joint remains at the same angle. It is commonly thought that the muscle stays the same length, but this is not true. When you contract the muscle (generate force) without changing the joint angle, the muscle shortens while the tendon lengthens. For example, say you're performing a hip thrust and I tell you to hold the top position while contracting your glutes as hard as you can. This is considered an isometric contraction because the glutes contract but the joint angle at the hips stays constant.

ISOMETRIC: HOLD THE BOTTOM OF A SQUAT OR TOP OF A HIP THRUST

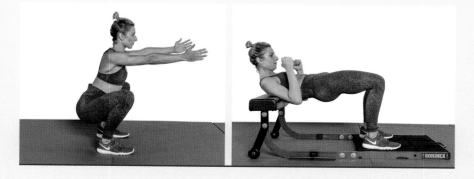

Eccentric muscle actions occur when muscles lengthen under tension. This type of action causes the most muscle damage because when a muscle contracts, it tries to shorten (pull itself together) while being stretched at the same time.

ECCENTRIC: LOWERING FROM A HIP THRUST OR SQUAT

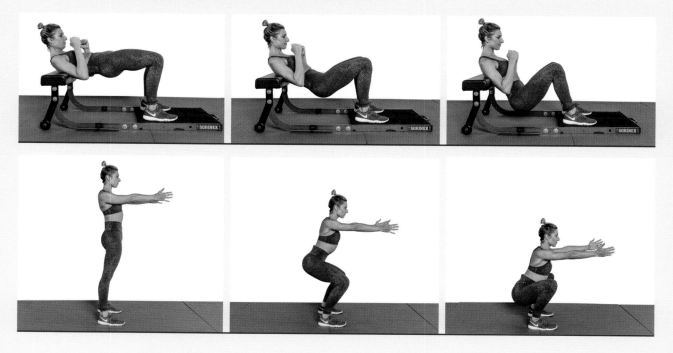

Concentric muscle actions involve the shortening of a muscle. In this case, the muscle contraction exceeds the force overcoming it in the other direction. For example, when you rise out of a squat or elevate your hips during a barbell hip thrust, you're creating enough muscle tension to turn your hips and knees into extension and overcome the downward force of gravity.

CONCENTRIC: EXTENDING YOUR HIPS DURING A HIP THRUST OR STANDING UP FROM A SQUAT

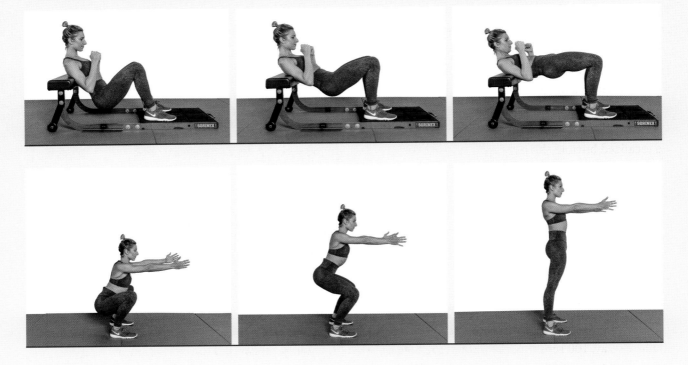

METABOLIC STRESS

Think about the feeling you get when you know you're really targeting a muscle—the burning sensation you elicit and the pump (muscle swelling) you achieve. These two mechanisms fall under the umbrella of metabolic stress.

Metabolic stress is brought about by several factors, including:

- **The occlusion (blockage) of veins by persistent muscle contractions, which prevents blood from escaping the muscle**
- **The hypoxia, or lack of oxygen supply, in the muscles due to the trapping of blood**
- **The buildup of metabolic by-products such as lactate and the increased hormonal surge**
- **The cell swelling or "pump" of the muscles, which is also due to blood pooling**

These factors are thought to aid in building muscle and to be synergistic with tension and progressive overload (doing more over time). They also help explain why Kaatsu training—lifting lighter weight with higher reps while restricting blood flow—is highly effective at inducing hypertrophy despite the lower levels of muscle tension compared to traditional resistance training. The fatigue also drives up muscle activation, which places greater tension on the individual muscle fibers.

To clarify, the pump—also known as *cell swelling*—involves blood getting trapped in the muscle, causing the cells to swell. For example, when you lift weights, your arteries pump blood to the muscle, but the muscle contractions obstruct the veins, trapping and pooling the blood in the muscle.

Most of the women I train love training for the pump because they like the way it feels and how it makes their glutes look. Some of my clients get up to a 2-inch glute pump, which means that their glute girth increases by 2 full inches following a workout. Training for the pump is also good for muscle development through the mechanical tension pathway, but in a unique manner. It puts tension on the cell structure, and then your body ramps up protein synthesis, which in turn develops a bigger muscle.

The burn is also associated with metabolic stress. You feel the burn when metabolic by-products like lactate, inorganic phosphate, and hydrogen ions accumulate in the blood, causing a localized burn in the muscle. In theory, this increases muscle growth through a variety of factors; most notably, it ramps up muscle activation and increases muscle contractions. As you perform more reps and start feeling the burn, you recruit more motor units, which increases tension in the muscle. But the metabolites themselves are thought to lead to growth, which is demonstrated by the fact that people see more muscle growth if they train in hypoxic chambers. (Imagine a gym that has a lower-than-normal oxygen level, which would cause the body to generate more metabolic by-products during training.)

When describing the glute pump and burn, I usually present it as the "burn/pump" because they are linked. But they are different, and you can have more of one than the other. For example, if I wanted the biggest glute burn, I might perform 1 set of high-rep frog pumps to failure—say, 100 reps. But if I wanted the biggest pump, I would perform multiple sets of lower reps, like 4 sets of 50 reps. Put simply, it's hard to get a good pump with a single set. For most people, it takes multiple sets to get good swelling in the muscle.

Scientists debate whether the pump and burn is good for hypertrophy, but I believe that it is. When you get a pump, fluid accumulates inside the cells, and there is a corresponding outward pressure or tension on the cell membranes (sarcolemmas). The cells perceive it to be a threat to the ultrastructure (structure within the cell) and respond by growing thicker, which in turn grows muscle. But this is purely theoretical, and it's difficult to prove or disprove because we don't have the technology to measure it. We have research showing that cell swelling can cause hypertrophy in different tissues, like liver tissue and mammary tissue. But does it work with the muscles? Is it enough? Is the swelling intracellular and not extracellular? Is the pressure sufficient? We don't know these things yet.

I believe that training for the pump and burn is good for muscle growth for the above-mentioned reasons, but that growth could also be due to a mechanism other than the pump and burn. It could just be that the fatigue associated with high reps and shorter rest periods drives up motor unit recruitment and slows muscle contraction speed, which allows for maximum tension in the glutes. Until we know more, I can't say for certain that training for the pump and burn is good for hypertrophy, but I currently believe it is, which is why I recommend it in my programming.

Exercise Strategies for Creating Metabolic Stress

There are many ways to create metabolic stress. The most straightforward strategy is to perform fast, high-repetition (20 or more) sets with short rest periods in between. You can also utilize several advanced training methods, which I cover in Part 3. Here are the best methods for creating metabolic stress:

- High reps at fast speeds
- Short rest periods
- Mind-muscle connection (page 93)
- Using bands and chains
- Kaatsu, or blood flow restriction (BFR) training
- Constant tension (isometric hold) (page 202)
- Partial reps
- Pyramids (page 205)
- Torque doubling (page 207)
- Dropsets (page 209)
- Supersets (page 213)
- Burnouts (page 213)

Here are three exercise examples of achieving high levels of metabolic stress:

1   Place a band around your knees and perform frog pumps for 4 sets of 50 reps.

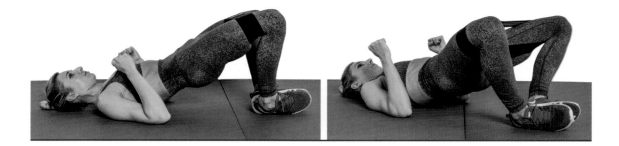

2 Place a band around your knees and perform 30 seated hip abductions while leaning back, then do 30 more reps with an upright torso, then do 30 more reps while leaning far forward.

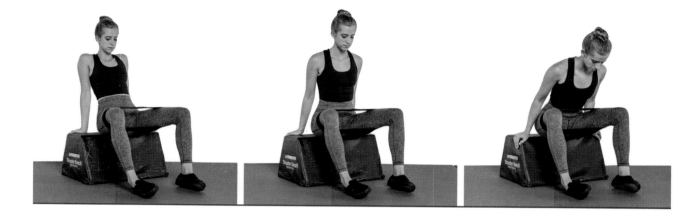

3 Perform a hip thrust dropset by loading a barbell with one 45-pound plate and three 25-pound plates on each side. This equates to 285 pounds. Perform 8 reps with this load, then immediately have a spotter strip off one 25-pound plate on each side. Without resting, perform 6 more reps with 235 pounds. Immediately after finishing that set, have your spotter take another 25-pound plate off each side. Again, without resting, perform 6 reps with 185 pounds. To complete the final set, have your spotter take off the remaining 25-pound plates and perform 10 reps with 135 pounds. In the end, you will have performed 30 total reps with loads ranging from 135 to 285 pounds in a relatively short time, creating a lot of metabolic stress.

MUSCLE DAMAGE

Approximately two days after a strenuous bout of exercise, your muscle soreness is likely to reach its peak. This soreness is somewhat indicative of muscle damage. Muscle damage is created by doing something unfamiliar, performing an exercise that stretches a muscle to long lengths, or accentuating the eccentric component of an exercise—slowly stretching a contracting muscle—which induces high amounts of strain. For example, lunges stretch the glutes while under tension, which is why people tend to get sore glutes from the lunge and squat movement patterns. Conversely, exercises that target the glutes at shorter muscle lengths (in a contracted position) not only build bigger glutes but don't leave you as sore.

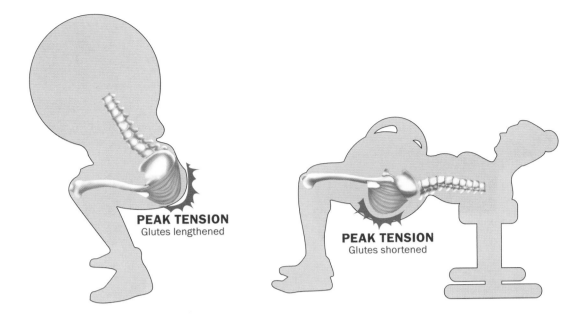

PEAK TENSION
Glutes lengthened

PEAK TENSION
Glutes shortened

The traditional thinking is that lifting weights tears muscles down and resting builds them back up, but, like a callus, the body supercompensates and builds the muscles back stronger. Muscle damage consists of microtears, lesions, and associated inflammation and exists at the sarcomeric, membrane, T-tubule, and fascial levels. It could be that muscle damage in and of itself doesn't build muscle, but the tension produced in the muscles through a full range of motion during a workout and the tension experienced inside the muscle cells in the days that follow due to cell swelling are responsible for the growth.

Whatever the case, most experts agree that damage is highly overrated and is the least important of the three proposed mechanisms. Yet the vast majority of people worship muscle soreness because they erroneously believe that they need to be sore to stimulate muscle growth. Not only is this thinking wrong, but it can easily do more harm than good. Imagine training really hard on Monday and then being too sore to train on Wednesday. Now you can't handle as much volume, and pain inhibits muscle activation, both of which are vital for growing muscle.

It is, however, important to factor in training frequency. If you're training only once a week, then you should train hard and not be too worried about soreness. But if you want to maximize your results, you need to train two or three times a week. Though there is little evidence in the literature to support this claim, I believe that training the glutes three days a week is ideal for most people. I've had the pleasure of working with half of the women with the best glute development on the planet, and they prioritize the glutes in their training and tend to work their glutes three to five times per week. (More on this in Chapter 12.) If you're training three days a week, you have to be careful not to overdo it. You want a little bit of soreness, but not so much that it interferes with your training frequency.

I also want to point out that I have clients who never get sore, and many of them see amazing glute development.

Exercise Strategies for Creating Muscle Damage

There are many ways to create muscle damage. When it comes to the glutes, the most straightforward strategy is to perform lunges and squats, which stretch the glutes. As a rule, any exercise that emphasizes the eccentric phase—that is, it stretches the muscle while under tension—is likely to create significant muscle soreness. You can also utilize several advanced training methods, which I cover in more detail in Part 3. Here are the best activities for creating muscle damage:

- Exercises that stretch the muscles, like squats and lunges
- Exercise variety, including new, unfamiliar movements
- Free weight (barbell, dumbbell, and kettlebell) exercises
- Enhanced eccentrics (page 206)
- Accentuated eccentrics (page 207)
- Forced rep negatives
- Cheat reps with good negatives
- Loaded stretching

Here are three exercise examples of creating muscle damage:

 Perform a 10-rep set of dumbbell deficit reverse lunges while standing on a 6-inch step.

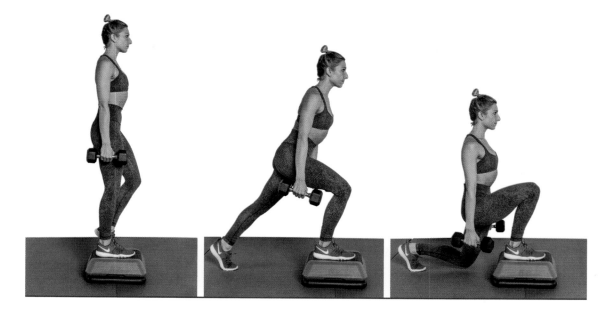

2 Perform a movement you haven't done in a while. For example, say it's been three months since you performed dumbbell between bench squats. Choose that exercise and perform 4 sets of 12 reps.

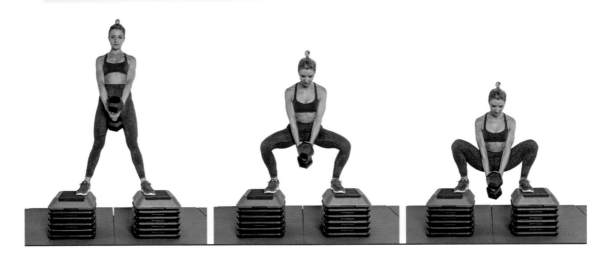

3 Perform enhanced-eccentric barbell hip thrusts. Have a training partner stand over you and push down on the barbell as hard as they can while you resist the load eccentrically during the lowering phase. Then they let up as you raise the load concentrically. Repeat this process for 10 reps. To clarify, your partner is placing an additional 100 pounds of resistance (it doesn't have to be 100 pounds, just additional weight based on what the person can handle) during the lowering phase of the movement so that there's a different load for the concentric and eccentric phases.

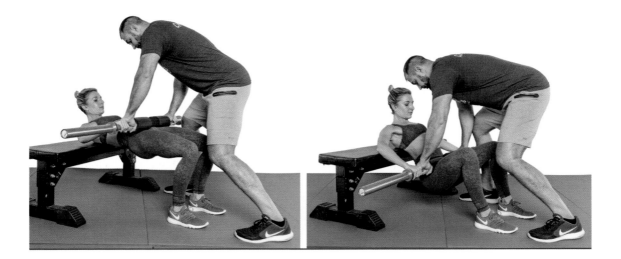

INTERRELATIONSHIP OF MECHANISMS

Mechanical tension, metabolic stress, and muscle damage are interrelated, and they signal hypertrophic responses through multiple, redundant pathways. For example, let's say you're performing knee-banded goblet squats. In this scenario, you're stretching your glutes while under tension, which creates muscle damage; you're carrying additional weight and pushing outward against the band, which creates mechanical tension; and, as you continue to perform reps, the prolonged muscle contractions create metabolic stress.

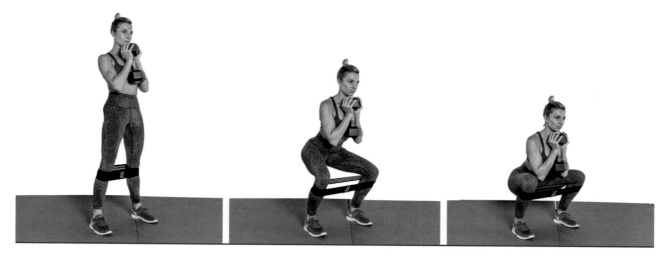

As you can see, the three mechanisms overlap. Although you can emphasize a specific mechanism with exercise selection, tempo, load, and effort, it's impossible to completely isolate one mechanism. At least this is the current thinking. We will home in on the individual signaling pathways over time as we learn more, but for now, we must cover our bases and target all three mechanisms by performing a variety of exercises, loads, and rep ranges at varying levels of effort. I call this the shotgun approach.

PICKING THE RIGHT EXERCISE FOR EACH MECHANISM

As you've learned, some exercises are better than others at eliciting a pump or burn, some exercises are better than others at creating tension in a muscle or a particular subdivision of a muscle, and some exercises are better than others at damaging muscle fibers. Let's bring all of this together with a quick recap.

Large compound movements like squats, deadlifts, glute bridges, and hip thrusts can be done with high loads, which maximizes mechanical tension in the involved muscle groups. Using relatively high loads with lower reps and longer rest periods (to aid in strength recovery) can help increase mechanical tension in these exercises. Because mechanical tension seems to be the biggest driver of muscle growth and lifting heavy requires the most focus and energy, I recommend prioritizing compound movements and performing them first in your workout.

Exercises that either place constant tension on a muscle or place the greatest tension on the target muscle at short muscle lengths (in a contracted position) are best for stimulating metabolic stress. For the glutes, this is hard to do without using a glute bridge or hip thrust variation. Using medium to high reps with short rest periods and multiple sets, glute bridges and hip thrusts can produce a serious burn and a skin-splitting pump that is ideal for enhancing the metabolic stress response. Taking this a step further, you can use bands or chains to make the loading more constant throughout each rep. I recommend performing these variations at the end of your workout in the form of burnouts (see page 213).

Movements that involve the greatest loading at long muscle lengths (in a stretched position) are best suited for creating muscle damage. Lunges, squats, Bulgarian split squats, Romanian deadlifts (RDLs), deficit deadlifts, and good mornings are good examples of exercises that cause damage to the glute muscles.

Pure eccentric, enhanced eccentric, or eccentric-accentuated reps can be used to increase muscle damage, but there's a fine line between optimal and excessive. Again, muscle damage is overrated and can easily do more harm than good if it interferes with strength gains and training frequency. Feeling a bit sore the next day is fine, but barely being able to sit down is overkill. For this reason, I recommend doing only one or two exercises that stress muscle damage in the course of a week, typically in the middle of a workout.

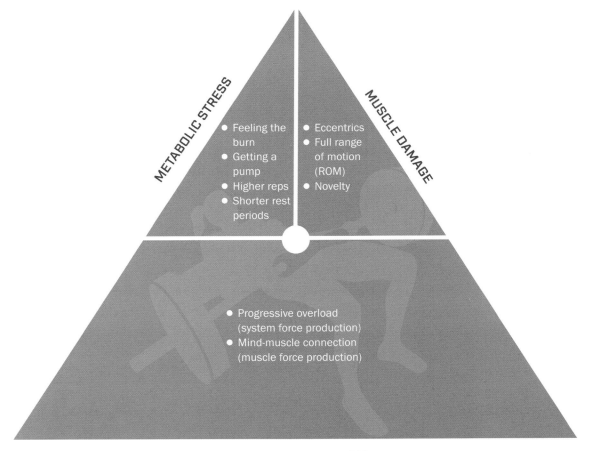

MECHANISMS OF HYPERTROPHY PYRAMID

METABOLIC STRESS
- Feeling the burn
- Getting a pump
- Higher reps
- Shorter rest periods

MUSCLE DAMAGE
- Eccentrics
- Full range of motion (ROM)
- Novelty

- Progressive overload (system force production)
- Mind-muscle connection (muscle force production)

MECHANICAL TENSION

In summary, the bulk of your muscle gains will come from placing increasing amounts of tension on your muscles. You achieve this by progressively overloading your training session (more on this in Chapter 9). Put simply, you need to do more over time—more weight, more reps, more sets, and so on—and focus on the most important aspects of muscle building, which revolve around creating mechanical tension.

But getting stronger doesn't always mean that the targeted muscle is receiving a greater tension stimulus. You could fail to create mechanical tension by altering your technique, using momentum, skimping on range of motion, and/or relying too much on other muscles to do the job. This is why you must utilize the mind-muscle connection in conjunction with progressive overload. One strategy without the other is inferior. You must mentally focus on the muscle you're training to grow in order to see hypertrophic results.

*

CONTINUED EDUCATION: MIND-MUSCLE CONNECTION

A number of studies have shown greater activation when you think about contracting the muscle you're trying to target, which is outlined in an article that I wrote with my good friend and colleague Brad Schoenfeld titled "Attentional Focus for Maximizing Muscle Development: The Mind-Muscle Connection." You can find it at bretcontreras.com/wp-content/uploads/Attentional-Focus-for-Maximizing-Muscle-Development-The-Mind-Muscle-Connection.pdf.

MIND-MUSCLE CONNECTION

For ages, bodybuilders have used the mind-muscle connection to bring attentional focus to the working muscle. *Attentional focus* is what you think about while performing a movement or exercise.

I'll use an example to help you understand how it works. Say you're doing barbell hip thrusts. As you perform the movement, you put all of your mental focus into squeezing and activating your glutes. As you lower the weight, you're tuned into the tension building in the muscle. As you elevate your hips to reach full hip extension, you're directing all of your attention into contracting the muscle to achieve maximum activation. This is the mind-muscle connection at work. It is also referred to as *internal attentional focus*.

The research is clear: you get more activation when you're thinking about the working muscle. By bringing consciousness to the area you're targeting, you're directing more neural drive to the muscle, which increases tension and activation. I've done a ton of EMG experiments on myself, and I can tell you that this works.

In addition to increasing activation, it increases metabolic stress. If you neglect the mind-muscle connection, meaning you're not thinking about activating your glutes when you perform exercises that involve the glutes, you work your glutes less, and other synergistic muscles, like your quads and hamstrings, compensate so that you can carry out the task (lift the weight).

When you're going for hypertrophy, you want to direct your attention inward toward the muscle, which, again, is the mind-muscle connection. But if your goal is to improve strength and performance, then you want to focus on something outside your body that is motivating (referred to as external attentional focus), not the muscle being worked. In other words, focusing on your glutes will improve your ability to grow bigger glutes. If you want to train your glutes so that you can jump farther or higher or lift more weight, then you don't want to focus on the muscle. Instead, you want to direct your attention externally, focusing on your environment and letting your body figure out which muscles to use at the right moment.

For example, say you're going for a one-rep max on a heavy back squat. In this situation, you don't want to focus on the muscles powering the movement, but rather on lifting the weight. So you might think about something that motivates you to get the weight up—like you're going to squat the bar through the roof. By focusing on the task and the environment, you rely on your body to sort out which muscles to recruit in order to carry out the task the most efficiently. In the research, this is known as *internal versus external attentional focus.*

I am not saying that you're not using your glutes or the working muscles. Whether you're squatting, hip thrusting, or deadlifting, you're still using good form and staying safe. But you're not trying to fire your glutes maximally the way you would if you were focusing on the mind-muscle connection for hypertrophic gains.

LONGITUDINAL EVIDENCE AT LAST!

Brad Schoenfeld and I recently got an experimental study accepted that shows evidence of the mind-muscle connection being superior for muscle growth. This is the first paper to examine this phenomenon. We knew that thinking about the muscle increased muscle activation, but now we know that it leads to more growth.

MAXIMIZE HYPERTROPHY

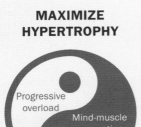

The next chapter covers progressive overload, which simply means doing more over time. Although progressive overload is important for muscle growth (if all you do is lift the same amounts of weight over and over again, you will have a hard time gaining muscle), it's also specific for developing strength. When employing the mind-muscle connection, on the other hand, you're trying to visualize and think about the working muscle and make sure your glutes are the primary mover.

Because both lifting heavier weight and focusing your attention on the muscle being worked are important for hypertrophy, you need to find a balance between the two methods. In Chinese philosophy, yin and yang describes how two seemingly opposite or contrary forces in the natural world may actually be complementary, interconnected, and interdependent and may give rise to each other as they interrelate. When training for maximum muscle growth, you need to get stronger over time with certain movements. However, sometimes you shouldn't concern yourself with quantity (progressive overload) and instead should focus on quality (the mind-muscle connection). Both are necessary to develop maximum muscle hypertrophy; one without the other would yield inferior results. I typically perform the first one or two exercises of the day with the goal of lifting heavy and then do the rest of my workout with a focus on the feel, not the weight.

Before I delve into progressive overload, there is one more important factor to consider when it comes to muscle growth, and that is muscle composition.

MUSCLE COMPOSITION

All of the muscles in your body are made up of muscle fibers, which are elongated cells that form the muscles, as shown in the illustration below. These muscle cells are designed to control movement by producing and absorbing force.

MUSCLE CONTRACTION

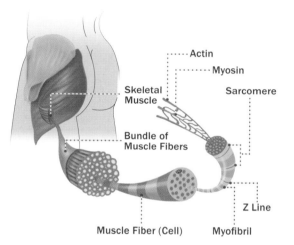

We commonly refer to two muscle fiber types: slow twitch (type I) and fast twitch (type II). You've probably heard that people have either predominantly slow twitch or predominantly fast twitch muscle fibers. Slow twitch muscle fibers are better suited for endurance efforts, like running marathons, whereas fast twitch muscle fibers are better suited for speed and power actions, such as sprinting and lifting. As the theory goes, a marathon runner has mainly slow twitch muscle fibers, and a sprinter has mostly fast twitch muscle fibers.

When you look at EMG research, it's common sense to think that the glutes are a fast twitch muscle group because they are not heavily recruited when you do things like stand up from a chair, climb stairs, walk at a normal pace, or perform activities of daily living that involve the glutes. But when you sprint, jump, or pick up something heavy, glute activation increases dramatically.

In this sense, the glutes are like sleeping giants that are called upon when you perform explosive and heavy movements. For this reason, everyone assumed that the glutes were comprised of predominantly fast twitch muscle fibers. However, two studies looked at the fiber type composition of the glutes. The first study showed that the glutes were 68 percent slow twitch and 32 percent fast twitch. The second study found that the glutes were 52 percent slow twitch and 48 percent fast twitch. To make matters more complicated, there is research indicating that the upper glute fibers have a little more slow twitch type composition than the lower glute fibers, which makes sense because the upper subdivision has more influence on the pelvis, controlling posture and other stabilization actions.

Whether the glutes are fast twitch or slow twitch, the question is, should we train them in a unique way?

This question has long been debated in the world of strength and conditioning. The idea is that you should train your muscles by following an exercise plan that is specific to your distinct muscle fiber type.

There are companies out there that will provide a vague reading of your muscle fibers. Your results might tell you that you have predominantly fast twitch or slow twitch fibers. Although this finding gives you some insight, it shouldn't influence how you train your glutes, because the only way to know whether your glutes are fast twitch or slow twitch is to perform a biopsy—that is, to stick a needle into the muscle, surgically remove a sample, and test the actual muscle fiber. In other words, it's hard to say whether your glutes are fast or slow twitch. And even if you did check them, the finding might not matter.

Here's the theory: if you're mostly fast twitch, you should perform explosive movements with fewer reps and heavier weight, and if you're predominantly slow twitch, you should perform more reps with lighter loads. My colleague Brad Schoenfeld and I are testing this theory with a training study (starting in 2019), so we'll know more in time.

While this approach might be helpful for people who are training for sport, it doesn't change anything when it comes to building the glutes, because we know that both high and low reps will result in muscle growth. What's more, if you train hard, you can't choose which fibers to activate during training. You will end up recruiting all of your muscle fibers. Proportions of muscle fiber types vary from person to person and from muscle to muscle, and motor units (groups of muscle fibers recruited by the nervous system to coordinate muscle contractions) are composed of a mixture of fibers. Furthermore, there is new evidence suggesting that you can alter your fiber type composition over time through vigorous training. So, as long as you train the muscle close to momentary failure—whether you hip thrust for high reps, for a one-rep max, or anywhere in between—you will activate all of the muscle's motor units and recruit both types of muscle fibers.

Remember, your glutes are incredibly unique and versatile in that they can operate effectively through long and short ranges of motion at both slow and fast speeds and resist fatigue during both long- and short-duration exercise—more evidence supporting the importance of exercise and training variety.

In conclusion, a genetic test that tells you your muscle fiber composition (fast or slow twitch) is fine, but it should not guide your training protocol when it comes to developing your glutes. For the best results, just follow the guidelines laid out in the final section of this chapter.

Muscle fibers can be classified into types by using a variety of methods, although the underlying principle across all methods is how fast the fibers can shorten. Fast twitch (also called type II or MHCII) muscle fibers contract much faster than slow twitch (also called type I or MHCI) muscle fibers.[1] Some researchers believe that training with lower loads and higher reps targets slow twitch muscle fibers while training with higher loads and lower reps targets fast twitch muscle fibers[2] on the basis of a small number of studies showing trends in this direction.[3, 4]

Only two studies have measured the muscle fiber type of the glutes, and unfortunately they came to different conclusions. One study found a 52 percent proportion of slow twitch muscle fibers in young male subjects.[5] The other reported a 68 percent proportion of slow twitch muscle fibers in elderly patients with hip osteoarthritis.[6] The higher proportion of slow twitch muscle fibers might have been due to the age of the subjects, although we can't know for certain. Either way, the glutes are not fast twitch; they are probably split evenly between slow and fast twitch fibers. Variety is key in glute training!

STRATEGIES FOR MAXIMIZING MUSCLE GROWTH

This chapter has covered a lot of ground, from the three mechanisms of hypertrophy to the mind-muscle connection and muscle fiber types. Consider the following a brief recap of the most important points of this chapter, as well as the key variables for maximizing muscle growth.

PERFORM EXERCISES CLOSE TO MUSCLE FAILURE TO INCREASE MUSCLE SIZE

Most of us want bigger muscles. To achieve that, we need to get stronger—much stronger. Gaining strength by lifting heavy weight places increased tension on the muscles over time, forcing them to adapt by growing larger. Heavier weights equal greater tension, which equals bigger muscles. Got it? Great!

However, heavier weight alone will not build the biggest muscles. Powerlifters lift more weight than bodybuilders, thereby placing greater tension on their musculature. Yet, despite this added tension, bodybuilders are generally more muscular. If tension were the be-all-end-all, powerlifters would have bigger muscles than bodybuilders. We can't say that it's the drugs, because natural bodybuilders are still bigger than natural powerlifters, and when powerlifters want to build muscle, they borrow methodology from bodybuilders by employing higher-rep assistance lifts with shorter rest times between sets instead of performing low-rep, heavy sets. Furthermore, bodybuilder workouts are more efficient because bodybuilders can handle more volume without getting as beat up. For example, powerlifters might max deadlift (lift heavy with longer rest periods) and then perform only 3 or 4 more sets in their workouts. In contrast, a bodybuilder would deadlift with less weight and shorter rest times and still be able to add in accessory exercises, such as hip thrusts or back extensions, because lifting to failure with less weight and shorter rest times is less taxing on the body.

What gives, then? There are two explanations. The first is that powerlifting techniques maximize the amount of weight you can handle, so you end up using more muscle overall and generating more ground reaction force. Bodybuilding techniques maximize the tension you put on the muscle, so you end up generating more muscle force mainly in the targeted muscle. Moreover, with lighter loads, the prevailing thought is that lighter loads end up placing sufficient tension on each fiber throughout the set due to Henneman's size principle. That is, as a muscle fatigues, the lower-threshold motor units can no longer carry out the task, so the higher-threshold motor units are called upon to pick up the slack and get the job done.

Although peak EMG activity never gets as high during sets with lighter weight as it does during sets with heavier weight, the sets take longer to carry out, and during this period, each muscle fiber ends up being recruited for a sufficient time to match the hypertrophy stimulus. This is evident from training studies comparing light versus heavy weight on muscle growth. There are more than 20 published papers on the topic, and the overwhelming consensus is equal growth between the two. In fact, an interesting study shows that muscle growth can be achieved simply by contracting the muscle with no resistance. The participants in one group squeezed their biceps with no load, and the other group did dumbbell biceps curls. The two groups saw similar hypertrophy. It could very well be that lighter loads cause slightly greater growth in slow twitch fibers while heavier loads cause slightly greater growth in fast twitch fibers, but total growth ends up being equal.

So, even though lifting heavy does build muscle and strength, you don't need to lift heavy to maximize glute growth. As long as you're carrying out the movement close to muscle failure using a load that's above 40 percent of your one-rep max (1RM) and moving through a full range of motion, you can get similar hypertrophy gains. Stated differently, you can achieve similar hypertrophy through a wide range of loads (even bodyweight training provides load in the form of your body weight as resistance against gravity) as long as you perform the exercise one or two reps shy of failure—that is, if you did another one or two reps, you wouldn't be able to perform the movement again without cheating the range of motion or compromising your form.

DO STIMULATING (EFFECTIVE, HYPERTROPHIC) REPS

The last 5 reps of a set to failure provide the majority of the muscle-building stimulus. If you do a heavy 1RM, even though it's brutal, it provides only one stimulating rep. If you do a set of 3 reps to failure, all three stimulate hypertrophy. The same goes for 5 reps. But once you exceed 5 reps, the number of stimulating reps doesn't increase. So let's say you perform a set of 20 reps to failure. Only the last five contribute meaningfully to muscle growth. What if you leave a rep or two in the tank and avoid training to failure? Then you subtract that from the 5 stimulating reps. Let's say you do a set of 10 reps with 2 reps in reserve (2 reps shy of muscle failure). This would amount to 3 stimulating reps. This example is grossly oversimplified, as each rep contributes a little to the muscle-building puzzle, but the reps closest to failure pack the biggest punch. And this is assuming your form and range of motion are stellar on every rep, because sloppy reps aren't as effective as pristine reps for building muscle.

In summary, you can essentially pick the rep scheme that you prefer as long as you follow the above protocol and perform a sufficient number of stimulating reps. Research needs to determine the optimal number of stimulating reps per week, and it likely varies from one person to the next. But you can see how 5 sets of 5 reps to failure would provide 25 stimulating reps,

8 sets of 1 rep would provide only 8 stimulating reps, and 3 sets of 15 reps would provide 15 stimulating reps.

Let's say you hate training to failure on certain exercises, like lunges or deadlifts. If you performed 8 sets of 8 reps to 3 reps shy of failure, this would amount to 16 stimulating reps. A pyramid involving 10/8/6/15 reps would amass 20 stimulating reps. Knowing this system helps you plan ideal training sessions.

We need more research to teach us how this system applies to certain exercises, such as high-rep bodyweight frog pumps. Say you do 4 sets of 50 reps and none of the sets is to failure. This system would indicate that it wouldn't stimulate any muscle growth, but this doesn't seem to be the case based on my anecdotal experience as a lifter and trainer. Models like these help us make sense of our methods and keep us on track, but they rarely withstand scientific scrutiny.

UTILIZE A SHOTGUN APPROACH AND EMPHASIZE VARIETY

One exercise can't be everything. As you have learned, you need to perform a variety of exercises with different loads and tempos and through varying ranges of motion to ensure that you target all three hypertrophy mechanisms and hit all of your muscle fibers. This is why I utilize a shotgun approach when it comes to exercise selection and program design, which you will learn more about on page 198.

HIGH ACTIVATION IS RELATED TO HYPERTROPHY, BUT YOU ALSO NEED SLOW CONTRACTION SPEEDS THROUGH A LARGE RANGE OF MOTION

Activation, as measured by EMG, is related to hypertrophy, but it is not perfectly linear, meaning that activation is not completely equal to muscle growth. You must consider other factors, such as the speed of the muscle contraction. For example, say you land from a jump. Your quad activation is through the roof, but you get only a brief spike.

To create adequate tension on the muscle fibers, you need a sustained contraction. More specifically, the contraction or activation needs to be slow enough to generate optimal tension throughout the muscle. It takes time for all of the possible cross-bridges to form—cross-bridges are the structures responsible for muscle tension to create the pulling forces on bones—which creates movement. This can be achieved either by lifting heavy or by lifting a light load to failure.

What's more, there is evidence that you need to create tension through a large range of motion to maximize hypertrophy in order to get the best of both worlds in terms of stretch and activation-related growth. Not all studies demonstrate this, however, so it likely depends on the muscle/muscle group and exercise in question. Isometrics don't seem to be as well suited for building muscle as dynamic exercises that move the muscles through their full ranges of motion.

So, while it's true that greater activation is better for hypertrophy, you need to create tension (activation) through a large range of motion with proper load, tempo, and effort to maximize muscle growth.

SQUEEZING YOUR GLUTES IS GOOD FOR HYPERTROPHY

When you're performing glute-dominant and certain hamstring-dominant movements, like the hip thrust, glute bridge, kickback, quadruped hip extension, and back extension, squeezing your glutes at the top of the movement is good for hypertrophy. Glute activation is very high with these exercises, which is why I recommend a one-second glute squeeze at end-range hip extension.

However, you have to be careful when squeezing your glutes at the top of a squat or deadlift. Most people squeeze their glutes naturally at the top of these movements to lock out their hips. But you have to avoid exaggerating the glute squeeze to the point where it compromises your form. For example, say you stand tall to finish a squat but squeeze your glutes so hard that you posterior pelvic tilt. In such a situation, your lumbar spine pulls into flexion and pushes your hips forward. If you have a heavy bar on your back, you're asking for trouble. You can't grow your glutes while injured, so exercise caution and prioritize form.

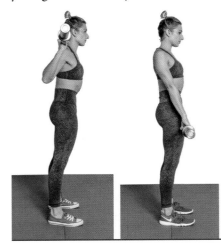 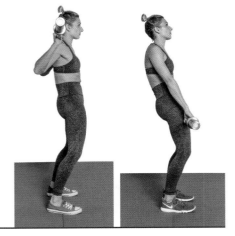

JUST ENOUGH GLUTE SQUEEZE   TOO MUCH GLUTE SQUEEZE

TRAINING FOR THE PUMP WILL MAKE YOUR BUTT LOOK BIG AND PROBABLY GROW MUSCLE

As I stated earlier, I believe that training for the pump is good for muscle growth, although we don't have concrete science to back it up yet. One thing is for sure: you will love the way your butt looks following a good pump workout, and there's a strong chance that it will help build bigger glutes as well.

HIP EXTENSION IS THE BEST JOINT ACTION FOR GROWING THE GLUTES

If all you ever did was hip extension exercises like glute bridge and hip thrust variations, you could probably achieve 90 percent of your maximum results.

Remember, maximum glute activation occurs at end-range hip extension, which is the shortest position for the glutes. It is for this reason (among others) that the glute bridge and hip thrust are considered great glute-building exercises. You can test this idea by sitting down or bending forward and then squeezing your glutes as hard as you can, which is similar to squatting and deadlifting. Although you can contract your glutes in this flexed position, you can't achieve peak tension; it feels like you're leaving room on the table in terms of maximizing glute density through contraction. But if you stand upright with your hips in full extension, you can squeeze your glutes maximally, which is similar to glute bridging and hip thrusting.

THINKING ABOUT THE WORKING MUSCLE INCREASES HYPERTROPHY

A ton of research shows that thinking about the working muscle—that is, using the mind-muscle connection—increases activation, and one study shows that it leads to greater hypertrophy. So there is no refuting this fact. Whether you're warming up using activation drills or you're trying to build muscle in a certain area, putting conscious effort into thinking about contracting that muscle will yield the best results.

PRIORITIZE RESISTANCE TRAINING AND AVOID SPRINTING AND PLYOMETRICS FOR GLUTE DEVELOPMENT

Although the glutes are highly involved in sprinting and jumping, I don't recommend plyometrics or sprinting as a strategy for building bigger glutes for two reasons. First, plyometrics and sprinting are risky in that they make you more susceptible to muscle strains and tears. Second, plyometrics and sprinting don't build muscle nearly as well as resistance training. Almost all of the best glutes in the world are built through resistance training because resistance training maximizes tension on the muscles—something that cannot be said of plyometrics or sprinting. Resistance training is also safer to perform and more predictable. Allow me to elaborate.

It is true that sport training builds some glute muscle (but doesn't maximize it) and improves neural output. When I work with athletes who have played ground sports (think soccer and football) but have never lifted weights, they see results much sooner than people who don't have athletic backgrounds. This is largely due to the fact that athletes have developed proficiency in utilizing their glutes explosively from every angle. In contrast, beginners who haven't played a lot of sports haven't yet developed the motor patterns and mind-muscle connection because they haven't been using their glutes in training.

But say I'm working with a beginner who has never played sports or done anything athletic, or even a former athlete whose goals have switched to aesthetics and maximizing glute development. In these situations, I don't recommend sprinting, jumping, or explosive training due to the risk of injury. Strength training is a better way to build muscle due to the slower contractions.

If you're an athlete and you're training for performance and function, on the other hand, then explosive and plyometric training is necessary, not because you're trying to build muscle but because you're trying to get better at your sport (think speed, power, agility, and coordination). You might be wondering, "Then why does [fill in the blank] athlete have such nice glutes?" It's true that numerous athletes have incredible glute development. However, this is likely due more to their strength training than to their sport training. Before weight training was popular, athletes' glutes weren't nearly as developed.

How to Gain Strength

One of my favorite experiences as a personal trainer is seeing the look on a client's face when they hit a new personal record on the hip thrust, squat, or deadlift. It's a joyful moment for everyone because it validates all of the training and hard work. The client is stronger than they were before, which is a clear measure of progress.

I encourage most of my clients to create strength-specific goals because it gives them something to come back to month after month. They get addicted to hitting new PRs. As a result, they work harder in the gym, and their training adherence improves. As they get stronger and more consistent, they start to notice more physique changes, which also encourages them to keep training.

Chapter 11 addresses specific strength goals that I expect all of my clients to achieve after training with me for six months. For now, I want to focus on the best strategy for improving strength. Although there is some overlap between training for strength and training for hypertrophy, it's not perfectly linear, as you might expect. In other words, you can gain size but not increase your strength and vice versa.

This is not to say that increasing muscle size won't increase strength or that improving strength won't facilitate muscle growth. Whether you're training for strength or training for hypertrophy, you will probably see gains in both departments if you're training properly.

But—and this is key—training for strength is not the same as training for hypertrophy. There is a specificity component that you have to consider. For example, as you will recall from the previous chapter, when you're training for hypertrophy, you don't need to lift heavy as long as you're carrying out the movement close to muscle failure. When you're training for strength, however, you need to lift heavy and utilize the progressive overload methodology.

PROGRESSIVE OVERLOAD

Progressive overload simply means doing more over time. This can mean more weight over time, more reps over time, or more sets over time, but if your goal is to gain strength, then more weight over time is your best bet. There are many other ways to progressively overload the body. For example, you can perform larger ranges of motion, use a smoother tempo, add a pause, or add an explosive element.

In a nutshell, the best way to develop strength—and, to a lesser degree, muscle size—is to do more over time to increase your work capacity and improve your form.

Although progressive overload is pretty straightforward, simply telling someone to add 10 more pounds or do two more reps with the same weight each week is not sustainable. There is a huge gap in fitness ability from one person to the next. If you're just starting your strength journey, you will see huge gains in the first few months of training, but as you start plateauing or reaching peak performance, the protocol gets a lot more complex. For this reason, it's nearly impossible to offer a blanket prescription. So, rather than try to give you an exact protocol, I've outlined 10 rules or guidelines to help you maximize your results using progressive overload.

1. PROGRESSIVE OVERLOAD STARTS WITH WHATEVER YOU CAN DO WITH PERFECT TECHNICAL FORM.

Let's say you're new to a particular exercise. You've seen all sorts of YouTube videos of strong lifters hoisting hundreds of pounds. You think you're a strong cat, so you load up the plates and find that the exercise just doesn't feel right. It feels awkward and unnatural, you don't feel the right muscles working, and it even seems jarring on your joints and potentially injurious. This exercise is definitely not right for you, right? Wrong! The exercise probably is right for you; you just need to approach it in a different way.

Do not concern yourself with what others use for loading (weight). When you begin an exercise, start out light and gradually work your way up. I'll provide two examples: the starting point for the weakest non-elderly and non-injured beginner I've trained, and the starting point for the strongest beginner I've trained. Chances are you'll fall somewhere in between these two individuals.

The weakest beginner I ever trained (a middle-aged woman who had been completely sedentary for around 15 years) had to start out with bodyweight high box squats on an adjustable step-up platform so that she was descending only about 8 inches before sitting on the box. This client also performed glute bridges, step-ups from a 4-inch step, and hip hinge drills—all with just body weight.

But she was squatting, hip thrusting, step-upping, and deadlifting. Granted, she was performing the most remedial variations of those exercises, but this was what was right for her at the time. Within six months, she was doing full-range goblet squats, barbell hip thrusts, Bulgarian split squats, and deadlifts from the floor with 95 pounds.

Conversely, the strongest beginner I ever trained—a high school wrestler—was able to use 185 pounds for full squats, 225 pounds for deadlifts and hip thrusts, and 155 pounds for bench presses and could do Bulgarian split squats, single-leg hip thrusts, and chin-ups with great form. Though he was an athlete, surprisingly he had never lifted weights before. Sports had strengthened his legs and upper body so that he was able to start out at a much more advanced level than most beginners. Even my (at the time) 13-year-old niece, a very good volleyball player, squatted 95 pounds, trap bar deadlifted 135 pounds, and single-leg hip thrusted (all with excellent form) in her very first weight training session.

But these people are not you. You'll find that due to your unique body type, you have an advantage with some exercises and a huge disadvantage with others. Long femurs? You probably won't set any squat records, but your weighted back extension strength is going to kick some serious butt. Long arms? You can kiss bench press records goodbye, but you will be a deadlifting rock star.

Figure out where you belong on the regression-progression continuum (basically a list of variations of an exercise from the easiest to the most challenging) and start getting stronger. This means staying conservative, not progressing too quickly, and letting your technique guide your progress. If your form starts to break down as you go up in weight, that's an indication that you're not strong enough to lift that much weight yet. In such a situation, you need to take a step back and build your body up to handle heavier loads.

Another mistake people make is following percentage-based programs—meaning they're lifting a certain percentage of their one-rep max—using a one-rep max from years ago. They're screwing themselves from the start because they're basing it on a one-rep max that they did when they were much stronger (and younger). If you are following a percentage-based program, it's important to retest your one-rep max and use that number as your starting point.

2. PROGRESSIVE OVERLOAD FOR BEGINNERS INVOLVES A FEW TENETS.

Progressive overload methodology is different for beginners than for more advanced lifters. It's also different for men than women and for those carrying a lot of muscle versus those not carrying much muscle. For example, I can't tell a woman who is new to strength training to add 10 pounds to the bar for squats and deadlifts each week. First, chances are some work has to be done just to get her to squat and deadlift properly before focusing on load. Some clients should start out with partial-range lifts, such as bodyweight box squats and rack pulls (deadlifting from an elevated platform), and simply work on progressive distance training, whereby the range of motion is increased slightly each week. If you keep squatting your own body weight (or rack pulling 65 pounds) for 3 sets of 10 reps, but each week you descend an inch deeper, that's progressive overload. Eventually you'll be using a full range of motion, and then you can concern yourself with adding weight.

With exercises that have you move a significant portion of your body, such as squats, hip thrusts, back extensions, and lunges, you must master your own body weight before adding load. As a general guideline, I like my clients to be able to perform 3 sets of 20 full-range-of-motion reps with bodyweight exercises before adding load.

What's more, many lifts require very small jumps in load over time, and attempts in these exercises usually involve jumps in repetitions instead of load. This applies to lifts that utilize smaller loads, such as cable kickbacks and cable standing hip abductions, as well as challenging bodyweight movements, such as skater squats, single-leg Romanian deadlifts, single-leg hip thrusts, and prisoner single-leg back extensions.

This is especially important for women and smaller men when it is not possible to access smaller plates (for example, 1.25 or 2.5 pounds) or make smaller jumps in dumbbell or kettlebell loads (say, 17.5 pounds). Think about it: going from 50-pound dumbbells to 55-pound dumbbells is a 10 percent jump in weight. However, going from 10-pound dumbbells to 15-pound dumbbells is a 50 percent jump in weight. You cannot expect to make a 50 percent jump in load and execute the same number of repetitions as the week before, but you can expect to get another rep or two with the same load.

Let's say that one week you perform ankle weight quadruped kickbacks with 10 pounds for 15 reps. The next week, rather than up the load to 15 pounds, try performing 20 reps with the 10-pound weights. When you can do 3 sets of 20 reps, increase the weight to 15 pounds.

3. PROGRESSIVE OVERLOAD CAN BE ACHIEVED IN A VARIETY OF WAYS—12 THAT I CAN THINK OF.

There are many ways to do more over time. I've already mentioned progressing in range of motion, repetitions, and load. In the beginning, you want to progress in range of motion and form. Yes, if you do the same workout you did the week before but with better form, you've made progress. You did more for your neuromuscular system in terms of motor patterning (developing coordination) and even muscle force because using better form involves relying more on the targeted muscles.

After you've established and ingrained proper form and full range of motion, it's time to worry about progressing in repetitions and load. But these aren't the only ways to progress. Here are all of the practical ways that I can think of:

- Lifting the same load for the same number of reps for increased distance (range of motion)
- Lifting the same load for the same number of reps with better form, more control, and less effort (efficiency)
- Lifting the same load for more reps (volume)
- Doing the same number of reps with heavier weight (load)
- Lifting the same load for the same number of sets and reps with less rest time between sets (density)
- Lifting the same load with more speed and acceleration (effort)
- Doing more work in the same amount of time (density)
- Doing the same work in less time (density)
- Doing more sets with the same load and number of reps (volume)
- Lifting the same workout more often throughout the week (frequency)
- Doing the same workout and maintaining strength while losing body mass (relative volume)
- Lifting the same load for the same number of reps and then extending the set past technical failure with forced reps, negatives, dropsets, static holds, rest pauses, partial reps, or a superset (effort)

Just remember, improvements in form and range of motion come first, and increases in reps and load come second.

4. PROGRESSIVE OVERLOAD WILL NEVER BE LINEAR.

Many strength coaches love to tell the story of Milo of Croton to illuminate the merits of progressive overload. Legend has it that Milo used to pick up a baby calf every day and carry it around on his shoulders. As the calf grew, Milo got stronger. Eventually, Milo was hoisting a full-sized bull and busting out sets of yoke walks like it was nothing. Pretty cool story, right?

Unfortunately, this story is a crock of bull (pun intended). First of all, a half-ton bull would be way too awkward to carry due to the lopsided nature and sheer size of the animal. But this is irrelevant.

No gains from weight training, be it in mobility, hypertrophy, strength, power, endurance, or fat loss, will ever occur in a linear fashion. The body doesn't work that way. Adaptations happen in waves. Sometimes you'll make big jumps in a single week in a particular quality, while other times you'll stall for three months in another quality. Over the long haul, everything goes up, but it's a windy road. There are physiological reasons for this phenomenon, which are highlighted throughout the book.

However, let's pretend for a minute that you could make linear progress for an entire year on a particular lift. A 10-pound jump per week equates to 520 pounds in a year. Even a 5-pound jump per week equates to 260 pounds in a year. Moreover, a one-rep jump per week equates to 52 reps

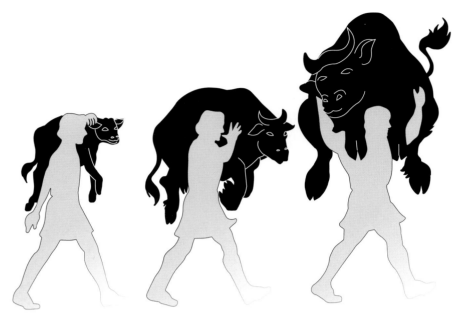

in a year, while a one-rep jump per month equates to 12 reps in a year. You won't gain 260 or 520 pounds in a year on any single lift. You won't gain 12 or 52 reps on most lifts, either. It's just not going to happen. In some sessions, you'll be surprisingly strong and make big gains; in some sessions, you'll simply tie your previous efforts; and in some sessions, you'll actually be weaker and go backward. But every six months, you'll likely be stronger and fitter.

The charts below depict a woman's progress in body fat percentage and lean body mass over a one-year period. Her transformation was the most dramatic I've seen to date, but notice the nonlinear adaptations. Also notice the drop in muscle, despite doing everything right. This woman gained a ton of strength on squats, deadlifts, hip thrusts, bench presses, military presses, rows, and chin-ups; she never missed a training session; and she ate perfectly for an entire year; yet she lost around 11 pounds of muscle during her yearlong pursuit of getting into contest shape of below 10 percent body fat. Nevertheless, she won her first figure competition and quickly became a popular figure competitor.

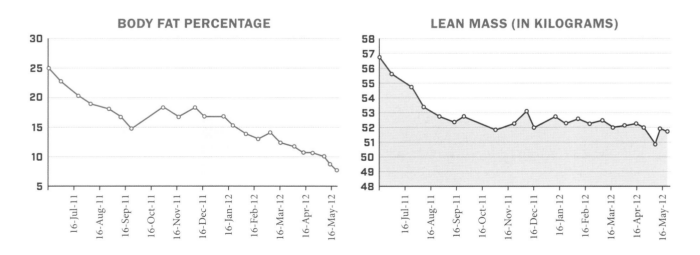

5. PROGRESSIVE OVERLOAD WILL NEVER BE AS FUN AS IT IS DURING YOUR FIRST THREE MONTHS OF LIFTING.

If you're a beginner, sit back and enjoy the ride! Your rate of strength gain during your first three months of proper weight training will be higher than at any other time in your life. Each week, you will slaughter personal records. Getting 15 reps of an exercise that you got only 10 reps of the previous week is not uncommon. This is mostly due to rapid gains in intermuscular coordination. Just don't get spoiled; your rate of gain will slow dramatically, and pretty soon you'll be just like the rest of us—fighting like hell for those gains.

6. PROGRESSIVE OVERLOAD FOR VETERAN LIFTERS REQUIRES SERIOUS STRATEGY AND SPECIALIZATION.

As a beginner, you can do pretty much anything and gain strength as long as you're consistent. After a couple of years of solid training, however, you have to be clever about your programming in order to continue to reach new levels of strength. You'll need to rotate your lifts, plan your program designs intelligently, fluctuate your training stress, specialize in whatever you're striving to improve most, and tinker with methodologies.

For example, one month you might have a deadlift focus, the next month a squat focus, and the next month a single-leg focus. However, you will be performing squat, deadlift, and hip thrust variations each month. By prioritizing one movement pattern, you will progress mostly with that lift. This is not to say you're neglecting the other movements, as maintaining strength is very easy. If you're following a squat specialization program, for instance, you might program that in the beginning of each of your workouts and then perform your glute-specific exercises afterward. Then the next month, maybe you follow a hip thrust specialization program, and then the month after that, you follow a deadlift specialization program. But you'll always include a variation of each exercise in your training. This is a great way to increase strength with specific lifts and progress your strength. Remember, building is hard; maintaining is easy.

Eventually, it becomes difficult to pack more pounds onto a particular lift or even gain another rep. In such a situation, you might need to give your body a chance to recover. When I program—whether it's for myself, for my Booty by Bret program, or for one of my clients—I typically have three hard weeks of training and then one deload week. Here's an example:

- Week 1 = 60 to 70 percent of overall effort
- Week 2 = 70 to 80 percent of overall effort
- Week 3 = 80 to 90 percent of overall effort
- Week 4 = 90 to 100 percent of overall effort

Then the cycle repeats. You can do three-week cycles or even six- to eight-week cycles, but I like four weeks because it fits within a calendar month.

7. PROGRESSIVE OVERLOAD IS MUCH HARDER WHEN YOU'RE LOSING WEIGHT.

Unless you're a beginner, increasing your strength while simultaneously dropping significant weight is challenging. In fact, simply maintaining your strength while losing weight is a form of progressive overload, as you'd be increasing your relative strength (strength divided by body weight) and therefore doing more over time.

Weight loss affects some lifts more than others. Squats and hip thrusts tend to take a dive, whereas deadlifts sometimes stay put and single-leg exercises may improve. You will see a huge jump in your strength and endurance on bodyweight exercises when you lose weight, so enjoy the boosts in reps on push-ups, chin-ups, dips, inverted rows, and Nordics.

8. PROGRESSIVE OVERLOAD SOMETIMES HAS A MIND OF ITS OWN.

Quite often, you'll do everything right, but you won't get stronger. The plan just doesn't work. You'll be lifting hard, adhering to an intelligent plan, eating well, and sleeping right, yet you still won't set any PRs. Other times, you'll do everything wrong and somehow gain strength. Your training can be derailed and your diet and sleep can go down the gutter, but you'll go to the gym and set a PR. This makes absolutely no sense and flies in the face of sports science. Nevertheless, this is how the body works sometimes. Physiology is tricky and multifactorial. Don't get cocky and think that you've stumbled upon some secret system that involves excessive partying, eating mostly junk food, and training sporadically. Engaging in these behaviors for too long will backfire on you, so stay on track to the best of your abilities.

9. PROGRESSIVE OVERLOAD SHOULD NEVER BE PRIORITIZED OVER PROPER FORM.

At any point, if you really want to set a PR, you can be lax on your form and likely set a record. For example, you could round your back excessively during deadlifts, let your knees cave during squats, skimp on squat depth or hip thrust lockout range of motion, or let your hips shoot up during lunges. However, this is a slippery slope that's best avoided. Progressive overload works only when you challenge your muscles to do more over time, and your muscles will not be forced to do more if your form gets sloppy. Moreover, you won't set any personal records if you're injured or constantly in pain.

10. PROGRESSIVE OVERLOAD REQUIRES STANDARDIZED TECHNIQUE.

The only way you will ever know whether you have gained strength is to perform the lifts the exact same way each time. In other words, true strength gains require proper depth, tempo, and execution. Many lifters lie to themselves and pretend that they've gotten stronger, but their ranges of motion diminish or their form goes out the window. These lifters didn't get stronger; they got sloppier. Federations in the sports of powerlifting, Olympic weightlifting, and strongman have created rules for their various exercises. It may be worth your while to learn these rules so that you always perform the lifts properly in training and when testing your max. Assuming you can perform the lifts properly, always squat to parallel or deeper, always lock out your hip thrusts and barbell glute bridges, and in general, always control the weight through a full range of motion.

My hope is that these 10 guidelines will help keep you on track and maximize your strength.

I have one more piece of advice to share with you. Even the most seasoned lifters often have to take a step back in order to take two steps forward. Sometimes we get caught up in chasing continuous PRs to the point of altering form, relying on the wrong muscles, skimping on range of motion, or training through pain.

Once a year, I recommend retesting your strength levels in your pursuit of progressive overload. Throw everything you've done out the window and start over using the best possible form through a full range of motion. This is your new baseline. Now work on adhering to that form while doing more over time. In the long run, your body will thank you for engaging in this simple yet effective practice.

MITIGATING RISK

Lifting heavy is dangerous if you don't exercise good form or follow a well-designed training program. For example, if you deadlift with an excessively rounded back, you might get injured. But if you keep your spine in the neutral zone—back flat with maybe a little bit of upper back rounding—then you're usually fine. The same is true for program design: If you try to deadlift heavy three times a week, you're setting yourself up for disaster. It's simply too much for your body to recover from. But if you're following a good program that takes into consideration recovery and you're deadlifting only once a week, you'll probably be fine.

It's like this: lifting heavy is inherently more dangerous than lifting lighter weights because you're putting more stress on your joints and you have less room for error. However, this shouldn't prevent you from lifting heavy or pursuing strength goals.

If you and your coach know what you're doing, you can mitigate a lot of the danger. Put simply, lifting heavy is safe as long as you listen to your body, follow an intelligent program, and prioritize good mechanics.

Exercise Categorization

When I start working with a client, I typically begin the conversation by asking about the client's training goals. The goals always vary, but more often than not, clients are seeking physique changes, trying to correct a gluteal imbalance or injury, or working toward a specific strength or performance goal.

Although their reasons for training are different, the underlying principles that I use to design their programs are the same, in that I select exercises tailored specifically to their experience, anatomy, and goals. Exercise selection, in other words, is crucial to ensure that my clients get the results they are looking for. If a client wants to develop the upper glutes, then I need to program exercises that primarily develop that area. If a client has one glute that is markedly larger than the other, then I need to select exercises that will help correct the imbalance.

Like a master carpenter, a good trainer has specific techniques and tools for every situation and circumstance. In most situations, trainers use the primary tools, like a barbell hip thrust or back squat, but in certain circumstances, they use a specialty tool, such as a single-leg foot-elevated banded glute bridge. And herein lies the point: to achieve training goals, you need to know how to select the right exercise for the job. And you can't select the right exercise for the job if you don't have a system for categorizing techniques. How else do you pick from the hundreds of exercises and variations? When you have a classification system for organizing and choosing techniques, you know why a specific exercise works and—equally important—when and how to apply it.

As you will learn, there are several ways to categorize glute training exercises, including planes of motion, force vectors, knee action, dominant muscle group, movement pattern, limb number, load position, and type of resistance (equipment). In this chapter, I cover only planes of motion, force vectors, and knee action because, when combined into one system, these classification methods create the most comprehensive and accurate categories.

In Part 5, I describe how to organize exercises based on the dominant muscle being worked, movement pattern, limb number, equipment, and load position (where on the body the equipment is placed). These methods are a great way to organize exercises into broad categories, and I use the same system in this book to make the exercises easier to navigate. But—and this is the crucial difference—it's not the most accurate way to categorize individual techniques.

To determine why certain exercises are well suited for specific goals and why certain exercises work the glutes better than others, you need to look at the position of your body relative to the load or weight you are moving. This is exactly what you will learn in this chapter. For instance, you will learn why squatting with a barbell on your back, which is a vertical load in a standing position, works your lower glutes and why hip thrusting with a barbell on your hips, which is a horizontal load in a supine position, works both your upper and lower glutes.

I believe this information is essential for anyone interested in learning how to fully develop their glutes. However, I realize that exercise categorization—especially planes of motion and force vector speak—is likely to make your head spin. So let me do you a favor and boil everything down to this: to get the most out of your glute training program, you need to target your glutes from a variety of angles in a variety of positions.

In this chapter, I describe those angles and positions in detail. This knowledge will help refine your approach to exercise selection and program design, which I cover in Part 4. If you're not interested in learning about the exercise categorization systems, or you just want a simple way to choose exercises based on how they work your glutes, you can refer to the Glute Exercise Categories chart on pages 124 and 125, which outlines all of the forthcoming information in one easy-to-understand infographic.

SCIENCE SPEAK: EXERCISE CATEGORIZATION

Exercise categorization is usually done for the purpose of figuring out which exercises transfer best to specific sports. Transfer of training is the extent to which an adaptation to a strength training exercise, such as maximal back squat strength, leads to an adaptation in a sporting task, such as vertical jump height. Done properly, an estimate of training transfer is achieved for a group of athletes by collecting data and then using the transfer effect coefficient (TEC) ratio. The TEC ratio takes the ratio of the gain in the sporting task performance after training (as an effect size: ESST) and the simultaneous gain in the exercise 1RM after training (also as an effect size: ESEX).[1] So TEC ratio = ESST / ESEX.

Less rigorously, training transfer can be predicted based on the similarity between the exercises and the sporting tasks. This is akin to the concept of "dynamic correspondence," which is "how closely the means of special strength preparation corresponds to the functioning of the neuromuscular system in a given sport."[2]

The extent to which dynamic correspondence of exercises is important depends greatly on the training status of the individual. For beginners, just about any exercise or activity will improve performance, as all of the muscles quickly gain in strength from being exposed to a novel stimulus. However, as the individual becomes more advanced, the need for greater specificity increases. In elite athletes, training has to be very specific to the task in which the athlete is trying to improve.

Exercises can display dynamic correspondence with sporting tasks across a broad range of domains. Specificity can encompass contraction types (concentric, isometric, or eccentric muscle actions), contraction speeds (explosive or controlled), loading (heavy, moderate, or light), force vectors (axial, anteroposterior, or combined), joint angles where peak contraction occurs, range of motion, time available for force development, stability requirements, posture, number of limbs acting, and many other factors.[3]

The trouble is, we don't know for sure which of these factors is most important when assessing each case!

Traditionally, when aiming to achieve better dynamic correspondence between exercises in the gym and sports performance, strength coaches focused on posture and stability requirements. There was a rush to the squat rack and away from the leg press, as the standing position and the need to stabilize the barbell were thought to more closely resemble the challenges of sport. Later, there was a move to single-leg movements, as running involves pushing off on one leg at a time, and many cutting and leaping movements also start from one leg or from a split stance. One factor that has taken a long time to come to the fore is the force vector, which is the direction of the force with respect to the body. And yet, this appears to be a mode of specificity that you do not want to ignore.

EXERCISE CLASSIFICATIONS

To reiterate, there are several methods of categorizing exercises. In this section, I focus on planes of motion, force vectors, and knee action. By themselves, these classifications are incomplete, but when you combine them into one system, you can effectively select exercises based on the movement and muscle you want to work—whether it is your upper glutes, lower glutes, both upper and lower glutes, quads, or hamstrings.

For instance, it's difficult to explain what a particular exercise is good for by looking only at where the movement occurs (plane of motion). To narrow down your options, you also need to know where the load is placed on your body relative to your position (force vector). And in order to know which muscle the exercise targets, you need to look at the motion of your knees (knee action) during the exercise.

To begin, I'll introduce and explain each classification method, and then I'll tie it all together and clarify how these methods are used to categorize glute training exercises.

PLANES OF MOTION

The first step in understanding how to categorize exercises is to get acquainted with planes of motion.

Plane of motion refers to the particular plane—front and back, left and right, top and bottom—in which movement occurs. To put it another way, when you lift weights, the motion usually occurs across defined planes of motion. This method of classification became popular with strength coaches because it helped describe movements in sport. Coaches would look at where the motion occurs (plane of motion) and then try to mimic that movement in a controlled environment to improve performance in a specific area or action. For example, if a movement occurred across the frontal plane of motion (side to side), then the coach might implement side-to-side or lateral movements in the gym.

In sports, movement involves a blend of planes, which is why so many coaches incorporate "multiplanar" exercises into their regimens. For the purposes of this book, I use planes-of-motion terms to label exercises and isolate certain movement patterns, such as frontal plane hip abduction and transverse plane hip abduction. To fully develop the different regions of the glutes, you must perform exercises from both categories. (More on this shortly.)

When it comes to human movement, there are three planes of motion: frontal, sagittal, and transverse.

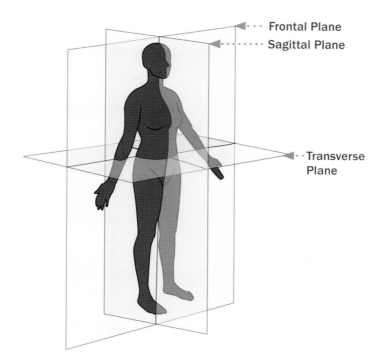

Frontal Plane divides the body into front and back halves. Examples include side-to-side or lateral movements and abduction exercises such as upright lateral band walks and side-lying hip abduction. Frontal plane exercises primarily target the upper glutes.

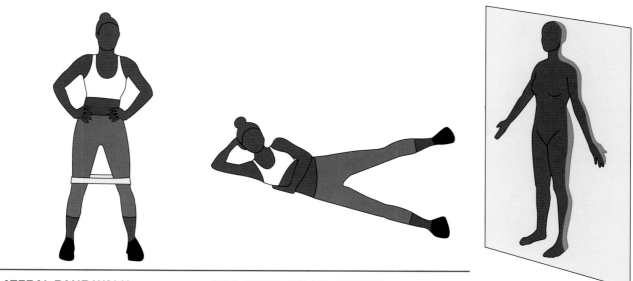

LATERAL BAND WALK   SIDE-LYING HIP ABDUCTION

Sagittal Plane divides the body into left and right halves. Examples include hip thrusting, squatting, deadlifting, and any exercise that is done with little to no side-to-side or rotational movement. Exercises in this category can be done with higher loads and typically comprise the main lifts.

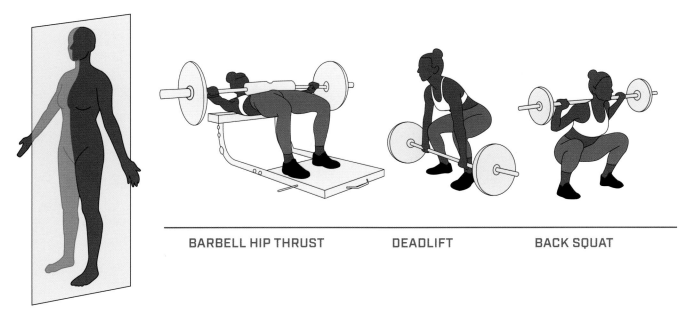

BARBELL HIP THRUST   DEADLIFT   BACK SQUAT

Transverse Plane divides the body into top and bottom halves. Examples include rotational exercises such as band or cable hip external rotation. Transverse plane exercises target both the upper and lower glutes.

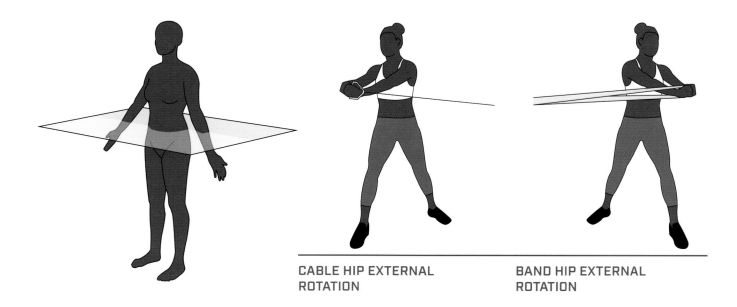

CABLE HIP EXTERNAL   BAND HIP EXTERNAL
ROTATION   ROTATION

Although categorizing movements using planes of motion tells us where the movement occurs, it doesn't paint a complete picture. In order to categorize glute exercises accurately, we must look not only at where the movement occurs, but also at the force vector, which is the line of resistance relative to the body.

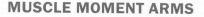

MUSCLE MOMENT ARMS

Muscle moment arms are measurements of leverage. If a muscle has a moment arm in a particular plane, then it causes the joint to turn in that direction when it is activated or stretched. Moment arms are often overlooked when determining the precise function of a muscle. However, they are essential for establishing how effective a muscle can be at producing a turning force at a given joint, at any given joint angle. Although we talk about muscles exerting force, we should instead refer to torque or "turning force," since limbs follow an angular path around the joint, which acts as a pivot. The amount of torque is calculated by multiplying the force by its perpendicular distance from the pivot (called the moment arm length, which is the amount of leverage that muscle has on the joint at that moment). The longer the perpendicular distance from the pivot, the larger the torque.

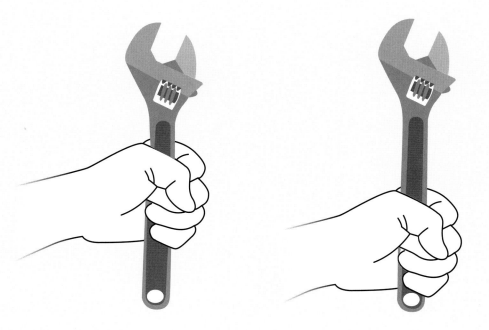

This is why holding a wrench lower down its handle is much easier than holding it farther up. The longer moment arm means that you can produce more torque when applying the same amount of muscle force to the lever.

PLANES OF MOTION

Muscles can have moment arms (leverage) in any of the three planes of motion: sagittal, frontal, and transverse. The glutes are fairly unique in that they have meaningful moment arms in at least two planes and almost certainly have a small moment arm in the third. This makes the glutes a key hip extensor, an important hip external rotator, and a minor hip abductor. You can see how the glutes stack up against the other hip muscles in each plane in the following chart.[4]

MOMENT ARMS OF HIP MUSCLES IN THE THREE PLANES AT NEUTRAL

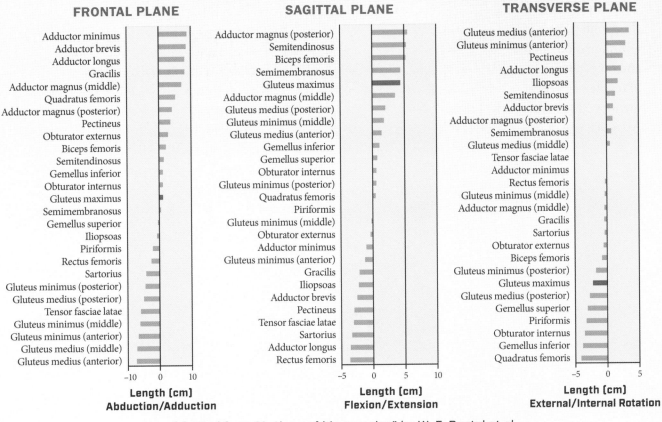

Adapted from "Actions of hip muscles" by W. F. Dostal et al.

LOAD/FORCE VECTORS

Organizing exercises based on the line of resistance adds another layer of accuracy when it comes to categorizing movements. In physics, a vector contains both magnitude and direction. But you can also think of vectors in terms of line of resistance, or the direction of loading relative to the body. For example, if you're performing a barbell back squat, the barbell on your back is considered a vertical load, which translates to an axial vector. However, the force vector changes based on body position. A vertical load in a standing position (back squat) forms an axial vector, but a vertical load in a supine position (barbell hip thrust) forms an anteroposterior vector. For this reason, I refer to movements with an anteroposterior vector as a *horizontal load* because—again—I'm taking into account the direction of load relative to body position.

Force vectors also help determine the level of glute activation while the hips are in motion. This measure of tension on the hips through flexion and extension range of motion is known as the *torque angle curve*. In addition to measuring the level of tension, you can think of the torque angle curve as measuring effort, as in being either harder or easier at certain phases of the movement. For instance, vertically (axial) loaded exercises, like squats, have a torque angle curve that is very hard at the bottom and easier at the top. Horizontally (anteroposterior) loaded exercises, like hip thrusts, have a torque angle curve that is flatter and more consistent throughout the range of motion. In short, a movement is either easier, harder, or consistent through hip extension range of motion depending on the force vector.

So, to determine the force vector, we must consider two things: the direction or line of the resistance (load position) and body position.

Direction of Resistance

There are four distinct types of force vectors in glute training: axial (vertical), anteroposterior (horizontal), lateromedial (lateral), and torsional (rotation). But just as movement occurs in a combination of planes, force vectors can blend together to form combination vectors. Axial anteroposterior vector (vertical-horizontal blend loading), for example, is a diagonal load or line of resistance. I cover many different blends of vectors in the pages to come, but the five I just mentioned are the most common.

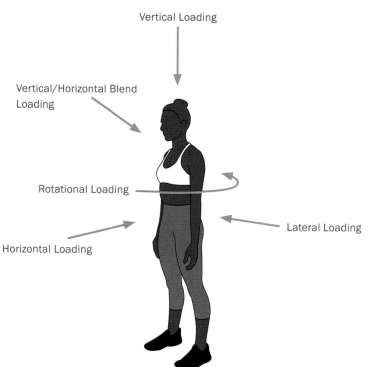

Vertical Loading

Vertical/Horizontal Blend Loading

Rotational Loading

Horizontal Loading

Lateral Loading

PRIMARY LOAD/FORCE VECTORS IN GLUTE TRAINING

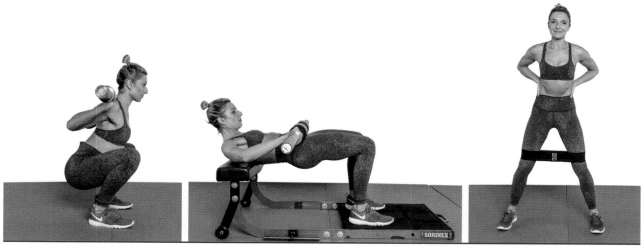

VERTICAL LOADING: SQUAT

HORIZONTAL LOADING: HIP THRUST

LATERAL LOADING: LATERAL BAND WALK

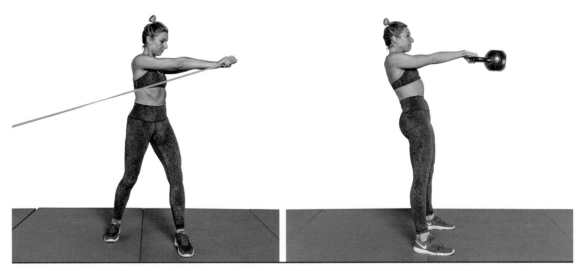

**ROTATIONAL LOADING:
HIP ROTATION**

**VERTICAL/HORIZONTAL BLEND
LOADING: KETTLEBELL SWING**

We've looked at force vectors in someone standing upright, but there are a lot of different positions in glute training, which include standing, seated, kneeling, supine (lying faceup), side-lying, prone (lying facedown), and quadruped (on hands and knees). Here is an exercise example of each:

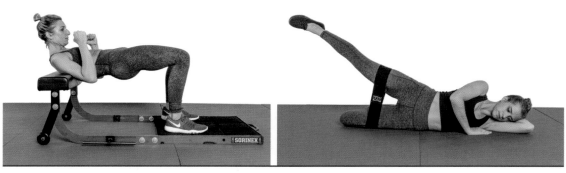

SUPINE

SIDE-LYING

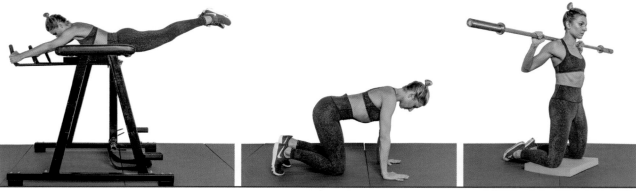

PRONE

QUADRUPED

KNEELING

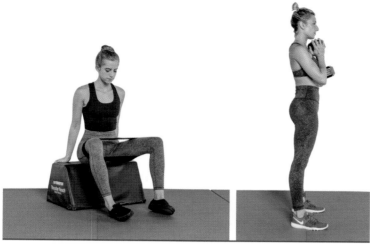

SEATED   STANDING

Once you understand planes of motion and force vectors, you can start to categorize glute training exercises based on the movement pattern and load position. This is exactly what I outline in the pages to come. But before I delve into the individual categories, it's important to understand why certain exercises work your glutes differently than others, which is determined by the action of the knees.

KNEE ACTION

If you've read the other chapters in this part, you know that squats and deadlifts stretch your glutes at peak contraction, while glute bridges and hip thrusts shorten your glutes at peak contraction. The former work more of your lower glutes but don't activate all of the muscle fibers and can leave you sore. The latter, on the other hand, work both your upper and lower glutes, maximally contract the muscle, and don't beat you up as badly.

Because hip extension is the joint action and movement pattern that primarily works the glutes, let's isolate knee action, which refers to the position and movement of the knees while the hips are in motion, during hip extension movements. By looking at hip extension knee action, you can start to connect the dots between which exercises develop certain areas of the glutes and why, as well as determine whether an exercise is glute dominant, quad dominant, or hamstring dominant. There are three main hip extension knee action categories: the knees stay bent as in a hip thrust, bend and straighten as in a squat, or stay straight or slightly bent as in a deadlift or back extension. Let's examine all three and plot where activation is highest and lowest while the hips are extending.

KNEES STAY BENT

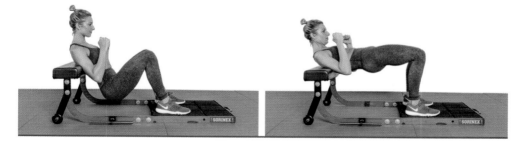

KNEES BEND AND STRAIGHTEN　　　　**KNEES STAY STRAIGHT OR SLIGHTLY BENT**

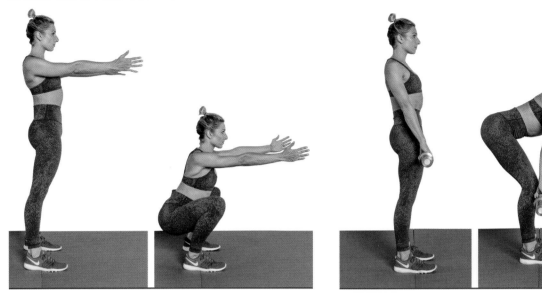

Research shows that the angle of the knee affects the gluteus maximus EMG amplitude when producing force to extend the hip.

Trying to perform hip extension with bent knees (in knee flexion) causes greater gluteus maximus EMG amplitude than trying to perform hip extension with straight legs (in knee extension).

For example, Sakamoto et al. (2009) investigated gluteus maximus EMG amplitude during four prone hip extension movements with varying joint angles. They tested prone hip extension in knee extension, in knee flexion, in hip external rotation and knee extension, and in hip external rotation and knee flexion. The researchers found that hip extension performed in knee flexion led to greater gluteus maximus EMG amplitude than hip extension performed in knee extension (23 percent versus 13 percent of maximum voluntary isometric contraction, or MVIC).[5]

Similar findings were observed by Kwon et al. (2013), who explored knee angles of 0, 30, 60, 90, and 110 degrees. Gluteus maximus EMG amplitude at 0 and 30 degrees of knee flexion was substantially lower (48 percent and 53 percent of MVIC, respectively) than in 60, 90, or 110 degrees of knee flexion (63 to 65 percent of MVIC).[6]

Knees Stay Bent (Glute Dominant)

When your knees stay bent as in a hip thrust or glute bridge, you have higher glute activation because your hamstrings, which are also responsible for extending your hips (referred to as a *hip extensor*), are less active due to the fact that they cannot produce maximal tension when they're shortened to that degree. This means your glutes have to do the lion's share of the work to extend your hips because they're not getting as much help from your hamstrings. What's more, there is constant tension on the glutes when your knees stay bent, which is to say that your glutes are highly activated as you flex and extend your hips. The movement is still harder at the top than at the bottom, but because hamstring activation is reduced, you maintain higher levels of activation throughout the entire range of the movement. This is why bent-knee hip extension exercises like the glute bridge and hip thrust are considered glute-dominant movements, because they primarily work the glutes.

Knees Bend and Straighten (Quad Dominant)

When the knees bend and straighten (flex and extend), the glutes stretch and reach peak contraction at the bottom of the movement. This means tension on the hips and glutes is highest at the bottom of the movement, and activation lowers as you reach the top position. Think of a squat or lunge. These exercises are hardest at the bottom when the glutes are stretched and get easier as you extend your hips when the glutes shorten. What's more, as you extend your knees and hips to stand upright from a squat, you get a ton of help from your quads, which further reduces glute activation. This is why squats and lunges are considered quad-dominant movements, even though the glutes are active and still play a role in carrying out the movement. Put simply, the quads are the prime mover, or the main muscle working during the exercise.

Knees Stay Straight or Slightly Bent (Hamstring Dominant)

When your knees stay straight or slightly bent, as in a deadlift, you get a ton of help from your hamstrings as you extend your hips and raise your torso to stand upright, which reduces glute activation. This is why deadlifts are considered hamstring-dominant movements, even though the glutes are active and still play a role in carrying out the movement. Put simply, the hamstrings are the prime mover.

FORCE VECTOR + KNEE ACTION

When you combine the force vector with the knee action categorization, you can more accurately predict how good an exercise is for building the glutes. This leaves you with seven categories for hip extension exercises:

HIP EXTENSION FORCE VECTOR + KNEE ACTION EXERCISE CATEGORIES

FORCE VECTOR (LOAD)	KNEE ACTION	EXERCISE EXAMPLES	MAIN MUSCLES WORKED
Anteroposterior (horizontal)	Bent	Hip Thrusts Glute Bridges	1. Glutes 2. Quads 3. Hamstrings
Anteroposterior (horizontal)	Straight	Back Extensions Reverse Hypers	1. Glutes 2. Hamstrings 3. Erectors (lower back)
Anteroposterior (horizontal)	Bend and straighten (flex and extend)	Donkey Kicks Pull-Throughs	1. Glutes 2. Quads 3. Hamstrings
Anteroposterior (horizontal)	Straighten and bend (extend and flex)	Glute Ham Raises Rolling Leg Curls	1. Hamstrings 2. Erectors 3. Glutes
Axial (vertical)	Semi-bent or straight	Deadlifts Romanian Deadlifts Stiff-Leg Deadlifts	1. Hamstrings 2. Lower glutes 3. Quads
Axial (vertical)	Bend and straighten (flex and extend)	Squats Lunges	1. Quads 2. Lower glutes 3. Hamstrings
Axial/Anteroposterior blend	Varies	45-Degree Hypers Walking Lunges	Depends

This is complicated, but it paints a comprehensive picture of the different types of hip extension exercises when you apply the force vector and knee action categories.

GLUTE EXERCISE CATEGORIES: PUTTING IT ALL TOGETHER

To ensure that your glute training program is both functional and balanced, you need to perform exercises from every plane of motion, force vector, and knee action. Combining all of these forms of classification provides five glute exercise categories: vertically loaded, horizontally loaded, rotary, transverse abduction, and frontal abduction exercises. It's important to point out that frontal and transverse planes are considered laterally loaded, but they work your glutes slightly differently due to body position. (More on this shortly.)

One of the biggest mistakes I see trainers, lifters, and athletes make is performing exercises from only one category. To ensure that my clients' programs are well balanced, I created the Rule of Thirds principle, which uses the load and vector classification: roughly one-third of glute exercises performed throughout the week should be horizontal, one-third vertical, and one-third rotary and lateral (which include frontal and transverse plane abduction exercises). I cover the Rule of Thirds in more detail on page 198. What's important to understand here is that the Rule of Thirds is a method for creating a balanced combination of loading and positions, ensuring that you target the glutes from every angle.

If you examine the glute exercise categories infographic that follows, you'll notice that each category works your glutes slightly differently based on the plane of motion, force vector, and knee action. You can use this infographic to select exercises for the Rule of Thirds program design template. However, it's important to realize that there are many more exercise options and even more categories (remember, there are blends) than are included in this chart. Continue reading to learn more about each category and which exercises fall into those categories.

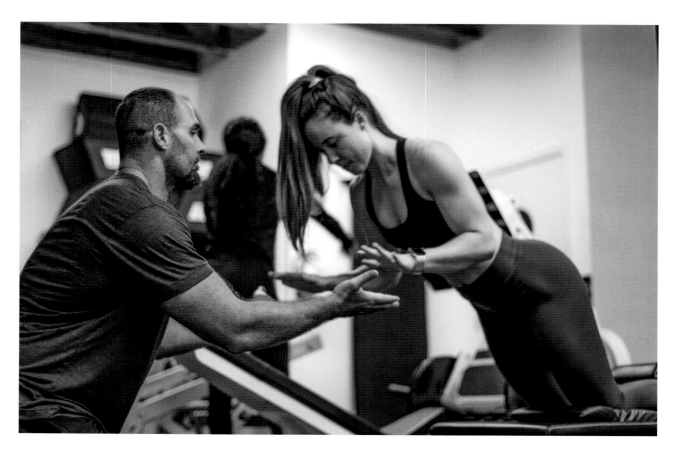

GLUTE EXERCISE CATEGORIES

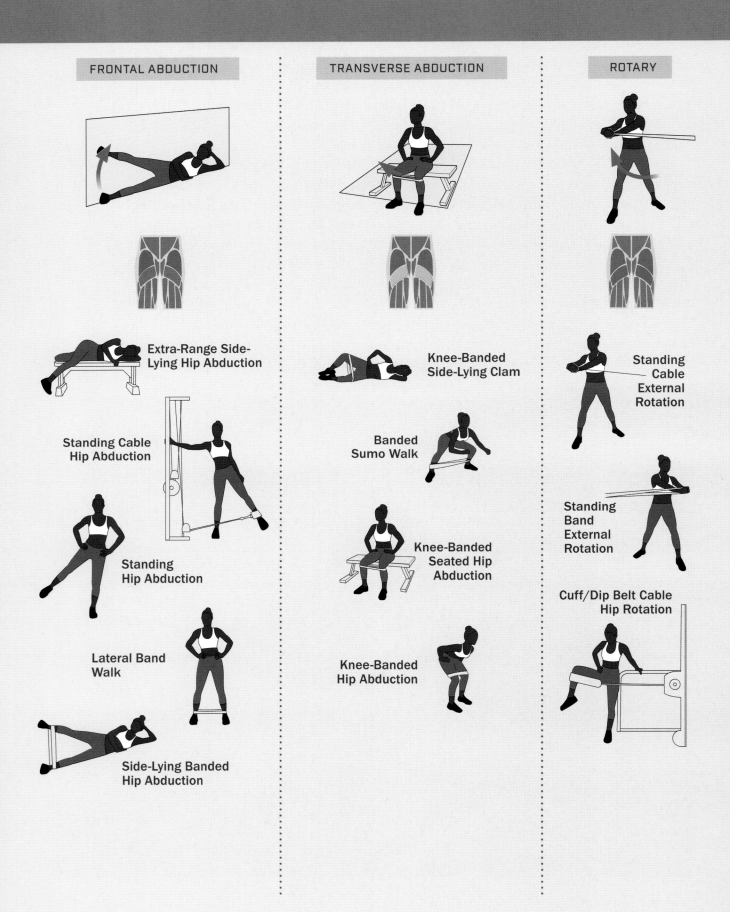

FRONTAL ABDUCTION

Extra-Range Side-Lying Hip Abduction

Standing Cable Hip Abduction

Standing Hip Abduction

Lateral Band Walk

Side-Lying Banded Hip Abduction

TRANSVERSE ABDUCTION

Knee-Banded Side-Lying Clam

Banded Sumo Walk

Knee-Banded Seated Hip Abduction

Knee-Banded Hip Abduction

ROTARY

Standing Cable External Rotation

Standing Band External Rotation

Cuff/Dip Belt Cable Hip Rotation

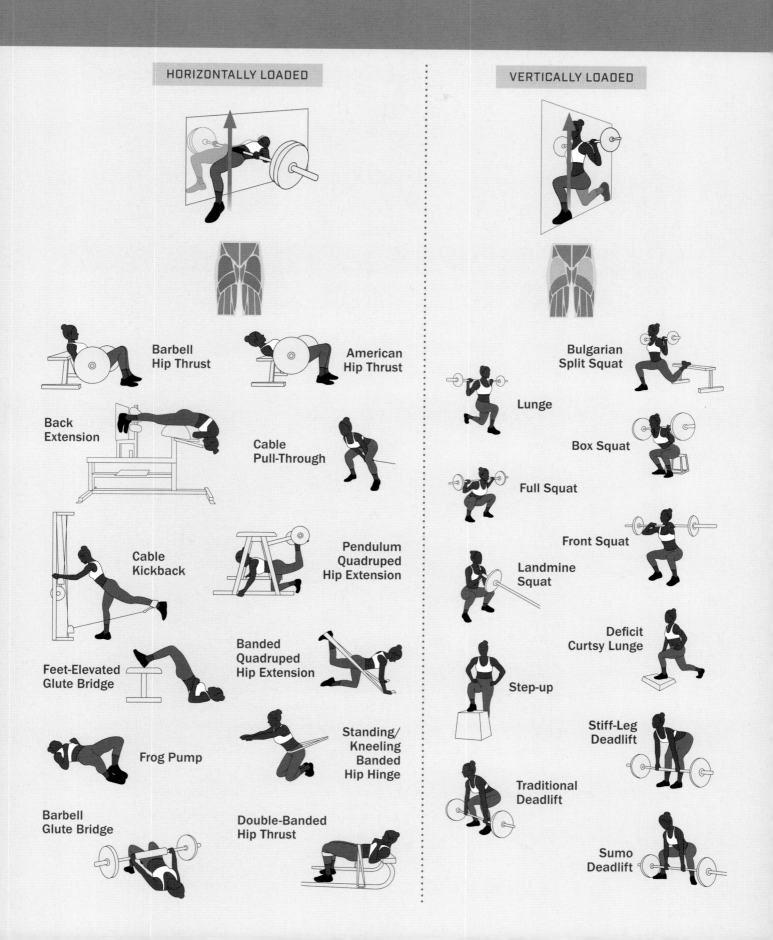

HORIZONTALLY LOADED

VERTICALLY LOADED

Barbell Hip Thrust

American Hip Thrust

Back Extension

Cable Pull-Through

Cable Kickback

Pendulum Quadruped Hip Extension

Feet-Elevated Glute Bridge

Banded Quadruped Hip Extension

Frog Pump

Standing/ Kneeling Banded Hip Hinge

Barbell Glute Bridge

Double-Banded Hip Thrust

Bulgarian Split Squat

Lunge

Box Squat

Full Squat

Front Squat

Landmine Squat

Deficit Curtsy Lunge

Step-up

Stiff-Leg Deadlift

Traditional Deadlift

Sumo Deadlift

VERTICALLY LOADED EXERCISES

Vertically loaded exercises are the hardest on the body and work more lower glute max than upper glute max.

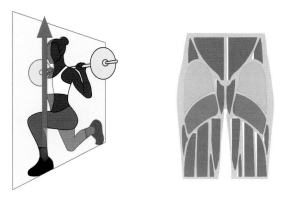

BODY POSITION	EXERCISES
STANDING	Squats, Deadlifts, Good Mornings, Lunges, Step-Ups and Step-Downs, Bulgarian Split Squats, Pistol and Single-Leg Box Squats, Skater Squats, Single-Leg RDLs and King Deadlifts, Olympic Lifts
SUPINE	Lying Horizontal Leg Press Machine
KNEELING	Kneeling Squats

HORIZONTALLY LOADED EXERCISES

Horizontally loaded exercises are less taxing overall and highly activate both the upper and lower glute max subdivisions.

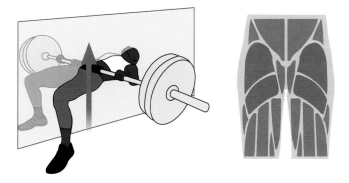

BODY POSITION	EXERCISES
SUPINE	Band, Dumbbell, and Barbell Single- and Double-Leg Hip Thrusts, Dumbbell and Barbell Single- and Double-Leg Glute Bridges, Band and Dumbbell Frog Pumps and Frog Thrusts
PRONE	Single- and Double-Leg Back Extensions, Single- and Double-Leg Ankle Weight Reverse Hypers
QUADRUPED	Pendulum Quadruped Hip Extensions, Quadruped Band and Cable Kickbacks
STANDING	Cable Pull-Throughs, Band and Cable Standing Hip Thrusts, Standing Band and Cable Kickbacks
KNEELING	Band and Cable Kneeling Hip Thrusts

COMBINED VERTICALLY AND HORIZONTALLY LOADED EXERCISES

Combined exercises contain a blend of vectors; they come at the body from more of an angle, or the vector is altered throughout the range of motion. For example, a 45-degree hyper can be thought of as a blend between a good morning (vertical) and a back extension (horizontal). Alternatively, they can just contain two forms of resistance. For example, a hip-banded Smith machine kneeling squat contains horizontal resistance in the form of a band pulling the hips rearward and vertical resistance in the form of a bar resting on the shoulders. This category works both the upper and lower glute max subdivisions.

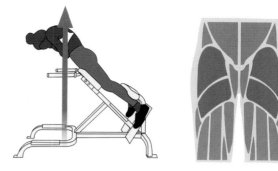

BODY POSITION	EXERCISES
STANDING	Kettlebell Swings, Sled Pushes, Walking Lunges, Hip-Banded + Barbell Romanian Deadlifts, Four-Way Hip Machine Hip Extensions
PRONE	Pendulum Single- and Double-Leg Reverse Hypers, Single- and Double-Leg 45-Degree Hypers, Reverse Hack Squats
SUPINE	Single- and Double-Leg 45-Degree Hip Sled (Leg Presses), Hack Squats
KNEELING	Hip-Banded + Barbell (or Smith Machine) Kneeling Squats/Thrusts, Quadruped Pendulum Donkey Kicks

FRONTAL PLANE HIP ABDUCTION EXERCISES

Frontal plane lateral exercises target the upper subdivision of the glute max.

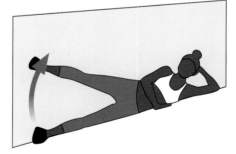 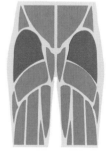

BODY POSITION	EXERCISES
SIDE LYING	Knee-Banded Side-Lying Hip Abduction, Ankle Weight Side-Lying Hip Abduction, Extra-Range Side-Lying Hip Abduction (Off Bench), Side-Lying Hip Raises with Top Leg Abduction
SUPINE	Knee-Banded Supine Bent-Leg Hip Abduction (Top Position of Glute Bridge)
PRONE	Ankle-Banded Hip Abduction
STANDING	Lateral Band/Sumo/X Walks, Long Band Standing Hip Abduction, Knee-Banded Standing Hip Abduction, Cable Standing Hip Abduction, Ankle Weight Standing Hip Abduction, Double Standing Hip Abduction, Lateral Sled Drags

TRANSVERSE PLANE HIP ABDUCTION EXERCISES

Transverse plane hip abduction and hip external rotation exercises work both the upper and lower fibers of the glute max.

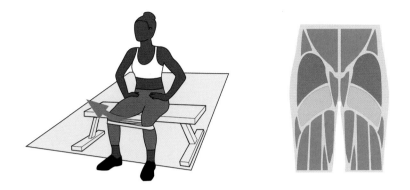

BODY POSITION	EXERCISES
SEATED	Machine Seated Hip Abduction (3-Level), Knee-Banded Seated Hip Abduction (3-Level)
HIP HINGE	Knee-Banded Hip Abduction
SUPINE	Knee-Banded Supine Bent-Leg Hip Abduction (Bottom Position of Glute Bridge) (3-Level), Band Supine Transverse Hip Abduction
QUADRUPED	Ankle Weight / Knee-Banded Fire Hydrants and Double Hip Abduction
SIDE LYING	Knee-Banded Side-Lying Clams, Bent-Hip Bent-Knee Raises, Extra-Range Bent-Hip Straight-Leg Raises (Off Bench)

COMBINED TRANSVERSE AND FRONTAL PLANE HIP ABDUCTION EXERCISES

The exercises in this category work both the upper and lower fibers of the glute max.

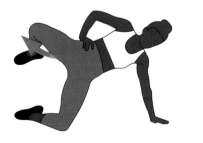
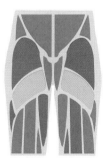

BODY POSITION	EXERCISES
STANDING	Knee-Banded Bodyweight Squats, Jump Squats, and Glute Bridges; Lateral Band Squat Walks; Forward/Backward Band Walks (Monster, Zigzagging)
SIDE-LYING	Bodyweight and Knee-Banded Side-Lying Hip Raises

COMBINED VERTICAL, HORIZONTAL, AND LATERAL EXERCISES

The exercises in this category work both the upper and lower fibers of the glute max.

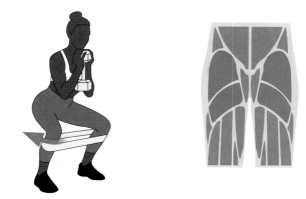

BODY POSITION	EXERCISES
VERTICAL AND LATERAL	Knee-Banded Goblet, Front, and Back Squats, Lateral Lunges and Step-ups
HORIZONTAL AND LATERAL	Knee-Banded Dumbbell, Hip Band, and Barbell Glute Bridges and Hip Thrusts

ROTARY EXERCISES

Hip external rotation exercises work both the upper and lower fibers of the glute max.

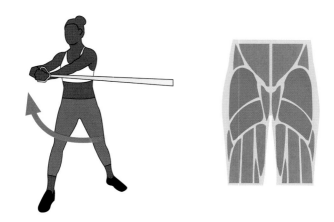

BODY POSITION	EXERCISES
STANDING	Cable and Band Standing Hip External Rotation, Cable and Band Standing Anti-Rotation Presses, Grappler and Landmine Rotations, Cuff/Dip Belt Cable Hip Rotation
HALF-KNEELING	Cable and Band Half-Kneeling Woodchops, Cable and Band Half-Kneeling Anti-Rotation Presses

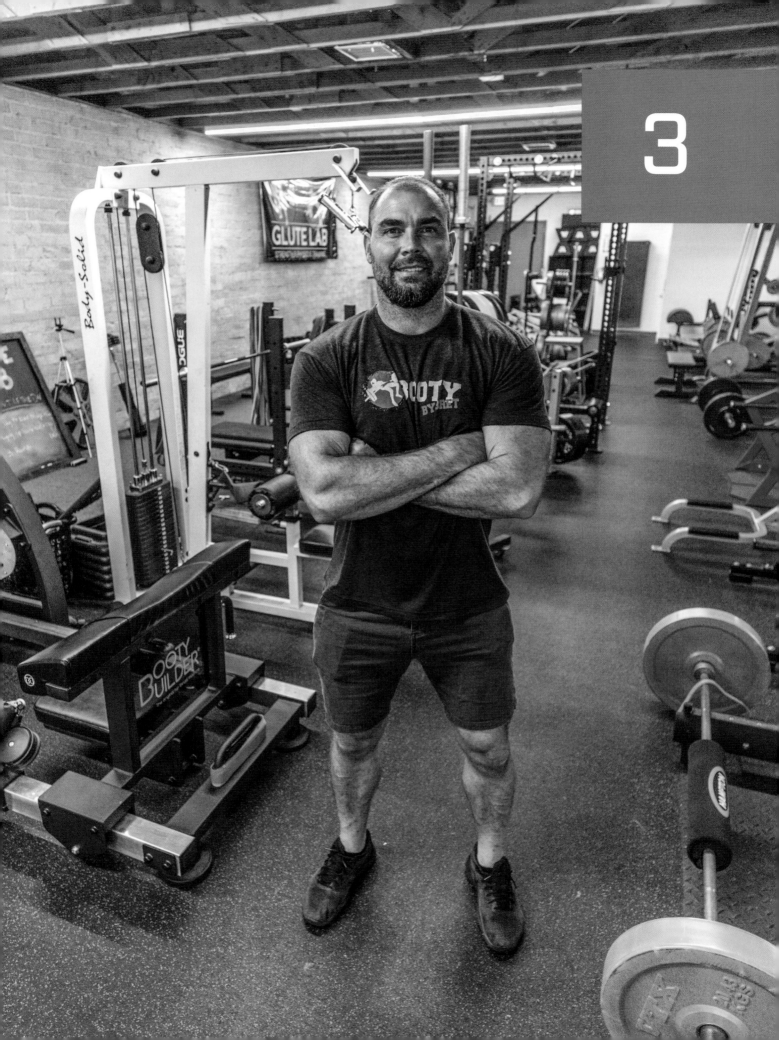

THE ART OF STRENGTH AND PHYSIQUE TRAINING

Glute training is a fringe benefit. Those of us who love to lift automatically assume that strength training is a well-funded and well-researched field. In a perfect world, we would have 50 published studies for every method on different populations and training regimens, and even have reviews and meta-analyses for each exercise.

Unfortunately, that is not the case. The subjects that get funded are the things that are killing us, like heart disease, cancer, obesity, and chronic illness. Strength training—and, as an extension, glute training—is considered a luxury. As a result, it doesn't receive the kind of funding required to carry out large, long-term training studies.

Although there is plenty of science to work with, it's far from conclusive. As we learn more, our methods will evolve alongside the research. In the meantime, we have to blend published research, scientific rationale, anecdotes, expert opinion, and tradition and then use logic and experience to weigh these various forms of evidence to create the best training plan, all while keeping an open mind and leaving no stone unturned. This means taking into consideration all of the variables, such as age, anatomy, injury history, goals, nutrition, mindset, lifestyle habits—the list goes on and on.

I think it's safe to say that we'll never have glute training down to an exact science due to the human factor. It'll never be as simple as: Jane Doe walks through the door, this is what she wants, and this is exactly how to get it.

Even if you have a specific goal, there is tremendous flexibility when it comes to designing a strength training program. As long as you're following evidence-based principles such as the ones covered in this book, you can achieve your desired outcome with very different training strategies. For example, you could give the top 10 trainers in the world the same client with the same goal, and each of them might implement different strategies and programs and get similar results.

For these reasons, glute training (and strength training in general) will always be more of an art than a science. By "art," I mean tying together evidenced-based science with program design and human variables. This is particularly important because there are many key questions that the current body of research cannot answer.

For instance, we still don't know which exercises are best for growing the glutes. In fact, we don't even know precisely how hypertrophy works. As of July 2019, only a few studies have measured gluteus maximus hypertrophy following a resistance training program, and they've examined the lying squat machine, leg press, stiff-leg deadlifts, and squats, all of which fall into the quad-dominant and hamstring-dominant categories and likely aren't the best exercises for gluteal hypertrophy. Based on the current research, we do not know the best training volume or how often you should train your glutes to get the best results. Can your glutes handle more volume, or do they follow the same typical pattern as other muscles? Should you implement more advanced training methods or stick to the basics? Is it better to train three days a week or five? These are questions you can answer only through solid coaching, consistent training, informed experimentation, and intelligent analysis.

We can extract certain nuggets of useful information from published research examining other muscle groups to home in on specific strategies, but there is still so much to learn, and a lot more research is needed before we can answer these questions with science. And even as we learn more from science, there will always be an art to training because research cannot tell us exactly how to blend the numerous variables. Science can guide us in certain ways, but we also have a lot of freedom.

As we learn more, our methods will become more refined, and we can use a rifle approach instead of a shotgun approach. In the meantime, we must base our methods on what we do know and apply the art of glute training so we can account for the many variables that science has not yet examined or explained.

In this part, you will learn the fundamentals of optimal glute training and how to design a glute training program. You will learn how to incorporate advanced methods to conquer plateaus and get the most out of your workouts, and how troubleshoot for the most common glute training mistakes and questions.

The information in this part takes into account what the scientific literature currently tells us, but it is also based on my experience: 28 years as a lifter, 23 years as a personal trainer, 16 years as a Certified Strength and Conditioning Specialist with Distinction (CSCS, *D), a PhD in glute training, dozens of published studies, virtual trainer to thousands, and coach to dozens of successful physique competitors and athletes.

As with any art form, mastery is achieved through passion, patience, consistency, and discipline. Once you understand how to blend all of the fundamental training principles and program design variables, you can apply the art of glute training to your physical practice and get the results you're looking for.

11 Fundamentals of Optimal Strength and Physique Training

When it comes to strength and physique training, it's hard to know which variable is most responsible for producing the desired outcomes—or for derailing progress. Genetics certainly plays a role, but so do training frequency, exercise selection, volume, and many other factors.

For instance, people send me amazing before-and-after photos of their glutes almost every day. These testimonials are great because they show that my methods work. But people are sending me before-and-after photos only when they get results. Even though these testimonials help validate my methods, they don't mean my methods are optimal. Maybe these people could've gotten even better results if they had tweaked their diet, training frequency, exercise selection, or some other crucial variable.

This is why glute training is an art. You have to be comprehensive, but also creative and attentive to the variables that have the biggest impact, which is extremely difficult to measure. You may not know which variable is most responsible because there are so many and they differ from person to person.

Think of it like this: people have a hard time taking care of houseplants, and for plants there are only three primary variables—light, water, and soil. If you want a plant to grow, you place it near a window so it gets enough sun and make sure it's getting enough water. But what if you're not getting the results you're looking for? Do you give it less light and more water, more light and less water, less light and less water, or more light and more water? Or do you need to give it nutrients to change the soil? To make matters more complicated, it's different for every plant and environment. Even though there are just three main variables, there are a lot of options.

Now imagine trying to grow muscle or reach a specific goal on a human when there are dozens of variables that can affect progress. You start to see why so many programs fail and why a comprehensive approach is so important.

In Chapter 12, you will learn about eight specific program design variables: training frequency, volume, effort, exercise selection, exercise order, load, tempo, and rest periods. To help you navigate these variables and get the most out of your workouts, I've devised some key principles for optimal glute, strength, and physique training. Think of them as general, all-encompassing guidelines, which include setting goals and expectations, understanding form and technique, accounting for injury and recovery, managing diet and lifestyle, and finally exercise variety and accounting for individual differences.

These are the big-picture variables that have the greatest impact on training. Consider the fundamentals covered in this chapter as the foundation of your training practice and the program design variables covered in the next chapter as the building blocks you will use to construct your training plan.

In this chapter, I offer general guidelines to help you maximize your training experience, most of which revolve around big-picture variables such as setting goals, prioritizing form, and managing your diet. In other words, they are not necessarily specific to glute training. Below, I highlight the most important and specific guidelines for optimal glute training. These guidelines include methods covered in Part 2 as well as strategies offered in the subsequent pages. If you want to get the most out of glute training, you need to not only follow the big-picture guidelines but also do the following:

- Build progressive overload on big lifts—squats, deadlifts, and hip thrusts—into the program (see page 102).
- Prioritize exercise variety by performing variations of squats, deadlifts, and hip thrusts, which include different stances, loading implements, rep ranges, tempos, and single-leg exercises. (This is the shotgun approach; see page 91.)
- Regularly utilize the mind-muscle connection (see page 93).
- Follow the Rule of Thirds (see page 198) for vector, load, and effort.
- Hit the upper glutes (for example, back extensions with a rounded upper back and lateral band walks), the lower glutes (deadlifts, squats, lunges, and single-leg hip thrusts), and both the upper and lower glutes together (glute bridges and hip thrusts).
- Focus on mechanical tension and plenty of metabolic stress, with a sprinkling of muscle damage.
- Listen to your body and allow for recovery and personal records (PRs).
- Include a deload (light training) week in your program cycles and fluctuate your training stress.
- Incorporate advanced training methods (see Chapter 13).
- Use the right exercise order for your goals by placing the most important exercises first in each workout.
- Aim for 30 to 36 sets of glute exercises over 3 to 6 workouts per week.

GOALS AND EXPECTATIONS

As with anything in life, setting goals and managing your expectations for training are bedrock to staying consistent, maximizing your results, and enjoying the process. When it comes to setting goals and expectations, it's important to keep a few key points in mind.

REGARDLESS OF HOW YOU LOOK, PRAISE YOUR EFFORTS

I'm proud of my progress because I train like a beast. Week in and week out, you'll find me in the Glute Lab hip thrusting, squatting, deadlifting, lunging, and frog pumping. Sure, I may not have the best glutes out there, but I don't have a pancake butt, either. If you think you'll be happy only if you have the most fabulous glutes in the world, then you will never be satisfied, because you will always be comparing yourself to someone else. Instead of focusing on the glutes you want, focus on training as hard as you can, and be proud of your glutes for how hard you train them.

MAINTAIN AN OPTIMISTIC MINDSET

I work with numerous women who look incredible and still are not happy with their physique. I'm the "Glute Guy," and I train my glutes as hard as anyone, yet I don't have the glutes of a linebacker and never will due to my genetics. Instead of letting this get me depressed and derail my training, I keep a positive mindset because I know that staying optimistic is the key to staying consistent. And staying consistent is the best way to make progress.

CREATE REALISTIC GOALS AND EXPECTATIONS BASED ON YOUR GENETICS AND EXPERIENCE

I touched on this subject in Part 2, but it's worth repeating: if you have poor glute genetics, you need to focus on what you can control, like your training strategies. Strength results will come, and physique gains will, too, just at a slower pace than genetically gifted individuals can expect.

I'm not saying you shouldn't set high expectations for yourself. To be clear, you should set high expectations, but they should be realistic—meaning that you can actually accomplish the goals you're working toward—and you need to believe wholeheartedly that you can accomplish them. If you don't believe you can accomplish the goals you've set for yourself, then you're setting yourself up for failure.

Even if your goals are realistic and backed by belief, remember that there will be periods when you will struggle to make gains. During these phases, you have to stay consistent and keep in mind that stalls are perfectly normal.

BE PATIENT WITH YOUR PROGRESS AND UNDERSTAND THAT PROGRESS HAPPENS IN WAVES

What many of my followers don't realize is that a lot of the women who post before-and-after photos have been training their glutes like crazy for four years or longer. It's not an overnight thing; developing the glutes takes time and patience.

Don't get frustrated with a bad workout, a bad week, or even a bad month. Instead, focus on your long-term progress. If you're training smart (and hard), you will continue to improve. Follow the programming and exercise guidelines that I outline in this part and the troubleshooting solutions offered in Chapter 14, and you will see results and conquer training plateaus.

Now, if you're new to glute training, it's a different story. In the beginning, growth is nearly linear, meaning that you get better day to day, week to week, and month to month. You hit a new PR every time you set foot in the gym. In this sense, you get spoiled because you become accustomed to steady gains. Eventually, though, you will plateau. Your body will not go up linearly forever. At a certain point, progress will start coming in waves: sometimes you beat your personal best, sometimes you tie your previous record, and sometimes you backslide a bit.

There will also be times when you stall in certain lifts and progress in others. It's like surfing: When you're in the wave, everything is awesome; you're making gains and loving every second. But when you're out of the wave and you're fighting the current trying to paddle back out, it's a lot harder and not as much fun. Enjoy the window when you're riding the wave of progress. Then, when you're out of the wave, maintain your discipline and do what's necessary to position yourself for the next one.

It's important to take pride in the small gains. Far too many of my clients are disappointed when they can do only one more rep or 5 more pounds. They expect more significant jumps because those are what they experienced during the developmental stage. When you've been training for a long time, however, one more rep or 5 more pounds is an amazing accomplishment.

BE PROUD OF YOUR PHYSIQUE BASED ON HOW HARD YOU TRAIN, NOT ON HOW OTHERS LOOK

I already touched on this point, but it's worth emphasizing. A lot of people get discouraged when they start glute training because they compare themselves to models with amazing glutes. If you go on my Instagram and check out the people I follow, you will see that every day I'm exposed to amazing lifters who look like Greek gods. If I compared myself to them, I would become discouraged and might give up on training. Instead, I get inspired by them.

You'll never be happy if you compare yourself to the top 0.1 percent. You have to compare yourself to you and work to beat your former self. I think that's why I'm happy with how I look. I grew up skinny and weak. True, I'll never be a powerlifting world champion or win a bodybuilding trophy, but I never thought I'd have a nice physique or hip thrust over 800 pounds. I'm proud of my physique, I'm proud of my training, and I'm proud of myself for sticking with it for so many years. If I can be happy with my results, you can be happy with yours, too!

SET AND PRIORITIZE STRENGTH GOALS OVER AESTHETIC GOALS

People often ask me what goals and expectations are realistic when it comes to glute training. Most of them expect me to outline specific goals related to aesthetics (think measurements and weight loss), but doing so would be disingenuous of me because everyone is different. Not only that, but judging your training results based solely on your physique is not always productive. Your glutes will look different from day to day, and your mindset has a lot to do with how you think you look on any given day. If you're hard on yourself or you don't see the results you're hoping for, it's easy to get discouraged. And when people get discouraged, they stop training.

For this reason, I prefer setting strength goals. As I said earlier, measuring strength is easier because most people get stronger as they progress through a program. If you're working toward a specific goal—say, a 225-pound hip thrust for a set of 10 reps—then you have something to focus on. Maybe your glutes aren't growing like crazy, but you're getting stronger. As your strength increases, so too does your confidence. And when you're confident and your training feels right, you look and feel better.

Although you should set your own strength goals based on your experience level, here's what I expect my female clients to be able to do if they train with me for six months or longer:

- Hip thrust—225 to 275 pounds for 5 to 10 reps
- Back squat—115 to 155 pounds for 5 to 10 reps
- Deadlift—135 to 185 pounds for 5 to 10 reps
- Bulgarian split squat—60 to 100 pounds for 5 to 10 reps
- Back extension—60 to 100 pounds for 10 to 20 reps

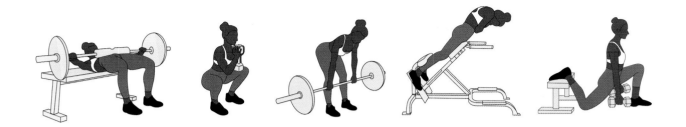

As a personal trainer, I'd be doing a huge disservice to my clients if I told them, "Eh, you're nothing special; you'll never get that strong." You have to push the envelope and let the chips fall where they may. I never knew if some of my clients would hit one of the above milestones or end up hip thrusting 400 pounds, but I certainly didn't let my preconceived notions stand in their way.

It's also important to point out that you can progressively overload repetitions, volume, and range of motion. In short, you don't always have to shoot for a one-rep max on big lifts. If chasing a one-rep max as a strength goal doesn't suit you, other options include doing more repetitions or sets or increasing the range of motion for a certain exercise (referred to as *progressive distance training*).

WHEN IT COMES TO YOUR RESULTS, CONSIDER ALL VARIABLES: YOUR STRENGTH, YOUR WEIGHT, YOUR SIZE, AND HOW YOU LOOK IN THE MIRROR

As I've said, how you look, how much you weigh, and how much you can lift will change from day to day. For this reason, you need to consider all indicators when judging the success of your training.

For example, a lot of my clients stay the same body weight for a whole year, but at the end of the year, their old jeans no longer fit because their glutes have grown and their waists have shrunk. Muscle is denser than fat, so if you're losing fat and gaining muscle, you might stay the same weight but shrink in overall size. I'm not saying you should be afraid of the scale, but it's just one indicator.

Change doesn't happen quickly, and a lot of times you can't detect progress visually. We look at ourselves in the mirror every day and don't notice the changes. Your perception also depends on your mood. If you're feeling down, you might decide that you look like crap even though you look better than you did a month ago. Like the scale, the mirror can be misleading. This is why it's helpful to take before-and-after photos or even take measurements so that you can accurately track your physique progress from month to month.

It's also important to listen to what other people are telling you. If you've been training hard, chances are your friends will start to compliment you on how you look. They might notice that your clothes fit differently. They'll ask what you've been doing. Don't ignore these compliments (or let them go to your head). Instead, take pride in knowing that your hard work is paying off.

FOCUS ON WHAT YOU CAN CONTROL

What you eat, the types of exercises you do, how you perform those exercises (your form and technique), your activity level, how you manage stress, and your quality of sleep can have a massive impact on how you look, feel, and think about yourself. I cover all of these topics in more detail in the following pages.

TREAT YOUR WORKOUTS AS IF THEY WERE MINI-COMPETITIONS

If I told you that in two days, you were going to compete in a race (or any type of event or lifting competition), you would immediately start mentally focusing on the task. You would prioritize your sleep, eat well, and avoid activities that might compromise your performance. The day of the event, you would make sure you ate just the right amount of food at the right time prior to your race to maximize your energy, you'd get a nap in (if you're a napper), and you'd show up early so you weren't stressed out. You definitely wouldn't try to squeeze in four workouts before the event, nor would you party the night before or do cardio immediately prior.

Doing these things gives you the best chance of performing well and setting a PR.

What does this have to do with working out, you might ask? Progressive overload is hard, especially after you've been training for several years. If you show up under-rested, under-recovered, underfed, or stressed out, you definitely won't get stronger, you won't put more tension on your muscles, and you won't improve your body composition or shape (assuming that your diet stays the same). But if you start treating your workouts like mini-competitions, focusing on what needs to get done and removing barriers and distractions, you will without a doubt see better results.

Strength and physique training is a 24-hour endeavor. You have to train smart and hard to maximize your gains.

FORM AND TECHNIQUE

Everyone agrees that moving with good form (also referred to as *technique, mechanics, motor control,* and *coordination*) is important and that moving with poor form is unsafe and counterproductive. You want to learn and practice good form for two primary reasons:

1. Focusing on form enables you to progress in your physical and athletic abilities over time. Using good mechanics ensures safe and effective movement patterns in life and sport, meaning that you activate the right muscles and align your body in positions that translate to similar movement patterns outside of training. For example, if you understand how to squat and deadlift correctly, you have a blueprint for getting up out of a chair and picking something up off the ground. You also know where you should feel tension in your muscles, which lets you know that you're using the right muscles for the job (for example, feeling your hamstrings and tension in your hips when you deadlift) and improves strength in the areas you're trying to develop. Now, this doesn't mean that every time you drop a pencil, you have to bend over and pick it up with perfect deadlift form; you have flexibility with your everyday movements and can condition your body to handle a variety of movement patterns. But it does mean that you should mind your spinal mechanics when lifting something heavy. You will learn the fundamentals of lifting with proper form for all of the exercises in Part 5.

2. Mastering good form helps prevent injuries. Numerous form-related guidelines and cues will help you maximize strength and muscle development and avoid injury in the gym, which I'll discuss in the coming pages. The main point I want to make here is that moving improperly—say, excessively rounding your back in a deadlift or allowing your knees to cave inward during a squat—puts unnecessary stress on your body. Moreover, you're not engaging the muscles needed to support the movement. And unnecessary stress combined with a lack of muscular support increases your chances of getting hurt. The solution, therefore, is to learn how to move with optimal technique and perform every exercise correctly.

GENERAL GUIDELINES FOR MOVING WITH OPTIMAL TECHNIQUE

I recommend four general technique guidelines for everyone. However, it's important to remember that everything must be individualized. This means modifying your stance, setup, and execution and tailoring your technique to your unique anatomy, goals, and experience. What's more, you need to listen to your body and develop the mind-muscle connection: if you're targeting your glutes with a specific exercise, then you should feel your glutes activate optimally without pain or discomfort.

With this in mind, you can use these four universal rules as a starting point when learning how to perform the primary glute training exercises. (*Note:* You will learn how these cues apply to the various exercises in Part 5.)

Keep Your Spine in the Neutral Zone

Keeping your spine in the neutral zone means keeping your back flat. Realize, though, that it's nearly impossible to keep your back perfectly neutral, especially when lifting a heavy load. This is why I don't like saying "neutral position" because it implies that your spine will not and should not move. Instead, I prefer to say "neutral *zone*" because there is some wiggle room: your spine will move, but it's still considered neutral. The idea, therefore, is to keep your back as neutral as possible. Hyperextending (overarching) or excessively flexing (rounding) your lower back is a recipe for tweaks and injuries when lifting heavy weight. This rule applies mostly to squats, deadlifts, and good mornings and not as much to pistol squats, hip thrusts, and glute-dominant back extensions.

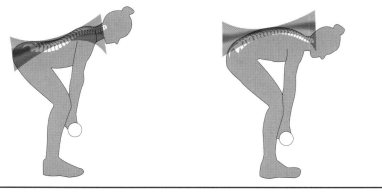

WITHIN NEUTRAL ZONE   EXCESSIVE SPINAL FLEXION

Adapted from Eugen Loki [@pheasyque], "Neutral Is a Range and Not a Fixed Position"

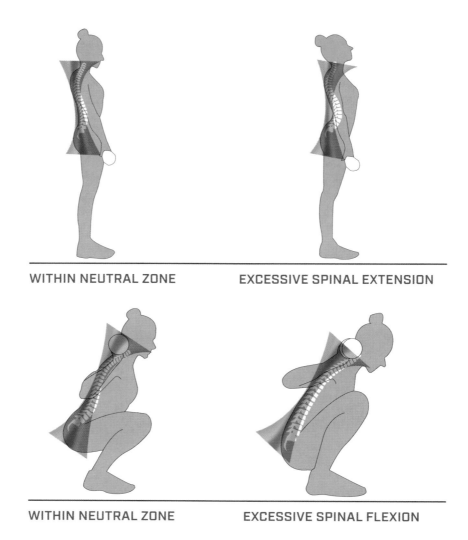

WITHIN NEUTRAL ZONE   EXCESSIVE SPINAL EXTENSION

WITHIN NEUTRAL ZONE   EXCESSIVE SPINAL FLEXION

Brace and Breathe

To keep your spine in the neutral zone and maximize your strength, you need to stabilize the position by bracing. That is, you need to take a big breath in and engage the muscles of your trunk to stabilize your spine in your neutral zone.

Your bracing and breathing strategy will change depending on the effort and duration of the lift. For example, say you're performing a one-rep max with a compound lift like a squat, deadlift, or hip thrust. To brace, you take a deep breath in (around 70 percent of max lung capacity) and then stiffen the muscles in your core (especially your diaphragm) to stabilize the position. Then you hold your breath until you pass the hardest part of the movement, referred to as the *sticking region*. If you're deep squatting, for instance, your sticking region probably starts at around one-third of the way up and ends at around two-thirds of the way up. Because the sticking region ends near the top of the movement, you can just hold your breath until you complete the rep.

If you're performing a max-effort lift for 2 to 5 reps, you can still hold your breath until you get to the top (or pass the sticking region), but you breathe out and then brace again after each repetition. Bracing can make you up to 10 percent stronger. It also creates intra-abdominal pressure (IAP), which helps stabilize the spine.

If you're doing a set of 10 or more reps, then you can breathe rhythmically, or breathe during the movement. Keeping with the squat example, you would breathe in during the eccentric, or lowering, phase and breathe out during the concentric, or rising, phase.

Drive Your Knees Out

Driving your knees out helps prevent knee valgus, also known as *medial knee displacement.* Allowing your knees to cave inward excessively can lead to ACL tears and other knee injuries when landing from a jump or to general knee pain during knee-dominant exercises, such as squat movement patterns. (*Note:* This cue applies more to squats—specifically in the bottom of the squat—than to hip thrusts and deadlifts.)

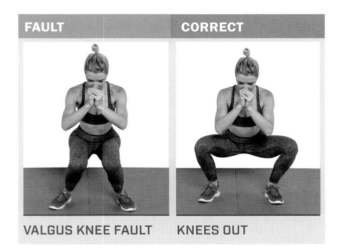

FAULT   CORRECT

VALGUS KNEE FAULT   KNEES OUT

Push Through Your Heels

Driving your weight through your heels keeps tension on your hips and helps you maintain a stable foot position. If you come up onto the balls of your feet, you rely more on your knees than your hips to carry out the movement. This can be a slippery slope if carried out for a long enough time.

It's worth repeating that there is some wiggle room with each of these four cues. For instance, some people can get away with (or, in certain cases, may even have to) rounding their backs a little bit when they deadlift or tilting their pelvises posteriorly (aka butt winking) to perform a squat. Though not ideal for the masses, it might be fine for certain individuals based on anatomy, mobility, soft-tissue strength, and muscle architecture. As long as you're not getting hurt and not feeling pain, there is an acceptable zone in which you can deviate from these cues and still be safe and effective.

As I said in Chapter 5, you should let your anatomy dictate how you move, and it's up to you to experiment and find the right stance, setup, and posture that allow you to move with good form.

FAULTS THAT COMPROMISE PERFORMANCE AND CAUSE INJURIES

Most technical faults occur on account of going too heavy or pushing a set too hard. However, often a person simply hasn't been taught how to lift optimally and isn't aware of what proper form looks like. Here are the top eight technical faults associated with glute training, along with tips to help you prevent them.

Lumbar Hyperextension (Commonly Associated with Excessive Anterior Pelvic Tilt)

Lumbar hyperextension involves overarching your spine while you're extending your hips. It most commonly happens at the top of a deadlift, hip thrust, or back extension. You do want some anterior pelvic tilt at the bottom of a deadlift, so lumbar hyperextension is not always a bad thing, as long as it's very slight and occurs at the right time during a lift. Regardless, it is common and can be due to:

- Ignorance, or simply not knowing it's wrong.
- "Cementing" an overarching movement pattern. This happens to people who have good spinal extension mobility and follow the "chest up" cue. Over time, overarching is how their bodies learn to carry out the motion.
- Not having enough hip extension range of motion to lock out your hips when squatting, hip thrusting, or deadlifting. In such a scenario, you hyperextend your spine in order to complete the movement.
- Trying to lengthen the hamstrings through anterior pelvic tilt so you're in a better position to contribute to hip extension, possibly to make up for weak glutes (but not always). For example, arching your back and tilting your pelvis anteriorly during a squat lengthens your hamstrings, which makes them stronger contributors to hip extension. If your glutes are strong, you wouldn't resort to this strategy unless it was a learned or compensatory movement pattern.

SPINAL HYPEREXTENSION FAULTS

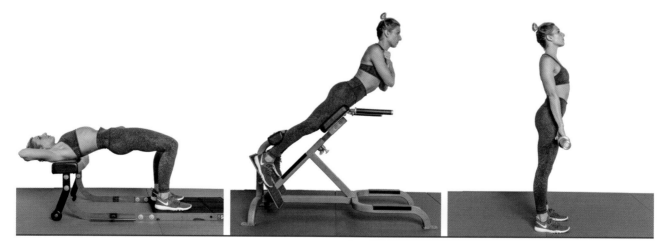

142

The correction to this fault is simply to learn proper and acceptable lumbopelvic (lower back and pelvis) hip complex mechanics. You need to extend your hips without overextending your spine at the same time. What's more, you need to do so when the weight gets heavy and when you take your sets close to failure. This requires a lot of discipline. Hip hinging, end-range hip extension, and glute-strengthening drills, as well as simply practicing proper form with lighter weight over and over, are the most common corrective drills that coaches use for this purpose.

Valgus Collapse (Excessive Medial Knee Displacement, Commonly Associated with Ankle Pronation, Hip Internal Rotation and Adduction, and Pelvic Lateral Drop)

Knee valgus occurs when your knees cave inward while you're extending your hips. This happens most often when rising from the bottom of a squat, but it can occur with other exercises, too, both bilateral (double leg) and unilateral (single leg). When I see people cave in slightly as they extend their hips during a hip thrust, I don't correct it, as I don't see it as problematic. Nevertheless, this fault is common, and it occurs due to:

- Ignorance, or simply not knowing it's wrong.
- Weak glutes and hip external rotators, or the hips being somehow stronger when you cave inward, possibly because it increases the leverage of the adductors.
- Putting the quads in a better position to produce force or torque.
- A lack of ankle dorsiflexion mobility, so the ankles pronate to allow for more forward knee migration.
- A combination of tight lateral leg musculature and weak medial leg musculature in the calves, quads, and hamstrings.
- A particular genetic shape and groove in the hip socket where the legs are forced into some caving when the musculature acting on the hips contracts forcefully.

Fixing knee valgus requires learning to keep your knees out during hip extension and cementing this pattern. Ankle mobility drills, transverse plane hip abduction exercises, doing squats with a resistance band around the knees, and just practicing proper form with lighter weight over and over are the most common corrective measures. It is also important to maintain discipline, because the tendency to cave will always be there when the weight gets heavy enough or the number of reps approaches failure.

Lumbar Flexion and Posterior Pelvic Tilt (aka Butt Wink)

The butt wink fault is characterized by rounding the lower back excessively, which can cause lower back tweaks and strains. You see this fault most often at the bottom of a deadlift or squat. Having a slight posterior pelvic tilt at the top of a hip thrust or back extension is actually a good thing, so it's important to be able to distinguish between proper utilization of different movement strategies. Butt winking is highly common and can happen due to:

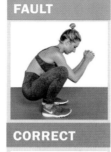

FAULT

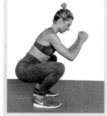

CORRECT

- Ignorance, or simply not knowing it's wrong.
- Poor hip flexion mobility, which differs depending on whether the exercise is a hip hinge or a squat pattern:
    a. In a hip hinge pattern such as a deadlift, tight hamstrings are usually the culprit.
    b. In a squat pattern, the culprit is often the skeletal anatomy of the hip. You see this at the bottom of a squat when a lifter reaches full hip flexion range of motion at around parallel and then continues to descend and go deeper by tilting their pelvis rearward and rounding their lower back.
- An attempt to make the movement more economical. When you fully round your spine, your erectors shut off (this is known as the *lumbar flexion relaxation phenomenon*), and you eventually stabilize your spine from rounding even further by being forcefully stretched rather than activated.
- Not being strong enough to carry out the task, so you shoot your hips up and round, which lengthens your hamstrings, shortens your quads, and slightly reduces the hip extension torque requirements by bringing your hips closer to the bar, allowing you to complete the lift.
- A combination of relatively long femurs and not enough ankle dorsiflexion range of motion, which causes you to round in order to maintain balance.
- Simply going too deep for your abilities (a combination of poor hip flexion mobility and attempting to make the movement more economical).

The solution is to extend your hips without flexing your spine. In most cases, you should simply not go as deep and opt for shallower squats and deadlifts such as parallel squats and block pulls. Hip flexion and ankle dorsiflexion mobility drills, including hamstring and calf stretching, hip hinging, erector strengthening, glute activation work, and just practicing proper form with lighter weight over and over will help prevent and correct this fault.

Pushing Through the Balls of the Feet

This fault most commonly occurs with squats and hip thrusts. You'll see lifters rise up onto their toes during a single-leg hip thrust, or you'll notice a forward weight shift at the bottom of a squat. Essentially, this amounts to pushing through the balls of the feet rather than the heels, which makes the movements slightly more quad dominant and diminishes the amount of gluteal recruitment. This fault occurs due to:

- Ignorance, or simply not knowing it's wrong.
- Having stronger quads relative to the hips.
- Poor ankle dorsiflexion mobility.

The solution is to set your feet properly and think, "Push through the heels," on each rep. You can also use glute-strengthening and ankle dorsiflexion mobility drills (see page 420) to improve your form. Elevating the heels onto a wedge, block, or plates helps dramatically with this fault, but it shouldn't be used as a crutch for someone who hasn't yet striven to build ankle mobility through stretches and drills.

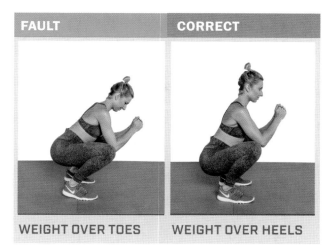

FAULT	CORRECT
WEIGHT OVER TOES	WEIGHT OVER HEELS

Shooting the Hips Up Out of the Hole

This fault happens during vertical hip extension exercises, including squats, deadlifts, lunges, Bulgarian split squats, and step-ups. The lifter descends with a particular torso angle and, as they initiate the concentric (rising) phase and rise up out of the hole, their hips shoot up and their torso becomes more horizontal. This fault can occur due to:

- Ignorance, or simply not knowing it's wrong.
- The hips being stronger relative to the quads.

Fixing this issue is a matter of practicing proper form with lighter weight and strengthening the quads over time to decrease the hip-to-quad strength discrepancy.

EARLY HIP DRIVE FAULT

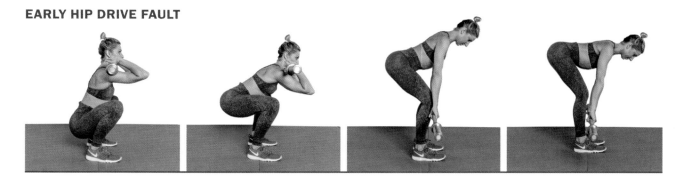

HIPS AND KNEES EXTEND SIMULTANEOUSLY

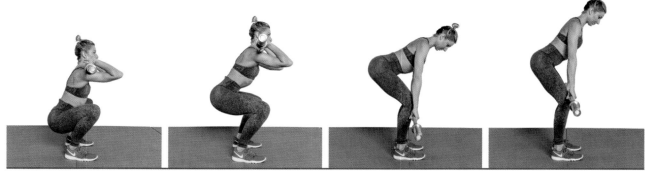

Failing to Use the Same Range of Motion and Form on Every Rep

When you observe advanced lifters, you'll notice that every rep tends to look strikingly similar. Even more common, advanced lifters have pre-lift rituals: they set up in their own unique ways and appear calm and confident. In contrast, beginners tend to be full of doubt: they set up differently each time, every rep in a set looks a bit different in form and depth, and their breathing is all over the place. This is due mostly to inexperience, but it also has to do with kinesthetic awareness and the desire to learn.

The solution is to set up correctly and pay close attention to your form on every rep. Don't just go through the motions; take your lifting seriously, just as any athlete does for their sport.

Setting Up Asymmetrically

You would think that the need to set up symmetrically would be obvious even to a beginner, but it's the most common error I see in my gym. It never ceases to amaze me how many lifters set up with the barbell off-center or with one foot turned out more than the other.

Now, some advanced lifters do this on purpose because they've learned that slight deviations in foot position aid their performance and comfort during a particular exercise, such as a squat or deadlift. But there's a huge difference between purposely setting up asymmetrically and doing so because you're oblivious. Your form is not going to be spot-on if you're off-kilter from the get-go.

Asymmetry happens due to carelessness and naivety. The solutions are to:

- Use the markings on the barbell to form a symmetrical grip and make sure that your feet are in line and flared outward to the same degree during squats.

- Make sure that the pad is on the barbell symmetrically and the bar is centered over your hips during hip thrusts.

- Make sure that your grip is symmetrical in terms of spacing and your feet are in alignment during deadlifts.

In addition, don't look to the side while you're training your glutes. Looking in the mirror is tempting, but cranking your neck to the side will cause your body to twist slightly, which isn't ideal. Instead, film yourself lifting and review the footage after each set.

Breathing Suboptimally

When you perform super high reps, as with frog pumps, you can breathe however you want. When you perform a moderate number of reps, you should breathe in during the eccentric (lowering) phase and breathe out during the concentric (rising) phase in a rhythmic fashion. When you lift heavy for low reps, you must learn how to brace your spine. You do so by taking a deep breath into your chest and belly and filling your lungs to around 70 percent of their capacity, then locking down the core musculature. It's mostly the diaphragm pushing down, but you also contract the pelvic floor, oblique, abdominal, erector musculature, and more. You hold this braced breath until you've carried out the concentric portion of the lift and then breathe out up top after locking out your hips. Repeat this sequence for each repetition. Research has shown that the hip extensors are stronger and the glutes activate more when the abdominal and core muscles are properly utilized during a lift.

IF YOU STRUGGLE WITH MOVEMENT, DEVOTE MORE CONSCIOUS EFFORT TO YOUR FORM

Some people need to be reminded to lift correctly every time they train, while others seem to move perfectly right out of the gate. Remember, exercise is movement, and movement is a skill. There are those lucky individuals who pick up on movement very quickly and others who have to work hard to get it right.

Motor learning—mastering a technique or developing coordination with a movement—takes a ton of practice and repetitions. So don't get frustrated if you don't pick it up in your first or even your twentieth training session. I still work on my form, and I've been lifting for 28 years. As long as I'm training, I will always work on maintaining good form.

DEVELOP THE MINDSET THAT ANYTHING THAT IS NOT GOOD FORM IS HURTING YOUR PROGRESS AND OPENING THE DOOR TO INJURY

In addition to mindful practice, you should work with a coach and film your movements. This is crucial. I routinely film my athletes so that they can see exactly what they're doing right and wrong. In my opinion, filming is one of the best ways to prevent, highlight, and correct movement errors. However, I don't want to make you so paranoid about your form that it prevents you from making progress. Initially, you have a lot of wiggle room because you're learning new movements and lifting lighter loads, which don't create a ton of joint stress. But over time, you will get stronger, and this is when poor form becomes dangerous.

FIND THE SWEET SPOT WHEN IT COMES TO FORM AND TECHNIQUE

If you're obsessed with perfect technique, you may never progress up in weight and get stronger. You might benefit from being less strict. And then there are people who pay zero attention to form and move with sloppy technique. These lifters get stronger and stronger, but they eventually break and get hurt. They would benefit from being much stricter with their technique.

The sweet spot is to care enough about your form that you stay safe and progress, but not be so strict that you never progress up in weight because you're obsessed with making your movement look pristine. If you wait until you can do everything perfectly, you will never advance. Remember, you have some wiggle room: you have to learn what you can and can't handle and what is acceptable and what is dangerous. This comes with experience, practice, coaching, and intelligent exercise selection and program design.

Instead of waiting until you can move with perfect form—which is never—wait until you are proficient. Being proficient means that you can move with a neutral spine (flat back) and maintain good body positioning throughout the entire range of the movement. Equally important, the movement should feel right and not cause you any discomfort.

STICK WITH BASIC VARIATIONS IN THE BEGINNING, THEN PROGRESS SLOWLY BY ADDING LOAD, VOLUME, AND RANGE OF MOTION

If you want to go from A to Z, then you need to go from A to B and then B to C. All too often, lifters and athletes try to go from A to M and then M to Z. The fact is, you have to progress gradually. As you become more proficient, challenge yourself accordingly by increasing the weight you're lifting (load), performing more sets of the exercise (volume), or increasing the range of motion. Just do so at your own pace. Believe me, you will see a lot of physique and strength changes along the way.

If you're having trouble performing a certain movement or you're consistently getting hurt or feeling pain, regress by reducing the load, shortening the range of motion, or changing the variation. For example, if you're having a hard time with the hip thrust, try glute bridging with your feet elevated. If you're struggling with the back squat, perform a high box squat, don't go as deep, or perform step-ups. If the deadlift is giving you trouble, reduce the range of motion by lifting from blocks (block pulls), start the movement from the top position by performing Romanian deadlifts (RDLs), or substitute single-leg RDLs. In short, there is always a modification that can be made.

IF YOU HAVE LIMITED RANGE OF MOTION, IMPROVING YOUR MOBILITY MIGHT ALSO HELP YOUR FORM

There are two kinds of mobility restrictions that may affect form. The first is a soft tissue–related restriction, meaning tight muscles are keeping you from accessing the normal ranges of motion that your body is capable of. You can improve this type of restriction simply by stretching and practicing the movements over and over.

The second kind of mobility restriction is skeletal or anatomical, meaning that your bone structure and anatomy won't allow you to move into certain ranges. For example, if you feel a pinch at the fronts of your hips every time you squat, it could be that your femurs are colliding with the ridge of your acetabulum (front of your pelvis). In this case, you may have to adjust the exercise and your setup to accommodate your unique anatomy.

EXPERIMENT WITH DIFFERENT STANCES AND SETUPS UNTIL YOU FIND THE POSITION THAT FEELS RIGHT, AND DON'T BE OBSESSED WITH RANGE OF MOTION

If your bone structure and muscle architecture are such that you can't squat to full depth or perform the full range of a movement, no problem. You can still perform the movement; you just have to limit the range or work within ranges that allow you to practice good form. I have clients who can't quite squat to parallel, and they still have amazing glutes.

If you're super tight, you may need to spend some time stretching to increase your range of motion. If you can't fully extend your hips because your hip flexors are tight, spend some time stretching your hip flexors—both the psoas and the rectus femoris (see page 156). If you can't get into a good squat position, use the techniques outlined on page 420 to improve your form.

MAINTAIN DISCIPLINE WITH EVERY REP

The reality is, your form will break down if you're training hard, going to failure, and lifting heavy weight. You have to stay disciplined. Maybe you need to cut the reps short or reduce the load. You have to listen to your body on a day-to-day and lift-by-lift basis. If you're not feeling it on any given day, roll with it and make the necessary adjustments.

Remember, the set stops when you can no longer carry out the movement with good form. Maybe you allow yourself a little bit of wiggle room, but it's up to you to stay disciplined and stop once your form degrades past a certain point.

In other words, every rep—regardless of load or the number of reps you're performing—should look relatively similar. Whether you're lifting 135 pounds for 20 reps or 225 pounds for 12 reps, all of the reps should look the same. If you start arching your back or not reaching full hip extension, stop your set. If you keep moving with bad form, you will not only ingrain poor movement patterns but also risk injury.

If you move with good form all the time, it will eventually become your default movement pattern. The same is true for moving with poor technique: if your reps are always sloppy, pretty soon you will always move with crummy form. Maintain discipline and focus on your technique, and you will know it the second your form starts to break down. The moment you don't come up as high or go as deep, or your knees cave inward, or your upper back rounds, or your lower back hyperextends, stop the set.

AS LONG AS A MOVEMENT DOESN'T HURT YOUR JOINTS, ALLOWS YOU TO GET MAXIMAL ACTIVATION, AND FEELS RIGHT—MEANING YOU'RE USING THE MIND-MUSCLE CONNECTION AND ENGAGING THE RIGHT MUSCLES— GO FOR IT

Remember, the technique guidelines that I have provided are exactly that—guidelines. They're general strategies for setting up and moving in a good position.

Some people I work with fit the mold perfectly and don't need to make many adjustments, while others stray far from the norm. For example, most of my clients adopt a slightly wider stance with their feet angled outward while hip thrusting. But I coached a client recently who prefers a narrow stance with her feet turned inward. I had never seen that stance before and never would have thought to make that adjustment. In fact, I did a study looking at different stances for glute activation, and a narrow stance activates the glutes the least of all of the stances. But not for her! She gets sky-high glute activation using that stance, and she has some of the best glute development I've ever seen. So who am I to tell her to do otherwise?

PAIN, INJURY, AND RECOVERY

When it comes to the glutes, any injury affecting the spine or lower body will result in some degree of gluteal inhibition (reduced activation and contraction), even stubbed toes and ankle sprains. It goes without saying—but I'm going to say it anyway—that if you want to maximize your glute gains, it's best to be free of pain and injury while you exercise.

In general, practicing good technique, following a well-thought-out and personalized program, and managing your diet and lifestyle—that is, adhering to the guidelines provided in this chapter—are essential to avoiding pain and injury. But pain is a complex topic, and it's not well understood. As with almost everything in the fitness world, there are many variables that can lead to pain and injury: anatomy, muscle architecture, soft-tissue genetics, program design (and all of the variables that influence program design), training experience, strength, flexibility, form, age, lifestyle habits, diet, hydration, substance use, previous injuries, fatigue, inflammation, stress, depression, anxiety, fear, beliefs about movement, pain, and the body—the list goes on and on.

The common reaction to pain is, "I did damage to my tissues and now I'm in pain." But you can have marked damage and no pain at all, or no damage and marked pain. You can also have referred pain—that is, pain in a part of your body other than its actual source. Stated differently, what you think is the source of your pain is often actually something else. For example, my brother was suffering from lower back pain, which he thought was from lifting, and it turned out that it was from GERD. He chewed tobacco for years and years and then moved to nicotine gum, and he ended up with some gastroesophageal reflux problems. When he resolved his GERD, his back pain went away. Then there is pain from an actual injury, like falling off your bike, and pain resulting from lifting with bad form (such as rounding your back during a max deadlift).

What's more, everyone interprets and experiences pain differently. This makes it impossible for me to provide an exact prescription or set of exercises for training around pain and injuries. The best I can do is to provide a set of guidelines that are universally well tolerated by most people and provide a blueprint for accelerating recovery post-injury.

It's as simple as this: if your pain doesn't inhibit glute activation and your exercise selection doesn't make the pain worse, then you can keep doing what you're doing. But if everything you do makes the pain worse, then you need to take a break until the pain subsides.

It's important to note that this section focuses on training around injuries and best practices for avoiding them. You will learn the best protocols for recovering from injuries in Chapter 14.

TRAIN AROUND PAIN, NOT THROUGH IT

Having enough discipline to self-regulate or make adjustments on the fly is a vital component of training over the long haul.

Every week you might have a little tweak or sore muscle that you have to train around. For this reason, you can't always just stick to your prewritten training program. You have to make adjustments according to biofeedback—that is, how you feel.

If you hurt your knee in training, for example, you need to adjust your program and choose exercises that don't make the problem worse. Common sense, I know, but one of the biggest mistakes people make is training through pain without making the necessary adjustments.

This is something that has taken me the better part of 20 years to implement. As a dedicated lifter, I always have something going on in my body that I need to work around. It's just part of lifting heavy weight, training hard, and aging. But I've learned to modify my program based on what is going on that day, and every aspect of my physical life is better when I adhere to this principle.

If something doesn't feel right to you, don't fall into the trap of thinking you're dysfunctional or some muscle is not firing correctly. More often than not, you just need to take a break, adjust your form, or modify your exercise selection and program design.

If I can impress this upon you, and you don't take 20 years to learn it like I did, then I will have provided a valuable service.

ALWAYS TAKE PRIOR INJURIES INTO CONSIDERATION

When I start working with a client—virtually or in person—one question I ask is if they have any prior injuries. This information is crucial for a couple of reasons.

First, it tells me the nature of the injury. Whether it's a genetic condition, the result of a catastrophic event like a car accident, or a factor that is within our control, like moving with proper form, I can construct a plan based on the nature of the prior injury. Second, and more importantly, it tells me which exercises to select. For example, if the client has a prior knee injury, I'll ask which movements cause them pain. If they say that the knee hurts every time they squat deep, I can formulate a plan for working around that issue. Depending on the injury, this might mean not performing certain squat patterns (such as lunges or pistols), reducing the range of motion, or adjusting the load (weight) and volume (number of reps they perform). Over time, I can usually get them doing most exercises pain-free, but I have to ease them into things, progress in a gradual fashion, and slowly increase the difficulty.

To train around prior injuries, you have to tinker around and figure out what you can and can't do. Chapter 14 provides exercise examples for training around specific symptoms, such as lower back pain and knee pain.

YOU DON'T WANT TO BE SO SORE (ANOTHER FORM OF PAIN) THAT YOU CAN'T TRAIN YOUR GLUTES FREQUENTLY OR HARD ENOUGH

It may surprise you, but many of my clients who see great results rarely get sore glutes. Everybody likes a little soreness the next day to remind them that they trained hard, but excessive soreness is counterproductive to growing the glutes.

Factors that contribute to soreness are:

- Novelty (doing something new or something you haven't done in a long time)
- Choosing exercises that stretch the muscle to a long length (for example, lunges)
- Purposely accentuating the lowering phase of an exercise
- Training your glutes infrequently

Factors that decrease soreness include:

- Consistency (performing similar movement patterns each week)
- Choosing exercises that stress short muscle lengths (for example, hip thrusts)
- Doing exercises that are more concentric in nature (for example, sled pushes)
- Training your glutes frequently

Research has shown that there's a huge genetic component to muscle damage. The same workout can produce markedly greater muscle soreness in some individuals than in others. If you're gaining strength and seeing results but rarely have sore glutes, just be happy. Sore glutes are a major inconvenience! It's no fun wincing in pain every time you stand up or try to walk. So take the above factors into consideration and try not to get too sore.

TO SHORTEN THE RECOVERY WINDOW BETWEEN WORKOUTS, ALLOW YOURSELF ENOUGH TIME TO REST AND RECOVER

You can also do things like foam rolling or get a massage, but don't fall for the hype and use these methods as a crutch. In other words, these practices should be supplemental and not a replacement for smart training and living.

The research is pretty clear that foam rolling is beneficial, but not for the reasons you might expect. Strength coaches commonly say that foam rolling improves tissue quality by realigning fascia, breaking apart scar tissue and adhesions, and releasing trigger points, but in reality, it likely works by reducing pain and stimulating mechanoreceptors within the muscles and fascia, which send signals to the brain to calm certain antagonist (opposing) motor units to "release the brakes" and stimulate agonist motor units to increase performance.

I think that if people knew exactly what was going on, they wouldn't be so paranoid when they go out of town and forget their foam rollers. Does this mean foam rolling is useless? Not at all. If it makes you feel better, by all means do it, especially before or after a workout or when you feel super tight. But understand that it's probably not doing all of the things that a lot of physical therapists are preaching. (To learn more about the science behind self-myofascial release and foam rolling, refer to the references section at the back of the book.)

Though you probably don't need to understand all of the mechanisms at work to reap the benefits of foam rolling, you shouldn't feel like it's a mandatory everyday practice, and you definitely should not use it as an excuse to avoid exercise.

It's the same with getting massages. I remember reading something about the Bulgarian weightlifting team's training schedule; they would train multiple times per day while getting a massage after each session. I thought, "Dang, if I could get multiple massages a day, I would recover so fast." But it's not true. Even though massage can be great—just like foam rolling—it doesn't greatly expedite the repair of muscle tissue.

Think about it like this. When you lift weights, you're breaking down muscle: you get popped sarcomeres, Z-line smearing, microlesions and tears in the T-tubules and sarcolemmas, and necrosis, all of which need to be repaired. In fact, this is one of the main reasons metabolism is elevated following high-intensity interval training and weight training—because of the damage and tissue repair that needs to take place. So there is a time component that you can't get around. Like me, people fall into the trap of thinking that if they just get a massage or foam roll, they won't be sore. But in reality, you just need to rest and let your tissues recover. Sure, if you perform some active recovery like walking, moving, and maybe foam rolling, you might feel better for an hour or two afterward, but once that feeling is gone, you'll notice that you go right back to being sore. These recovery activities help a little bit, but they don't rid you of the soreness altogether, especially if the delayed-onset muscle soreness (DOMS) is severe.

Don't get me wrong; massages and foam rolling definitely have their place, especially if you enjoy them and they make you feel better. However, they don't greatly accelerate healing. Sometimes you should just sit out a workout, rest, and relax so that you can recover and get back to setting PRs.

USE ACTIVATION DRILLS TO WARM UP FOR STRENUOUS EXERCISE

Glute exercises such as the glute bridge and quadruped hip extension can be done at the beginning of a workout as a way to prep the glutes for more strenuous exercise. These are referred to as *activation drills*. Strength coaches commonly call glute activation "low-load glute activation" because the goal is to stimulate, not annihilate. More specifically, you want to wake up the muscles, not fatigue them. For example, if you're doing an activation drill, you might perform 3 sets of 10 glute bridges and quadruped hip extensions with each leg in the warm-up. Now, you probably could perform 100 glute bridges if need be, but you stop at 10 while squeezing your glutes maximally at the top of each rep. As you proceed to the strength portion of the session, you'll use your glutes more during complicated compound movements, which will support better form and prevent breakdown. But the caveat is that you cannot fatigue your glutes, or else you'll use them less during subsequent movements, not more.

Here's a sample glute activation routine that you can perform as a warm-up to a lower-body training session or anytime you want to "wake up" the muscles—say, after extended periods of inactivity:

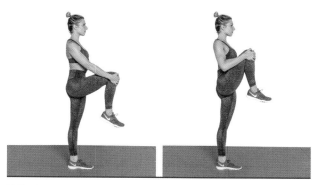

WALKING HIGH KNEES: 20 TOTAL STEPS

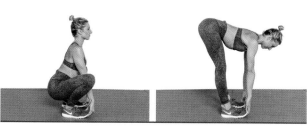

SQUAT TO STAND: 10 REPS

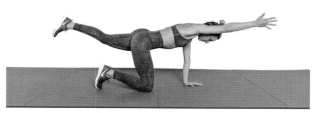

BIRD DOG: 10 REPS EACH SIDE

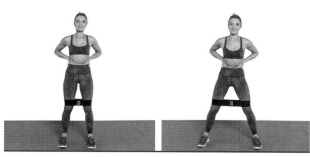

LATERAL BAND WALK: 10 STEPS EACH DIRECTION

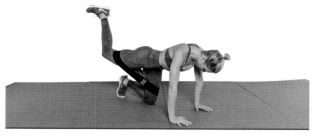

KNEE-BANDED QUADRUPED HIP EXTENSION: 10 REPS EACH SIDE

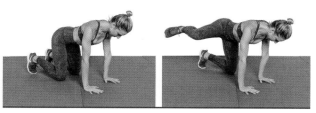

FIRE HYDRANT: 10 REPS EACH SIDE

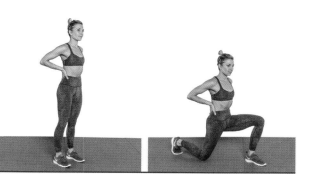

REVERSE LUNGE: 10 REPS EACH SIDE

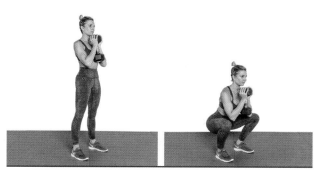

LIGHT GOBLET SQUAT: 10 REPS

RANGE OF MOTION AND MOBILITY

There is evidence that you need to create tension through a large range of motion to maximize hypertrophy, but this is not to say that exercises with shorter ranges of motion don't have their place. The glute bridge—and to a lesser degree, the hip thrust—usually has a shorter range of motion than squats and lunges but is better for developing the glutes. So this rule does not always apply to glute growth.

It's also worth mentioning that the studies looking at range of motion and muscle growth mostly examine other muscle groups. To date, there is only one study looking at range of motion as it relates to glute growth, which showed that deeper squats lead to greater glute hypertrophy compared to shallower squats. But the fact that the gluteus maximus has a unique EMG-angle curve in that it achieves its highest activation at the shortest possible muscle lengths (in contrast to most muscles, which display their highest activation at mid-range or longer lengths) casts doubt on the research involving other muscles.

PERFORM BOTH FULL-RANGE AND SHORTER-RANGE-OF-MOTION EXERCISES

One exercise can't be everything. Sometimes you need to reduce the range of motion until you develop the strength, coordination, and mobility to perform a movement properly. Don't think there is something wrong with you just because you can't perform all of the exercises included in this book. If your goal is to maximize glute growth, you should perform both full-range and shorter-range-of-motion exercises. This means you should perform hip thrusts, glute bridges, back extensions, lunges, squats, deadlifts, lateral band walks, and more.

IMPROVE YOUR RANGE OF MOTION THROUGH RESISTANCE TRAINING AND STRETCHING

Although stretching is good for improving joint range of motion, and I do provide some basic stretches, it's important to understand that performing strength training movements will improve your mobility as well. Squats, deadlifts, lunges, hip thrusts, back extensions, and lateral band exercises will improve mobility throughout your lower body. There's been a lot of research comparing strength training and stretching for improving joint range of motion, and the results are similar. In fact, strength training is arguably more beneficial because in addition to improving mobility, it also develops strength throughout those ranges of motion.

This is not to say that stretching doesn't work, because it does. But stretching doesn't change the mechanical properties of the muscle like strength training does. You're not lengthening your muscle or becoming more elastic. All that's happening is that your brain is recognizing that the position isn't causing your body harm, so your nervous system releases tension, allowing you to go a little deeper into the stretch.

A lot of stretches are good for improving flexibility in your hips and legs. I've provided a few that specifically target the glutes, along with two that target the hip flexors. Consider the stretches provided here as a starting point—there are a lot of great stretches that might suit your individual needs better.

I also want to point out that there are many different ways to stretch. For example, you can perform a stretch dynamically (referred to as *dynamic stretching*) or statically (referred to as *static stretching*).

Dynamic Stretching: This form of stretching is performed with movement. You're not holding the stretch; you're pulsing or moving in and out of the stretch. The idea is to momentarily move a particular body part to the limits of its range of motion (referred to as *end range*) and then back away. This process is typically repeated for 3 to 10 reps. For the best results, perform dynamic stretching before a workout as a warm-up or between sets of an exercise.

DYNAMIC DEEP LUNGE STRETCH

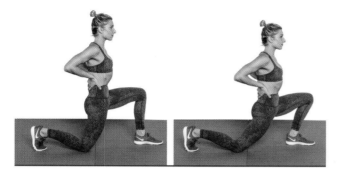

Let's say you're warming up to squat. In this situation, you can perform a dynamic deep lunge stretch by getting into the deep lunge position and then pulsing in and out of the stretch by dropping your hips, lowering your torso, and pushing your knee forward for 3 to 6 reps.

Static Stretching: This form of stretching is performed without movement, meaning that you hold the stretch at the limit of your range of motion for an extended period. Unlike dynamic stretching, which is done before a workout, static stretching should be done after a workout as a cool-down or later in the evening as a way to relax and promote better sleep. Static stretching momentarily weakens the muscle being stretched, so never do it before a big lift like a squat, deadlift, or hip thrust. If you stretch your hamstrings and then immediately try to deadlift, for example, you'll notice that you aren't as strong. If you are hell-bent on stretching before exercise, you can perform a dynamic stretch or stretch the antagonist muscle. For instance, if you're performing a hip thrust, you can stretch your hip flexors but not your glutes.

To improve your flexibility and get the best results from static stretching, keep the following in mind:

- Hold each stretch for 30 to 60 seconds and repeat two or three times.
- Breathe rhythmically (don't hold your breath).
- Warm up before you stretch.
- Most importantly, stretch only to the point where you feel tension in the muscle; never stretch beyond what is comfortable or where you feel excessive pain.

STATIC DEEP LUNGE STRETCH

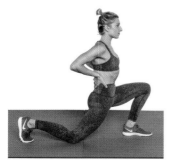

To perform s static deep lunge stretch, simply get into a deep lunge so that you feel tension in your muscles, making sure to stay below the pain threshold, and then hold that position for 30 to 60 seconds.

Whether you're trying to improve your range of motion or get into better positions or you simply like the way stretching feels for recovery, the following are great options.

DEEP LUNGE STRETCH

Good for:

- Stretching the psoas and hip muscles
- Improving hip extension, deep squats, and split squat range of motion

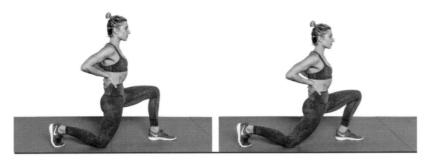

Get into the bottom of a lunge, place your hands on your hips or on the ground in front of your knee for balance and stability, and then extend your rear leg behind your body, keeping your quad square with the floor. You can either position your rear foot flush with the ground or remain on the ball of your foot. To drop into a deep lunge, lower your hips, then shift your weight forward. You can also push your lead knee forward and/or out to the side.

RECTUS FEMORIS STRETCH

Good for:

- Stretching the rectus femoris and psoas muscles
- Improving hip extension and hip thrust range of motion

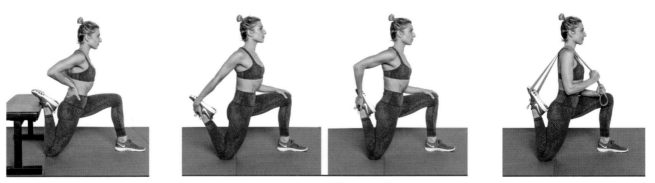

OPTION 1   OPTION 2   OPTION 3

There are several ways to perform the rectus femoris stretch. You can place your lower leg flush against a wall or on a bench (option 1), then raise your torso; you can grab your foot and pull your lower leg toward your butt in a lunge position (option 2); or you can hook a band around your foot, drape it over your shoulder, and then use the band to pull your grounded knee into deeper flexion (option 3).

HIP EXTERNAL ROTATION STRETCH

Good for:

- Stretching the glutes and hip external rotator muscles
- Improving hip external rotation range of motion

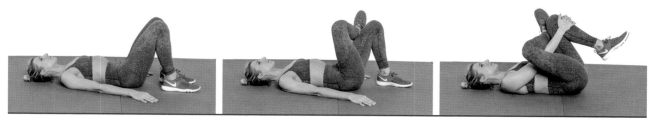

OPTION 1

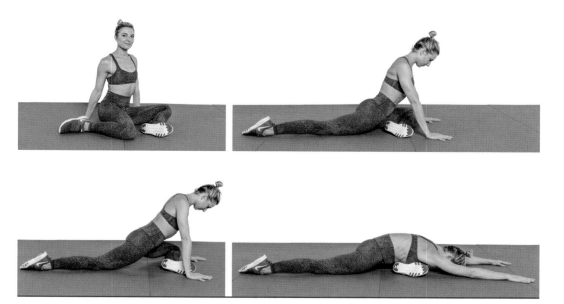

OPTION 2

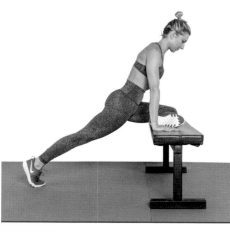

OPTION 3

The easiest variation of the hip external rotation stretch is to lie on your back with your knees bent and your feet flat on the floor as if you were performing a glute bridge. Cross one foot over your other knee, then pull your knee toward your chest using both hands (option 1). You can also perform the pigeon pose. To set up for this variation, sit on the ground with one leg curled in front of you with the outside of your thigh and lower leg flush with the floor. Extend your other leg behind your body, keeping your quad square to the ground. If you lack flexibility or you're tight, keep your front foot close to your hip and your torso upright or slightly leaning (option 2, top). For a deeper stretch, position your lead shin so that it is perpendicular to your body and lean your torso forward (option 2, bottom). If these variations are too intense, try placing your lead leg on a bench and using your rear leg to support your weight (option 3).

TWISTING GLUTE STRETCH

Good for:

- Stretching the gluteus maximus
- Improving hip external rotation and hip flexion range of motion

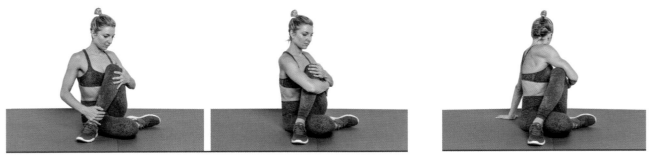

OPTION 1   OPTION 2

Sit on the floor with your legs straight out in front of you. Cross one leg over the other, positioning your foot as high up your thigh as possible. You can keep your grounded leg straight or bend it as shown. Wrap your arms around your top knee, then pull it toward your chest (option 1). To increase the stretch, you can twist slightly toward your top leg, placing your arm in front of your thigh and looking behind you (option 2).

IF SOMETHING IS GOING ON IN YOUR BODY OR SOMEONE POINTS OUT A WEAKNESS, REMEMBER THAT YOU'RE NORMAL

Just because something is going on in your body—whether it is a muscular imbalance, a minor injury, or limited mobility—doesn't mean that something is wrong with you. Imbalances are normal, pain is normal from time to time, and most people have limited mobility somewhere in their bodies.

There's a growing trend among sports doctors, physical therapists, chiropractors, manual therapists, athletic trainers, personal trainers, and strength coaches to label minor problems as dysfunction. This labeling has far-reaching and broad implications. Words matter. If you go to someone for help and they tell you that you're dysfunctional, you might interpret that literally and think you can't do anything.

Think about it: *dysfunction* implies that you're not functioning properly. Well, we're not at 100 percent all the time, especially when we're training hard. This "dysfunctional" mantra is a scare tactic, using labels to get customers to keep returning for business. If all you have is a hammer, everything looks like a nail. If you're looking for a "syndrome" in the body, you'll find it. Some practitioners are taking advantage of their customers' naivety while raking in the dough. This practice purposely keeps people dependent and weak in order to make those professionals more money. Luckily for me, in my profession, we make more money when our clients get stronger.

I am a strength coach, and I have no place for labeling clients. My job is to strengthen people's bodies, minds, and spirits and to instill confidence and improve self-esteem. I've never told a client that they have dysfunctional glutes or that their glutes are not firing optimally, because I don't want them to develop phobias that they can use as a crutch. Instead, I build confidence by starting my clients off with rudimentary exercises. Then I move them to more advanced exercises, complimenting them along the way. And I assure them that the human body is amazingly powerful, versatile, and resilient. This builds a healthy relationship with strength training based on empowerment, not fear or doubt.

If something is causing you pain, it's usually not that you're dysfunctional or you need corrective exercise; you just need to take some time off and avoid the insulting exercises. Then you need to practice better form, listen to your body, and pay attention to program design (make sure you're performing the optimal exercises with the right amount of volume and frequency for your body).

There's risk associated with lifting weights, and it's natural to push the envelope with training. You want to get stronger, bigger, and leaner, so you train hard. And sometimes you train too hard and get hurt. Minor tweaks, aches, and pains are part of the process of lifting weights. Obviously, you should try to avoid getting hurt, and I've provided plenty of guidelines to help prevent injury and pain. But it's a delicate balance between training hard and staying pain-free. Listening to your body and knowing when to push yourself and when to back off is an art in and of itself.

For instance, some people have poor soft-tissue genetics in certain areas, leaving them susceptible to injuries. If you're constantly battling lower back pain, maybe you need to adjust your range of motion or select exercises that don't put a ton of strain on your back, like lunges and lateral band walks. In other words, your lower back is not hurting because you have a dysfunction; it's hurting because you did something that didn't agree with your body.

The bottom line is that fitness professionals need to stop telling people they are dysfunctional. In addition to fearmongering, it creates a "nocebo effect." The nocebo effect is the opposite of the placebo effect, which is when something fixes an issue but has no therapeutic value. For example, I give you a sugar pill and tell you it will cure your headache, and it works. The nocebo effect works in exactly the same way, but in reverse. Imagine if I said, "Oh my, look at your glutes! You have no muscle. Do you have back pain? You don't? That's shocking, because I would think that with your pathetic glutes, you would have a ton of back pain. Wow, you're lucky."

Now, all you're going to think about is how you should have back pain because you have no glutes. Every time you lift, you'll be thinking, am I going to get back pain? And then, all of a sudden, you manifest back pain because that is what you've been told. Then you start hunting for a solution.

Just as there are lousy personal trainers and strength coaches, there are lousy rehab specialists. Few of them will ask you to see a video of your lifting form or a copy of the training program you've been following. Put simply, many lack the knowledge and experience to understand strength training. A chiropractor will say that you need to get adjusted and crack your bones. An acupuncturist will want to put needles in you to make you feel better. A massage therapist will tell you how tight you are and massage your stiff muscles. A physical therapist will tell you how dysfunctional you are and give you corrective exercises.

Clearly, there is a place for chiropractors, acupuncturists, physical therapists, and massage therapists. These are well-intentioned practices that help a lot of people. Furthermore, many of these practitioners are studying strength training and pain science and learning more about the power of their words and labels, and they're getting better at helping people. But you have to use common sense, realize that you're rarely going to feel perfect, and understand that you are stronger than you think. And when it comes to recovering from pain (muscle soreness) or injury, time is the most important variable. Sure, it feels good to get adjusted and massaged, and corrective exercise might help. But what a lot people fail to realize is that while they're getting treated, they're avoiding the things that caused the problem in the first place. Time, in other words, heals all wounds. As the famous French philosopher Voltaire said many years ago, "The art of medicine consists in amusing the patient while nature cures the disease."

This resonates with me because—like many of you, probably—I've been labeled as dysfunctional. When I was 15, I was in a bad car accident, and the doctor evaluating me said that I had the spine of a 90-year-old. He told me I had the worst case of disc degeneration he'd ever seen in someone my age and advised me never to lift heavy weight or my spine would break. Yet I went on to deadlift 620 pounds and hip thrust 815 pounds, and my spine is just fine.

I'm not saying that you should lie to yourself and pretend you don't have an issue. If you have scoliosis, I'm not going to try to convince you that you don't have scoliosis. But I would point you to an article on Lamar Gant, who is one of the strongest deadlifters of all time and had severe scoliosis. His scoliosis actually provided him with an advantage, and he credited lifting and stretching with keeping him healthy.

My point is this: following the guidelines in this chapter and the program design variables in the next chapter is not only the best way to avoid pain and injury while training hard, but also the best way to recover. Unless you don't push yourself in training, it's inevitable that you will experience pain or discomfort. You shouldn't think, "Oh no, I'm ruined!"

Everyone has inherent strengths and weaknesses. You're going to be good at 10 exercises and mediocre or poor at 5 others. And we all are going to have exercises that don't feel very good and others that do based on our individual anatomy. Instead of thinking that you're dysfunctional, remember that pain is just a part of training hard and aging, and use logic and experience to address the issue so that you can resolve it without fear or worry.

DIET AND LIFESTYLE

It should come as no surprise that what and how much you eat can have a massive impact on the appearance of your glutes and overall physique. Just as there is no one-size-fits-all approach to program design, what and how much you should eat depends on your goals and individual needs. Some people need to eat more, while others need to eat less. Some need to avoid certain foods, while others do not. For this reason, I'm reluctant to offer specific advice. Outlining a comprehensive approach to eating and body composition is a book in and of itself.

Rather than delve into the minutiae of dieting, my intention is to summarize general guidelines related to nutrition and glute appearance. When it comes to losing weight through dieting, you need to keep four things in mind.

ALL WEIGHT LOSS DIETS WORK BY CREATING A CALORIC DEFICIT

Let me begin by stating that if your goal is to lose weight, then what you're really trying to do is lose fat. You want to keep your muscular shape and burn fat for energy, which you can do by being patient, consuming ample protein, and lifting weights, but I digress.

It is commonly said that you need to cut 500 to 1,000 calories a day to lose 1 to 2 pounds a week (since 3,500 calories equals about 1 pound of fat). This would all be well and good if the body didn't lose metabolically active tissue or become lethargic, but it does. Therefore, you will have to keep readjusting your calories and macros to make sure you stay on track and continue losing weight at the proper rate. And the rate is different for different people; larger individuals need to be more aggressive with fat loss initially.

For example, if you have 40 percent body fat, then you need to be in a huge caloric deficit or be at a caloric deficit for an extended period to lose ample weight. If you have 20 percent body fat, then maybe you can keep your diet the same and focus on getting stronger. This is known as *body recomposition, or recomp* for short. It means that you stay at the same weight but gradually increase your muscle and decrease your fat so that your body composition improves. But make no mistake about it: being in a caloric deficit—that is, burning more calories than you're consuming (eating less and moving the same amount, eating the same and moving more, or eating less and moving more)—is the only way to lose weight. All popular diets work by getting you to consume fewer calories by sticking to various rules. This is true for the ketogenic diet, the Paleo diet, the Zone diet, Weight Watchers, the South Beach Diet, intermittent fasting, and the list goes on and on. The key is to find a balance where you're eating enough to fuel your workouts but not so much that you gain weight or fail to lose fat.

It's worth mentioning that if you diet to lose weight, your butt will shrink (unless you're a beginner). Every bikini competitor I've worked with has had this complaint. These women have big butts when they weigh 150 pounds, but when they compete at 120 pounds, their glutes are much smaller.

The best way to keep most of your glutes is to lose weight gradually. The more gradually you drop weight, the more muscle you will retain. If you lose 20 pounds in a month, you'll lose a lot more muscle than if you lose 20 pounds over the course of five months. Make sure you strive to maintain (or even build) as much strength as possible during the cut and consume adequate protein.

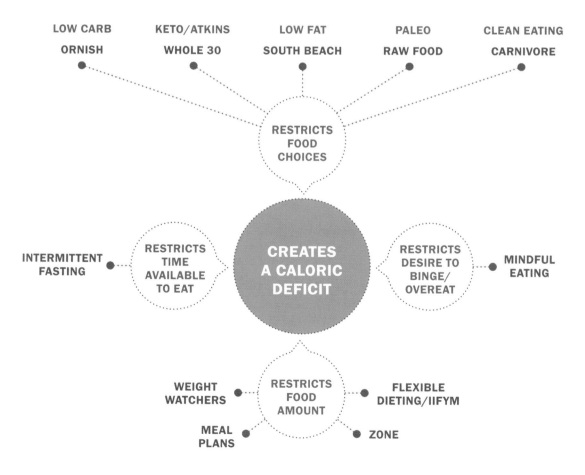

Adapted from Marie Spano (@mariespano)

CONSUME ABOUT 1 GRAM OF PROTEIN PER POUND OF LEAN BODY MASS PER DAY

If you have 20 percent body fat and you weigh 150 pounds, your lean body mass is 120 pounds. You want to consume about 120 grams of protein per day, broken up into several feedings. You could also just multiply your body weight by 0.8 and consume that number of grams of protein per day.

Consuming enough protein not only ensures that you maintain the muscle you have but also helps regulate your appetite. Protein is satiating, which might help you eat less. What's more, protein has a high thermic effect, so you burn more of what you consume compared to carbs and fat. As long as your protein intake is sufficient and you remain in a caloric deficit, you can choose how much fat and carbohydrates to consume and still lose weight.

Although eating enough protein is important, don't freak out if you don't reach your protein target. Your metabolism is flexible, and you won't lose a ton of muscle in one day. It's also important not to worry if you eat too much protein in one day. As long as you stay close to your caloric target, it won't derail your progress. The point is that you have wiggle room and you shouldn't obsess about protein. In addition, going over the protein recommendation will not cause you to build more muscle. So the remaining calories should come from fat and carbs, which are not only tasty, but also good for hormone production, micronutrient absorption, energy levels, and more.

CALCULATING LEAN BODY MASS

1 Figure out your body weight and fat percentage.

2 Multiply your body weight by your fat percentage.

3 Subtract the result of Step 2 from your body weight.

Body weight: 150 pounds

Fat percentage: 20 percent

150 x 20% = 30 | 150 – 30 = 120 (lean body mass)

FOLLOW THE FLEXIBLE DIETING MODEL

When it comes to dietary guidelines, I recommend the flexible dieting approach, which is based on the idea that 85 percent of your calories should come from whole, minimally processed foods, and the other 15 percent are discretionary.

The discretionary part is crucial because we all crave things from time to time, and you're probably not going to stick with something if you constantly feel deprived. As you diet down and get to lower levels of body fat, you stray from your natural "set point," and it becomes harder and harder to stay on track. Your body responds by becoming lethargic and hungry. This is where diet breaks can come in handy, which is the whole point of flexible dieting: it increases adherence and enables you to stay on track. It doesn't matter how great a diet is if you fall off the wagon. As you lose weight, you get hungrier and it becomes more difficult to stay the course. By allowing yourself small amounts of foods you crave, you don't feel as deprived, and you therefore won't slip up and binge or give up altogether. I also want to caution you not to become overly obsessed with the 85/15 percentages. You don't need to split hairs over whether some food is considered discretionary as long as the majority of your food comes from nutrient-dense sources. However, it's important to realize that the more you rely on processed foods and dip into discretionary calories, the harder it is to stick to your caloric goals.

Interestingly, you can eat junk food and still lose weight as long as you're following the first two guidelines. Conversely, you can gain weight when eating healthy food if you overeat. Health and longevity are important, though. If you want to look and feel your best, eating nutrient-dense food is better than eating junk, as long as you can stick to your weight loss goals without being neurotic about your food choices.

I follow the flexible dieting model and recommend it for most people. But you must adjust your caloric intake and macros (protein, carbs, and fat) based on your body weight, genetics, daily activity, and goals.

It's also important to point out that there are different levels to flexible dieting. You may choose to weigh and track your food intake and make sure your daily consumption meets your targets. For example, let's say you weigh 150 pounds at 20 percent body fat and can be in a caloric deficit that has you losing weight at 1,800 calories per day. Your target will be 120 grams of protein per day (480 calories), with the remaining calories coming from some combination of carbs and fat. Carbs and fat are roughly interchangeable, so the remaining 1,320 calories could come from 105 grams of carbs and 100 grams of fat, from 218 grams of carbs and 50 grams of fat, or anywhere in between. In general, it's a good idea to consume at least 0.4 gram of fat per pound of body weight per day, but you don't have to reach this target every single day.

Other approaches include just tracking calories but sticking to foods you know will generally get you close to your targets, just tracking calories and protein intake, or just roughly tracking protein intake but making sure you consume a consistent number of calories each day.

Remember, you have to match the intervention to the individual. Some people should not weigh and track their macros because it creates neuroses around food. Instead, they should focus on creating good eating habits. Conversely, some people are fine counting calories and macros, and they're better off because of it.

Ultimately, the idea is to get to a point where you can eat fairly mindfully and stay at your target weight and physique. In other words, you eat based on how you feel while maintaining habits that keep you on track. Some days you eat more and some days you eat less, but you always look and feel good. That's the goal!

MEAL TIMING IS IMPORTANT, BUT NOT AS IMPORTANT AS THE OTHER GUIDELINES

As with all of the dietary guidelines for weight loss, when and how often you should eat (known as *meal timing*) depends on your specific performance and health goals. While you should probably split your daily protein consumption into three or four different feedings in order to maximize muscle growth, meal timing is otherwise largely overrated. We used to think that eating frequently—six times per day, for example—would "stoke the metabolic fire" and keep the metabolism revved all day long, but now we know that this is not the case.

We also used to think that eating immediately following a workout was mandatory. People used to obsess about eating within an hour of working out. This is referred to as the *anabolic window*—that is, you have an hour to eat protein and carbs to maximize protein synthesis (the process of creating proteins to repair muscle tissue) and recovery. But with regard to protein, you have roughly a five-hour window, and what you ate before also matters. So, if you eat a meal two hours before your workout, that food is still being digested and absorbed, meaning you don't have to eat again post-workout to maximize protein synthesis.

When it comes to carbohydrates, it's more circumstantial. If you're just interested in building muscle and you lift only one hour a day, four days a week, then carbohydrate timing doesn't matter. But if you're an athlete who plays sports or you're training multiple times a day, then you should consume carbs immediately following a workout to accelerate recovery. Even then, it's not something you need to obsess over.

What's vital is how many calories and macros you consume on a daily basis, not so much how you arrange your meals and feedings throughout the day. However, you want to make sure that you are energized for your strength workouts. This is very important, and not taking it into consideration can hinder your results.

There is a happy medium for most people, which is to eat an hour or two before a workout. Some folks can train fasted, but I'm not one of them, and most of the women I work with have lackluster workouts if they're hungry. Obviously, being overfed or full is not great, either, because it's uncomfortable. So make sure to consume the proper amount of food at the ideal time prior to your workout, but also make sure to consume the right types of food for your body. Nobody enjoys gastrointestinal discomfort while training.

NUTRIENT TIMING
HOW IMPORTANT IS IT?

NOT VERY IMPORTANT FOR...	POSSIBLY IMPORTANT FOR...	REALLY IMPORTANT FOR...
• Weight loss or general health in overweight/obese	• Extreme fat loss in advanced exercisers	• Competition with more than one glycogen-dependent event
• Body composition in novice exercisers	• Extreme muscle or strength gain in advanced exercisers	• Competition with minimal time between events
• Non-fasted strength exercise lasting less than 1 hour	• Exhaustive training done after an overnight fast	• Exhaustive/continuous training lasting more than 2 hours
• Goals that don't include endurance competition	• Continuous training done after an overnight fast	• Competition events lasting more than 2 hours
• Goals that don't include extreme muscle gain	• Exhaustive/continuous training lasting more than 1 hour	
• Goals that don't include extreme fat loss		

The majority of people fall into the left-hand category and don't need to worry too much about nutrient timing.

Adapted from Alan Aragon's Continuum of Nutrient Timing Importance (alanaragon.com)

TO IMPROVE BODY COMPOSITION WHILE STAYING THE SAME WEIGHT (KNOWN AS RECOMPING), FOLLOW A CALORIE MAINTENANCE STRATEGY

Recomping (n): the act of improving body composition while staying the same body weight by simultaneously increasing muscle mass and decreasing fat mass.

Several years back, I worked with a client for an entire year. She was roughly 5-foot-6 and weighed 132 pounds. She was already eating in a healthy manner (around 1,600 calories and 110 grams of protein per day), so I told her to keep eating the same way.

Over the course of the year, her body weight never fluctuated by more than a few pounds. She went from squatting 65 pounds to 215 pounds, deadlifting 65 pounds to 275 pounds, hip thrusting 95 pounds to 365 pounds, and bench pressing 45 pounds to 105 pounds, and she was able to perform three bodyweight chin-ups. Her physique improved markedly despite zero change in body weight and caloric intake, and she looked lean and athletic. She put on a pair of pants she had worn before she started lifting, and there was a 4-inch gap in the waist, but they were very tight in the glute area. This is a perfect example of recomping.

When you recomp, you lose overall body volume because muscle takes up less space than fat at equal mass. Moreover, you add shape to the right areas and whittle shape from the "problem" areas, which results in a much more aesthetically pleasing appearance. In short, you gain lean muscle, lose a little bit of fat, and get stronger while sticking to the caloric intake that maintains your body weight (referred to as *calorie maintenance* or *maintenance calories*).

This is what happens with many of my clients. Every few months, their body composition improves. Obviously, individuals who are overweight or underweight are placed on a calorie deficit or calorie surplus, respectively. But many can keep their caloric intake the same (though typically increasing protein intake) while utilizing progressive overload on a variety of lifts in a variety of rep ranges and become stronger and fitter. I've demonstrated this over and over, even with advanced lifters.

Bulking and cutting is a popular strategy. However, you do not always have to increase caloric intake to gain muscle, nor do you always have to decrease caloric intake to lose fat. You can maintain caloric intake while training like a beast—this is recomping. It's important to know about this option so you're not under the false impression that your body weight has to fluctuate drastically to improve your body composition. You can also "gaintain" by eating at a very slight calorie surplus and moving up in weight gradually over time—for example, adding 1 to 3 pounds a year.

To summarize, here's how to recomp:

1. Eat at a calorie maintenance level (the total number of calories required on a daily basis to maintain your body weight with no gain or loss in fat and/or muscle tissue) and consume around 1 gram of protein per pound of lean body mass per day.

2. Get way stronger and fitter.

3. Do this for months on end until you are too lean for your liking and would prefer to gain some extra body weight.

Here are four ways to calculate your maintenance calories, from least to most accurate:

1. Multiply your body weight (in pounds) by 14 or 15 (for example, 150 pounds x 15 = 2,250 calories per day).

2. Use the Mifflin-St Jeor equation to determine your resting metabolic rate, or RMR (the energy your body expends while at rest) with activity variables: RMR (kcal/day) = 10 x (weight in kg) + 6.25 x (height in cm) – 5 x (age in years) + 5 (for men) or – 161 (for women).

3. Eat only prepackaged foods for one day and add up the number of calories consumed (try to match your normal daily intake).

4. Weigh everything you eat on a food scale and track your calories over a seven-day period, then average it out (make sure your body weight doesn't change over the week).

CALORIES BURNED AND CONSUMED OVER A 24-HOUR PERIOD

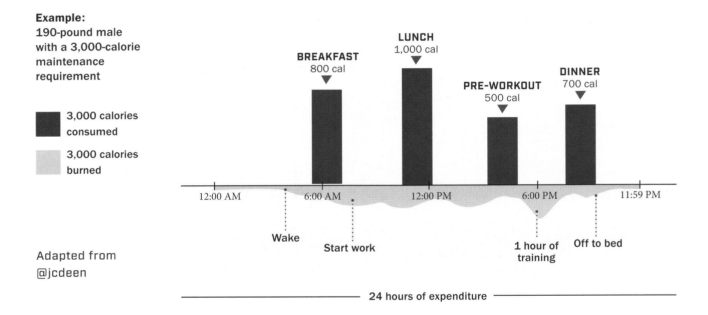

Example:
190-pound male with a 3,000-calorie maintenance requirement

3,000 calories consumed

3,000 calories burned

Adapted from @jcdeen

You will use maintenance calories if you are recomping. If you are striving to lose weight, use a 10 to 12 multiplier on method 1; if you're trying to gain weight, use a 16 to 18 multiplier. In some cases, I've had to go down to an 8 multiplier for fat loss, and I've had to bulk up some people at a 25 multiplier, but these ranges work decently well for the masses.

I haven't found much difference between using the simple multiplier in method 1 and the more complicated equation in method 2. The first approach assumes that you are moderately active and lift for an hour a day, three or four days a week. Of course, there are large individual variances in metabolism and NEAT (non-exercise activity thermogenesis). If you run around all day at work, train twice a day, and fidget nonstop, then your maintenance needs will be markedly higher. I work with people who are at a 23 multiplier, and I've worked with sedentary people who maintain at a 10 multiplier. It's important to note that methods 1 and 2 are just estimates.

Most of you will never use a food scale, so method 3 is a viable strategy. You'll need to eat foods such as yogurt, meal replacement shakes, small boxes of cereal, and anything that is small and prepackaged and has nutrition information on the label. If you are willing and able to weigh and track, then taking a seven-day average while making sure your body weight stays relatively stable will give you the most precise measurement.

You just need a starting point from which you can adjust. Plan on taking a month to dial in your precise maintenance number. For example, say your true maintenance number is 1,600, but you start out at 1,900. In this scenario, you would gain scale weight, so drop 100 calories three weeks in a row so that you end up at the true number within a month. No biggie; you may be up a couple of pounds, but you'll have had great workouts during this time because you were fueled up, and your strength and muscle will be slightly higher. Now you've established a baseline that you can begin to adjust depending on your goals.

TRACKING MACROS IS A GOOD WAY TO DETERMINE HOW MUCH PROTEIN, CARBS, AND FATS YOU SHOULD CONSUME EACH DAY

When it comes to managing your weight—whether you're trying to lose weight, recomp, or bulk—monitoring your calories is the most important variable in achieving the physique you desire.

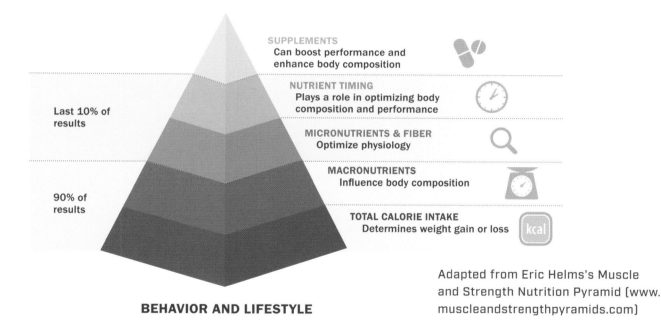

SUPPLEMENTS
Can boost performance and enhance body composition

NUTRIENT TIMING
Plays a role in optimizing body composition and performance

MICRONUTRIENTS & FIBER
Optimize physiology

MACRONUTRIENTS
Influence body composition

TOTAL CALORIE INTAKE
Determines weight gain or loss

Last 10% of results

90% of results

BEHAVIOR AND LIFESTYLE

Adapted from Eric Helms's Muscle and Strength Nutrition Pyramid (www.muscleandstrengthpyramids.com)

As a quick recap, if you want to lose weight, you have to be in a caloric deficit, meaning that you are eating fewer calories than your body burns each day. If you want to recomp, you eat at a calorie maintenance, which is the total number of daily calories required to maintain your body weight. And if you want to gain weight, you need to eat at a calorie surplus.

In each scenario, monitoring how much you eat by counting calories is a vital part of reaching your physique goals. Tracking your macros by calculating the number of grams of protein, carbohydrates, and fat that you should consume based on your caloric needs takes it one step further.

There are several reasons for tracking macros. In addition to gaining a better understanding of how much of each macronutrient you should eat (which mainly ensures that you're getting enough protein), the process brings a greater sense of awareness to the quality of the food you're eating. The fact is, not all calories are created equal. We're surrounded by hyperpalatable foods that are easy to overconsume. In most cases, people are eating too much and don't even know it. For example, you might eat a small portion thinking it's not high in calories, when in reality it is. Not only that, but different foods have different effects on the body. A 200-calorie portion of vegetables is larger and more nutritious than a 200-calorie snack bar.

Though tracking macros gives you control over the food you eat and can help improve your body composition, there's a huge psychological component that is important to consider. Some people get stressed out by the idea of weighing and tracking or become neurotic about it, while others prefer to track because it gives them control. Whether it's for you or not, tracking macros is a delicate balance of learning how much you should eat based on your preferences, goals, and genetics and not getting overly obsessed to the point where it creates anxiety. You should be able to go out for a nice dinner and not feel guilty about deviating from your plan. And you should be able to track to get a baseline without feeling stressed or overwhelmed.

If you do well when you track your calories and macros, then by all means keep doing it. But if you're the type of person who gets stressed out about it, then perhaps a better approach is to do it just for a week to determine your baseline so you can figure out what adjustments you need to make. You might realize that you're eating way too much and that is the reason you're overweight or not reaching your body composition goals. Or you may realize that you're not getting nearly enough protein to support your goals, or that you're going overboard on fat. Sure, eating intuitively might be the goal, but you might intuitively eat more based on your genetics, the type of training you enjoy doing, and your appetite. This is why tracking calories and macros—even for a week, or periodically throughout the year—is a good idea. The goal is to get good at tracking mindfully, but you need to actually weigh and track for a while in order to get good at estimating calories and macros based on portion sizes. I've seen even highly experienced weighers-and-trackers grossly misjudge the macros in a particular meal.

As management guru Peter Drucker said, "What gets measured gets managed." If you never track your workouts or exercises, it's a lot harder to know what works for you and what doesn't. But when you follow a program and do it for a long enough period, you can begin to train intuitively by adhering to a protocol. It's the same with tracking your food, sleep, activity, or weight: you measure to figure out where you are, increase awareness, and determine what adjustments you need to make, and then you manage the protocol to stay on track.

Here's how I set up macros. Other coaches use different methods, but this approach works well for the masses.

Step 1: Calculate maintenance calories.

Start out by determining your caloric intake. As already discussed, I prefer to use the simple equation over the more complex Mifflin-St Jeor formula, which is to multiply your body weight (in pounds) by 14 or 15, which represents a moderate activity level. If you're more active, use a higher multiplier, and if you're more sedentary, go with a lower multiplier.

Example: | 150 lbs x 15 | 2,250 calories per day |

Step 2: Calculate protein intake.

Option 1: 0.8g x body weight in pounds
Option 2: 1g x lean body mass

Next, figure out your protein intake. Using 1 gram per 1 pound of body weight per day tends to overestimate requirements for obese subjects; the 0.8 gram per pound of lean body mass per day is more accurate. But the former is quicker.

Option 1 Example:

0.8g x 150 lbs	120 grams of protein per day

Option 2 Example:

150 lbs x 20% (body fat)	30
150 – 30	120 lbs (lean body mass)
1g x 120	120 grams of protein per day

Step 3: Calculate fat intake.

After that, you figure out your fat intake by multiplying your body weight in pounds by 0.45.

Example:

150 lbs x 0.45	67.5 grams of fat per day

Step 4: Calculate carb intake by subtracting protein and fat calories from maintenance calories and then dividing by 4.

Now that you have your calories, protein, and fat intake set, the next step is to figure out your carb intake. You do that by multiplying protein grams by 4 and fat grams by 9, then subtracting the sum of the two from your total calorie intake and finally dividing by 4.

Example:

120g (protein) x 4 calories per gram	480 protein calories
67.5g (fat) x 9 calories per gram	608 fat calories
480 (protein calories) + 608 (fat calories)	1,088 protein + fat calories
2,250 (total calories) – 1,088 (fat/protein calories)	1,162 carb calories
1,162 / 4 calories per gram	290.5 grams of carbs per day

So a person who weighs 150 pounds would eat roughly 120 grams of protein (480 calories), 67.5 grams of fat (608 calories), and 290.5 grams of carbs (1,162 calories).

Step 5: Adjust based on satiety responses, physiology, goals, taste preferences, etc.

The last step is to fine-tune everything over time. These numbers are merely a starting point. You may see better results if you eat more protein. Some people see good results when they go very high on fat and keep carbs to a minimum (keto). It should be noted that the leanest physique competitors tend to go with higher carbs and lower fat. Carbs and fats are roughly interchangeable, meaning that you can get more of your calories from carbs and less from fat or vice versa. You can also fluctuate your carbs and fat in a strategic (or nonstrategic) fashion; some people like to cycle their carb intake or have refeed days. If you're simply trying to be healthy, your protein requirements are much lower. Moreover, your caloric needs may change over time, depending on your muscle mass, activity level, fitness level, and goals. This is where working with an experienced coach comes in handy—they can help you make the proper adjustments.

The bottom line is this: you don't need to calculate your macros to reach your physique goals. For the vast majority of people, following a flexed dieting protocol and periodically tracking calories to make sure you are on target is perfect. If you have specific weight-related goals, monitoring your caloric intake is the next logical step. And if you really want to make sense of your diet, you enjoy weighing and measuring, or you are training for an event or want to ensure the best possible body composition results, then tracking your macros might be for you.

IT'S COMMON TO UNDERESTIMATE CALORIC INTAKE AND OVERESTIMATE PHYSICAL ACTIVITY

I'd venture to guess that a fourth of my fat loss clients over the years have thought they had some type of metabolic disorder that was preventing them from losing weight. Numerous studies have shown this not to be true. The culprit is a simple case of people eating more and exercising less than they think.

In one study, researchers examined the discrepancy between the actual number of calories consumed and exercise performed and the reported number of calories consumed and exercise performed by obese subjects who were struggling in their weight loss endeavors. The results were shocking. The researchers found that all of the participants (obese subjects who believed that they had "diet resistance") in fact had normal metabolisms.

What, then, was causing their alleged diet resistance? It turns out they were underestimating/underreporting their caloric intake by a whopping 47 percent and overestimating/overreporting their physical activity by 51 percent! To elaborate, the subjects thought that they were taking in 1,028 calories per day, but actually were consuming 2,081 calories per day. Moreover, they thought they were expending 1,022 calories per day when they were really expending just 771 calories per day. It is quite obvious why these subjects were failing to see results.

In other studies, lean subjects tended to underreport by 30 percent, and even nutritionists underreport by 20 percent. As soon as people learn how to track their calories and macros accurately, voilà!—they start making progress. If you are spinning your wheels and just guessing with regard to your caloric intake and energy expenditure, it would be a good idea to start tracking your caloric and macronutrient intake and activity levels. There are many free phone apps that you can use.

YOU DON'T NEED TO BULK UP TO GROW YOUR GLUTES

I've been helping people achieve their fitness goals for 23 years as a personal trainer, and during this time, nobody has ever said to me, "I want to be 30 pounds overweight for the majority of the year and then use extreme methods for a few months to get temporarily chiseled so I can take a bunch of pictures during the lean months and use them throughout the year, pretending that this is the way I look year-round."

Bulking and cutting started with male bodybuilders who would get down to 6 percent body fat onstage. Not only is this unsustainable, but it's not ideal for muscle-building physiology. So they'd bulk up during the off-season with the intention of packing on as much muscle mass as possible by pushing themselves year-round. When they'd diet down again, they'd usually be rewarded with a slightly better physique than the last time around.

Having worked with hundreds of professional bikini competitors, I can say with great confidence that most of them aren't getting too low in body fat to where they can't build muscle, most let their body fat get way too high during the off-season, most do not like the way they look during the off-season, and most do not train hard during the off-season and "turn it on" only when they're in prep. In short, they hate how they look during the bulking cycle and like how they look only during the latter stages of the cutting cycle.

If you genuinely love the way you look while you bulk and cut, have at it! But a better approach for the general population is to get to a body weight you're comfortable with, then stay within 10 percent of that weight and gradually recomp. This is what the vast majority of my clients did before I moved to San Diego. They trained hard year-round and looked better and better every few months. They didn't live off throwback Thursdays and flashback Fridays and could post a bikini shot any day of the week.

I'm not aware of any research on bulking and cutting. A moderate approach is just as effective as an extreme one but without the drawbacks—which include psychological distress, increased appetite, reduced insulin sensitivity, increased numbers of fat cells, and having to buy a new wardrobe.

NUTRITION AND EXERCISE STRATEGIES FOR PHYSIQUE TRAINING

I have worked with hundreds of bikini competitors, and one thing that fascinates me is the varying types of approaches they take to prep. Different physique coaches have different methods, yet each method can lead to pleasing results onstage.

Nevertheless, there are many misconceptions associated with bulking and cutting. There's a belief that when bulking, you should stick to the basics, doing less training volume and performing more compound exercises with heavier weight for lower rep ranges with longer rest periods. In contrast, when cutting, many people believe you should perform more single-joint exercises with less weight for higher reps with shorter rest periods and include more variety.

These notions are false. There will be some differences in training, but for the most part, the only necessary changes are related to diet. You need to reduce calories in a prep. Some research indicates that you should slightly elevate your relative protein intake, and cardio might increase depending on the rate of progression. I've trained several high-level competitors who did zero cardio during prep and ended up looking their all-time best—even some who competed on the Olympic stage.

If you've been training hard consistently for a long time, your strength levels will indeed change. Absolute strength on common barbell lifts will drop, whereas relative strength on common bodyweight exercises will increase. You probably won't set any squat or hip thrust PRs, but you'll become a boss at bodyweight movements like chin-ups and Nordic ham curls.

Think about it like this: what builds muscle best in a surplus maintains muscle best in a deficit. Resistance training methods for improving your physique do not need to vary much when you're bulking or cutting. There may be some merit to training in higher rep ranges or doing more isolation work or machines as a way to prevent injury. For example, my PRs in all of the main lifts have occurred when I weighed between 240 and 250 pounds. If I wanted to get fairly shredded, I'd have to get down to 215 pounds, and my absolute strength would necessarily plummet over the course of the prep. If I kept attempting to deadlift 545 pounds for 7 reps or military press 205 pounds for 6 reps, I'd eventually hurt myself.

The main point is, you don't have to switch the exercises or the set and rep schemes and rest periods as long as you're aware that strength will diminish and you know to stop the set once stellar form is no longer possible. For example, you don't need to go from doing 5 sets of 5 reps with 3-minute rest periods in a calorie surplus to doing 3 sets of 20 reps with 1-minute rest periods in a calorie deficit. You can and should hit all of the rep ranges as you diet down.

Many people mistakenly believe that they should do pure powerlifting when bulking and transition to circuit training when cutting. This is not the case. You will lose more muscle when dieting down if you abandon all of the methods that helped you build the muscle in the first place than if you stick to tried-and-true principles and strive to maintain as much strength as possible on the big lifts that suit your body best.

	GAINING/BULKING	RECOMPING/ MAINTAINING	LOSING/CUTTING
Calories	▲	Same	▼
Protein	▼	Same	▲
Cardio	▼	Same	▲
Exercise selection	Same	Same	Same
Exercise order	Same	Same	Same
Frequency	Same	Same	Same
Volume	Same	Same	Same
Load	▲	Same	▼
Effort	Same	Same	Same
Rest periods	Same	Same	Same
Rep ranges	Same	Same	Same
Tempo	Same	Same	Same
Advanced techniques	Same	Same	Same
Personal record attempts	▲	Same	▼

EAT ENOUGH CALORIES TO FUEL YOUR WORKOUTS

Remember, food fuels good workouts, so you need to eat sufficient calories to get bigger glutes. With good workouts comes more calories from the training session and more muscle damage, which requires energy to repair. Muscle damage will elevate your metabolism, and if you're training hard on a consistent basis, you will always be using up energy for regeneration. Of course, you must pay attention and make sure your workouts aren't making you lethargic by making you too sore—remember, there's a sweet spot with soreness, and too much is counterproductive. In addition, a good diet keeps your energy levels high so that you stay active throughout the day. Dieting down too aggressively or performing excessive cardio can backfire. That is, you can become run-down to the point where you lie around all day, drastically reducing your normal activity.

So, if you're trying to put on weight around your butt, don't be afraid to eat, focus on strength training, and avoid doing excessive cardio—see page 219. Although diet plays a big role in your appearance and performance, you must consider other lifestyle factors, too, such as hydration, daily activity, sleep, and stress management.

NO SUPPLEMENT IS MANDATORY FOR BUILDING MUSCLE AND STRENGTH

Many people think that supplements are magical, but in terms of importance for developing a strong, muscular, and lean physique, supplements pale in comparison to proper training, eating, sleep, and stress management. If you're eating nutritiously and getting ample sunlight, you probably don't need any supplementation. But things are rarely perfect in the real world, and supplementing can help you cover your bases; just don't expect it to work miracles.

For example, there is a ton of evidence for using creatine for strength and muscular development, but there are nonresponders to creatine, and many of my fittest clients don't take it. Like creatine, beta-alanine has a good amount of research supporting it, but it's not vital, so don't worry about taking it if you're strapped for cash or don't like spending money on supplements.

Branched-chain amino acids (BCAAs) are another supplement that has a lot of support in the scientific literature. But when you compare people who eat enough protein to people who take BCAAs, the research shows no measurable benefit. So, if you eat protein from real-food sources or drink whey protein shakes, both of which have tons of BCAAs, then BCAA supplementation won't accelerate your recovery or do any of the things it claims to do. However, if you don't eat adequate protein, then BCAA supplementation might be beneficial, which is what the maze of research suggests. My recommendation is not to spend your money buying BCAA supplements (which typically taste terrible and are rather expensive) and instead spend that money on whey protein or high-protein foods.

There are, however, circumstances in which supplementation is necessary. If you have a deficiency in a particular vitamin or mineral, for instance, supplementing can be a game-changer. For this reason, I recommend that you get blood work done regularly to see where you are. For example, I recently found out that I was low in magnesium, so I began supplementing. I noticed immediate improvements in my sleep. Many people don't get ample sunlight and are low in vitamin D, and they benefit greatly from supplementation. It's a good idea to take a good-quality multivitamin/mineral just for "insurance," but you don't have to take one every day. If you eat healthy, you can take one every two or three days.

Please understand that going overboard on antioxidants interferes with muscle growth and strength. Yes, that's correct: people who consume too much beta-carotene, vitamin C, and vitamin E actually sabotage their muscle-building efforts. The same goes for cold water immersion and cryotherapy and pain medication (specifically nonsteroidal anti-inflammatory drugs, or NSAIDs). Inflammation is important for neuromuscular development, and you don't want to minimize it. There's a sweet spot that maximizes your results. Too much chronic inflammation is also problematic and is characteristic of both overtraining and frailty syndrome seen in the elderly.

COLD WATER IMMERSION AND CRYOTHERAPY FOR ATHLETES

While cold therapy might not be the best for muscle growth, it can help with recovery, and it certainly has a place for athletes who train frequently. So, if you're an athlete, cold water immersion or cryotherapy might be helpful for you. But if you're more concerned with putting on muscle and you're not training multiple times a day, then it might be counterproductive.

I supplement with whey protein because I don't cook meat and eggs often enough. I'm always too busy taking on projects, like writing this book! So every morning and evening, I mix two scoops of whey protein with skim milk. This gives me an extra 100 grams of protein and helps me meet my 190-gram daily target. (I weigh 240 pounds, so 0.8 x 240 = 192 grams of protein per day.) But if I made eggs in the morning, grilled chicken for lunch, ate a steak for dinner, drank a couple of glasses of milk, and had a couple of containers of Greek yogurt per day, I wouldn't need to supplement with whey protein. I should mention here that I don't technically consider whey protein to be a supplement. To me, it's food, but I digress.

If you eat fish that is high in omega-3 fats (mainly salmon) a couple of times per week and consume walnuts regularly, then you probably don't need to take fish oil capsules. But if you're like me and you don't, then you should probably supplement with good-quality fish oil capsules. Greens powder may be a good idea, too, if you don't eat your veggies regularly.

Caffeine is another supplement worth noting. It can boost workout performance, but don't go overboard to the point where it interferes with your sleep, and don't use it as a crutch for lack of sleep. The same goes for pre-workout supplements and energy drinks; they can be a slippery slope. Of course, there are hundreds of supplements with some evidence supporting their inclusion, and in certain situations you might benefit from taking supplements like alpha lipoic acid, quercetin, pycnogenol, resveratrol, grapeseed extract, coenzyme Q10, niacin, NAC, and glucosamine or chondroitin. But know that the populations that live the longest on this planet don't take a lot of supplements. I recommend you read up on the Blue Zones (regions of the world where people tend to live the longest) and note the importance of low stress, social support, ample walking, and quality nutrition for longevity and vitality.

In summary, no supplement is mandatory for building muscle and strength. But, depending on your situation, you may benefit from taking creatine, whey protein (or other protein powder), fish oil, beta-alanine, and a multivitamin/mineral.

SHOOT FOR SEVEN TO NINE HOURS OF SLEEP PER NIGHT

Getting quality sleep is one of the most underrated performance-enhancing habits. If you're like me, you want to believe that you can get a bad night of sleep and still perform at your best. But we're lying to ourselves. There is a ton of research linking poor sleep to decreased insulin sensitivity, increased fat mass and obesity, increased rate of injury and illness, and decreased performance.

Obviously, there will be times when you don't get great sleep. During these times, you should carefully consider modifying your workouts. You also want to pay close attention to your diet. Whenever I get a bad night's sleep, I am more susceptible to eating junk food.

If you find yourself struggling to get adequate sleep, try some of these tips:

- Use white noise to block out ambient noise, such as a sound machine or fan.
- Darken your bedroom with blackout curtains or wear a sleep mask.
- Set the temperature of your room to 67 degrees Fahrenheit.
- Create a calming bedtime routine and consider meditation or guided imagery.
- Wear blue light–blocking glasses while using electronics (or stop using electronics) within two hours of bedtime.
- Go to bed and wake up at the same time each day.
- Avoid caffeine consumption at least six hours prior to bedtime.
- Get some sunlight each day.
- Consider supplements such as magnesium, melatonin, and CBD oil.

IF YOU'RE STRESSED OUT, CONSIDER TAKING THE DAY OFF OR LOWERING YOUR TRAINING VOLUME

When I got dumped by my girlfriend in college, my strength dropped rapidly. My training routine didn't change, but I was so weak because I was depressed and stressed out. The constant stress impacted my attitude, my sleep, my diet, and my energy levels and recovery. All this added up to poor training results.

If you do not see good progress in your training, perhaps it's due to stress, sleep, or your diet.

You also need to look at your program design and exercise selection. You might think you're doing everything right, but in fact, you may be doing too much or not enough. If you believe your lifestyle and diet are optimized, consider reducing or increasing your training volume or simply designing a new program to keep experimenting.

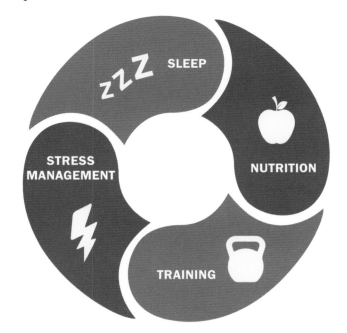

EXERCISE VARIETY AND INDIVIDUAL DIFFERENCES

Throughout this book, I've hammered home the importance of exercise variety and individual differences, so I won't go too in-depth here. Consider this section a brief recap and summary.

TO MAXIMALLY DEVELOP YOUR GLUTES, YOU NEED TO HIT THEM FROM EVERY VECTOR WITH A VARIETY OF LOADS AND TEMPOS

In Part 5, I cover hundreds of exercise variations. I did this because I want to give you as many options as possible and because—as I covered in Part 2—you need to hit your glutes from a variety of angles to ensure maximal development. Sure, you can probably get 80 percent of your potential glute gains by performing glute-dominant exercises (beginning on page 304) that stress the muscle fibers at shorter muscle lengths, but the remaining 20 percent might come from quad- and hamstring-dominant exercises that stress the muscle fibers at longer muscle lengths.

In the next chapter, I cover the Rule of Thirds (see page 198), which provides a template for programming exercise, load, and effort variety. To learn how to target your glutes from every load vector, refer to Chapter 10. In Part 5, you will learn how to perform all of the different exercise variations, as well as learn more about how different exercises work your glutes in slightly different ways, which ensures optimal development.

CHOOSE EXERCISES THAT YOU ENJOY DOING AND FEEL GOOD

It's important to figure out which exercises you like and dislike so that you enjoy the process of training. They all work, but it's up to you to figure out what works best for you through experimentation and practice. As long as you're following the guidelines outlined in this chapter and you take into consideration all of the program design variables provided in Chapter 12, you will be able to design a program and select exercises that are well suited to your goals and individual needs.

VARIETY IS ESSENTIAL, BUT YOU SHOULD PRIORITIZE THE EXERCISES THAT WORK YOUR GLUTES THE BEST

When it comes to glute development (or muscle development in general), I could make a convincing argument for performing only your top glute exercises, as well as for performing a variety of glute exercises.

For instance, say there is a glute exercise that targets your entire gluteal region, meaning it targets your upper and lower glutes to a high degree. Let's also assume that you tend to get hurt easily, you have a history of injuries, and other exercises consistently cause you problems. In this case, prioritizing one exercise is not a bad idea, especially if you're getting the results you're looking for.

I can also make a case for performing a variety of exercises, even if you feel your glutes activate more with one particular exercise over all others. Remember, different exercises stretch and activate the muscle fibers in unique ways. And it's nearly impossible to stretch and target all of the muscle fibers with one exercise. For example, one exercise might be better at hitting the upper subdivision than another exercise.

You shouldn't just vary the exercises; you should vary the loads, too. Heavier loads may work the type II muscle fibers slightly better, whereas lighter loads might be slightly better at hitting the type I fibers. Exercises that stretch the glutes, like lunges and squats, might be better at creating muscle damage, especially in the lower subdivision of the glutes, while exercises like the hip thrust and glute bridge are better for creating mechanical tension and metabolic stress.

Because there's no research on variety in training involving the glutes, I can't say with any degree of certainty what the best practice is, so I have to use my best judgment. It's definitely an interesting concept to ponder, however. One study compared variety versus just the squat for quad development. Interestingly, total quad hypertrophy was similar between the groups that performed only squats and the group that performed a variety of exercises. But when the researchers looked at the individual regions within the quads, the variety group displayed better results. Obviously, we need a study looking at the glutes to make definitive conclusions.

Here's what I can say, though: if you feel good when performing one particular lift and you tend to get hurt when you perform other lifts, then you might see better results by sticking to that one exercise that doesn't beat you up and working on getting really strong and fit at it. As I discussed, if you're hurt or in pain, you will not develop your glutes maximally. Pain inhibits muscle activation, which diminishes the results you will see from your training. You may see 80 percent of your results from that one movement, while the other 20 percent comes from variety in rep ranges, loading patterns, stance setups, and so on.

While variety may be important, you must know how to go about it. What you absolutely do not want to do is go to the gym, aimlessly throw together some exercises at random, and go through the motions. You want to perform some big movements that feel right for your body first, and you want to stick with those for several weeks at a time, utilizing a progressive approach and aiming to set PRs. Then switch to new exercises and variations (or just new set and rep schemes or tempos) and repeat the process of setting a baseline and trying to go up in weight, reps, or sets for a few weeks. The latter portion of the workout can be more random and based on feel. In other words, you shouldn't try to set records and utilize progressive overload on every exercise in the workout. After you've gotten the big stuff out of the way, you can have some fun, focus on quality and not quantity, and really home in on feeling your glutes and utilizing the mind-muscle connection with higher rep ranges and less rest time between sets.

In the next chapter, I discuss all of this in much greater detail. You will learn about program design variables and how each plays a role in creating a safe and effective individualized training program. You will learn the best methods for determining training frequency, structuring a workout, selecting exercises, and much more.

HOW TO ACHIEVE YOUR
BEST PHYSIQUE

IMPORTANT ✓

- Choosing 6 exercises to progressively overload that feel good and combine to work your entire body
- Being flexible with your diet and eating nutrient-dense foods roughly 85% of the time
- Training hard 3 to 5 times a week for 45 to 90 minutes
- Training consistently year-round while fluctuating training stress
- Building a proper foundation of form and range of motion for each exercise
- Enjoying your program and adjusting it based on biofeedback
- Consuming an average daily number of calories that aligns with your goals
- Consuming 0.8 gram of protein per pound of body weight spread out over 3 or more feedings per day
- Staying in eustress (beneficial stress) and out of distress (negative stress)
- Feeling recovered from your workouts
- Getting good sleep (quality and quantity)

NOT IMPORTANT ✗

- Doing every exercise imaginable—even ones that don't feel right
- Rigidly sticking to a training plan that doesn't feel right
- Training through instead of around pain
- Training to failure on every set
- Training hard 52 weeks a year
- Getting sore, feeling the burn, getting a pump, and feeling exhausted after every workout
- Doing tons of cardio year-round
- Being overly restrictive with your diet and fighting cravings at all costs
- Hitting precise macros every single day
- Eating 6 to 8 meals a day
- Getting protein within an hour of your workout
- Taking a lot of supplements

Program Design Variables

Once you understand the fundamentals of optimal strength and physique training—how to create goals, move with good form, train around injuries and pain, manage diet and lifestyle, and account for individual differences—you can start getting into the particulars of program design.

As you will learn, designing a program can't be boiled down to a one-size-fits-all, cookie-cutter approach. To make any program work, you need to take into consideration eight program design variables. Those variables are the focus of this chapter.

LOAD

Load is the weight you use. If you're performing a bodyweight exercise, then your body weight is the load. If you're lifting a 135-pound barbell, then the weight of the barbell (plus the plates) is the load. You can also use a percentage of your one-rep max (1RM), which is referred to as *relative load.*

As you become proficient with an exercise, meaning that you can execute the movement with good form, it might be a good time to start adding load. It's especially important to add load to the main lifts, which for glute training are the hip thrust, squat, and deadlift. However, you don't necessarily need to focus on lifting as much weight as possible with just the barbell variations. You can work on getting stronger at bodyweight, machine, band, dumbbell, and kettlebell exercises as well.

If you train long enough, however, you will reach a point where most bodyweight exercises are too easy. Unless you want to perform hundreds of reps of each exercise, adding load, even if it's just a little bit of resistance, is necessary to maximize strength and, to a lesser degree, muscle growth.

LIGHT VERSUS HEAVY LOADS

You might recall from Chapter 8 that lifting heavy is not mandatory for hypertrophy. As long as you utilize good form, train hard, and go close to muscle failure, you can build muscle just the same as if you were lifting heavy.

However, there might be a small benefit to lifting heavy. It may be only a 5 percent advantage, but that's a lot if you're an advanced lifter. And it's different for everyone; some people might benefit more or less from going heavy than others based on their genetics, anatomy, and training goals.

For instance, if you have relatively long femurs or relatively short arms, you will have to lean forward more when you squat and deadlift, respectively, which might put more stress on your lower back. Or, if you have poor hip flexion mobility, you might round your back as you deadlift. This is not necessarily a bad thing if you're keeping the weight light, but going heavy in this situation puts a ton of compressive and shear forces on the structures in your lower back, which increases your chance of injury. In this sense, going heavy might hurt your hypertrophy gains. If there are lifts that don't feel right when you go heavy (meaning you can't do more than 5 reps) but feel fine when you go light, then you will see better results by staying light and performing high reps to failure. For example, you may find that heavy squats and deadlifts aren't good for your body, but heavy hip thrusts and leg presses are fine. Everyone must experiment to figure out the lifts that suit their bodies best.

Having said that, I believe that you can and should go heavy on the lifts that feel good for you. In addition to improving strength and hypertrophy, it gives you strength goals to shoot for. What's more, if you're trying to improve your strength, heavy loading is essential. There's a skill and specificity component, so you need to lift heavy and follow the progressive overload method (see page 102). If you want to get strong at squats, for example, you have to program heavy squats.

In general, I believe there is an advantage to programming a combination of loads in your training—see the Rule of Thirds section later in this chapter. However, the added benefit is probably very small. This is purely theoretical and depends largely on the individual, but you could probably stick to a range of 8 to 12 reps—which would be medium to heavy weight—and reap around 95 percent of your hypertrophy results. So, if your goal is simply to put on muscle, then you can basically pick the rep ranges and loads you like most, as long as you're pushing some of your sets close to muscle failure.

FINDING YOUR SWEET SPOT

Whether you're lifting heavy or light, the key is to find your sweet spot with loading where you get maximal glute activation. For example, you might feel your glutes activate higher when you barbell hip thrust with 185 pounds, but any heavier and you start to feel it more in other areas, like your quads or hamstrings. In such a situation, you might consider working within your sweet spot and then every once in a while venturing out and adding a little bit of weight for variety.

In most cases, this approach will increase your sweet spot rep range. For example, let's say you can perform 8 barbell hip thrust reps with 185 pounds, and you mix in one heavy day on which you perform 2 or 3 reps with 225 pounds. After a few weeks, you might notice that you can perform 10 to 12 reps with 185 pounds because you're a little bit stronger, pushing your sweet spot to 190 or 195 pounds. And remember, even if you're not feeling it in your glutes when you go heavier or lift outside your sweet spot, you're still working your glutes. You're just not feeling it as much because your quads and hamstrings are also working hard to carry out the task.

LOAD AND TRAINING FREQUENCY

Load is also important when determining your optimal training frequency. For example, some exercises induce a lot of overall fatigue and muscle damage when you lift heavy: performing a heavy back squat, deadlift, or even barbell hip thrust can wipe you out, which affects how often you can train. In other words, if you're lifting heavy every time you exercise, you might be able to train only once or twice a week because the heavy load is taxing your body. Conversely, if you use lighter weight and perform more reps, you might be able to train three to five days a week. Although high reps are actually more damaging to the muscles than low reps, heavy weight is more damaging to the joints because form deteriorates more. This scenario rings true especially for those who struggle to keep their form solid on the big lifts when they work in low rep ranges.

TEMPO

Tempo is your cadence. More specifically, tempo encompasses the amount of time it takes you to lower the weight, the amount of time you spend in the bottom position, the amount of time it takes you to raise the weight, and finally the amount of time you spend in the top position. So there are four timed phases. For example, a typical tempo for squats and deadlifts is two seconds down, no pause at the bottom, one second up, and no pause at the top. This is noted as 2/0/1/0. Sometimes you tinker with tempo by prolonging (accentuating) the lowering phase or pausing at the bottom or top position.

Different lifts tend to have different inherent tempos based on their strength curves and range of movement. For example, because a hip thrust is easier at the bottom of the lift, you can lower and reverse it more quickly. Common tempos for the hip thrust are 0.5 to 1 second on the way down and 0.5 to 1 second on the way up. People typically do 10 reps in under 15 seconds (unless they're purposely slowing down the negative phase or incorporating a pause at the top). So hip thrusts are usually around 0.75/0/0.75/0. It's strange to use decimals with tempos, but we have to do it if we want to represent how an exercise is done in the real world.

To learn more about tempo and the various strategies you can implement, flip to Chapter 13.

REST PERIODS

Rest periods refers to how long you rest between sets. Typically, you rest longer for bigger lifts, 2 to 3 minutes being the general recommendation for lifts that focus on progressive overload (the barbell hip thrust, squat, and deadlift). You can shorten your rest periods to 30 to 60 seconds toward the end of a workout when you're focusing on metabolic stress (pump and burn). In other words, rest longer when you're focusing on quantity and rest less when you're drilling quality.

Although 2 to 3 minutes is the general recommendation, there are times when you might vary your rest time depending on what you're doing. For example, if you're going for a one-rep max, then you might rest for 5 minutes, whereas if you're performing a burnout or trying to get a pump, you might take brief rests of about 20 seconds.

I typically rest for 2 minutes or longer for heavy lifts at the beginning of a workout. Sometimes I'll rest for up to 10 minutes if I'm going for a big PR. As I progress through the workout, my rest periods get shorter, especially toward the end, because I'm focusing on the mind-muscle connection and trying to get a pump and feel the burn (metabolic stress). If I'm performing frog pumps or lateral band walks, for example, I might rest for a minute or less.

Two minutes of rest is a good reference point, but you still want to listen to your body, meaning that you may need a shorter or longer rest period depending on your capacity to recover. There's a great study on this concept. One group rested for exactly 2 minutes after each of 3 sets of various upper and lower body exercises, while the other group listened to their bodies and chose their own rest periods. Both groups performed 3 sets with the same weight, but the group that chose their own rest periods had different rest splits. For instance, one participant may have rested for 2 minutes 13 seconds after the first set and 1 minute 45 seconds after the second set.

What's interesting is that the group that selected their own rest times finished a similar number of reps but took less time.

So, if you're wondering what the right amount of time is, 2 minutes is a good guideline. If you're going heavy, the idea is to fully recover before starting your next set. Sometimes this may require 3 to 5 minutes depending on how strong you are and how quickly you naturally recover. If you're going for a pump or burn, then a full recovery is not necessary; you can shorten the rest time to 1 minute. Whether you're lifting heavy or going for reps, your body will let you know when you're ready for the next set if you're paying attention.

EXERCISE SELECTION

Exercise selection refers to the exercises you choose to include in your program. The exercises you select should match—you guessed it—your goals, experience, anatomy, and injury history.

For example, if your goal is to build your upper glutes, then the idea is to select exercises that target the upper glutes, like hip thrust, back extension, and hip abduction variations. If you're primarily concerned with building your lower glutes, then you want to select exercises that primarily target the lower glutes, like lunge, squat, and deadlift variations. This holds true for all areas of your body. You want to choose exercises that target the region you're trying to develop and strengthen. Similarly, if you play sports and want to develop speed and power, then you need to select explosive movements like squat jumps and employ banded hip thrusts because you can perform these movements with speed.

In addition to evaluating your goals, you have to experiment. When I start working with clients, I throw a lot at them in the first few training sessions and then pay close attention to their feedback. This is how I determine which exercises they like and, equally important, which exercises are well tolerated. If I'm working with a client who is new to lifting weights, I generally start with body weight and dumbbells, introduce the different stances, and then layer on more advanced variations.

For instance, say I have a client who wants to strengthen their hamstrings, glutes, and erectors and improve their deadlift. In such a situation, I might take them through the good morning variations. First, I'll introduce the basic technique and stances. If they can perform the movement with good form and enjoy doing it, I will experiment with banded good mornings and then move on to the barbell variation, eventually adding plates to the bar. Conversely, if they don't like the good morning, it doesn't align with their physique goals (maybe they have overdeveloped erectors), or they have a history of lower back pain, then we won't do it.

The real question is, how do you find the best exercises for you? As I said, this requires a ton of experimentation, not only with different exercise variations but also with different loads, stances, setups, and postures. You might stumble upon a little tweak to your form that works for you and nobody else, which you can figure out only through experience and testing.

You can try to narrow down the exercise category that works best for you by using a couple of experiments. In a perfect world, you could walk into the gym, get hooked up to an EMG device, and put yourself through a bunch of different exercises to determine what gives you the most activation in the upper and lower gluteus maximus subdivisions. Because that is not possible, I recommend trying the prone bent-leg hip extension and the standing glute squeeze and then assessing by feel which exercise activates your glutes more.

The idea is to use the mind-muscle connection to determine which position gives you more activation. You can also use palpation, simply feeling with your hands to determine where your glutes activate more in these two positions.

If you get a higher level of glute activation with the standing glute squeeze, perhaps straight-leg exercises like back extensions and reverse hypers are better for your glute development. If you get a higher level of glute activation with the prone bent-leg hip extension, then hip thrusts, glute bridges, and quadruped hip extension exercises might be better for your glute development.

PRONE BENT-LEG HIP EXTENSION

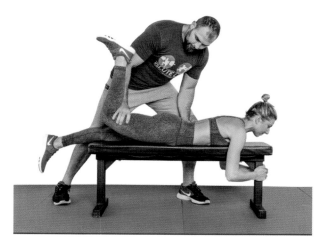

Lie facedown, bend your leg, and then extend it upward while your training partner or coach manually pushes down on your lower hamstrings. If you don't have a partner, simply extend your hip upward as high as possible and squeeze your glute as hard as you can.

STANDING GLUTE SQUEEZE

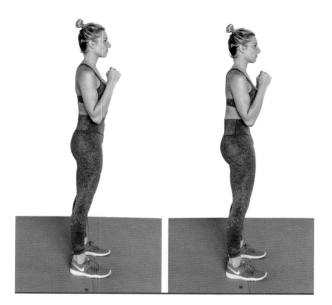

Stand upright with your feet slightly wider than hip width apart and slightly turned out, then squeeze your glutes as hard as you can.

SEVEN STRATEGIES FOR DETERMINING EXERCISE SELECTION

Here are seven ways in which lifters, coaches, and scientists can determine which exercises are best for the task at hand:

1. Exercise Performance: Do a few hard sets of the exercise with different levels of resistance and see where you feel the exercise working and at which ranges it produces the most tension and metabolic stress. (See if you get a pump and/or "feel the burn.")

2. Biomechanical Analysis: Consider the various muscle origins and insertions, the lines of pull on the muscle fibers at various joint angles throughout the range of motion, the number of joints and total muscles involved, the torque angle curves of the involved joints, and so on.

3. Functional Analysis: Consider the movement pattern, load vector, number of limbs utilized, muscles worked as prime movers and stabilizers, type of resistance, level of stability and support, system center of gravity, muscular transfer through the core, muscular transfer through the feet, kinetic chain type, multiplanar stabilization requirements, similarity to sport actions, "joint-friendliness," coordination requirements, requisite levels of joint mobility, and so on.

4. Muscle Palpation: Use your hands to feel the muscles on yourself or another person throughout the exercise.

5. Delayed-Onset Muscle Soreness: Do a bunch of sets and see where you feel sore in the next couple of days.

6. Feedback: Analyze what other lifters, coaches, trainers, and athletes have to say about the exercise.

7. Research: Read acute (e.g., EMG) and/or longitudinal (e.g., training) studies on the exercise.

Ideally (I know I keep bringing up this gluteal utopia, but please bear with me), so many mechanistic and training studies would be conducted on every exercise that we'd have review papers and meta-analyses to inform us as to exactly how the exercise works biomechanically, how it transfers to everyday life and sport performance, how the body adapts on a neuromuscular level as a result of performing it, and how best to prescribe it in terms of program design variables. Unfortunately, we don't have enough studies to be confident one way or another. Until we know more, we have to blend the available forms of aforementioned evidence and formulate an opinion using an evidence-based approach.

FINDING THE PERFECT GLUTE EXERCISE

In theory, a perfect glute exercise would meet the following criteria:

- The exercise has to fully stretch the glutes in a deep hip flexion position while slightly adducting and internally rotating the legs (think of a curtsy lunge). This is impossible to accomplish with both legs simultaneously, so the exercise would have to be unilateral.

- You need to be able to externally rotate and abduct your hips as you move them into extension.

- Your knees must stay bent to somewhat remove your hamstrings from the equation and maximize glute activation.

- You need to keep fairly constant tension on your glutes through the full range of motion—meaning you don't have a period of unloading where it's markedly easier at the bottom and harder at the top (like a hip thrust) or easier at the top and harder at the bottom (like a squat).
- The exercise must be comfortable, convenient, stable, and easy to coordinate, control, and progressively overload over time.

The problem is, you can't combine all of these elements to form one exercise. I've tried using biomechanics to figure out the perfect, all-encompassing glute exercise, but I don't think it's possible. It's hard to scientifically engineer an exercise based on theory. We usually learn the other way around: we find the best exercises in the gym and then try to better understand their utility using biomechanics.

There is no one perfect exercise for glute development because it's impossible to stretch, pump, and activate the glutes to the highest degree with just one movement. Though the hip thrust might be the best all-around glute exercise, it's not perfect because elements are missing, such as stretching the glutes through a full range of motion under tension, which is better accomplished with squat and deadlift variations. This is yet another reason why you need to perform a variety of exercises to ensure that you hit all of the muscle fibers and stress your glutes from all angles.

As mentioned previously, the best way to figure out the optimal glute exercises for you would be to conduct a thorough EMG analysis of your glutes by putting yourself through 100 different exercises and experimenting with different postures and stances to find the exercises and positions that elicit the highest EMG ratings (activation). Then I'd program and prioritize the exercises that activated your glutes to the highest degree and omit the ones that didn't. This would be the ideal method for customizing a program. I've had incredible success using this exact process with my real-life clients. Unfortunately, this approach is not possible for the masses, and I'm aware of no such company that offers this service.

So here's what I recommend instead. Use the mind-muscle connection model, in which you consciously think about the muscle being worked, and experiment with different stances, pelvic positions, postures, and ranges of motion to find the movement patterns and variations that give you the most glute activation. Put simply, you have to feel it out. You can also feel or have someone else feel the muscle and communicate which variations create the most tension in the muscle, but this requires some skill. My most advanced clients with the greatest gluteal development have unique ways of performing their favorite exercises, which is another way of saying that they take the time to figure out what works best for their particular anatomy.

EXERCISE SELECTION AND TRAINING FREQUENCY

The exercises you choose to perform highly influence how often you can train your glutes. For example, exercises like squats, weighted lunges, and Bulgarian split squats create more muscle damage and typically leave your glutes very sore. This soreness might limit how often you can train because if you're beat up, you can't train as frequently. Similarly, if you perform a number of sets of heavy deadlifts, you'll feel like a truck hit you the next day, which would affect your training frequency. If you did only heavy squats, deadlifts, lunges, and good mornings, you might be able to train your glutes hard only once or twice a week.

Then there are movements like hip thrust and glute bridge variations that maximize glute activation but don't leave you beat up or as sore the next day. Banded variations and hip abduction exercises also fall into this category. If you're doing a lot of glute-dominant movements, you can probably train more frequently because you're not too sore to train. If all you did was glute-dominant variations and banded exercises, you might be able to train your glutes three to six days a week and be just fine.

How many exercises you can perform per training session also depends on your training frequency, or how often you train your glutes. For example, if you train your glutes five days a week, you can't or shouldn't perform as many exercises as you could if you trained your glutes only two or three days a week.

Most people train their glutes three days a week, so I recommend around four exercises per training session, and I follow the Rule of Thirds: one or two horizontal exercises (hip thrust and glute bridge variations), one or two vertical exercises (squat and deadlift variations), and one or two lateral/rotary exercises (hip abduction or hip external rotation).

This gives you a lot of options. One day you might perform two horizontal exercises (single-leg hip thrust and back extension), one vertical exercise (goblet squat), and one lateral/rotary exercise (knee-banded seated hip abduction), and then the next day you might perform one horizontal exercise (barbell hip thrust), two vertical exercises (Bulgarian split squat and single-leg Romanian deadlift), and one lateral/rotary exercise (side-lying hip abduction). Note that one session involves a transverse plane hip abduction exercise and the next session involves a frontal plane hip abduction exercise.

If you're training more than that—say, five days a week—then you might choose only three exercises per session. And if you're training less than three days per week—say, just once—then you might choose six exercises per session. But again, in my experience as a lifter and a coach, three days a week seems to be best. (More on this shortly.)

EXERCISE ORDER

Exercise order refers to how you sequence the exercises in your workouts. What's programmed first in a workout gets the best results. So, as a general rule, you want to prioritize the exercise or area that you want to improve first. For instance, if you have a glute imbalance or a weak area that you need to strengthen, you should prioritize and work just the weak side first. Otherwise, I recommend prioritizing your primary lifts, which might include barbell hip thrust, squat, and deadlift variations.

After the primary lifts, I recommend accessory work. This could include anything from upper-body exercises to single-leg variations, or maybe just another variation of the hip thrust, squat, or deadlift. For example, if you hip thrust first and that is your priority for the day, then you might choose a bilateral or unilateral squat or deadlift variation next.

Typically, you want to do high-rep or metabolic stress training (training for the pump and burn) as a finisher. For burnouts, I love performing hip abduction exercises, frog pumps, back extensions, and reverse hypers, but you can get creative and use the exercises and methods that you feel and enjoy the most. To learn how to construct your own burnout workouts, flip to page 213.

Here's what a typical glute workout might look like:

Sample Workout Exercise Order

Primary Lift	Hip Thrust 3x10
Accessory Work	Single-Leg RDL 2x10, Back Extension 3x30, Walking Lunge 2x20
Burnout	Knee-Banded Hip Abduction 30 seconds, Standing Kickback 30 seconds, Lateral Band Walk 30 seconds, Knee-Banded Supine Hip Abduction 30 seconds, Banded Glute Bridge 30 seconds, Banded Half Squat Isohold 30 seconds

VOLUME

Volume is the number of hard sets you perform, usually measured on a single-workout or weekly basis. It can be considered per muscle group (for example, weekly glute volume) or per lift (for example, weekly squat volume).

Like all of the other program design variables, determining how much volume you can handle depends on how often you train, your genetics, the exercises you perform, how hard you push yourself, and a number of other factors.

For example, if you perform 30 sets in one training session, which is a ton of volume, you might be able to train your glutes only once or twice a week. But if you perform just 15 sets in one session, then you might be able to train your glutes three days a week. Many years ago, I coined the phrase "not all volume is created equal." This is obvious if you lift weights. On the systemic front, deadlifts will beat you up much more than lateral band walks, and from a muscular standpoint, lunges will beat you up more than glute bridges. Accommodating resistance such as bands and chains can be carried out for more sets than using straight weight on the bar because it's not as challenging in a stretched position. And you can perform more volume with exercises that work less overall muscle mass and with exercises that stress short versus long muscle lengths.

If you're looking for a general guideline to follow, then 16 total hard sets per workout—hard sets representing compound exercises performed to or close to failure—is a good upper limit. But you want to split up the sets among different exercises. Unless you're trying to get stronger at a certain lift, you should perform 3 or 4 sets of each exercise.

In other words, I would rather see someone perform 3 sets of 5 exercises or 4 sets of 4 exercises than 5 sets of 3 exercises or 6 sets of 2 or 3 exercises, because each exercise hits you from a unique angle and targets different muscle fibers.

Proponents of high-intensity training (HIT) will wrongly tell you that HIT is the best method for building muscle because you're performing one all-out set per exercise. But they are right about one thing: we know that you get your best exercise stimulus from your first set. Probably 80 percent of your results come from that first set, with each subsequent set delivering diminishing returns. So you can see how some people might think HIT is an optimal way to build muscle. And a lot of studies show that you can get great results from training that way. It's definitely the most time-efficient method for muscle building. However, virtually all bodybuilders and bikini competitors perform high-volume training with multiple sets per exercise. What's more, my friends Brad Schoenfeld and James Krieger have published meta-analyses showing better growth from performing multiple sets. (See page 97 for evidence-based training guidelines for hypertrophy.)

My personal belief is that you should perform multiple sets and then throw in a high-intensity workout from time to time if it's something you enjoy. Sometimes it's fun to perform one all-out set of 6 to 10 glute exercises each because the overall volume is kept low, but you get in a high-quality set for each lift. This can be beneficial because, normally, when you get to certain lifts, you're fried.

But this isn't the case when you perform only one set of an exercise. I have some of my clients train in this manner, but they train with higher frequency. For example, they might perform one all-out set of 6 glute exercises per day and train 5 or 6 days a week, which comes out to 30 to 36 total weekly sets of glute exercises. Close-minded individuals would never consider this a viable method. However, even though no particular session is high in volume, you get in all of your volume throughout the course of the week—and this is high-quality volume with no "junk" sets. This strategy isn't in line with my Rule of Thirds model, but it seems to work very well for certain people. You have to experiment and be open-minded about different training strategies if you're going to figure out the best system for you.

SET AND REP SCHEMES

When it comes to set and rep ranges—regardless of the exercise—I recommend following the Rule of Thirds, which states that one-third of your sets should be done with heavy weight between 1 and 5 reps, one-third of your sets should be done with medium weight between 8 and 12 reps, and one-third of your sets should be done with light weight over 20 reps. Like the number of reps, the number of sets you do depends on your goals and the amount of volume you can handle. In general, I recommend 3 to 5 sets unless you're performing a burnout set, in which case maybe you do only 1 or 2 sets with high reps.

I'm also a big fan of the pyramid structure. For example, you might perform a set of 10 reps, add some weight and do a set of 8 reps, add some more weight and do a set of 6 reps, and then drop the weight and do a set of 15 reps. Here are some of the set and rep schemes that we use at the Glute Lab with common exercise examples:

SET AND REP SCHEME	EXERCISE EXAMPLES
1 set of 20 reps	Squat, Hip Thrust, and Deadlift variations
2 sets of 20 reps	Goblet Squat, Kettlebell Deadlift
3 sets of 1 rep	Squat and Deadlift variations
3 sets of 3 reps	Squat, Deadlift, Hip Thrust, Nordic Ham Curl
3 sets of 5 reps	Squat, Deadlift, Hip Thrust
3 sets of 8 reps	This works well with the majority of exercises
3 sets of 10 reps	This works well with the majority of exercises
3 sets of 12 reps	This works well with the majority of exercises

SET AND REP SCHEME	EXERCISE EXAMPLES
4 sets of 8 reps	This works well with the majority of exercises
4 sets of 10 reps	This works well with the majority of exercises
5 sets of 3 reps	Squat, Deadlift, Hip Thrust, Nordic Ham Curl
5 sets of 5 reps	Squat, Deadlift, Hip Thrust, Nordic Ham Curl
1 set of 10 reps, 1 set of 8 reps, 1 set of 6 reps, 1 set of 15 reps	Hip Thrust, Leg Press
1 set of 15 reps, 1 set of 10 reps, 1 set of 5 reps, 1 set of 20 reps	Hip Thrust, Leg Press
3 sets of 20 reps	Knee-Banded Glute Bridges, Glute-Dominant Back Extensions
3 sets of 30 reps	Knee-Banded Glute Bridges, Glute-Dominant Back Extensions
4 sets of 30 to 50 reps	Frog Pumps*

*With frog pumps, we often employ even higher reps, like 2 sets of 100 reps.

Here are a few things to consider when structuring your set and rep schemes:

- As previously mentioned, the first set gives you the greatest growth stimulus, with each successive set giving you a slightly lesser stimulus.
- For building strength, keep the sets and reps at or below 5.
- For hypertrophy, reps can range from 5 to 100, with 8 to 12 typically being the sweet spot.
- Sometimes you want to perform 3 sets of as many reps as possible (AMRAP) with a particular load and strive to improve your 3-set total over time. For example, say you can do 95-pound back squats for 8, 6, and 5 reps for a total of 19 reps. In a month, maybe you get 10, 7, and 5 reps for a total of 22 reps. This is progressive overload at its finest, and it's great for both strength and hypertrophy. You can also employ high-intensity training (HIT), which involves performing 1 set to failure. To learn more about HIT and how I implement it, check out the "High-Intensity Training" sidebar on the next page.
- For strength and hypertrophy, you want a balance of low-, medium-, and high-weight reps, but you should perform your heavy lifts at the beginning of the workout. For example, you can perform a pyramid set with the following reps: 15, 10, 5, 20. You will learn more about the pyramid method in Chapter 13.
- For a pump and burn, I've found that multiple high-rep sets are ideal. So you could do 10 sets of 10 reps with a lighter load, 4 sets of 30 reps, 3 sets of 50 reps with body weight, or even a long burnout set of 100 reps. If you're working for a pump, performing more sets with rep ranges of between 20 and 50 is probably your best bet, but the ideal rep range varies according to the exercise.

In the year 2000, I stumbled across a couple of websites that promoted something called HIT. Not to be confused with HIIT (high-intensity interval training), HIT stands for *high-intensity training,* which involves performing one set to failure on a handful of exercises per session on nonconsecutive days. For the eight years prior, I'd been performing high-volume body part split training. To go from four sets of an exercise to just one set and perform fewer exercises less often seemed ludicrous, yet I couldn't stop wondering if there was any merit to this method.

I gave it a go, but I opted for two sets per exercise because I felt like I wasn't doing anything, and it was such a departure from what I was used to. I wasn't very good at doing one all-out set to failure, which I didn't realize at the time, because you don't know what you don't know.

Just like everything else, you get better with practice. After about a month, I was seeing such good results that I dropped from two sets to one. After several months, my brief workouts were brutal.

To this day, the eight-month period of HIT represents my greatest period of muscle growth and strength development. Perhaps it was the novel stimulus, or maybe I was overreaching with high-volume training and was finally recovering. Regardless of the mechanism, it worked wonders for me.

As with any program, the gains eventually tapered off, and I moved on to lower/upper splits, total-body training, and more. These days, I have an open mind with strength training and incorporate the knowledge I've gained from every system.

I meet so many lifters who will never stray from what they've done their whole lives and are so set in their ways that it negatively impacts their results. I'm not suggesting that everyone should do just one set to failure. However, many individuals would see better results if they reduced their volume, but they'll never try other methods to figure out if they're overdoing (or underdoing) it.

You have a lifetime of weight training ahead of you; don't be afraid to experiment along the way.

LESS IS SOMETIMES MORE

Far too many people are obsessed with volume. They brag about their brutal 40-set sessions but are weak and have little to show for it. In fact, most of the women who come to me for personal training are doing way more than what I ultimately program. They wonder, "How can I see results by doing less volume?" But here's the deal: even though they may be programming more exercises and sets, they are not pushing themselves sufficiently during each set, meaning that they're using volume instead of effort as their main driver.

In most cases, women who prioritize volume over effort never get stronger and plateau in their training, which is why they seek my coaching. Once they start putting more effort into their sets and resting properly, they can't do as much volume, but they see better results. The point is, volume is a good thing only if you can recover from it and continue to make progress in the gym. Most experts recommend 10 to 20 sets per week per muscle, but the glutes can handle a bit more than other muscles. Again, this is highly individualized.

HOW MUCH VOLUME PER WEEK SHOULD I DO FOR GLUTES?

Many of my clients and followers want to know how many sets they should perform per week for glutes. Again, I can't provide a blanket recommendation because, when it comes to program design, the answer depends on a number of variables. Some of my followers with amazing glute development perform just 10 sets a week, whereas others do more than 40 sets. This discrepancy has a lot to do with genetics and the other program design variables.

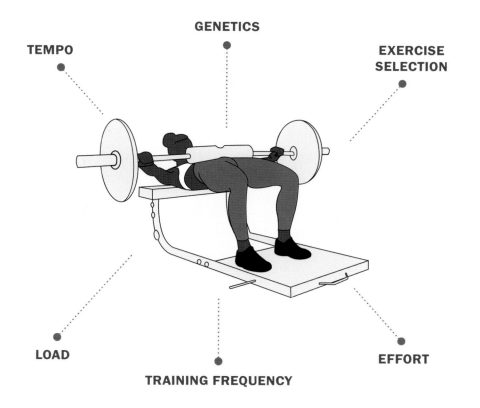

How much VOLUME per week should I do for glutes?

TEMPO

GENETICS

EXERCISE SELECTION

LOAD

TRAINING FREQUENCY

EFFORT

Perform 10 to 40 sets of glute exercises per week depending on:

- Tempo: The speed at which you perform an exercise determines volume. For example, if you stop a set and then perform additional reps in a rest-pause fashion, you can't do as many sets compared to the traditional way.

- Genetics: There is a huge genetic component to the amount of muscle damage you experience, as well as how efficiently you recover.

- Exercise Selection: Some exercises beat you up and leave you sore, while others do not.

- Effort: You won't be able to perform nearly as much volume if you carry out every set to muscle failure.

- Training Frequency: Increasing training frequency can up your volume as well, as there's only so much you can do in a given day.

- Load: Heavier loads tend to cause more form degradation and therefore greater joint stress.

EFFORT

Effort is how hard you push yourself during your sets. If you perform a set of hip thrusts to failure, meaning you can't perform another rep without compromising your form, going to failure is your level of effort. Most novices don't know how to push themselves to muscle failure; effort is a teachable and learnable skill that should be mastered over time.

Now, it's important not to confuse effort with intensity. Intensity can involve load or effort, so I refrain from using the term *intensity* when referring to effort. Effort is often measured on a scale of 1 to 10 in terms of RPE, which stands for *rate of perceived exertion,* or RIR, which stands for *repetitions in reserve.* For example, if you performed 7 reps with a load that you could have lifted 10 times, you lifted with a 3 RIR.

So, if you perform an exercise to muscle failure, then you hit a 10 RPE or a 0 RIR. Some exercises require a lot of effort and leave you sore and fatigued, while others don't. For example, if you perform a max-effort deadlift, chances are you will be crushed the next day. But if you perform a max-effort set of lateral band walks, you'll be fine. Just as load and volume affect how often you can train your glutes, your effort as it relates to exercise selection also factors into the training frequency equation.

For instance, if you're training to muscle failure with every set of every exercise, you won't be able to handle as much volume or train as frequently. But if you perform only one-third of the exercises to muscle failure and the rest of your effort is moderate to easy, then you can handle a lot more volume and train more often throughout the week. To determine how much effort you should put into your workouts during the week, I recommend that you follow the Rule of Thirds, which is covered a little later in this chapter.

FREQUENCY

Frequency can be broken down into three categories:

- **The number of times you train per week**
- **The number of times you perform a certain exercise in a week**
- **The number of times you train a particular muscle group in a week**

For example, you have your overall (whole-body) training frequency, your hip thrust frequency, and your glute training frequency.

Like all of the program design variables, determining your optimal training frequency takes a bit of experimentation. It's also important to take into account your genetics and the other program design variables, such as exercise selection, volume, load, and effort, all of which will help you determine how often you can train your glutes.

Even though genetics is perhaps the most important variable, it's an area that many strength and conditioning coaches and practitioners fail to factor into their program design strategy. Some people experience less muscle damage—this has been demonstrated extensively in the scientific literature—and can recover faster than others, and therefore they can handle more training volume. Some people get the best results from training their glutes twice a week, while others get the best results from training six days a week. This largely depends on their genetics. Obviously, knowing what you can and can't handle requires experience and practice. You have to listen to your body and tinker with different program design templates to find the best match for your genetic profile.

In general, most of the women I coach see the best results from training their glutes three days a week, but it's all relative. Let's say, for example, that 60 percent of your gains come from training once a week, training two days a week gives you 90 percent of your gains, and training three days a week gives you 98 percent of your gains. Adding a fourth and fifth training day might help you or hurt you depending on whether you can recover and feel recharged by the next training day.

If you train your glutes three days a week, you could do three similar lower-body days, or you might have one quads and glutes day, one hamstrings and glutes day, and one glutes-only day. For example, on your quads and glutes day, you would focus on squats and lunge variations; on your hamstrings day, you would focus on deadlifts and back extensions; and on your glutes day, you would focus on hip thrusts and glute bridges. And you would still be hitting your abduction work and glute burnouts toward the ends of your workouts. This is how I program for the majority of my clients who prefer adhering to body part split templates.

If you have great glute genetics, you can certainly see good results from training your glutes just once per week. But, in my opinion, two days a week is a lot better than one, and three days a week is marginally better than two.

Many people ask me if they can train their glutes every day. The answer is yes, but only if you choose exercises that don't beat your body up and you don't perform every set to muscle failure. In other words, you have to focus on the mind-muscle connection and train for the pump and burn, which typically doesn't create as much muscle soreness. For example, if you do dumbbell hip thrusts, knee-banded glute bridges, and hip abduction work and stick primarily to body weight, band, and light dumbbell and/or kettlebell movements, training your glutes every day is possible. However, if your goal is to maximize glute development and strength, this might not be the most effective approach.

As I said, three days a week is ideal for most people. You don't need to add or subtract days unless your schedule demands it or you want to switch things up. Change is not mandatory. If you have a well-designed program, you can train three days a week (or however often you decide is best for you) for the rest of your life and be just fine. Sometimes mixing it up is good psychologically because it keeps you motivated to train hard. Sometimes it's nice to train more frequently but spend less time in the gym per session, or to do the opposite and train longer, but condense your training into fewer total training days. It's nice to know that you have some flexibility with your training schedule to accommodate life's demands; you just have to adjust your volume and the other aforementioned variables to optimize your training.

The amount of time you spend training your upper body largely depends on your physique, training goals, and level of fitness. Most of the women I train who split up their workouts do two upper-body and core sessions a week. If your goal is to maintain upper-body size, then you could do just one day per week and be fine. But if your goal is to get bigger arms or gain muscle, you need to push yourself harder in your upper-body workouts and consider adding an extra day or more of upper-body sets to your weekly regimen. If you train full body, you can include a compound upper-body press and a compound upper-body pull and then throw in some accessory work, like different delt raises, at the end of the workout. You will learn more about how to incorporate upper-body training into your workouts and programs in the next part of the book.

Example Session 1 (Upper Body Only):

Pause Push-up 3x AMRAP (1-second pause at bottom)

Feet-Elevated Inverted Row 3x AMRAP

Eccentric-Accentuated Push Press 3x6 (4-second lowering phase)

Seated Face Pull 2x15

EZ Bar Curl 2x12

V-Bar Triceps Extension 2x15

Example Session 2 (Full Body):

Dumbbell Bulgarian Split Squat 3x8

Dumbbell Seated Shoulder Press 3x10

Constant-Tension Knee-Banded Barbell Hip Thrust 3x20

Underhand Grip Lat Pull-Down 3x10

Braced Single-Leg Romanian Deadlift 3x8

Seated Row 3x10

Banded Seated Hip Abduction 3x30

Lateral Raise 2x15

Front Raise 2x12

Prone Rear Delt Raise 2x12

INTERRELATIONSHIP OF VARIABLES

All of the program design variables are interrelated. To design an optimal program, you need to not only take into account all of the variables, but also understand how each variable affects the others. That is, your training frequency must jibe with your exercise selection, volume, and effort. For example, if you train two days per week, you'll have more time to recover. In this situation, you can perform full-body workouts involving mostly compound movements with around 16 total sets per session—anywhere from 10 to 22 sets is fine depending on the exercise selection and your capacity to recover—while training close to failure on each set.

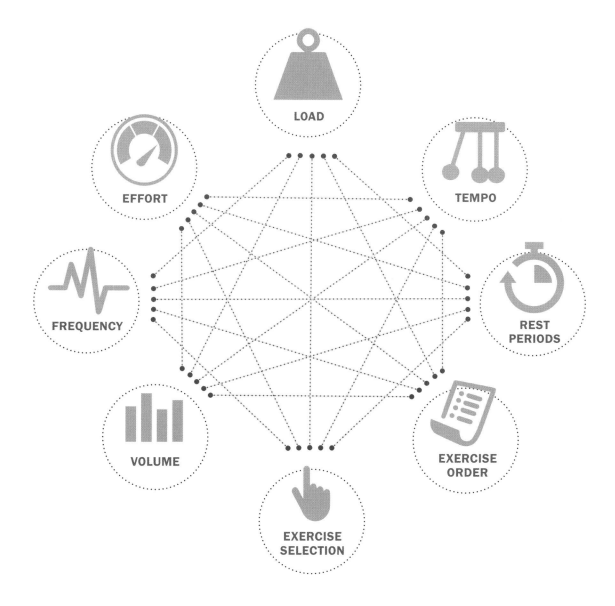

Another approach to help you determine your training frequency is to consider volume, exercise selection, and effort. For example, if you prefer to perform 30 sets per session and work your entire body hard without going heavy or quite to failure, you could hit two lower-body sessions and two upper-body sessions throughout the week and perform a variety of compound and single-joint lifts for higher reps with shorter rest periods. Just know that you need to set personal records—even if they're high-rep PRs (such as hip thrusting 135 pounds for 30 reps) or volume PRs (performing 135-pound sumo deadlifts for 3 sets of 10 reps). The point is, you can tailor your training to your preferences and still see great results by manipulating the variables. But there are still rules and margins to abide by.

Here are some more general relationships pertaining to programming. Volume is inversely related to effort: 2 sets of 8 reps with a 10 RPE is probably equal to 4 sets of 8 reps with a 7 RPE in terms of taxing the body and muscles. Load and effort impact tempo in that executing a true 1RM or the last rep of a set to failure will necessarily be relatively slow compared to a 3RM or a rep at the start of a set. Exercise selection impacts frequency in that some exercises can be performed nearly every day while others cannot.

And there's more. If you do 4 sets of heavy deadlifts (load) and to failure (effort) with each set, you'll likely be able to do it only once per week. But if you avoid going to failure, or if you take only the last set to failure, or if you reduce the number of sets to three, you might be able to do it two times in a week. But you could do 3 sets of knee-banded glute bridges close to failure four days per week and be just fine. Doing loaded walking lunges to failure four days per week would be counterproductive due to the damaging element and associated time required for recovery, but once or twice per week for 4 total sets would be reasonable.

What's more, you can't program three heavy lifts like deadlifts, squats, and barbell walking lunges with high volume and effort on the same day unless you train your lower body only once per week, for the same reason—you'll beat yourself up and risk injury during the following day's workout. You can train high frequency, high volume, or high effort, but trying to do all three simultaneously is a recipe for disaster. Something's got to give, whether it's the number of days you train per week, the number of sets you perform per week, or how hard you push each set relative to failure.

As you can see, designing a program is not as easy as it may seem. The good news is that you don't have to worry about getting everything perfect. There are many, many ways to make a program work as long as you take into account the eight program design variables. But this is easier said than done. To make designing a program easier to manage, it's helpful to use a basic template. The Rule of Thirds is the template I use for training the glutes, which I cover over the following pages. If you need a simple full-body template, use the Basic Strength Training Template that follows. And if you want more comprehensive programs, turn to Chapter 18.

BASIC STRENGTH TRAINING TEMPLATE

Many people ask me for a basic strength training template that they can easily follow. I've given this Basic Strength Training Template to my mom, my dad, and the rest of my family and friends who need a sound training program and can commit to two or three training days per week. I figure the rest of you are in the same boat—either you need it for yourself or you have friends and family who go to the gym but may not be performing well-rounded programs. This simple template ensures balance and comprehensiveness, and, most importantly, it works for everyone. But don't mistake this approach for something that's only for beginners. It also works very well for advanced lifters as long the principle of progressive overload is utilized.

Pick one hip-dominant exercise, one upper-body pull, one knee-dominant exercise, one upper-body press, and one core exercise. Perform 2 or 3 sets of each exercise in the 8 to 12 rep range and call it a day. Repeat this two or three times a week consistently, and you'll get great results.

The various categories encompass many other exercises, but I show only three of each below. Feel free to modify the exercise selection and order based on your preferences. You can also sprinkle in some single-joint exercises or burnouts at the end of the workout if you'd like.

Most people neglect certain movements and fail to train their entire bodies intelligently. Adhering to this template prevents that while allowing you to use your time in the gym wisely and focus on the most important movements.

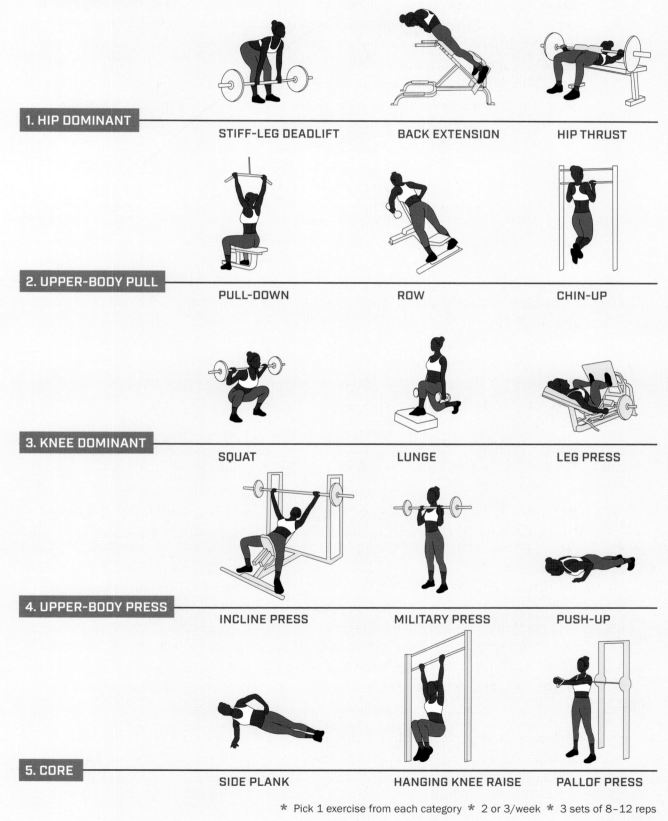

1. HIP DOMINANT

| STIFF-LEG DEADLIFT | BACK EXTENSION | HIP THRUST |

2. UPPER-BODY PULL

| PULL-DOWN | ROW | CHIN-UP |

3. KNEE DOMINANT

| SQUAT | LUNGE | LEG PRESS |

4. UPPER-BODY PRESS

| INCLINE PRESS | MILITARY PRESS | PUSH-UP |

5. CORE

| SIDE PLANK | HANGING KNEE RAISE | PALLOF PRESS |

＊ Pick 1 exercise from each category ＊ 2 or 3/week ＊ 3 sets of 8–12 reps

THE RULE OF THIRDS

When it comes to programming—as previously stated—I use a shotgun approach, which is to say that I emphasize variety in all aspects of training. I take into consideration the levels of mechanical tension, metabolic stress, muscle damage, and cell swelling in my programming for the upper and lower gluteus maximus subdivisions, which require different training methods to cover all of the bases. As the science evolves, I will start dialing in the specific methods that build hypertrophy and eliminating methods that are redundant or not fruitful. I hope that down the road I can use a rifle approach, but until then, we'll have to blast a big area, leave no stone unturned, and hope for the best results.

The Rule of Thirds ensures that your strength and physique training program is productive, efficient, and well balanced. It provides structure and organization for the program design variables and exercise selection by taking into account vector, load, and effort.

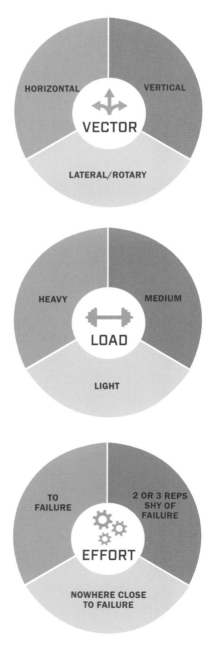

VECTOR (DIRECTION OF RESISTANCE RELATIVE TO THE BODY)

To develop your glutes maximally, you need to perform exercises from each of three vectors. Approximately one-third of the glute exercises you perform should be horizontal (thrust and glute bridge variations), one-third vertical (squat and deadlift variations), and one-third lateral/rotary (lateral band walks). To see precisely which exercises fall into each vector, flip back to page 123.

LOAD

Although you can choose your ideal loading and still get great results if your effort is high, I believe there is an advantage to programming a combination of loads in your training.

Roughly one-third of the loads you use should be heavy for low reps (1 to 5), one-third should be medium for moderate reps (6 to 12), and one-third should be light for high reps (13 to 50). If you loathe a particular rep range, you can omit it and still see excellent results as long as volume and effort are sufficiently high.

EFFORT

It's important to vary your level of effort throughout the week. Effort is a lot harder to program because it is a perceived exertion. In general, you want to push big lifts like the hip thrust, squat, and deadlift to failure or 1 rep shy of failure; accessory lifts to 2 or 3 reps shy of failure; and burnouts or banded abduction exercises nowhere close to failure. It's important to point out that when you perform high-repetition burnouts, your glutes will burn and you will feel like you're going to failure, but you're actually not. Again, *failure* means that you can't possibly do another rep. When it comes to high-repetition burnouts, you're limited by your motivation and mind, not your muscles. If you're performing bodyweight exercises or banded abduction work, for example, you could probably do another 10 reps if you really had to, but if you are performing a max-effort deadlift or hip thrust, no amount of motivation would enable you to get another rep.

Around one-third of your sets should be carried out to failure or 1 rep shy of failure, one-third of your sets should be performed to 2 or 3 reps shy of failure, and one-third of your sets should be taken nowhere close to failure. By programming your glute training this way, you will:

- Fully develop the upper and lower subdivisions of the gluteus maximus
- Fully develop the type I and type II muscle fibers
- Hit the glutes from every angle/vector and joint action, thereby transferring optimally to sports performance and functional activities
- Be able to tolerate higher workloads without accumulating excessive fatigue

Sample 1-Week Program

Here is an example of a one-week Booty by Bret program that emphasizes the hip thrust using the Rule of Thirds. As you can see, there are three full-body days and two additional glute workouts that can be done at the ends of the full-body workouts or on the off-days. There is a well-balanced mix of vertical (goblet squat and good morning), horizontal (hip thrusts), and lateral/rotary exercises (extra-range side-lying hip raise and seated hip abduction). The exercises you push to failure are the hip thrust, squat, and deadlift variations. You don't go to failure with the other exercises programmed near the end of the workout, like the B-stance good morning and single-leg Romanian deadlift, and you go nowhere near failure with the separate glute workouts. *Note:* This is a one-week program that is repeated for one month.

DAY 1	
Hip Thrust Pyramid	12/8/4/20
Military Press	10/8/6
Goblet Squat	3x8
Inverted Row	3x AMRAP
B-Stance Good Morning	3x8
Extra-Range Side-Lying Hip Raise	3x10

DAY 2	
Pause B-Stance Hip Thrust	3x6 (3-sec pause)
Close-Grip Bench Press	10/8/6
Reverse Lunge Isohold	2x 1 min
Neutral-Grip Pull-up	3x AMRAP
Single-Leg RDL	3x8
Nordic Ham Curl	3x3

DAY 3	
Hip Thrust Dropset	2x10/10/10
Push Press	3x6
Back Squat	3x5
Chest-Supported Row	3x10
Deadlift	3x3 (ramp up)
Seated Hip Abduction	2x30

GLUTE WORKOUT 1	
Frog Pump	80
Extra-Range Side-Lying Hip Abduction	30
Frog Pump	60
Extra-Range Side-Lying Hip Abduction	25
Frog Pump	40
Extra-Range Side-Lying Hip Abduction	20
Frog Pump	20

GLUTE WORKOUT 2 (DO 3 ROUNDS)	
Lateral Band Walk	20
Standing Knee-Banded Hip Hinge Abduction	20
Banded Standing Kickback	20
Standing Knee-Banded Hip Abduction	20
Standing Glute Squeeze	20

When implementing the Rule of Thirds, it's important not to obsess about your programming and make sure every week and session is in perfect balance. The idea is simply to keep your overall plan in check. In this way, the Rule of Thirds is a template that is meant to be modified.

In Part 4, I discuss how to create programs with a specific goal in mind. As you will see, I use the Rule of Thirds to help structure and organize the workouts, but I modify the overall program to focus on certain areas of training.

For instance, when I create programs that span several months or even a year, I switch the focus of the plan every 4 to 12 weeks. One month I might follow a hip thrust specialization program, which emphasizes the hip thrust 3 days a week, and the next month I might switch to a squat or single-leg specialization program. You will learn more about how to structure training cycles based on a specific goal (*periodization* is the term used to describe this programming strategy) on page 296, and I provide several sample programs to get you moving in the right direction on page 292.

Here's my point: by routinely switching up the focus of the program, you will not only get better at certain lifts and movement patterns but also avoid hitting plateaus. If you do the same exercises all the time—even if you're using the Rule of Thirds—you'll eventually get bored, and your progress is likely to stall. Most people want to get stronger at all of their favorite lifts and exercises, but you can't go up linearly forever. Once you get the basics down and move past the novelty phase, progress slows. At this stage, strength training becomes a juggling act. To get stronger and reach your physique goals, you have to focus on certain areas of your training while maintaining the other areas of your training. And you have to be strategic and utilize different methods—that is, switch up the focus of the program by emphasizing a certain lift, movement pattern, or body part, as well as implement more advanced methods.

EVIDENCE-BASED TRAINING GUIDELINES FOR HYPERTROPHY

The chart on the next page summarizes what we currently know about building muscle. It's based on hundreds of randomized controlled trials, review papers, and meta-analyses.

While we need much more research to be more certain about various topics, this table looks very different than it would have looked 10 years ago. In other words, muscle scientists—like my good friends Brad Schoenfeld and James Krieger—have done a great job of conducting meaningful experiments and expanding our knowledge base.

TRAINING GUIDELINES FOR HYPERTROPHY

⚡	**FREQUENCY**	Training a muscle group twice a week is better than once a week. There isn't much evidence in support of training more often than that except to split up volume when specializing.
📊	**VOLUME**	10 to 20 sets per week per muscle is ideal based on individual recovery. Some evidence suggests you can go higher for short periods, especially if specializing.
🎛	**EFFORT**	Most sets should be carried out close to muscle failure, but reaching actual failure is not necessary and can be counterproductive if not kept in check.
🏋	**LOAD**	All loads build muscle. Heavier loads require greater training durations and can beat up the joints, and lighter loads can be nauseating, so bodybuilders tend to prefer moderate loads. Performing a combination of rep ranges might lead to better results.
👆	**EXERCISE SELECTION**	Both multi-joint and single-joint exercises build muscle. Multi-joint moves should be prioritized in training, but you cannot neglect single-joint exercises if you are seeking maximum muscle growth, as they are necessary for building certain muscles and subdivisions.
📋	**EXERCISE ORDER**	Muscles targeted earlier in a workout will see slightly better gains than muscles targeted later in the workout, so prioritize exercise order according to your preferences.
🎏	**TEMPO**	Faster and slower tempos lead to similar levels of muscle growth, but you must control the eccentric phase and not let gravity do the work for you, and you can't do super slow reps that last 10-plus seconds. Anywhere from 2 to 6 seconds per rep yields similar results, but definitely focus on the muscle while lifting.
⏱	**REST PERIODS**	2 to 3 minutes of rest between sets appears to maximize muscle growth, but you can go by feel and listen to your body. It may be optimal to rest more for big lifts performed earlier in a workout (3 minutes) and less for smaller lifts performed later in the workout (90 seconds).
🥧	**TRAINING SPLIT**	Nearly all bodybuilders perform body part splits. However, all popular splits can be effective for muscle building. Total-body training has been shown to be equally effective for hypertrophy as body part splits.
📅	**PERIODIZATION**	Having a plan is more effective for building muscle than winging it. However, there is no single best way to periodize a program, and many methods are successful at building muscle. Strategize, but allow for some flexibility based on how you feel from day to day.

13 Advanced Training Methods

When you start glute training, you will see big gains right out of the gate with just basic programming (progressive overload and mind-muscle connection). The first couple of months are fun because you can do almost anything and see rapid results. But there comes a point when your body starts to adapt to the training stimulus; this usually happens 3 to 6 months into training. At this stage, following a loosely structured program might not be as fruitful. To overcome plateaus and ensure continual progress, you have to be more strategic. This is where advanced methods come into play.

Advanced methods are thought to maximize results by recruiting more motor units. As a quick recap, a motor unit is a group of muscle fibers recruited by the nervous system to coordinate a muscle contraction. According to Henneman's size principle, an easy task recruits the lower threshold motor units. As you get fatigued or you lift heavier weight, your nervous system recruits the larger motor units.

To maximize hypertrophy, you have to recruit all of the motor units for a sufficient period of time. Stated differently, you have to get tension on all of the different muscle fibers. And in order to do that, you have to go heavy or carry out your sets close to failure. All of these methods place more tension on the muscles by overloading a particular aspect of the lift. It's important not to abandon progressive overload using traditional straight sets like 3 sets of 8 reps. When the time is right, you'll want to sprinkle in a couple of advanced methods each month and maybe do a burnout at the end of each session. Don't go overboard, though.

In this chapter, you will learn all of the advanced methods used in glute training and how to incorporate them into your exercise routine.

CONSTANT TENSION REPS

Constant tension reps are exactly what the name implies: you create constant tension by not resting at any time during the set. Think of going up and down like a piston. You still use a fairly full range of motion on each rep, but you reverse the movement as soon as you reach end range. The reps are performed fairly rapidly, but smoothly and fluidly. This leads to high levels of metabolic stress.

In glute training, this technique is typically used with squat and hip thrust variations. With a squat, you can omit the last little bit of range of motion at the top just to keep better tension on your hips. You accomplish this by lowering into a full squat and then moving up and down with no rest at the top or bottom. With the hip thrust, don't touch the bar down at the bottom of the rep. Instead, let the bar come very close to the ground and then reverse it in midair as you work to fully extend your hips to lockout. Don't pause at the top even for a moment; just go right back down into your next rep. One rep typically takes one second to complete, so you'll get 20 reps in about 20 seconds.

In general, I use lighter loads and shoot for sets of 20 to 30 reps. I know this doesn't seem like a lot because your time under tension isn't as high as it is with normal sets, but believe me, it is brutal—like all of the advanced techniques. You'll be amazed at how much lighter you initially have to go in order to carry out a full set.

REST-PAUSE REPS

Rest-pause reps are a type of cluster set in which you perform one continuous set with predetermined rests or pauses between reps. For example, say you're hip thrusting a lot of weight. For your first attempt, you can get only 6 continuous reps (you're using a 6RM load). Instead of performing more reps with crummy form and questionable range of motion, lower the bar to the floor, pause, and take a few big breaths. This is your rest-pause moment. After a very brief recovery—maybe five breaths—perform 2 more reps and then rest-pause again. After another brief recovery, get one more. You're nearly finished, but you still have one more left in you, so you finish strong.

To summarize, instead of performing 6 straight reps, you do 6 reps, rest for around 10 seconds, then 2 reps, rest for around 10 seconds, 1 rep, rest for around 5 seconds, and then one more rep to finish. There are an infinite number of ways to perform rest-pause reps considering the number of reps and the amount of rest between reps, but at the Glute Lab, we typically stick to this pattern of 6/2/1/1 for 10 total reps when we use the rest-pause method.

ISOHOLDS

Isoholds are the same as isometric training in that you're holding a static position in a range that creates tension in the muscles. For example, you can perform an isohold at the top of a hip thrust or the bottom of a squat. You can hold the position for max time or for a predetermined period, like 30 seconds. This creates high levels of tension and generates high levels of metabolic stress while building strength primarily in the position you're holding for time. This translates to better strength out of the hole with squats and better lockout strength during hip thrusts.

I also recommend sometimes using a resistance band (Glute Loop) or using a mini band around your knees with squats and hip thrusts to create more tension in your glutes. For example, say you're squatting. By wrapping a mini band above your knees and holding the bottom of the squat for 30 seconds, you're not only increasing your hip extension strength in the position but also drilling in good form and building hip abduction strength. Normally, when you perform a movement, you're in the bottom and top position for only a second or two. But when you isolate the position, you're forced to spend time working on your mechanics in that one position, which can carry over and improve your overall technique.

At some point, every lifter needs to try the 20-rep squat routine. I did it back in the day and saw impressive results in terms of repetition strength, thigh mass, and mental fortitude.

I promise you this: after this protocol, you'll never begrudgingly perform a heavy set of lower-body training ever again. Sets of 5 and under are hard, but they don't hold a candle to 20-rep squats performed according to the protocol's standards.

How to Do It:

The 20-rep squat routine is essentially a rest-pause squat for 20 reps. Here's how it works: Take your 10RM load and squat it for 20 reps by refusing to rack the bar and continuing to produce reps in a rest-pause fashion. After the first 10 reps or so, stand with the bar on your back and rest, get another rep, and repeat—performing reps and resting accordingly—until you get to 20 reps. They're commonly referred to as *breathing squats* because you end up breathing so hard during the set.

Nineteen years ago, I increased my 20RM from 135 pounds to 275 pounds over the course of a few months. The set of 275 pounds lasted 9 minutes. Yes, I had the bar on my back for 9 whole minutes.

The first 10 reps were probably performed in one minute, and the remaining 10 reps took an additional 8 minutes. The typical protocol is 6 weeks, but I continued with it until I never wanted to perform another 20-rep set of squats for the rest of my life. (I still haven't.) Give it a shot.

It's important to mention that we don't do isoholds often because I believe that the other methods are better for growing muscle. However, isoholds are great if you are injured and can't perform certain ranges of motion for an exercise. For example, maybe you can't squat to full depth, but squatting halfway is fine. In this scenario, you can perform an isohold in the half squat position. Isoholds are also great for training weaknesses. For instance, say you're strong in the bottom of the hip thrust but have problems locking out your hips. Performing isoholds at the top where you're weak for a sustained period will help you develop strength in that position.

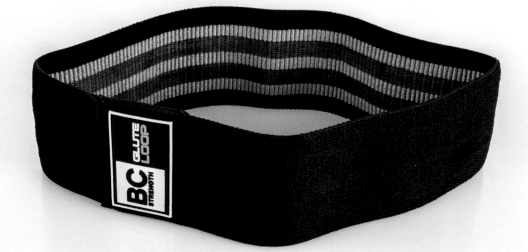

PYRAMIDS

The pyramid protocol has been around for ages and was popularized by the late Vince Gironda (aka the Iron Guru) with his 10/8/6/15 pyramid. It's a great method that allows you to hit the entire repetition spectrum for an exercise, meaning that you're performing low, medium, and high reps within one workout. This not only helps you get stronger in a variety of rep ranges but also ensures that you target all of the muscle fibers in one session.

Say you're applying the pyramid protocol to the hip thrust, for example. Here's how to approach the exercise. Warm up first, and then perform a hard set of 15 reps. Add some weight, rest for a couple of minutes, and then perform a set of 10 reps. Add more weight, rest for a couple of minutes, and then perform a heavy set of 5 reps. For your last set, reduce the weight significantly, rest for only a minute, and perform a final set of 20 reps. You might consider adding a mini band or resistance band around your knees on the last set to finish off your glutes. This is how we do it at the Glute Lab.

BC PYRAMID	
Set 1	Select a load that you can perform for around **15 reps**.
Set 2	Select a load that you can perform for around **10 reps**.
Set 3	Select a load that you can perform for around **5 reps**.
Set 4	Select a load that you can perform for around **20 reps**. *Add a resistance band or Glute Loop.

It's important to mention that there are numerous ways to set up a pyramid. For example, you could do 10, 8, 6, 15 or maybe 10, 8, 6, 4, 2, 20. The goal is to stick with the pyramid for 3 to 4 weeks and strive for progressive overload using the same load on the bar but trying to beat your reps. For instance, here is what a sample month might look like:

BC PYRAMID SAMPLE MONTH

	SET 1 225 lbs	SET 2 275 lbs	SET 3 315 lbs	SET 4 185 lbs	TOTAL REPS for the week
WEEK 1	15	10	5	20	50
WEEK 2	17	12	5	20	54
WEEK 3	18	13	7	20	58
WEEK 4	20	14	8	22	64

ENHANCED ECCENTRICS

Enhanced eccentrics require you to use a heavier load during the eccentric phase (muscle lengthening while contracting: think lowering into the bottom of a hip thrust) than during the concentric phase (muscle shortening while contracting: think locking out your hips in the hip thrust). There are several ways to do this in strength training. The first is to perform the two-legs-up/one-leg-down method. Say you're doing single-leg hip thrusts and you lift the weight up with two legs, then lower slowly with one leg.

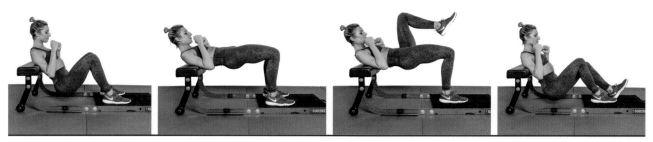

TWO UP / ONE DOWN METHOD

The second way is to use weight releasers, which attach to the end of the barbell and release at the bottom of the movement, but this method only allows you to overload the eccentric phase for one repetition. The third way is to utilize a flywheel, which is a specialized device that works like a yo-yo. And the fourth way is to have a trainer or training partner provide manual resistance on the way down during an exercise.

Using the hip thrust as an example, say you're coaching someone who is hip thrusting 135 pounds. To enhance the eccentric phase, you would lean over them and push down on the bar, which might add another 80 pounds as they lower into the bottom position. So they are lifting 135 pounds on the way up and 215 pounds on the way down. Have them reverse the movement right before the bar touches the ground so that they perform all of the work to absorb and transfer the motion.

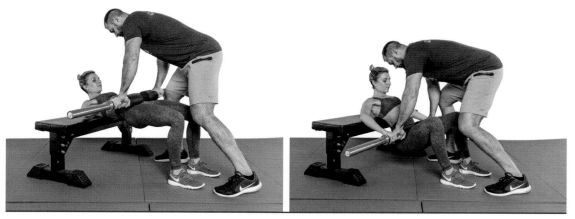

MANUAL RESISTANCE HIP THRUST

Although enhanced eccentrics are effective and great for variety, we don't utilize them that often because they are more challenging to perform, require the help of a coach or training partner, and can only be done with certain movements. So we might implement them every few weeks, and we typically do them only with the hip thrust, leg press, 45-degree hyper, reverse hyper, seated hip abduction machine, side-lying hip abduction, Nordic ham curl, leg extension, and lying leg curl exercises.

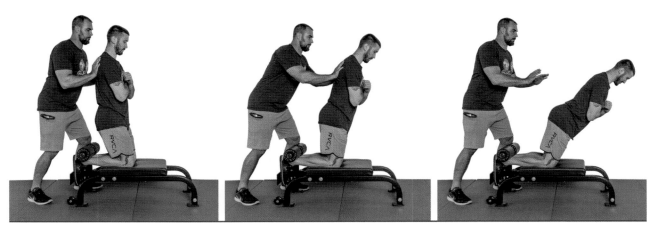

MANUAL RESISTED NORDIC HAM CURL

ACCENTUATED ECCENTRICS

With accentuated eccentrics, you slow down or accentuate the eccentric phase of a movement. For example, say you're performing a barbell hip thrust. To accentuate the eccentric phase, you extend your hips as you normally would into the top position and then lower into the bottom position very slowly. Normally, it would take you one second to lower your hips. But in this scenario, you take four to six seconds to lower the weight.

Although accentuated eccentrics offer a different training stimulus that can certainly improve strength and hypertrophy, they are especially great for training around injuries, like muscle strains or tweaks. Realize that many muscle strains are not that bad. You can still train around them, but you don't want to push yourself too hard or lift too heavy, or you risk making it worse. But with accentuated eccentrics, you can use a lighter load and still spark muscle growth because you're spending more time under tension during the all-important negative phase without exacerbating your injury.

TORQUE DOUBLING

Torque doubling involves wearing a mini band or resistance band (Glute Loop) above or below your knees while performing hip extension movements. Knee-banded glute bridges, hip thrusts, and squats are considered torque doubling techniques. Now, I know the name makes it sound complicated and technical, but I didn't know what else to call it.

You can think of torque doubling as making the glutes pull double duty. You're working your glutes through hip extension, and by pushing your knees outward into the band, you're also working your glutes through hip abduction.

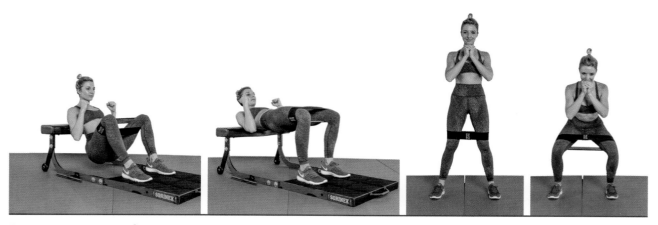

TORQUE DOUBLING (KNEE-BANDED HIP THRUST AND SQUAT)

I've found that torque doubling dramatically increases tension in the glutes. It's a great way to increase the difficulty of bodyweight variations. And if you love the glute pump and burn, then torque doubling is where it's at. Interestingly, torque doubling is unique to the glutes in that it's the only muscle where you can easily challenge two joint actions that work the same muscle simultaneously.

PULSES

With pulses, you're just moving up and down in a small range at the hardest part of the movement. For example, with a squat, you lower all the way into the bottom of the movement, come up a quarter of the way, and then go back down. You can repeat this cycle—going down and a quarter of the way up—over and over again until you have completed the desired number of reps. With a hip thrust, you come up to the top of the movement, go down a quarter of the way, and then rise back up.

My favorite exercise for pulses is the heels-elevated goblet squat. For this exercise, I like to perform sets of 30 reps. I lower into the bottom of the squat and then perform 6-inch pulses, moving up and down within that zone. You get a lot of metabolic stress, and it's a killer glute burn.

1¼ REPS

A 1¼ is a full rep combined with a pulse. We do these a lot with hip thrusts (both double and single leg), squats, and Bulgarian split squats. Using a Bulgarian split squat as an example, you go down all the way, come up a quarter of the way, go back down, and then rise up to the starting position. That's one rep.

CLUSTERS

Clusters are groups of reps with shorter rest windows. There are numerous ways to organize a cluster, but let's say you can hip thrust 315 pounds for 3 sets of 10 with a 2-minute break between sets. If each set takes you roughly one minute, then it will take you about 9 minutes to complete the exercise. To make it a cluster set, you could hip thrust the same weight, but instead of performing 3 sets of 10 with a 2-minute break, you would perform 6 sets of 5 reps with a 1-minute break. You're still performing 30 reps within the same window of time, but it's not as fatiguing.

> Typical set: 3x10 with a 2-minute break between sets
>
> Cluster set: 6x5 with a 1-minute break between sets

Although you don't build up the same amount of metabolic stress, you get the same amount of volume. This is great for a couple of reasons. For one, it's easier on your body. You're not pushing yourself to fatigue, which doesn't beat your body up as much. This makes clusters a great method for people who play sports and need to keep their bodies healthy for other activities. Second, it helps develop power. You're still working with heavy weight but keeping the reps explosive because you won't be grinding any reps out. The caveat is that it's not as good for muscle growth because you're not pushing yourself to fatigue.

DROPSETS (STRIP SETS)

To perform a dropset, you start out with a heavy weight and then drop or reduce the weight so that you can keep performing more repetitions. The idea is to perform the exercise until you are close to muscle failure with each attempt or drop. The dropset, specifically, is a method for extending your sets beyond failure.

In the Glute Lab, we primarily perform dropsets with hip thrusts, leg presses, and the seated hip abduction machine. Generally, we stick with a triple dropset, meaning you drop the weight twice for a total of 3 sets. Here's an example of what it might look like with a barbell hip thrust.

Say you start with 235 pounds—that's two 45-pound plates and four 25-pound plates. You set up the bar with four 25-pound plates because they're easy to strip off. On your first attempt, you get 6 reps. Once you reach muscle failure and can't do any more full-range reps, you lower the weight and have your training partners peel off the 25-pound plates. This is the drop. Now you have 185 pounds on the bar, and you go again immediately, lifting until you're just short of failure.

Suppose you get 10 reps for the first drop. Once complete, you lower the bar and have your partners peel off the other two 25-pound plates. There's now only 135 pounds on the bar, but you haven't rested, and your glutes are on fire. For your last set, you get 12 reps, bringing your total to 28. This is your new benchmark. Next week, try it again and strive to beat this number. It's important to mention that in this particular example, this type of set is also commonly referred to as a *strip set*.

The idea is to limit your rest time between sets. As soon as the plates are stripped off, you start again immediately with the lower weight.

If you don't have any training partners with you, you can still do a hip thrust dropset. You can either lean over and push the plates off or get up and pull them off and then get back into the starting position. You can also use bands. I like to use a thick band, a medium band, and a thin band. Like the weights, you perform the first set with all three bands, and then you take off the thick band for your second set, and then you take off the medium band for your third set. You can wear a band around your knees for torque-doubling as well.

Dropsets are also great on machines, and they're easy to perform; all you have to do is move the pin up the stack of weight. This is why they're so conducive to seated hip abductions.

Make no mistake about it: dropsets will have your glutes screaming for mercy! But they are the most efficient practice for increasing muscle size, as one all-out dropset per exercise is all you need to spark growth.

PAUSE REPS

Pause reps have you pause at the bottom or top of a movement during each repetition. For glute training, we typically do pause reps with squats and hip thrusts. With squats, for example, you pause at the bottom, when your glutes are stretched, for 3 to 5 seconds. With hip thrusts, you pause for 3 to 5 seconds at the top of the movement, when your glutes are at peak tension. You can also pause at the bottom of a hip thrust to remove the stretch reflex, which I often prescribe for bodyweight foot and shoulder elevated single-leg hip thrusts where the buttocks actually rest on the ground for a 1-second count. This method, which is also used with deadlifts, where you touch down with the barbell and reset, is referred to as *dead stop reps*. Powerlifters prefer dead stop deadlifts because they are more specific and are better suited for building maximal strength. I prefer "touch-and-go" deadlifts, where you tap down but don't reset with each rep.

If you're implementing the pause rep technique, you have to go lighter than you normally would. For instance, if you usually lift 225 pounds for 8 normal reps, you should lift only 185 pounds for 8 pause reps. I also employ pause reps to make bodyweight training workouts more challenging.

When you pause, you want to truly pause for the prescribed amount of time. In my experience, most people pause for 1 second when they are supposed to be doing 3-second pause reps, and they pause for 3 seconds when they're supposed to be doing 5-second pause reps. They count too quickly, so sometimes I add 2 seconds to my clients' pauses to ensure that they hold the position for the desired amount of time.

ACCOMMODATING RESISTANCE

Accommodating resistance involves using bands or attaching chains to the barbell to make it harder at lockout. As you rise upward, the bands stretch or the chains lift off the ground, increasing the difficulty of the movement as you reach the finish position. I love bar-plus-band hip thrusts and deadlifts, and I prefer chains with squats and bench presses. But to use bands for deadlifts or hip thrusts, you need a place to attach them. The Hip Thruster works well for this purpose, but you can also crisscross dumbbells or hook bands around the base of a power rack or machine. When using accommodating resistance, you might have 185 pounds in the bottom position and 245 pounds in the top position depending on the exercise and the amount of band or chain resistance used.

Accommodating resistance is great for producing good amounts of tension and high amounts of metabolic stress while minimizing muscle damage (because there is less loading in the stretched position).

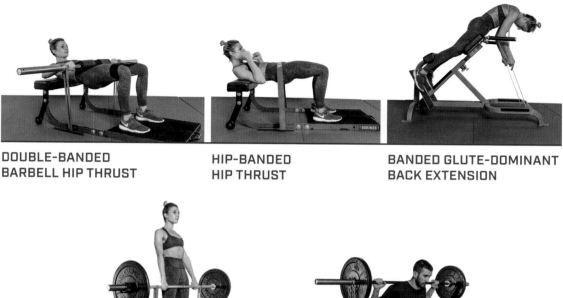

DOUBLE-BANDED BARBELL HIP THRUST

HIP-BANDED HIP THRUST

BANDED GLUTE-DOMINANT BACK EXTENSION

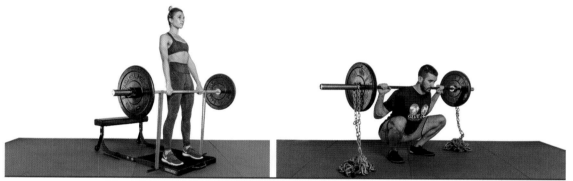

BANDED DEADLIFT

CHAIN BACK SQUAT

DYNAMIC EFFORT REPS

Dynamic effort reps are performed with lighter loads but with maximum acceleration and speed. They are not intended to build strength or muscle hypertrophy; they are used to develop power and athleticism. You can perform variations of squats, deadlifts, hip thrusts, glute bridges, and back extensions with dynamic effort. Exercises like kettlebell swings, reverse hypers (off the pendulum machine), and of course Olympic weightlifting variants like power cleans are naturally performed explosively in a dynamic effort fashion. Sled pushes can be utilized in this way as well.

It's sometimes hard to distinguish between dynamic effort reps and plyometrics/ballistics in situations where the lifter leaves the ground or projects the implement into the air. For example, if you explode in a hip thrust with maximum acceleration at submaximal loads, the bar will lift off the hips into the air. With the dynamic effort method, you keep the reps low and aim for maximum speed. So even if you could perform 20 to 30 reps, you stick to sets of 3 to 5 reps because you're striving to build power, not endurance.

LADDERS

We perform descending ladders at the Glute Lab primarily with knee-banded glute bridges and supine hip abductions. We have beginners start at 12 and work their way down, but our advanced clients start at 15. It goes like this: You perform 15 knee-banded glute bridges and then 15 banded supine hip abductions. Then 14 of each, then 13 of each, then 12 of each, until you get down to 1. You can rest as needed throughout the process, but the goal is to eventually be able to perform the whole ladder with no rest. It's brutal and develops considerable metabolic stress in the glutes. This method is generally performed at the end of a workout as a burnout.

PRE-EXHAUSTION

Pre-exhaustion is a method whereby you fatigue one muscle with a certain exercise and then perform another exercise in hopes of getting more activation out of the muscle you want to target. For example, bodybuilders would "pre-exhaust" a muscle to make sure it gets fully worked during compound movements. At least that was the original idea, but studies have shown the opposite. If you perform flies or cable crossovers prior to bench presses, your pecs don't activate more, but your triceps do. Put another way, if you fatigue your pecs and then bench press, you end up using your pecs the same and your triceps more—great if you want to target your triceps, but not if you want to target your pecs.

This is what's great about research; it gives you something to work with. After these studies were conducted, researchers flipped the scenario and found that if subjects fatigued the triceps and front delts and then did bench presses, they ended up using their pecs more. Unfortunately, there aren't any conclusive studies on the glutes. One promising study conducted on elderly subjects fatiguing the quads prior to standing from a chair did show greater glute activity. And we've been experimenting in the Glute Lab gym by having people do Nordic ham curls before 45-degree hypers, and they typically report feeling higher levels of glute activation. I also tested this idea by performing leg extensions and leg curls before frog pumps and got the biggest glute burn of my life.

What am I getting at here? All of these things have me thinking about potentiation and inhibition during resistance training. We need research to pinpoint the precise mechanisms that contribute toward these sensations. The nervous system can detect fatigue and steer neural drive to synergistic muscles. Pumped-up muscles that are engorged with blood can alter mechanics. Pre-activation can acutely increase EMG activity or diminish it if too much fatigue sets in. Simply performing an exercise before a compound lift can make that lift "feel better" by increasing body temperature and mobility. Some of this could also be due to the placebo effect.

I encourage you to experiment along these lines. If you haven't already, try performing low-load glute activation or leg curls prior to squats, deadlifts, or back extensions. Try fatiguing the hamstrings, quads, and/or adductors prior to frog pumps or glute bridges. Try performing hip thrusts last in a lower-body workout in a fatigued state with lighter loads. See if any of these tricks helps you feel your glutes more.

It's important to point out that pre-exhaustion is not to be confused with glute activation. With glute activation, you're doing low load with low reps; you're just waking up the muscles and priming them for more strenuous work.

SUPERSETS

A superset combines two exercise sets back to back. So you perform one set of one exercise immediately followed by one set of another exercise, and then you rest. Traditionally, there are two main types of supersets: agonist (primary muscle working to carry out the movement) and antagonist (opposing muscle to the agonist). With agonist supersets, you perform two exercises that target the same muscle; with antagonist supersets, you're targeting opposing muscles. An example of an agonist superset is one set of lateral band walks right into a set of goblet squats. The agonist superset is good for variety and fatiguing the muscle. An example of an antagonist superset is performing leg extensions, which target the quads, followed by a set of leg curls, which target the hamstrings.

After some experimentation in the Glute Lab, I created another category: synergist supersets. With synergist supersets, you're fatiguing the synergist (the muscle that helps facilitate the action carried out by the agonist) so that the prime mover (agonist) does more work. An example of a synergist superset is a set of Nordic ham curls right into a set of back extensions (as described in the pre-exhaustion section, opposite). The idea is that the Nordic ham curls fatigue the hamstrings, so when you perform back extensions, you feel your glutes more during the exercise.

Another popular paired superset is upper/lower. To perform upper and lower supersets, you do one set with your lower body and one set with your upper body, such as a squat set and then a set of pull-ups, or a set of deadlifts immediately followed by a set of bench presses. Notice that the exercises in these examples don't compete with each other. For example, if you paired a deadlift with a pull-up, the pull-up would be negatively impacted, as your grip would be fried. This is why deadlifts are paired with bench presses instead. As with the antagonist superset, upper and lower supersets are great for people who don't have a lot of time to work out. It's difficult to get a hard full-body workout and work multiple muscle groups in one hour, making these supersets a time-efficient strategy for people who have a small training window.

BURNOUTS

A burnout involves performing nonstop glute exercises for a predetermined period of time, say two or three minutes. We do these at the ends of our workouts at the Glute Lab, and they are brutal. They are best done with a resistance band (Glute Loop), but they can be done with body weight, a mini band, or ankle weights as well. The idea is simply to keep tension on the glutes in some capacity for two to three straight minutes by alternating through different glute exercises—see the "Burnout Template" sidebar below. For example, you might perform 30 seconds of lateral band walks, 30 seconds of knee-banded hip abductions, 30 seconds of banded glute bridges, 30 seconds of banded quadruped hip extensions, 30 seconds of banded fire hydrants, and 30 seconds of banded wall sits. These are great for metabolic stress and hitting the glutes from all angles to stimulate all of the fibers.

Though burnouts are fun and provide a good glute pump and burn, there is no evidence to support that placing burnouts at the end of your workouts does anything for muscle growth. I suspect that it plays a small role, but we don't have research or studies to back up that claim. What I can say is that people love the way it makes them feel. My clients get in their cars with their glutes still burning; it feels like they have finished off their glutes, and they leave the gym feeling like they got a great glute workout.

There are many ways to construct a glute burnout, such as ladders, timed rounds, and high-rep sets. Below, I provide a sample three-minute glute burnout template. Based on my experience, I feel that three straight minutes of work is the right amount of volume. Any more and it turns into an endurance effort; any less and it's too easy. Three minutes seems to be the sweet spot. The only piece of equipment you need is a resistance band, such as a Glute Loop or mini band.

You can perform this burnout in any order—the key is to hit each category. And you're not going for PRs, so don't bother counting reps. The idea is just to maintain good form and to try to move the entire time. If your form breaks down, take a few breaths, recover quickly, and get back to work.

3 minutes:

60 SECONDS (30 SECONDS EACH SIDE/LEG): HIP EXTENSION	
Exercise examples:	Single-Leg Glute Bridge
	Quadruped Hip Extension
	Standing Kickback

30 SECONDS: FRONTAL PLANE HIP ABDUCTION	
Exercise examples:	Lateral Band Walk
	Side-Lying Hip Abduction
	Standing Hip Abduction

30 SECONDS: TRANSVERSE PLANE HIP ABDUCTION	
Exercise examples:	Hip Abduction
	Seated Hip Abduction
	Side-Lying Clam
	Supine Hip Abduction

30 SECONDS: COMBINED HIP EXTENSION AND ABDUCTION	
Exercise examples:	Squat Isoholds
	Glute Bridge Isoholds

30 SECONDS: RANDOM	
Exercise examples:	Cha-Cha
	Standing Glute Squeeze
	Side-Lying Hip Raise
	RKC Plank
	Monster Walk

SAMPLE BURNOUT	
60 seconds	Single-Leg Glute Bridge (30 seconds each leg)
30 seconds	Lateral Band Walk
30 seconds	Seated Hip Abduction
30 seconds	Squat Isohold (hold the bottom of the squat)
30 seconds	RKC Plank with maximal glute squeeze

INCORPORATING ADVANCED METHODS

How you incorporate advanced techniques depends largely on your training frequency. For example, if you train your glutes only once per week, you should stick with straight sets (no advanced techniques) or possibly use the pyramid method, which involves performing about three sets with progressively heavier weight and then a final back-off set with lighter weight for higher reps (12, 8, 4, 20).

But if you train your glutes more frequently—say, three days a week—you have more opportunities to experiment and program many of the advanced techniques into your training. For example, you might perform hip thrust dropsets on day one, constant tension hip thrusts on day two, and maybe a single-leg hip thrust variation with pause reps on day three. The idea is to mix in a different method on each day. However, don't overload or overcomplicate your training by incorporating too many advanced methods into one session.

In my opinion, the more variety you have, the better it is for glute growth, as long as you're sticking to the same movement patterns and focusing on gaining strength on a couple of big lifts involving the glutes each month. At most, do two per day, with the last being a burnout. Although the muscle confusion concept is a bit overhyped, there are benefits to changing it up and adding variety in terms of loads, postures, tempos, and strategies.

There are so many ways to write a good glute training program, but understanding your primary goal will provide a solid template. For example, if you're trying to build power, then the methods that build power should go first in the workout. This applies mostly to athletes. If you're striving to increase strength, the methods that build strength should be placed at the beginning of the workout. Methods that build hypertrophy can be placed anywhere in the workout, but if they also build endurance, then they should go at the end. Endurance methods should always go last. Some methods can be used for multiple purposes, but the loads should vary depending on the goal. For example, if you are performing enhanced eccentrics to build strength or power, you want to perform low reps (such as 4 sets of 5 reps). But if the goal is to build hypertrophy, you can go heavy, medium, or light as long as you rep out close to failure.

METHOD	STRENGTH	HYPERTROPHY	ENDURANCE	POWER
Constant Tension Reps		*	*	
Rest-Pause Reps	*	*		
Isoholds	*		*	
Pyramids (10/8/6/15)	*	*	*	
Enhanced Eccentrics	*	*		*
Torque Doubling	*	*	*	
Pulses		*		
1¼ Reps		*		
Clusters	*			*
Dropsets (Strip Sets)		*	*	
Pause Reps	*	*		
Accommodating Resistance	*	*		*
Dynamic Effort Reps				*
Ladders		*	*	
Pre-Exhaustion		*	*	
Supersets		*		
Burnouts		*	*	

For the third and final time, I want to caution you not to get overzealous and overcomplicate your workouts by trying to incorporate more than two advanced methods per session. The reality is, advanced workout routines have not been shown to be superior to basic workout routines. Remember, advanced methods are great for keeping things interesting, making training fun, overcoming plateaus, and training around injuries, but you still need a good foundation. The basics form the foundation of every good program, and the advanced methods should be considered supplemental. In fact, I would rather you stick to a basic routine with no advanced methods and focus on pushing yourself with each set than try to come up with crazy variations and advanced methods just for novelty.

When I write programs for people, I have a goal in mind. If I'm training someone who has not mastered the art of pushing themselves to failure and they don't understand how to properly implement progressive overload, then I use the advanced methods sparingly or not at all. The bottom line is this: every exercise and method has its place, but you should never underestimate the basics.

ADVANCED ROUTINES VERSUS BASIC ROUTINES

One of the most annoying aspects of my job involves trying to convince people that "advanced" routines aren't necessarily better than "basic" ones. Trust me, if I wanted to razzle-dazzle someone, I easily could. No one is more skilled than I am at coming up with crazy variations, different tempos, dropsets, supersets, and burnouts. However, the basics form the foundation of every good program.

The routine shown at the bottom of the chart on the next page is an amazing lower-body workout. If you think that this workout is too "basic" for you, then, quite frankly, you don't know how to push yourself in the gym. Yes, it's "only" 12 sets, but if you know how to push yourself and you've built up your strength, it will crush you. A workout that combines hip thrusts, squats, and deadlifts is very demanding. Getting stronger at these lifts will build your entire lower body.

The problem is, many lifters don't know how to push themselves, don't understand how to properly implement progressive overload, and overvalue variety and novelty. As I said, I write programs for people with a goal in mind. If I write you something like what's shown in the bottom workout, it's because I want you to build your compound bilateral strength. If your coach prescribes something similar, don't second-guess. Don't get me wrong, the top workout is great, too, but it's not necessarily better than the basic workout.

Pause Single-Leg Foot-Elevated Hip Thrust (3-sec pause)	3x8
Dumbbell Deficit Curtsy Lunge/Step-Down Machine Superset	3x12/8
Single-Leg Sideways Leg Press Dropset	2x20/20/10
Lateral Band Walk/Knee-Banded Hip Abduction Superset	3x20/20
Cable Kickback 21s*	2x7/7/7
Rounded Back Extension	2x30
Knee-Banded Glute Bridge	3x30

"ADVANCED" ROUTINES HAVE NOT BEEN SHOWN TO BE SUPERIOR TO "BASIC" ROUTINES

Barbell Hip Thrust	3x8
Back Squat	3x6
Stiff-Leg Deadlift	3x10
Seated Hip Abduction Machine	3x20

*7 bottom half partial reps, 7 top half partial reps, 7 full-range reps

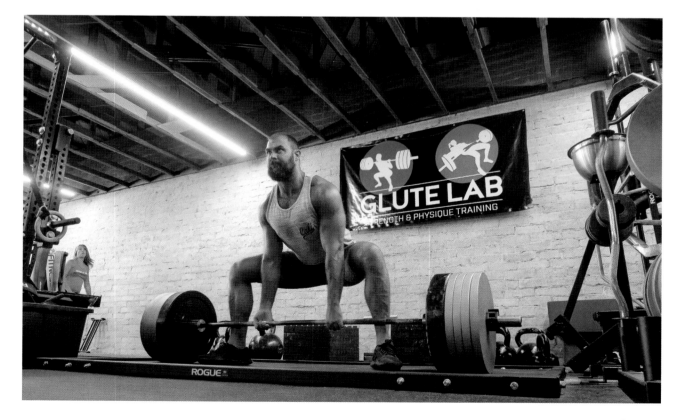

14 Troubleshooting Solutions

Everyone makes mistakes and encounters barriers in training. I've been lifting for nearly three decades, and I still make mistakes and face problems that flatline my progress. The great thing about making mistakes and hitting obstacles is that it provides valuable insight. You learn what you're doing wrong, how to correct it, and more; you also learn unique strategies for dealing with specific problems, such as recovering from an injury. The point is, obstacles and setbacks provide opportunities for growth. The process of overcoming obstacles is how we turn weaknesses into strengths.

In this chapter, I summarize the most common mistakes people make with glute training, such as performing only squats or doing excessive cardio as a strategy for optimizing glute growth. I also provide simple guidelines for overcoming common obstacles in training. You will learn strategies for training around and recovering from specific injuries and excessively sore muscles, conquering training plateaus, and minimizing gluteal imbalances.

In addition, I offer troubleshooting solutions for the most common glute training hurdles: getting started, being strapped for time, being too embarrassed to hip thrust, and not having access to equipment. (*Note:* I covered the most common form-related faults in the previous chapter, and I address specific technique errors alongside the exercises in Part 5.)

Lastly, I address some of the most frequently asked questions pertaining to glute appearance and physique training, such as how to grow your glutes without growing your legs and waist, whether certain aesthetic features like hip divots and cellulite can be corrected, and how to train through pregnancy.

It's human nature to seek an easy way out. But I'm here to tell you that the easy way out is, more often than not, a justification that creates guilt. And that guilt is harder on your psyche than just putting in the work. As you will learn, it's better to find the solution, which this chapter provides, than to let your excuses or lack of knowledge get in the way of your progress.

THE MOST COMMON GLUTE TRAINING MISTAKES

Even if you know how to train your glutes optimally, it's helpful to know what not to do so you can avoid making errors that might negatively impact your training goals. And if you're a trainer or someone people look to for training advice, knowing what not to do is even more important, because people will ask you if they can do certain things, and it's up to you not only to steer them in the right direction but also to educate them as to why certain training strategies are not productive and fruitful. Glute training has come a long way in the last decade, and I've learned a lot. Here I outline the most common mistakes that I see people make and that I have made in the past and explain why they're not ideal for maximizing glute training results.

MISTAKE #1: JUST SQUATTING

As you've learned, squat variations work the glutes in a unique way in that they stretch the glutes while under tension. Stated differently, you get maximal glute contraction at the bottom of a squat when the glutes are fully lengthened, which hits the lower subdivision of the gluteus maximus. For this reason, squats (and deadlifts) are a primary movement pattern that is essential for developing the glutes.

But here's the rub: if all you're doing is squatting, you'll never develop your glutes to their full potential. Squat variations don't work the upper glutes that much, they don't produce a lot of metabolic stress, and they don't get you maximal glute activation. You might recall from Part 2 that bent-knee hip extension movements such as the hip thrust and glute bridge activate the glutes maximally and target both the upper and lower subdivisions. This makes them, along with all of the other glute-dominant exercises, more effective at developing and strengthening your glutes than just squatting.

MISTAKE #2: TRAINING THE GLUTES ONLY ONCE PER WEEK

Many people think they can train their glutes once a week and get great results. If you've been lifting properly for a while and have built up your glute strength, you might be able to maintain what you have, and if you're genetically gifted, you might even see slight gains. But for most of us, and for those who want bigger, stronger glutes, one day a week won't cut it. The glutes are large and robust muscles that can take a beating. For the best results, you need to train your glutes at least twice a week, with three days probably being optimal for the vast majority of people.

MISTAKE #3: NOT DOING ANYTHING FOR THE UPPER GLUTES

This ties in with Mistake #1. If all you do is squat, deadlift, and lunge, you're primarily working your lower glutes. To work your upper glutes, as well as your upper and lower glutes combined, you need to perform glute-dominant movements such as glute bridges, hip thrusts, kickbacks, pull-throughs, and abduction variations.

MISTAKE #4: NOT DOING ANTEROPOSTERIOR (HORIZONTALLY LOADED) GLUTE EXERCISES

If you want to develop your glutes maximally, then you need to perform horizontally loaded exercises like the glute bridge, hip thrust, and 45-degree hyper. These exercises produce a ton of tension and metabolic stress, keep your glutes under fairly constant tension throughout the movement, and strengthen the zone of hip extension range of motion that maximizes activation, which is important.

MISTAKE #5: THINKING THAT CARDIO WILL YIELD GOOD GLUTE DEVELOPMENT AND WEIGHT LOSS

Make no mistake: cardio is great for your heart and overall health. However, people think they need to do cardio (cycling, running, swimming, elliptical training, stair climbing, and so on) to burn fat and lose weight, but in truth, you mainly just need to follow a good resistance training and diet plan. (Remember, diet is the key factor that determines whether you're gaining, maintaining, or losing weight.) Sure, cardio can help, especially if it blunts your appetite, but if you can stick to your diet and create a calorie deficit by eating less while still training hard, you'll lose weight. In other words, cardio as a weight loss strategy is highly overrated. You might notice that doing cardio helps you lose weight, but it might not be the cardio; it could be the effect that cardio has on your appetite. It can either make you hungrier or decrease your appetite, depending on your genetics and the type of cardio you perform (such as HIIT training; see sidebar, opposite). And there's more: people overestimate how much cardio helps with fat loss because they believe the monitors on the machine are accurate. But they are not accurate, especially if you are already lean. The monitor might say you burned 800 calories when you actually burned only 300.

But enough about fat loss. How effective is cardio for building the glutes?

If you're training your glutes as I outline in this book, it's not necessary to perform cardio for your glutes. Now, if you're a novice or a sedentary person, you may experience some glute growth in the first few months of doing cardio. But if you're an advanced practitioner or you've been training for several months, especially if you're following my system, then you will not get any additional glute growth from doing cardio.

It's important to realize that cardio pulls from the same overall recovery pool as glute training, meaning that you're accumulating physical stress. If you're trying to condition your body for endurance efforts, cardio is necessary because it's sport and task specific. If you're training for overall health, then doing cardio is beneficial. But if you're hitting the stair stepper hard in hopes of growing your glutes, you're wasting your time. You're better off focusing on resistance training and doing cardio that you enjoy and doesn't interfere with muscle development, such as walking.

When it comes to strength and conditioning, you can't be the best at both. In other words, you can be very strong and conditioned, or you can be strong and very conditioned, but it's hard to be very strong and very conditioned. So you'll never squat the most weight and run your best marathon at the same time. This implies that training for multiple qualities can compete with one another. Scientists have coined this the "interference effect." While you shouldn't be afraid of performing some cardio, doing too much can hamper your glute training gains.

If you're hell-bent on doing cardio, you simply enjoy it, or you're getting the results you desire, then I recommend prioritizing your strength workouts first and then doing your cardio afterward. But understand that too much cardio will likely interfere with your glute growth. For example, if you go for a long, hard run, chances are you will get fatigued and potentially sore. And if you're drained and beat up, you can't hit the weights as hard.

Here's what I want you to understand: Cardio does burn more calories than lifting weights, but lifting weights builds and maintains muscle, whereas cardio doesn't. So, if you're striving to lean out and you want bigger, stronger glutes, cardio isn't mandatory. It is useful and necessary if you are concerned only with losing fat and you don't want to maintain or put on muscle. But remember this: You need to lift weights to maintain the muscle you have underneath the fat. If you enjoy doing cardio and cardio suppresses your appetite, you might benefit from lifting weights and then doing cardio afterward. But if you want to get lean, you need to keep your muscle and lose just fat for weight loss. This is best achieved through intelligent weight training and proper nutrition.

MISTAKE #6: ENGAGING IN HIGH-RISK TRAINING ACTIVITIES

Although the glutes are highly involved in activities such as plyometrics, sprinting, and most sports, doing these activities is not the best way to develop your glutes. Again, resistance training reigns supreme for building muscle. The best glutes in the world are almost all built by placing maximum tension on the muscles (strength training), something that cannot be said of sprinting and plyometrics, since the contractions are too fast for the muscles to generate maximum force. Resistance training is also safer to perform and more predictable. But allow me to elaborate.

It is true that sport training builds some glute muscle (but doesn't maximize it) and improves the functioning of the nervous system in terms of recruiting the gluteal muscles. Athletes who have played ground sports (think soccer and football) but have never lifted weights tend to see results much quicker than people who don't have athletic backgrounds. This is largely due to the fact that they have developed proficiency in utilizing the glutes explosively from all of the aforementioned vectors (vertical, horizontal, lateral, and rotary). In contrast, beginners who haven't played a lot of sports haven't developed the motor patterns and mind-muscle connection because they haven't been using their glutes in their training.

But let's say I'm working with a beginner who never played sports or did much of anything athletic—or even a former athlete whose goals have switched to aesthetics and maximizing glute development. In these situations, I don't recommend sprinting, jumping, or dynamic training due to the risk of injury. Strength training is the best way to build muscle due to the slower speed of muscle contractions. The slower contraction in weight lifting produces maximum tension on the muscle and therefore leads to greater hypertrophy.

If you're an athlete and you're training for performance and function, on the other hand, then explosive and plyometric training is necessary, not because you're trying to build muscle but because you're trying to get better at your sport (think speed, power, agility, and coordination).

FACT VERSUS FALLACY

If you enjoy doing cardio and engaging in activities like core training, HIIT (high-intensity interval training), and stretching, then by all means have at it. Cardio is good for your heart, stretching is good for your mind, and it's good to have strong abs.

But it's important to realize that strength training does all of this and more. For instance, resistance training is a form of HIIT. It burns fat, reshapes your body, and is great for your heart. What's more, resistance training is a form of loaded stretching, which increases flexibility. And nice abs are achieved by having low body fat levels, which are mainly influenced by your body composition and diet. Remember, abs are made in the kitchen and glutes are made in the gym.

The point is, for physique purposes, strength training is the cake and the rest is the icing on the cake. And you can go overboard with the icing and interfere with the taste of the cake. If you do too much cardio, stretching, or core work, you might compromise the positive adaptations that straight training produces, so you have to prioritize accordingly.

FACT VERSUS FALLACY

MISCONCEPTIONS:

REALITY:

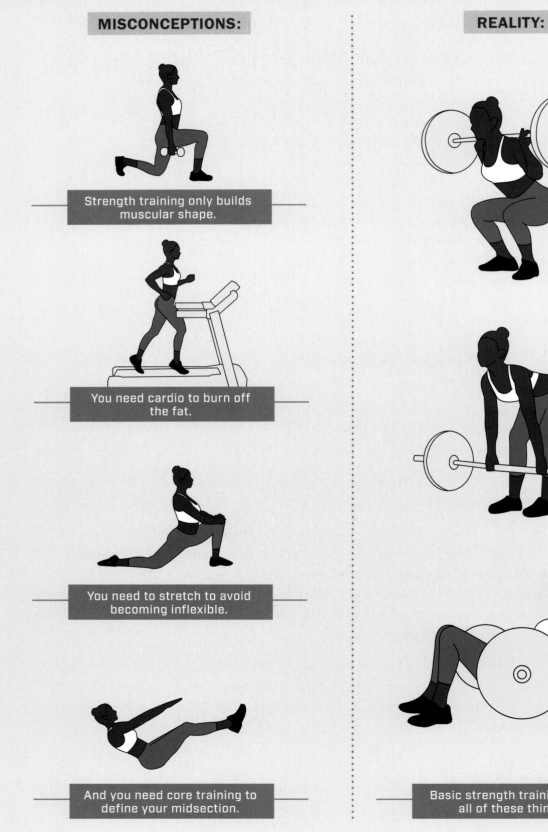

Strength training only builds muscular shape.

You need cardio to burn off the fat.

You need to stretch to avoid becoming inflexible.

And you need core training to define your midsection.

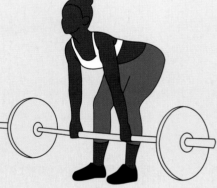

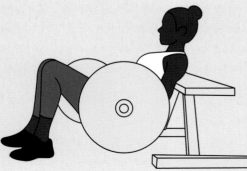

Basic strength training does all of these things.

MISTAKE #7: NOT HAVING FUN

If you're not having fun with your training, then you will have a hard time staying consistent. Adherence is the name of the long-term game, and you won't stick with your training if you don't enjoy it. Find the exercises and program design that you enjoy the most and avoid exercises and training routines that you loathe. It's that simple.

TRAINING AROUND DISCOMFORT AND SORENESS

If you train hard day in and day out, issues will arise within your body. It's unrealistic to assume that you will always feel perfect, especially if you're chasing strength goals. Most of the people I know who have trained progressively for years (myself included) always have something they need to train around. To stay on track with your goals, you can try many different strategies, such as working on your form, reducing your training volume, improving your sleep, decreasing your stress levels, doing more foam rolling or stretching, trying corrective exercises, or improving your hydration (to mention a few ideas).

However, it's important to point out that if you are injured, you may need to take special precautions and follow a strategic protocol to improve and accelerate your recovery. I cover the difference between being hurt and injured, as well as how to shorten the recovery window following a serious injury, in the pages to come. What I want to convey here is that if you have a minor tweak or you are sore in one area, chances are you can train around the discomfort without making the problem worse.

The key is to listen to your body and make the necessary adjustments based on how you feel. In some cases, you should rest and take some time off to heal. In other cases, you can train around the issue and be fine. It's impossible for me to tell you one way or the other unless I'm working with you one on one. Put simply, only you or your coach can determine what you can and can't do based on the level of discomfort and soreness you're experiencing.

It's important not to get discouraged. Think of training around soreness and discomfort as a learning experience. First, you learn which exercises are damaging, which exercises are well tolerated, how often you should train, and how much volume, load, and effort you can handle. Second, you learn new techniques and training strategies as a result of training around issues. You're forced to do something different—something you're not used to doing—and inevitably you will stumble across new or neglected techniques that are actually great for you.

Assuming you're not too banged up or at risk for injury, don't use discomfort or soreness as a crutch not to train, because you might find an exercise or training method you enjoy that you otherwise never would have done.

BACK ISSUES

It is very likely that at some point during the year, your back will hurt—maybe your lower back is fried from a long flight or a heavy deadlift day—but you still want to train your glutes. In this situation, you might want to consider sticking with bodyweight exercises like deficit reverse lunges, step-ups, or Bulgarian split squats and exercises that don't fire up your back musculature too much, like knee-banded glute bridges, frog pumps, and abduction variations.

It's important to realize that different mechanisms are responsible for back discomfort. Issues may arise from your lower back, or your back could be perfectly fine but your nervous system is sending out false alarms. In other situations the pain may stem from your SI joint, in which case hip abduction exercises might exacerbate the problem. Again, you need to listen to your body and figure out which movements you can perform without discomfort.

You have to tinker around and figure out what you can and can't do. I wish I could provide a universal, concrete list, but I can't, because back soreness is subjective and unique to each individual. Most people tolerate the above-mentioned exercise examples well, but it's up to you to figure out your ideal protocol. Sometimes all you need to do is tweak an exercise or use a slightly different stance, posture, or exercise variation.

HIP ISSUES

For the majority of people who have hip discomfort, deep hip flexion (bottom of the squat) is the primary culprit. Sometimes full hip extension (top of the hip thrust) bothers people, but this issue is much rarer. This situation doesn't leave you with a ton of options, but you can still perform partials or limited-range-of-motion movements. For example, you might be able to squat or bridge through the mid-range portion of the movement. You can also perform isometric holds, like wall squats, and of course abduction movements that feel okay. Sometimes you just have to change up your stance or posture, and the issues clear up right away. You can also use this time to focus on leg strength by performing leg extension, leg curl, and Nordic ham curl variations.

KNEE ISSUES

Like back discomfort, training around knee issues largely depends on where you feel the soreness. If you have pain around the front of your knee, which is sometimes related to your quads, there's a good chance that you can perform abduction exercises and straight-leg hip hinging variations like 45-degree hypers. If you have pain around the back of your knee, however, you should probably steer clear of straight-leg hip hinging variations and focus on high-rep knee-dominant exercises like goblet squats, along with abduction movements that don't cause you problems.

In general, when you have knee discomfort, you want to avoid knee-dominant exercises like squats, lunges, step-ups, and Bulgarian split squats and focus either on techniques that don't require a lot of knee motion or on single-joint techniques for the hamstrings, such as stiff-leg deadlifts, Romanian deadlifts, lying leg curls, glute ham raises, Nordic ham curls, back extensions, and reverse hypers. In some cases, you can still do feet-elevated bridging, frog pumps, and thrusting variations.

ANKLE AND FOOT ISSUES

Sprained or sore ankles and injured feet are quite common, especially if you are highly active and play sports. If you have an ankle or foot injury, you can still perform open-chain glute exercises such as quadruped hip extension and side-lying hip abduction movements. Athletes I've worked with are often amazed at how great of a lower-body workout I can give them even if they have injured themselves during their sport. Other open-chain glute exercises include cable kickbacks, cable hip abduction, and reverse hypers. Often, back extensions and bridges can be performed without discomfort as well, and in some cases Romanian deadlifts or box squats may be tolerated.

EXCESSIVELY SORE GLUTES

If your glutes are super sore, then you need to back off and give your body a chance to recover. Excessive soreness tells you that you did too much. You're not going to spark growth when you're overly sore. You can, however, train other areas of your body. This might be a good time to do some isolation work on your legs, like leg extensions or leg curls, or maybe do an upper-body day. Or perhaps you can just go for a long walk in the park and get some extra sleep so you can resume your normal training the following day.

EXCESSIVELY SORE ERECTORS

If you overdid it with deadlifts, good mornings, or even squats, you might end up with excessively sore erector muscles. To train around the soreness, try high reps of the following exercises using just body weight or holding onto light dumbbells: walking lunges, step-ups, Bulgarian split squats, and single-leg Romanian deadlifts. Depending on how sore you are, you might be able to perform glute bridges and frog pumps, as well as lateral band work and other abduction exercises.

EXCESSIVELY SORE ADDUCTORS

The adductor muscles usually get sore from different squat and lunge variations, but you can probably still perform squats, deadlifts, and hip thrusts with a very narrow stance. You can also do partials, meaning that you perform only the top half of the movement, such as a high box squat with a narrow stance. Another option is to focus on upper-body training and perform isolation leg exercises like leg curls and leg extensions, as well as lateral band work and other abduction exercises. Knee-banded glute bridges tend to work well in this scenario, too.

EXCESSIVELY SORE QUADS

If your quads are smoked, the squat movement pattern is pretty much off the table, which includes all double-leg squat variations and single-leg variations like lunges, split squats, pistols, and step-ups. The hip thrust ties in quite a bit of quads, so hip thrust variations should also be avoided. But you can still train your glutes and posterior chain. All hip hinging exercises, like deadlifts, Romanian deadlifts, back extensions, swings, reverse hypers, good mornings, and pull-throughs, work the glutes without targeting the quads. You can also play around with feet-elevated bridging patterns (elevating your feet transfers tension from your quads to your hamstrings), kickback variations, lateral band work, and abduction exercises for the upper glutes.

EXCESSIVELY SORE HAMSTRINGS

If your hamstrings are sore, you want to avoid hip hinging movements and single-joint knee flexion exercises that target your posterior chain. This means no leg curl or deadlift variations. Your hamstrings are also involved in hip thrusts and glute bridging, so knee-dominant squatting movements performed with an upright torso, like heel-elevated goblet squats and front squats, are excellent options. Short-stride single-leg variations such as lunges and Bulgarian split squats are great, too. You can also perform an ample volume of lateral band work and abduction exercises.

RECOVERING FROM INJURY

It's important to realize that there is a difference between being hurt and being injured. When you are hurt, you can still exercise. You might have to train around the site of pain, but you can still train. For example, say you experience discomfort stemming from a minor tweak or an excessively sore muscle. As you just read, training around discomfort and soreness helps you stay consistent in the gym and may even open your eyes to new techniques and training strategies. More importantly, the problem tends to go away quickly without special treatment.

When you are injured, on the other hand, you might have to abstain from training altogether, and you should employ certain protocols to accelerate the healing process. For example, say you experience a severe muscle strain, joint sprain, or bone fracture. Depending on the nature and location of the injury, you might be able to perform certain exercises and train around the pain, but doing so won't dramatically improve your situation. In short, training around the injury doesn't do much to accelerate healing at the site of the injury, which is typically drawn out over several weeks or months.

So the question is, what strategies can you implement that will shorten your recovery window after you sustain a serious injury?

Fortunately, I endured a severe glute tear while writing this book. I've never heard of anyone tearing their glutes, and there are no studies or literature on glute tears, which turned out to be a blessing in disguise because it forced me to come up with my own approach using the best scientific practices. Although the protocol I implemented—which I outline over the coming pages—was focused on rehabilitating my glutes and getting me back to training as quickly as possible, the strategies and methods I used can be applied to any type of injury. First, I'll explain how the tear happened, and then I'll describe what I did to accelerate my recovery and retain as much strength as possible as my body healed.

As with most injuries, my body was trying to tell me that I was not at 100 percent. I could feel a flu coming on, but I wanted to train my glutes, so I ignored those signals. I did a light glute workout consisting of two sets of bodyweight back extensions, frog pumps, extra-range side-lying hip abductions, and machine seated hip abductions. In hindsight, I should have taken the day off, because when I woke up the next morning, not only was I sick, but I also had a hard lump spanning laterally across my upper left glute. Over the next 10 days, I couldn't do any training due to illness. When I started feeling better and was ready to train again, the swelling in my glute still hadn't subsided, but I tested the waters and found that I could squat and deadlift without pain. I did two leg workouts and ended up sumo deadlifting 585 pounds with ease, leading me to believe that whatever was going on in my glute would be fine. Then it happened.

Two days later, thinking my glutes were good to go, I did two sets of hip thrusts on the Nautilus Glute Drive. Immediately after finishing my second set, I knew something was off. I was in pain and couldn't walk properly. Over the next several days, my left glute swelled to what seemed like double its normal size. Realizing that something was seriously wrong, I got an MRI, which showed a severe tear in the upper gluteus maximus with a giant hematoma and hemorrhaging.

What's interesting is that squats and deadlifts were fine because they work the lower glute max, but hip thrusts were not because they work the entire glute. If I had trained intelligently around the minor strain that had occurred just before I got sick, I probably would have been fine. But I decided to push through the discomfort and hip thrust, which ultimately caused the injury.

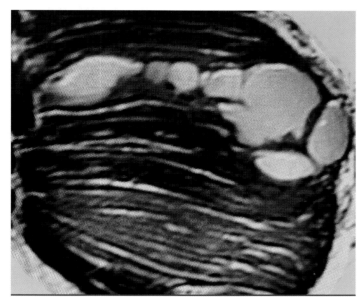

MRI IMAGE OF MY TORN GLUTE

Although tearing my glute was unpleasant, I say that it was fortunate because it forced me to examine and put into practice evidence-based protocols that not only shortened my recovery window and helped me retain strength and muscle size but also enabled me to strengthen my mind-body connection. Having gone through the protocol, I feel more in tune with what is going on in my body post-injury than I was pre-injury. It's hard to quantify the efficacy of the protocol, but according to the medical feedback that I received from doctors, 12 weeks is the standard recovery time for the type of injury I sustained, and I was back to full strength in less than six weeks. Here's what I did and what you can do, too, should you experience a serious muscle strain injury.

MENTAL IMAGERY TRAINING

Mental imagery training has been used for ages as a tool for improving performance. Think of a musician visualizing hitting all of the notes, a golfer imagining the perfect putt, a combat athlete mentally chaining together techniques, a public speaker envisioning every aspect of a speech, or an athlete picturing a flawlessly executed lift. In every example, the person visualizes in their mind the action they want to polish. These mental repetitions have been shown in the research to be almost as effective as physically performing the action; you're activating the same part of your brain as if you were actually doing it.

When it comes to strength training and exercise, there are two mental imagery strategies. The first is a supplement to training for performance and usually involves compound and more technical lifts. For example, visualizing yourself over and over completing a max-effort squat the week before a powerlifting meet or a clean and jerk before an Olympic weightlifting meet might increase your chances of successfully completing the lift.

The second strategy is centered around maintaining strength and function while you are injured. For example, visualizing yourself performing workouts while you are immobilized might accelerate your recovery and minimize or prevent muscle atrophy. With this strategy, you can imagine strength training workouts and actual muscle contractions such as those that occur during single-joint exercises or when flexing the muscle as hard as possible isometrically.

You can visualize in the first person or the third person. When you visualize in the first person, you imagine yourself performing the action through your own point of view. When you visualize in the third person, you imagine yourself or someone else doing it from an outside perspective. According to the research, visualizing in the first person gives you better results; some estimate that it's three times more effective than third-person mental imagery. However, there is research showing different nervous system adaptations between the two. For this reason, the general recommendation is to do it both ways, even though first person has been shown to be more effective.

When I tore my glute, I prioritized first-person mental imagery training and then supplemented with short periods of third-person visualization as I progressed through the protocol. Here's what I did.

First, I set myself up for success by lying in a dark, silent room. Having eliminated all external stimuli that might distract my focus, I pulled my attention inward. I pictured myself in the gym going through the motions as if I were actually working out. I imagined the situation as vividly as possible. I grabbed my energy drink, turned on all of the TVs in the Glute Lab, cranked up the music, and got warmed up. Then I started my workout:

Hip Thrust	3 sets of 10 reps
Squat	3 sets of 10 reps
Lunge	2 sets of 12 reps
Back Extension	2 sets of 12 reps
Seated Hip Abduction	1 set of 20 reps

Even though the entire training session took place in my mind, I tried to make it as detailed as possible, from loading the weights, setting up in the right position, and executing each movement to imagining the muscles contracting during the exercise and resting between sets. I braced and breathed the same way I would when performing each exercise and imagined the feeling of finishing a hard set. Initially, I was immobilized, so I wasn't maximally contracting my muscles or moving my body, but just by imagining the resistance, my muscles activated to a small degree. By the time I finished, I was sweating, my heart rate was elevated, and I felt like I had done an actual workout. The best part is, the entire drill took only 10 minutes because I wasn't resting for long periods between sets. (I let my mind rest for only about 20 seconds between sets to allow my brain to "recover" and maximally focus.)

I did this mental imagery training every day during my recovery, slowly working up to a 12-minute and eventually a 15-minute session employing both first- and third-person visualization. After about a week, I could implement small amplitude movements into the mental imagery training. From a kneeling position, I'd move my torso and hips through a small range of motion while I imagined myself doing the workouts. After two weeks, I could do the workouts more realistically, setting up against a couch for hip thrusts and standing for squats and deadlifts. By week 3, I was moving through a much greater range of motion.

About two weeks into my mental imagery training, I realized that I was not only getting better at the visualization component but also starting to feel a lot better. My glute wasn't nearly as sore, and I could do a lot more in the gym, such as upper-body movements and leg extensions and leg curls, which didn't flare up my injury. After only five weeks, I was back to glute training, and all of the swelling, bruising, and discomfort were gone. What's more, when I returned to training, I was moving with good form, and I didn't lose much strength or muscle size. (All of this may have been due to the other strategies I implemented, which I cover shortly.)

Seeing just how effective mental imagery training is, I plan to use it at important times throughout the year even when I'm not injured, such as in the week prior to going for a big PR. If you play sports or do a complex activity like Olympic weightlifting, then you would benefit from performing a mental imagery workout every week or even every day.

Even if you don't make mental imagery training a weekly or daily practice, it's nice to have a chip in your pocket to use when the time calls for it, such as when you are injured or sick. Or maybe you're on vacation and don't have access to a gym, or you're feeling beat down, and you want to be productive and not feel guilty for not doing anything. In such a situation, you can do a mental workout and reap the nervous system benefits of a real workout in a fraction of the time.

CROSS-EDUCATION TRAINING

Cross-education was first described in the research in the late 1800s. The researchers found that when you train only one side of your body, the other side gets stronger, even though you didn't train it. This is due to the nervous system adaptations that are generated through strength training and work bilaterally even if you train just one side.

Because only one side of my glute was torn, I could perform a lot of movements on the opposite side. It took some experimenting to figure out which exercises I could and couldn't do without causing further discomfort. For example, I found that I could do bodyweight Bulgarian split squats and dumbbell single-leg Romanian deadlifts with my right leg. I took it easy and kept the sets and reps low: 2 sets of 8 reps. As I progressed through my recovery, I increased the volume, load, and effort and started employing different single-leg exercises that felt good.

Eventually, I started doing enhanced-eccentric single-leg hip thrusts involving the two-up/one-down method (see Chapter 13).

To get the best results from cross-education training, I recommend following the same protocol. Start out doing just body weight, perform only exercises that feel right to you, and progress according to how you feel. Just remember that if you feel pain, then you're only slowing down your recovery. You have to select exercises that don't cause you discomfort or make the problem worse.

ISOMETRIC CONTRACTIONS

Doing isometric contractions during times of injury can help you retain strength and muscle mass, but it's a risky endeavor for many people because they end up overdoing it. At first, it works by keeping the nervous system adaptations established, not allowing coordination to erode, and preventing type I muscle fiber atrophy, but over time, as the effort becomes sufficiently high, it also prevents type II muscle fiber atrophy. (These are the larger fibers that are more responsible for your overall shape and come into play only with very hard or fatiguing contractions.)

To employ the isometric contractions strategy, you contract the muscle involved in the injured area for 10 seconds, rest for 10 seconds, and then repeat for 3 minutes. For example, I contracted both glutes, making sure to stay under my pain threshold. In other words, if I squeezed any harder, I would feel a little bit of pain. At first, I could contract at only about 10 percent of my maximum voluntary isometric contraction (MVIC), but after a few weeks, as my glute healed, I was contracting at about 60 percent. I also performed maximum isometric contractions with just my right glute since it wasn't injured.

Just like the other protocols, the idea is to steadily ramp up both the level of contraction and the amount of time you spend performing the drill. By the end of my recovery period, I was performing up to six minutes of isometric contractions. After four weeks, I could maximally contract my left glute with no discomfort. I always paid close attention to the lump in my glute the next day to note whether it seemed to be getting smaller. Only one day did I do a bit too much and feel the lump get bigger instead of smaller, which served as a reminder not to be overzealous. I took a day off from isometrics and then got right back on track, making sure to train in a more gradual fashion.

ECCENTRIC CONTRACTIONS

I didn't employ eccentric contractions during my rehab, but I want to mention them because they have a ton of support in the literature. When I started feeling better, I could have had a partner help me perform manual-resisted eccentric hip extensions while lying prone with my leg hanging off a bench by pushing against the back of my thigh. Or I could have bridged up and had my partner provide resistance on the way down. I did use the two-up/one-down method, but I could have done much more in the form of eccentric training. For hamstring injuries, the use of Nordic ham curls is an essential component of rehabilitation and fast return-to-play for athletes.

ALTERNATIVE METHODS: LIGHT MASSAGE, HOT AND COLD THERAPY, AND SO ON

In addition to mental imagery training, cross-education training, and isometric and eccentric contractions, you can employ methods like light massage, foam rolling, very light stretching, and hot and cold therapy. For instance, I lightly massaged my injured glute for about five minutes each night, which seemed to help. Maybe these activities brought fresh blood to the area and assisted my immune and lymphatic systems in clearing debris and restoring balance to the swollen and bruised tissue, or maybe they helped me solely via the placebo effect. Either way, I wasn't spending too much time or money on it, so I figured it couldn't hurt to try.

Many people use hot and cold therapy to treat pain and injuries. Cold therapy such as icing, cold baths, and cryotherapy reduces blood flow, inflammation, and pain, while heat therapy such as a sauna or hot bath increases blood flow and connective tissue elasticity while decreasing pain. I didn't undergo hot or cold therapy to treat my glute injury, but they're worth mentioning, and in some situations, they're very important.

Even though these alternative methods may not work miracles, they are simple, cheap, and—when done correctly—safe strategies to implement while your injured body part heals. Plus, they make you feel good because you're being proactive instead of sitting around doing nothing. The key is not to try to do too much.

A lot of people mistakenly think that recovery has to be a demanding activity. As a result, they push themselves too hard, too fast (aggressively stretching, doing too much soft-tissue therapy, or exercising through the injury), and they never fully heal. It's the same with training. People assume that they have to train an hour a day, six days a week, or they'll lose everything. But you can probably get away with training twice a week for 40 minutes and maintain your physique and strength, assuming that you keep your diet and other lifestyle factors in check. I realized this while I was injured. I can't remember ever doing such low volume and having my physique and strength stay the same. However, if I had done nothing and just allowed myself to be a couch potato for six weeks, then I would have probably lost around 30 percent of my strength and muscle size.

To state the obvious, you still need take care of your body by eating well, getting adequate sleep, and performing activities of daily living that don't make your injury worse. And you need to progress according to how you feel. The protocol I just outlined was for a glute injury, but it should serve you well if you strain a different muscle (assuming it's not torn off the bone). It's easy to maintain and stick to a schedule. You can do it every day and gradually ramp it up as you heal. If you feel better every day, you know you're doing it right. If you feel worse, then you know you're doing too much. Find the right balance, stay consistent, and you might return to training with new tools that you didn't have before the injury.

GLUTEAL IMBALANCES

Contrary to popular belief, gluteal imbalances are common and should be thought of as a normal human phenomenon. While you should strive to normalize your imbalances, you should not expect perfect symmetry, nor should you freak out if you feel one glute working harder than the other. Almost all of my clients shift slightly to one side when squatting, have one glute that seems to activate higher during various glute exercises, and possess one glute that is slightly larger than the other. There are a few factors that can cause these imbalances.

One, as I just mentioned, is that no human being is perfectly symmetrical. Most people have a dominant hand or leg that they favor during movement. Right-handed people typically jump off their left leg, so the left hip extensor tends to be stronger than the right, while the right hip flexor tends to be stronger than the left. This should be considered normal.

Imagine telling a golfer to take 100 practice swings and then switch to the other side and take another 100 swings to avoid gluteal imbalances. That would be less time with specificity, meaning less time honing their movement patterns and motor control for their sport. This would be bad advice because in both life and sport, you're generally more effective having a preferred, stronger side.

The second factor that can cause imbalances is a preexisting injury, pain symptoms, or poor rehabilitation following an injury. There's research showing that the glutes are inhibited after a sprained ankle, for example. It's important to realize is any kind of pain signal will inhibit the muscles responsible for carrying out motion. This is likely a self-protective mechanism to allow the body to heal and prevent you from continuing to injure the area, and it actually alters your movement patterns. This change can cause imbalances over time, and it's not uncommon for people never to rehabilitate an injury properly, so they're left using one side more than the other for many years.

Think about how many times you jumped back into training post-injury as a kid or teen without rebuilding the muscles that had atrophied during your recovery period. Here's an example to help you understand how this might play out. Say you sprain your ankle and you don't train or play sports for six weeks. You've been limping and favoring one side of your body. The healthy side, which has been bearing most of your weight for six weeks, stays strong, while the weak side loses a bit of size and strength. When you get back to training, are you focusing on redeveloping the weaker side? Probably not. You just go about your training as you normally would and assume that it will rebalance. Sometimes it does, but a lot of times it doesn't, creating a more pronounced imbalance over time. Eventually, you have one glute that is a lot bigger than the other, and you favor it throughout your life.

The third factor could be an injury to the nerves supplying the glute. Sometimes this can be improved upon and fixed and sometimes not, depending on the severity.

The fourth reason is simply anatomical variation. We see case reports on this in the literature sometimes, where people have different-shaped muscles, attachment points, or nerve supplies. Heck, one report discusses an individual who had an additional muscle belly in their gluteus maximus—something that had never been seen before!

The bottom line is that you will never have perfectly symmetrical glutes, but you can prevent or normalize them by employing the strategies described on the following pages.

HOW TO PREVENT GLUTEAL IMBALANCES

You can't completely prevent glute imbalances, but you can get close simply by recognizing that you have a dominant side and trying to balance your training by working the weaker side of your body harder. This is the value of strength training: you can focus on and isolate one side of your body with specific exercises without compromising sport-specific mechanics. For instance, to help prevent glute imbalances, you can work your weaker side first. If you're performing single-leg hip thrusts and your right leg is dominant, start your set using your left leg.

Another helpful strategy is to film your bilateral lifts and then watch to make sure you don't shift too dramatically to one side or the other. For example, say you film yourself deadlifting from directly behind and notice that you shift a little to your left side. Now you can cue this and bring some consciousness to your movement to prevent it from happening again. Filming yourself also gives you a framework to work with and lets you know where your weaknesses lie.

I also recommend balancing your training by using free weights because they force you to use both sides equally. If all you do is train with machines—like the leg press and Smith machine—then you might push more with one leg and not even know it because the weight moves just the same.

HOW TO NORMALIZE GLUTEAL IMBALANCES

My current favorite method for normalizing glute imbalances is to perform single-leg reverse hypers with 5- to 10-pound ankle weights for women or 10- to 20-pound ankle weights for men with only the weaker side. You can do 2 or 3 sets up to 5 times a week.

I like the single-leg reverse hyper because it's the best hip extension exercise for isolating the glute. Of course, numerous hip abduction exercises would work here, but they typically work the upper glutes much better than the lower glutes. You really want a hip extension exercise that works well, and most single-leg movements work too many other muscles. Think about it: single-leg squatting exercise variations like lunges, step-ups, split squats, and pistols work the quads incredibly well, so if you went with those for minimizing imbalances, you might develop a quad imbalance in the process. Single-leg hip hinging exercises like single-leg Romanian deadlifts and single-leg 45-degree hypers involve a ton of hamstring contribution, so you may overdevelop the hamstring by working only the weaker side. Even single-leg hip thrusts involve a lot of quad, hamstring, and adductor muscles. However, the single-leg reverse hyper mostly involves the glute (some hamstring, too), especially if you don't go too heavy and you focus on isolating the glute via a strong mind-muscle connection.

If you don't have a reverse hyper machine, you can use a bench, a glute ham developer, or any elevated and stable flat surface, such as a countertop or table, to perform the reverse hyper exercise. And if you don't have anything at all upon which to position your torso, you can simply post up against a wall, lean over, and perform ankle weight bent-over single-leg kickbacks, which mimic the reverse hyper motion.

In addition, you want to make sure that your bilateral training is symmetrical, meaning that you're not shifting to one side or the other. You also want to perform isometric contractions with the weaker glute throughout the day and do an extra set of unilateral exercises with the weaker side when they appear in your program.

FIX FOR GLUTE IMBALANCES

Do 3 sets of 12 reps of ankle weight single-leg reverse hypers or bent-over single-leg kickbacks prior to each training session for the weaker glute only.

EMG ACTIVITY of 10-pound ankle weight single-leg reverse hyper (mean, normalized to MVIC)	
GLUTE	50%
QUAD	10%
ADDUCTOR	15%
HAMSTRING	50%

OVERCOMING PLATEAUS

To reiterate, if you're new to strength training, chances are you will see great results right out of the gate. If you train smart, lift with good form, and follow an intelligently designed program, you will see better and better results. The problem is, this upward trend won't last forever.

Some of my new clients add 5 pounds or an extra rep per week for most of their big lifts and exercises, but after a few months, their rate of progress slows. They still make gains, but not as quickly, and then they start to plateau. Some weeks, they even drop a few pounds in some lifts. As I said, progress always happens in waves, especially as you start to reach the limits of your physical potential.

Once you reach the stage at which you start to plateau, it's even more important to optimize your training and other aspects of your life, like diet, sleep, and stress management. The fact of the matter is, the longer you've been training, the more plateaus you'll hit.

On the following pages, you'll find a comprehensive list of strategies to implement when you've plateaued in your training.

Create a Personalized Program. A lot of lifters can get away with following universal training templates or tried-and-true programs for the masses and make them work for a while. But once you stop making progress, you should consider creating a program that is specific to your goals, fitness level, and body type. I've had to stray from the norm with the way I train certain clients, but by paying close attention to what they respond to best and how they recover, I've been able to help expedite their results substantially.

Follow a Specialized Program. I put my advanced clients on specialized programs, focusing on one lift or movement pattern at a time. Instead of trying to get stronger at the squat, deadlift, and hip thrust simultaneously by training them all three days a week, we focus on just one (say, the hip thrust) for a four-week cycle. Maybe we go with a DUP approach. We still hit the other movement patterns, but we emphasize one in particular so that the client can focus on getting stronger in that area.

Include a Deload Week. This is another tip that ties into program design. I have clients who do not work hard enough and need to up their volume or effort, although this is rarer than you might think with advanced lifters. Most of my advanced clients, or people who come to me with a lot of training experience, are doing way too much volume. What's more, they've been hitting it hard for way too long. Simply dialing it back a little bit and giving their bodies a chance to recover and adapt provides a nice bump in their training performance.

Perhaps we can "resensitize" our bodies to volume by unloading for a week. It may even be beneficial to deload for a few weeks a couple of times per year. Let me clarify that when you deload, you're not taking time off from the gym. You still go to the gym and go through the motions, but you don't push it hard. Your workout might be a 6 out of 10 in terms of overall effort. You may do just 5 reps of an exercise you could do 10 times. It may seem like you're not doing anything, but this approach is better for strength and muscle growth. But you have to know that you're stimulating gains by training moderately; otherwise, you'll be tempted to stray from the plan and train too hard, in which case you're not really deloading.

Reduce Your Glute Training. At any point, your level of readiness is determined by your fitness and fatigue levels, which are always changing. You spark fitness gains by finishing a smart and hard training session. In doing so, however, you also fatigue your body, and the amount of fatigue is determined by the exercises you perform, how hard you push them, and how many sets you do. Some people are always masking their fitness because they're constantly fatigued, and they never gain because they can't put more tension on their muscles when training in a fatigued state.

Let's say you've been training your glutes 4 times per week, doing an average of 15 sets per day for a total of 60 sets per week, and you've been plateaued for many months. You may benefit from training your glutes just twice per week with 12 sets per session for a total of 24 sets per week. You should be fluctuating your training stress by deloading regularly and gradually ramping up your effort and volume and then bringing it back down. But many people have way too high a baseline in terms of dedication to glute training, and they're never truly recovered when they train.

Change It Up. As Albert Einstein famously said, "Doing the same thing over and over again and expecting different results is the definition of insanity." Experiment with different exercises, tempos, training frequency, and set and rep schemes. Variety can be a great thing, especially if you've been practicing the same variations and programs for long periods of time. In my opinion, it's best to create a new plan every three to six weeks.

Sometimes you just need a change in environment. I recently started training at a new gym in San Diego, and there are jacked and swole dudes walking around and tossing around heavily loaded barbells like it's nothing. While this may intimidate some people and be the wrong type of training facility for many, it's a great environment for me right now. I consider myself a total bro, just one with a PhD, which I pursued simply due to my extreme curiosity. Being surrounded by fit, strong people motivates me to train harder. If you're not seeing results, you could be training at the wrong gym or in the wrong environment, and a simple switch could be all you need.

Consider Working with a Coach or Trainer. Everyone can benefit from working with a coach. Even coaches need coaches. If you've plateaued and you're training yourself, find a coach who can help highlight weaknesses in your workouts, program design, and form and push you in the gym. Or maybe you simply need to pair up with an awesome training partner who pushes and focuses you. It's in our nature to assume that we're in tune with our bodies, but many times we're blind to our own weaknesses, even if we are well read, have a lot of experience, and are good at helping others achieve their goals.

Implement Advanced Training Methods (see Chapter 13). Advanced lifters can benefit from advanced techniques and methods. Check out the advanced methods outlined in the previous chapter and start implementing them into your training. Doing so will add variety and new training stimuli to your workouts. But don't abandon basic training!

Clean Up Other Areas of Your Life. As I've said, there are many variables that can influence your training. In order to optimize your training, you have to get good sleep, eat well, and manage your stress. You don't want to minimize stress outright, though; you want to optimize it by staying in eustress and out of distress. It's good to challenge yourself in life. Just don't take on too much too often. Life is a game of sweet spots, and it's your job to figure those out.

Find the Fun in Training. Getting bored with exercise goes hand in hand with stalled progress. Following these guidelines might help you break this cycle. Or you may want to reassess your goals and expectations. Sometimes you just need to change your mindset around training. For instance, if you've been focusing primarily on building bigger glutes (which is an aesthetic goal), perhaps you should shift your focus to trying to get stronger at certain lifts (which is a performance goal).

Don't Put a Timeline on Your Progress. Although creating goals is important, realize that you will go up and down—that's just the way it is. In order to maintain a positive mindset around exercise, it's better to imagine the goal and work toward it with the understanding that it might take months or even years to reach. Rather than focus on a specific timeline, think about staying consistent, having fun, and playing around with different training strategies.

NOT SEEING RESULTS

So you've been following the strategies and advice offered in this book, but you're not seeing any results, and you're thinking, what the hell?

Unless I'm training you one-on-one, it's difficult for me to know what you're doing right or wrong. Here's what I can say: often, people think they're doing everything right when in fact they are doing a lot wrong. If you're self-trained, then there is a lot you might be missing. Your form might be off, or your diet might be affecting your fat loss goals. Perhaps you're training too much or not enough, you have poor muscle-building genetics, or you're stressed out and not sleeping enough.

This is the real value of working with a coach or personal trainer. Even if you're following a customized program that I wrote for you online, I still can't see how you're lifting, your tempo, your range of motion, or whether you're going hard or heavy enough. I can't make adjustments based on how you feel and how you're responding to the program because I'm not there with you in person.

Even if you trained with me at Glute Lab and I personally coached you for every training session, I still can't be with you 24 hours a day to see how you handle the other 23 hours. Bodybuilding is a 24-hour sport, and everything you do affects your results.

If you're training yourself, you have to be objective and understand that there might be something you're missing or not doing right. And that's perfectly normal. I've been lifting for nearly 30 years, and I still make mistakes. But luckily, I'm surrounded by great coaches, and I'm constantly learning, tweaking, and adapting.

If you feel like you're following everything to a T and still not getting results, take a step back and consider the following:

- Are you sleeping enough?
- Are you training hard enough? Or are you running yourself into the ground?
- Do you need to switch up your program?
- Is your diet affecting your physique?

Evaluate yourself as you would assess someone else. If possible, find a coach you respect and consult with them. Find your weaknesses and correct them.

OVERCOMING COMMON OBSTACLES

Whether you are new to glute training, you are strapped for time, you lack access to equipment, or you are having trouble activating your glutes, there are solutions to these and other similar problems.

NEW TO GLUTE TRAINING

For most people, the most difficult obstacle is getting started. Not knowing what to do or where to start is overwhelming and can prevent you from training before you even begin. There are a few important truths that every beginner should realize.

As any trainer will tell you, the most important step is starting. You don't need to jump right into barbell hip thrusts. Don't overthink your training and overwhelm yourself. You're on the ground floor, and you can only go up. Have a positive outlook and say to yourself, "I am on my way to getting better glutes, and everything I do from here on out is better than what I was doing before," which might have been nothing. Sure, you have a lot to learn, but simply familiarizing yourself with the squat, lunge, hip hinge (deadlift), glute bridge, and hip thrust movement patterns is a giant step forward. Keep an optimistic mindset and follow the protocol outlined in this book, and you will rise to the top floor before you know it.

A lot of people wrongly assume that they need to become experts before they begin. They use this as a crutch to avoid training. Think about a person who says they need to get in shape before joining a gym. Everyone is new at first, so put your ego aside and just start training.

If you're new, begin with bodyweight movements (see page 277 for a basic bodyweight program), prioritize glute-dominant exercises like hip thrusts and glute bridges, and sprinkle in some squat and deadlift movement patterns. Take the time to learn proper form and try not to overthink what you're doing. Realize that this is a new system of training that takes time to learn. As you get more coordinated and comfortable, slowly add more complex variations and increase your load and volume. If you've been following the old way of glute training, meaning only squatting and deadlifting, add in the hip thrust and other glute-dominant movements and go from there. A sample program template might look something like this:

Monday, Wednesday, Friday:
3 sets of 20 bodyweight squats, hip thrusts or glute bridges, and Romanian deadlifts
Finish with a hard set of lunges and a few minutes of lateral band work

Consistency is crucial. Most people fail to get bigger, stronger glutes because they are not following a program or training their glutes enough. It might take you several years to reach your physique goals, and that is just fine. The more consistent you are, the better you will get at the movements. As your form improves, so too will your strength. Before you know it, you will have a bigger, stronger butt that you can be proud of.

You also need to embrace experimentation. You need to keep learning and tinkering. If you're reading this book in the hopes of expanding your glute training knowledge, then you're on the right track. But you have to keep experimenting to find the exercises and program design that work best for you. Understand that if you are at point A and you want to get to point Z, you won't go from A to Z overnight. By going from A to B to C, you will see results. Then, by going from C to D to E, you will see more results, and so on.

Finally, have fun. In my experience as a personal trainer, the clients who get the best results and stay consistent are the ones who are having fun with their training. If you're not having fun, then something needs to change.

EMBARRASSED PERFORMING HIP THRUSTS AND OTHER EXERCISES

A lot of people get embarrassed or shy when performing barbell thrust or bridge variations because it's a relatively new exercise. It is true that the bodyweight variations of these movement patterns have been popular for ages, but the barbell versions have been around only since 2006. Although the hip thrust is becoming more and more popular, it still resonates as a sexual movement to some people, especially those who have never seen it before. Imagine being the first person ever to perform a Romanian deadlift or stiff-leg deadlift. You're essentially sticking your butt out and bending over as far as you can. That's about as sexual as it gets, yet nobody bats an eyelash anymore because it's an accepted lift. The same is true for the adduction and abduction machines. You're actively spreading your legs, but the action is not shocking because we see it all the time.

As the hip thrust grows in popularity, it will become less awkward. Soon, it will be no different than performing any other exercise. My first reaction when people come to me with this excuse is to say, "Get over it!" But I know that is not an empathetic response, so here are a couple of recommendations that I hope will help you feel less self-conscious:

- If you're working out in a busy gym, try to position yourself so you are facing a wall.
- Find a quiet corner or area that is secluded from the rest of the gym, like an empty aerobics room.
- Do a lot of your glute training at home.

You have options, and you definitely don't need to avoid glute training because you're embarrassed.

STRAPPED FOR TIME

Almost everyone I know is extremely busy, yet many still find time to exercise and eat well. I get it. Getting to the gym can be tough, especially if you don't particularly enjoy working out. If you fall into this category, consider a two- or three-days-a-week training schedule. If you don't have a ton of time to spend at the gym, there's a lot that you can do at home with minimal equipment.

Even if you work out only twice a week, it's only two hours a week, which everyone should be able to manage. You can also spread your training throughout the week. For example, instead of doing two one-hour training sessions, consider four 30-minute sessions. The reality is that the time it takes to exercise and see good results is minimal when you think about how much time you have throughout the week. In other words, the time excuse falls flat once you consider how much bang for your buck you get out of two full-body workouts.

Remember, exercise is good for your health. Sure, you probably train your glutes and exercise because you want a better butt and body, but it's important to realize the long-term health benefits of training. When it comes to scheduling time to exercise, you have to create habits that enable you to stay healthy. If you can't find time, then that is a failure in time management, and you need to reconsider your priorities. I get it, you may have a family and you need to work, but you'll be a better worker and a better friend and family member if you're healthy and feeling good, which is the primary benefit of exercise.

At times it's been hard for me to train three days a week, so I understand. But you have options. If you work all day, try training first thing in the morning. Yes, getting up early takes discipline, but once you ingrain the habit and commit to taking care of your body, it becomes second nature, something you do without even thinking about it.

Learn to train from home, learn how to perform bodyweight movements, and pick up a mini band and Glute Loop. If, on top of that, you can make it to the gym a couple of times a week, that is way better than not going at all.

LACKING ACCESS TO EQUIPMENT

If you lack access to equipment or cannot make it to the gym, you can still get a lot of work done by performing high-rep bodyweight exercises. If all you ever did was bodyweight glute exercises, you could still see great results from performing advanced exercises like pistol squats, dead-stop single-leg hip thrusts, and side-lying hip raises while carrying out your sets to muscle failure. That said, I recommend that, at a minimum, you pick up a resistance band (or any thick band to wrap around your knees, such as a Glute Loop). It is inexpensive, doesn't take up a lot of space, and will make your at-home bodyweight workouts a lot more effective. Over time, you can add more equipment, like some dumbbells, kettlebells, and maybe even a barbell and bench.

The bottom line is this: you have a ton of options, so not having equipment or being unable to make it to the gym is not a legitimate excuse.

PHYSICALLY DEMANDING JOB

If you have a physically demanding job, chances are it will negatively affect your training. As a personal trainer, I'm on my feet all day sometimes, demo-ing movements and walking around. By the time I get to my own workout, I'm cooked. If you fall into this category, it might be better to perform your workouts in the morning. Or try to take a quick nap, get a meal in you, and relax for an hour before your workout.

GLUTE TRAINING WHILE TRAVELING

There are a ton of glute exercises that you can do while traveling. Essentially, all bodyweight glute exercises are available to you, including free squats, split squats, Bulgarian split squats, lunges, skater squats, step-ups, pistols, single-leg hip hinging variations, and side-lying hip abductions. You can also perform glute bridge, hip thrust, and frog pump variations—feet elevated, wide and narrow stance, single leg and double leg.

The Glute Loop, which is small and portable, opens up a ton of abduction exercises and, again, is an easy way to add resistance to bodyweight movements. If you have access to a hotel gym, that opens up even more options. Most gyms have dumbbells, so you can perform goblet squats, dumbbell single-leg deadlifts, dumbbell reverse lunges, and dumbbell single-leg hip thrusts. And many gyms have cable columns that allow for kickback variations, cable hip abductions, and pull-throughs.

At the end of the day, you should never fear missing a glute workout when on vacation because there are so many options. Here is a sample hotel workout using a couch and ottoman:

- Feet-Elevated Hip Thrusts: 20 reps
- Single-Leg Foot-and-Shoulder-Elevated Hip Thrusts: 12 reps each leg
- Alternating Over Bench Bird Dogs: 20 reps
- Frog Pumps: 50 reps
- Deficit Reverse Lunges: 20 reps each leg
- Extra-Range Side-Lying Hip Abduction: 30 reps each leg

Perform 3 rounds with a 1-minute rest between sets.

NOT FEELING YOUR GLUTES ACTIVATE

Human physiology is strange. Sometimes you get sky-high glute activation with a certain exercise, and other times you don't. Sometimes you go to the gym and your glutes burn like crazy and you get an insane pump; other times you perform the exact same workout and don't feel anything.

First things first: Some people are much better at activating their muscles than other people. It tends to be muscle-specific, too. For example, some people can feel their glutes working hard on everything but have trouble activating their lats or hamstrings. Others feel most of their muscles activating except their glutes.

Don't fret. I haven't noticed a linear relationship between glute size and shape and the perception of activation. Some of my clients with incredible glute development seem to have trouble activating their glutes, while others feel their glutes activating like crazy but don't have glutes that are as big.

Many people find that their glute activation improves over time through training. One study indicates that low-load glute activation improves the brain's ability to target the glutes (via corticospinal pathways). But not everyone will feel their glutes working hard during every glute exercise. Frog pumps burn my glutes so bad that it brings tears to my eyes, but I don't always feel my glutes activate during heavy hip thrusts, and I always get sky-high levels of glute activation when measured via EMG.

Sometimes you shouldn't worry about feeling it in your glutes; you just want to use good form. For example, if you feel your quads a ton in the hip thrust, it doesn't necessarily mean that your glutes are not working; it just means that the feeling of your quads activating overpowers your glute activation signal. (*Note:* I offer specific tips for increasing glute activation in the glute bridge and hip thrust in the next section.)

If a failure to feel your glutes ruins your training experience and causes you to have a pessimistic outlook, you will not see results. Stay positive and focus on getting stronger while using good form and performing a variety of movements in a variety of rep ranges. In most cases, you just need time to develop a better mind-muscle (or mind-glute) connection.

NOT GETTING A PUMP AND BURN

Some days, the stars will align, and you will achieve high levels of metabolic stress. Other days, you won't achieve even the slightest pump or burn despite your best efforts. This is just the nature of the iron game. Don't sweat it! Keep a long-term perspective.

With that said, you should feel the burn and get a nice pump at least once a week. If not, address the following factors that contribute to the pump and burn:

- Hydration
- Supplements (such as creatine)
- Carbohydrate ingestion prior to training
- Sodium and electrolyte balance
- Full systemic recovery
- Full specific muscle recovery from the previous training session
- Novelty
- Exercises that stress short muscle lengths (such as the lateral band walk)

- Exercises that place consistent tension on the muscles (such as the hip thrust)
- Constant-tension repetitions in a rapid, pistonlike fashion
- Rep ranges
- Rest periods

PHYSIQUE TRAINING SOLUTIONS

I field a lot of questions on social media and my blog, mostly related to glute appearance. These are the most common questions I receive: "How do I grow my glutes without growing my legs?" "What needs to happen for my glutes to look perky and strong?" "Why do my glutes look good one day and not the next?" "How do I get rid of cellulite, saddlebags, and hip divots?" I provide the answers in this section.

MY GLUTES ARE SAGGY AND WEAK. HOW DO I MAKE THEM LOOK PERKY AND STRONG?

Many people, especially women, fail to think logically about this question. This much is apparent: for the woman asking this question, her ideal glutes are leaner and more muscular than her current ones. However, when she looks in the mirror, she tends to notice only the fat that she carries in her gluteal region. She ignores the muscle-building component and instead tries to shed body fat through excessive cardio and calorie restriction. This approach leads to a skinny-fat appearance, preventing her from achieving the results she desires.

There's no getting around it: to gain muscular shape in your glutes, you have to train hard. Except for the genetic elite, a nice booty is a strong booty. So, to make your glutes look perky and strong, you have to stick to a glute training program and follow the guidelines offered in this section.

WHY DO MY GLUTES LOOK GREAT ONE DAY AND NOT THE NEXT?

A lot of variables determine how your glutes look from day to day. Stress, sleep, carb and salt intake, hormone levels, muscle damage—all of these factors can affect how much water your body is holding and ultimately how pronounced your glutes look. If all of these factors align in just the right way, your glutes might be filled out and look amazing. If one or more of these factors is off—say, you had a bad night of sleep, or you're sore from the previous day's workout, or you didn't take in enough salt, or you're dehydrated—then your glutes might look a little flatter than they did the day before. If you're a woman, your menstrual cycle plays a big role here, too.

So don't get discouraged if your glutes look good one day and not as good the next. Progress is never linear. You may experience daily or weekly development and then all of the sudden hit a plateau. It happens to everyone.

When evaluating your glute training progress, you have to look at the big picture. You can't let an occasional, improperly perceived setback derail your progress. Having good days and bad days is part of the game.

HOW DO I GET RID OF HIP DIVOTS?

Everyone will develop hip divots (see page 52) if they get lean enough. Some individuals have more pronounced divots than others. Your genetics, hip anatomy, and gluteal attachment points are the primary factors that determine the shape of your hip divots. As I said in Chapter 5, you may be able to affect your curves through training, but hip divots are determined mainly by your skeletal anatomy and body fat percentage. You may find that there is a body fat level that optimizes the way your glutes look according to your preference. Some women are happier with their butts when they're a little heavier, while others prefer a leaner look. This might take some tinkering. The key—as I say throughout this book—is not to get hung up on things you cannot change. Hip divots are not a bad thing and shouldn't be thought of as a problem that needs to be fixed.

HOW DO I GET RID OF SADDLEBAGS?

Just as your genetic muscle architecture and bone structure affect how your hips look, your fat storage sites are determined mainly by your genetics. Men and women store fat differently, due mostly to hormonal differences. However, some women can be lean all over but still store fat around their hips, commonly referred to as *saddlebags.* While it is possible to spot enhance by adding muscle to specific areas, it is very difficult, if not impossible, to spot reduce (lose fat only in a specific area). What's more, your overall body fat percentage largely dictates the amount of fat you store in your problem areas. Some women can have 30 percent body fat and look phenomenal because of the way their fat is distributed, while others can have 15 percent body fat and still possess glaring "stubborn areas" (pockets of stored fat in undesired regions).

The solution is straightforward: build as much muscle as possible underneath that area through resistance training (using the guidelines outlined in this book), adhere to sound dietary principles, and stay active to promote overall fat burning. As you lose fat and build muscle, your glutes will gain shape, you will lose fat in your problem areas, and your appearance will improve dramatically.

A lot of women make the mistake of dieting down too aggressively and doing a ton of cardio in an attempt to lose fat. Sure, you might lose fat if you follow this approach, but your butt will lose its shape, too. A round butt makes your thighs look less pronounced. To put it another way, the bigger your butt, the smaller your thighs appear. For this reason, I recommend building as much muscle as possible in your glutes and sticking with a specialized glute training routine.

How to Get Rid of Saddlebags:

- Prioritize glute-dominant exercises (like hip thrusts)
- Perform a variety of lower-body exercises
- Build muscle under problem areas
- Adhere to sound dietary principles
- Work out consistently
- Be active throughout the day
- Don't replace strength training with cardio (spinning, jogging, and so on)
- Have patience

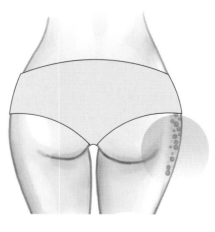

HOW DO I GET RID OF CELLULITE ON MY GLUTES?

First of all, cellulite is a natural physiological occurrence in the thighs and buttocks of women. Every woman I've ever trained has had some degree of cellulite.

Cellulite is incredibly stubborn and resistant to a vast array of treatments. No single method in the research has been shown to be highly effective in combating cellulite. A lot of people mistakenly think that liposuction will get rid of cellulite, but it doesn't. Cellulite is an infiltration of fat into the connective tissue, as shown in the illustration below. Liposuction decreases fat storage, which may reduce the appearance of cellulite but will not remove it completely.

So, while certain tools, devices, therapies, supplements, and creams have been purported to rid the body of cellulite, the best approach is a holistic one: train hard, create a caloric deficit (if you're trying to lose fat), get some sun, sleep well, eat a nutritious diet, and manage stress.

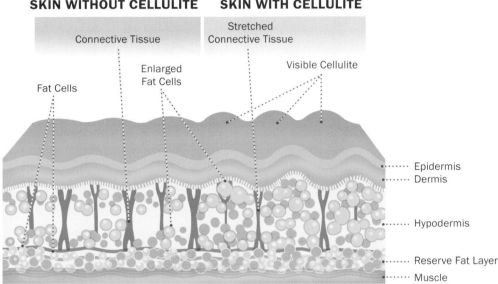

HOW DO I GROW MY GLUTES WITHOUT GROWING MY LEGS?

Men tend to want to build their legs, whereas many women think their legs are too bulky and want to avoid training them hard. This is unfortunate, because the problem is not that these women carry too much leg muscle, but that they have too much fat surrounding their leg muscles. You need to train your legs hard to keep the muscle but also dial in your diet and perform some cardio after weight training—as long as the cardio doesn't increase your appetite or compromise your resistance training routine. Nevertheless, some women develop leg muscles that are too big for their liking, and they need a special strategy.

The truth is, most great glute exercises also highly activate the leg muscles. The hip thrust, for example, works the quads, hamstrings, and adductors a ton. In other words, it's challenging to work the glutes without working the legs as well.

As you already learned, muscle grows from low reps (1 to 5), medium reps (6 to 12), high reps (13 to 20), and even really high reps (21 to 50). As long as the sets are carried out close to muscle failure and the intensity of effort for the session is sufficiently high, you can choose your ideal rep scheme and still build muscle. So avoiding a particular rep range or avoiding heavy weights is not the solution.

This leaves you with two options:

1. Avoid exercises that highly activate and stress your quads, hamstrings, and adductors.
2. Perform exercises that highly activate and stress your glutes.

If you want your legs to stop growing, you need to reduce or eliminate movements that highly activate your quads and hamstrings. This means no squat variations, no single-leg squat variations like lunges, step-ups, and pistols, and no quad-dominant movements like leg presses, hack squats, and leg extensions, because these lead to high levels of quad activation. It also means no hip hinging variations like Romanian deadlifts (RDLs), back extensions, and good mornings and no knee flexion movements like leg curls, Nordic ham curls, and glute ham raises because these lead to high levels of hamstring activation.

Although this takes a lot of exercises off the table, there is still a lot you can do:

*   Low-Load Glute Activation Work: There are lots of drills that you can and should do to shuttle the focus toward your glutes and away from your quads and hamstrings. A sample glute activation sequence might look like this: side-lying clams, banded glute bridges, bird dogs, and quadruped hip extensions.

*   Hip External Rotation Movements: Cuff/dip belt hip rotations are the best, but you need to learn how to use your glutes during these movements by rotating your hips with your rear glute while keeping your torso rigid instead of rotating your torso with your obliques.

*   Hip Abduction Movements: Focus on extra-range side-lying abduction, banded standing hip abduction, band seated hip abduction, band walk variations, and hip abductor machines.

*   Barbell Glute Bridges: Glute bridge variations reduce much of the quad activity that the barbell hip thrust produces. The glute bridge will be your money exercise—the exercise at which you want to keep getting stronger over time. Strength creates curves, and without it, your glutes won't grow. You can pull double-duty on your glutes by wearing a resistance band around your knees during this exercise.

*   American Deadlifts: These are a better option than RDLs due to the increased glute activation. To avoid an increased hamstring stretch, you should decrease the range of motion (that is, don't go too low).

*   Pull-Throughs, Reverse Hypers, and Kettlebell Swings: The key is to make sure you're feeling your glutes do the work.

*   Feet-Elevated Hip Thrusts: You can do these with one leg or two, and you can wear a mini band around your knees if you like. And you can perform them with body weight, dumbbells, or band resistance.

*   Frog Pumps: Two-thirds of people tend to like frog pumps. If you're part of that majority, flare your knees out, place your heels together, and pump away. If you're among the one-third who don't like frog pumps, skip them.

HOW DO I GROW MY GLUTES WITHOUT GROWING MY WAIST?

If you're training your glutes the way I recommend, meaning you're performing a variety of lower-body exercises such as deadlifts and squats, then there's a chance your erectors will grow. This is a concern for some women who want their butt to grow but their waist and trunk (erectors, abs, and obliques) to remain slim.

Some people develop muscle easily in certain areas. If you fall into this category, you should avoid exercises that build muscle in areas where you don't want muscle. This means avoiding exercises that activate your abs and obliques, like crunches and sit-ups.

Squats and deadlifts don't effectively build your abdominals and obliques (you use your diaphragm to create intra-abdominal pressure, which is mistakenly interpreted as core activation), but they do hit the erectors. Depending on the individual, reducing squat and deadlift volume might be worth considering.

Here are six tips for growing bigger glutes without growing your waist:

1. Prioritize hip thrusts (don't have high core activation) and focus on keeping your ribs down (don't hyperextend your lumbar spine).
2. Avoid excessive squat/deadlift volume.
3. Avoid all abdominal/oblique exercises.
4. Prioritize single-leg exercises (bilateral or double-leg exercises stress your core to a higher degree).
5. Perform bodyweight, band, cable machine, and ankle weight abduction work.
6. Stick to higher reps and use pristine form.

I WANT MY BUTT TO GET SMALLER, NOT LARGER. WHAT SHOULD I DO?

I have never met a woman who says that her glutes are too muscular when she's truly lean. When someone wants smaller glutes, it's usually because they are storing fat around the hips, and this fat is what they really want to lose. The logic that follows is far from optimal. They stop training their glutes because they think it will cause their butt to grow, and instead, they starve themselves and do a ton of cardio. Sure, they lose fat, but they also lose shape.

Even if you want your butt to get smaller, you should train your glutes the way you would if you wanted them to grow. You're trying to lose fat, not muscle, and working the area will help you do precisely that. What's more, if you stop training your glutes, you'll lose muscle, and muscle is what gives the glutes shape.

So, if you want your butt to get smaller, not larger, here's what you can do:

1. Continue training your glutes to keep your muscle and shape.
2. Avoid doing too much high-intensity cardio, which will strip muscle off your body. (Thirty minutes of steady-state low-intensity cardio three to five days a week is fine.)
3. Keep your diet in check. Reducing calorie intake and making sure to consume ample protein while striving to retain your strength in the gym is the best way to lose fat without affecting your physique.

Now, there are people who are fairly lean and have glutes that are too muscular for their liking. What should you do if you fall into this category? Well, this isn't the best book for you, since *Glute Lab* is mostly about strength training. If you want to rapidly shrink your glute size, you need to quit highly activating your glutes and avoid all movements that work them thoroughly. You want to avoid nearly every glute exercise mentioned in this book. To shrink them, you could run for long durations every day for a couple of months and decrease your protein intake during this time. If you want to grow other muscles while shrinking your glutes, keep your protein intake high and don't run, but avoid all glute exercises and perform only leg extensions, leg curls, core exercises, and upper-body work. If you want your glutes to stay strong while shrinking, do 3 singles (3 sets of 1 rep) of hip thrusts, and that's it for glute training.

I'M EXTREMELY OVERWEIGHT, AND I WANT TO LOSE 70 POUNDS. WHAT DO YOU RECOMMEND?

If I were training a woman who weighed 200 pounds and she told me she wanted to lose weight, I would ask her, "What does your dream body look like?" If she pointed to a woman who was about the same height and weighed around 130 pounds, this would mean that my client would need to lose 70 pounds. In her mind, if she starved herself and did a ton of cardio, she would lose the weight and achieve her ideal physique. But her dream body has shape and curves. I would tell her that in order to accomplish her goal, she has to keep muscle (and maybe even build more in some areas) and lose fat.

This is where it gets tricky. To lose 70 pounds, she would have to be at a serious caloric deficit for a long time. This makes it hard to maintain muscle, let alone put on muscle.

How do you maintain as much muscle as possible while losing quite a bit of fat? There are four important guidelines to follow:

1. Prioritize progressive overload (see page 102). In other words, work on getting stronger and building muscle with strength training. As you lose weight, your muscles will give your body shape, not to mention that lifting weights and strength training will help burn fat off your body.

2. Consume adequate amounts of protein. The general rule is to consume 1 gram per pound of lean body mass. The woman in this example may have only 120 pounds of lean body mass, which equates to 120 grams of protein per day. To get more specific numbers, she would need to measure her body fat percentage.

3. Remain in a caloric deficit. This should be calculated by a professional and should be individualized, but as long as you are burning more calories than you are consuming, you will lose weight.

4. Lose weight gradually. Taking your time helps you retain muscle. If you lost 70 pounds in 3 months, you would lose too much muscle to have the shape you desire. If possible, it would be great to drop 25 pounds in the first month, 10 pounds in the second month, and then 35 pounds over the course of the next 10 months. In addition to being easier to sustain, this approach would give your skin and body an opportunity to adapt to the body composition changes.

GLUTE TRAINING AND PREGNANCY

A lot of women falsely assume that training the glutes and hip thrusting during pregnancy are dangerous. I've trained a lot of women during pregnancy, and although there are some general guidelines to keep in mind, you can still train your glutes and perform most exercises. In the first trimester, you might experience morning sickness and nausea. In the second trimester, you'll probably feel like Wonder Woman, and you'll be able to resume normal training. In the third trimester, you'll likely start to feel achy, and you'll have good training days and not-so-good training days. Just do the best you can.

It's easy to let yourself go during pregnancy, but it's hard to get your body back if you take a year off of training, especially after you've just delivered a baby. Plus, having a newborn to care for creates a time management issue, and you are getting less sleep. If you break the habit of training, not only do you have to work harder to get back in shape, but you also have to create a new habit around training with a more demanding schedule.

IS IT SAFE TO TRAIN WHILE PREGNANT?

Not only is it safe to train while pregnant, it's healthy. But it's crucial to listen to your body. Don't force yourself to perform exercises that you could do before you were pregnant but feel awkward or uncomfortable now. And what does and does not feel comfortable is likely to change throughout the course of your pregnancy. You shouldn't avoid training because you think it's dangerous, but you do need to be smart and pay attention to the signals your body is sending. You have a lot of options to choose from, so stay consistent and keep training. You and your baby will be better off because of it.

HOW SHOULD TRAINING CHANGE DURING PREGNANCY?

Some women have to modify or avoid certain exercises that feel uncomfortable, while others feel fine performing all of the same movements they did before becoming pregnant. It largely depends on how you feel each day and how your body responds to the training stimulus. Almost without exception, though, most women should reduce the load as they progress deeper into their pregnancy.

To state the obvious, your body weight will increase, which adds load to your movements. For this reason, I recommend lifting lighter weight and performing higher reps, especially during the latter stages of pregnancy. This is not to say that you can't or shouldn't lift heavy, but it's something to approach carefully, because lifting heavy places more stress on your joints.

With regard to training volume and frequency, not much needs to change. For instance, if you're used to training four days a week for an hour, you can still do that as long as it feels right. Again, you might need to modify the exercise variations and rep ranges.

CAN I STILL HIP THRUST DURING PREGNANCY?

The short answer is yes; you can still hip thrust while pregnant. Some doctors advise women who are pregnant to avoid supine exercises, which includes the hip thrust and glute bridging patterns. What you have to remember, though, is that doctors are primarily concerned with keeping you alive, so they give you extra safe advice. Now, if you agree with their advice and hip thrusting feels sketchy, then you should absolutely take their advice and avoid supine movements. But all of the pregnant women I've trained have been fine with, and loved, hip thrusting (and glute training in general).

What's more, I looked into the research, and it's not conclusive. One well-conducted study showed that supine exercises didn't decrease blood flow to the fetus, and a recent review paper concluded that there is insufficient evidence to deduce that supine exercise during pregnancy is unsafe. Therefore, I wouldn't worry about doing a few sets of hip thrusts a couple of times per week.

However, you will need to modify your setup and execution of the hip thrust in four ways:

1. Place your feet slightly farther away from the bench than normal.
2. Don't go as deep as normal.
3. Place the barbell (or other loading implement) lower on your hips so that it's not putting pressure on the fetus.
4. Push the bar forward to create more space between the bar and your abdomen.

WHAT ARE SOME GOOD EXERCISES TO DO DURING PREGNANCY?

Like I said, the exercises you select largely depend on how you feel. You might find that all exercises are fine, but you need to make some small adjustments, such as reducing the load or altering the band and/or bar position. If certain exercises don't feel quite right, try experimenting with different variations. You might find that by adjusting your stance or modifying the movement, you can still perform the exercise. For example, if deadlifts are uncomfortable, you don't necessarily need to throw out all hip hinging movements; instead, try performing dumbbell Romanian deadlifts or dumbbell stiff-leg deadlift variations.

With regard to specific exercise recommendations, pretty much all bodyweight exercises are on the table unless they don't feel right to you. Then you can scale up from there and experiment with bands and perhaps a dumbbell, kettlebell, and barbell. Some of my clients like wide-stance leg presses, dumbbell sumo squats, knee-banded glute bridges, and lateral band walks, for example. You don't have to do a million glute exercises to stay strong and maintain your muscle. If there are five you can do that feel right, that's plenty.

ARE THERE ANY EXERCISES I SHOULD AVOID WHILE PREGNANT?

I want to be careful not to make a blanket statement because exercise varies so much from one woman to the next, especially during pregnancy.

I will say that I have trained women who couldn't do single-leg exercises because it caused them discomfort. This could be due to a hormone that is released during pregnancy called *relaxin,* which causes the ligaments to become more elastic. Perhaps their pelvises were looser and slightly unstable, causing them pain. But I've also trained pregnant women who had zero issues performing single-leg movements, so it depends on the individual.

Obviously, I can't say, "Avoid this, this, and that." But there will be some exercises that don't feel right, and those are the ones to avoid. You have to pay attention and listen to your internal signals because your body changes a lot during pregnancy, and you can't predict what is going to feel comfortable and what isn't.

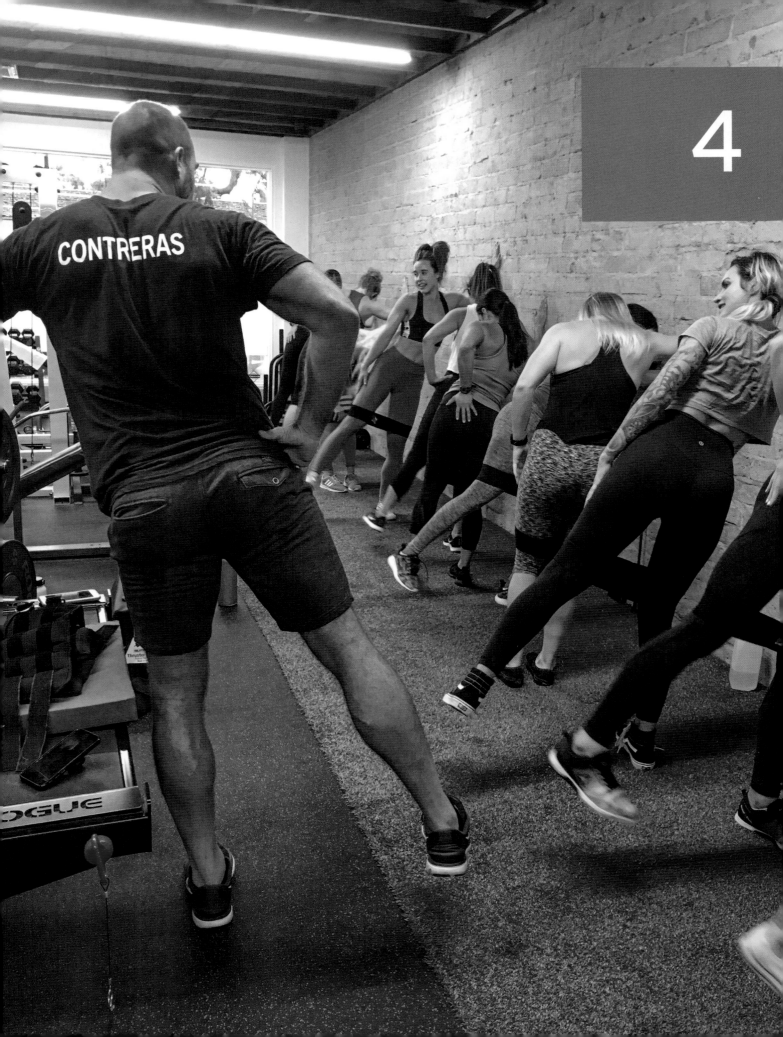

4

PERIODIZATION AND PROGRAMS

In Part 3, I provided the foundational knowledge needed to construct your own individualized training program. You learned about the eight variables used to determine program design, as well as other factors, like fitness level, diet, and genetics. You also learned how to use the Rule of Thirds to create a well-balanced weekly glute training template that balances load, effort, and exercise selection.

Here, I take it a step further by elucidating how I create a comprehensive training plan, referred to as *periodization.* I explain how I program for my clients, how I structure long-term training strategies based on movement patterns and goals, and how to organize those strategies into programs. I also provide several templates for structuring workouts and training splits that cater to a wide range of preferences, as well as how to apply glute training to other fitness modalities, like sports, CrossFit, powerlifting, and bodybuilding.

Although my goal is to equip you with the tools you need to design your own programs, it's helpful to have sample programs to follow, especially if you're a coach looking for basic templates, you're new to strength and physique training, or you simply want a progressive and sequential plan that integrates all of the methods, principles, and techniques covered in this book. That's why I offer three 12-week sample programs in Chapter 18 that take you from beginner to intermediate to advanced.

Regardless of your background, goals, and experience, it's important to understand not only how to build your own training plan, but also why being able to do so is important and what a good program looks like. This is exactly what you will find in this part.

Periodization

In a nutshell, periodization is planning. It's how you logically organize and manipulate each of the program design variables in a sequential fashion in order to bring about a certain physiological effect—gaining strength on a particular lift, putting on muscle, losing fat, peaking for an event, and so on. Think of *periodization* as another term for planning different training strategies and phases (also referred to as *cycles* or *periods*) to maximize the likelihood of achieving the desired fitness results while minimizing the risk of burnout and overtraining. You can organize the phases or cycles of training into individual workouts, which combine to make up the microcycles (usually a week long), which combine to make up the mesocycles (usually around four weeks long), which combine to make up the macrocycles (usually around 16 weeks long), which combine to make up the annual or multi-year plan.

Consider an Olympic athlete who has to peak at different times throughout the year for world championship competitions and every four years for the Olympic Games. To ensure peak performance leading into competition, the athlete needs to fluctuate training stress in a strategic manner and implement a plan that is specific to their sport, the timing of each event, and their unique physical attributes. In other words, performing the same exercises and workouts every week, month after month and year after year, is not an effective strategy. Therein lies the value of periodization. It's necessary, especially when you're shooting for a specific performance goal.

But here's the rub: Some of the foundational beliefs inherent to periodization are based on outdated and incomplete assumptions. In addition, periodization began as a way to train Olympic athletes (very logical), and then it was adapted to fit the needs of powerlifters (still logical) and eventually bodybuilders (not as logical in the traditional sense). And there hasn't been much thought or clarification when it comes to adapting periodization strategies to different training goals, types of athletes, and individuals.

As someone who works primarily with people interested in strength and physique training, I have always viewed long-term periodization as a necessary strategy reserved mainly for serious and specialized athletes. The average personal training client might stick with me for only six months, so sketching out a yearlong periodized plan would not be practical or fruitful. Furthermore, personal training clients aren't as consistent with their training as Olympic athletes, so I can't assume that my clients will show up to every session. However, this is not to say that trainers and self-trained strength and physique enthusiasts can't use some of the principles inherent in different periodization systems to their benefit.

Over the years, strength coaches have borrowed a lot of periodization strategies developed by coaches and athletes to maximize results and minimize the risk of overtraining. In fact, if you create a training program or strive to improve a certain aspect of your game, you will implement some form of periodization whether you know it or not. For this reason, it's important to understand the terminology and acquire a basic foundational knowledge so that you can make sense of the different systems, understand how they work, and figure out how you can use them to create an effective and successful training program.

In this chapter, I break down the terms, principles, strategies, and phases of periodization and explain how to integrate the program design variables to create a well-rounded and systematized training plan specific to strength and physique training. In short, you will learn my unique approach to periodization, which will also help clarify the structure and organization of the three 12-week programs offered in Chapter 18.

PERIODIZATION STRATEGIES

Periodization is complex. To create the best training plan, you need to not only factor in all of the program design variables but also take into account your goals, training experience, fitness level, lifestyle, age, and genetics.

What's more, there are numerous forms or systems of periodization, such as linear, block, undulating, conjugated, and concurrent, each of which has strengths and weaknesses and caters to different training objectives. To make things even more complicated, most training programs incorporate a variety of periodization strategies.

Because this is a book about strength and physique training—or, more specifically, glute training—I'm going to cover periodization only as it pertains to building a bigger, leaner, stronger physique. My intention, in other words, is to explain the primary forms of periodization and how we use them to create well-rounded strength and physique training programs.

There are four periodization strategies that I use when creating a training plan: linearity, undulation, conjugation, and block periodization.

LINEARITY IS PROGRESSING A FITNESS QUALITY OR TRAINING STRESSOR IN A LINEAR FASHION.

Traditionally, linear periodization involves performing fewer reps over time while using greater loads. For example, on the squat and bench press exercises, you might progress from a month of 3 sets of 12 reps with 135 pounds to a month of 3 sets of 8 reps with 155 pounds to a month of 3 sets of 4 reps with 175 pounds. This is the classic method of utilizing linearity. However, there are many other ways to periodize a training plan linearly.

For example, all intelligently structured training programs utilize a form of progressive overload. Progressive overload in and of itself is a linear strategy because you're attempting to increase volume, load, or range of motion linearly over time. Let's say you want to increase your volume each week for a month. You could perform one more rep or one more set or lift 5 more pounds. Each of these is a linear strategy aimed at increasing volume. You could also increase range of motion linearly over time—for example, performing two weeks of block pulls or high box squats, then two weeks of deadlifts or parallel box squats, then two weeks of deficit deadlifts or low box squats.

UNDULATION IS FLUCTUATING THE TRAINING STRESSORS IN A STRATEGIC FASHION.

The traditional method of utilizing undulation in a training program is to vary set and rep schemes on a particular exercise over time. For example, you might hip thrust three times a week for a month, once going for 4 sets of 8 reps, another time going for 5 sets of 6 reps, and another going for 3 sets of 10 reps. This method would be considered *daily undulating periodization*. You could also utilize *weekly undulating periodization* by performing hip thrusts twice a week for a month with 4 sets of 8 reps in weeks 1 and 3 and 5 sets of 6 reps in weeks 2 and 4. (We use this strategy frequently with our Glute Lab clientele.)

Most programs involve an element of undulation because you perform similar movements but in different set and rep schemes throughout the week. For example, performing heavy deadlifts or squats on Monday and lighter stiff-leg deadlifts or goblet squats for higher reps on Thursday is an undulating strategy. And if you're utilizing progressive overload and training to failure and going up in weight over time, your reps will likely be undulated. Even though the goal is to increase linearly, it doesn't happen that way in real life. Take the hip thrust, for example. One week you might hip thrust 225 pounds for 12 reps, then 9 reps, then 7. The next week you might up the weight to 235 pounds and get 10 reps, then 8 reps, then 7. Maybe you stick with 235 pounds for another week and get 12 reps, then 10 reps, then 6. If you go to true failure on all of your sets, then the reps are never nice and neat like 3x8. (I'm not saying you should go to failure on every set; the point is that strength adaptations are never perfectly linear. Human physiology doesn't work that way.)

CONJUGATION IS COMBINING MULTIPLE METHODS THROUGHOUT THE TRAINING WEEK.

If a training program prescribes a wide variety of rep ranges each week, which most programs do, it falls into the conjugate periodization category. For example, you might perform heavy military presses one day (5 sets of 3 reps), seated dumbbell shoulder presses on another day (4 sets of 8 reps), and light high-rep dumbbell lateral raises on another day (3 sets of 15 reps). In this scenario, you're targeting delt strength, hypertrophy, and strength endurance all in the same week. And you'll likely switch up the exercises regularly, which is also considered a conjugate strategy.

BLOCK PERIODIZATION INVOLVES FOCUSING ON DIFFERENT QUALITIES OF TRAINING DURING SPECIFIC PERIODS.

Block periodization is hard to define because it encompasses different types of training. In general, the blocks of time are organized in a manner that supposedly allows for continuous positive adaptation. When it comes to the duration of each phase or block, three to six weeks is the norm. But I program every four weeks, or month to month, which I will elaborate on shortly.

Now that you're familiar with the basic periodization strategies, let's talk about how to incorporate the program design variables into these systems to create the best possible training plan.

PERIODIZING THE PROGRAM DESIGN VARIABLES

Although periodization usually involves tweaking sets, reps, and loads, I want to emphasize that any training and program design variable can be strategically manipulated. This is the main criticism I have with popular forms of periodization: the programs are often generic and lack creativity, manipulating only a few of the program design variables—specifically volume, load, and effort—instead of taking into account all eight program design variables, which also include training frequency, exercise selection, exercise order, tempo, and rest periods.

To create a well-rounded periodization program for people interested in strength and physique training, you could fluctuate the effort in a weekly fashion by training progressively harder for a few weeks in a row and then having an easy week (referred to as a *deload week*). You could get creative with your exercise selection by performing progressively harder exercise variations—for example, push-ups for three weeks, then dips for three weeks, then handstand push-ups for three weeks. You could also rotate exercise order by performing squats last in the workout in a fatigued state for two weeks, then in the middle of the workout for two weeks, then first in the workout while fresh for two weeks. You could periodize tempo by picking a lift and performing eccentric-accentuated reps one week, then pause reps the next week, then constant tension reps the following week. Perhaps you perform the same sets and reps with the same load for four weeks in a row but decrease rest periods between sets, thereby increasing training density.

As you can see, the possibilities are endless when it comes to periodizing the program design variables using the principles inherent to periodization. The point is that you need to factor in all of the variables, not just two or three of them, when creating a training plan. What's more, there are an infinite number of ways to create a program when you take all of the training variables into account.

However, some strategies pan out better than others when put to the test in the real world. Although periodization is very popular among strength coaches and its classic schemes are used almost predominantly in the training of athletes, it's been widely criticized in the literature for various reasons. This is not to say that periodization isn't beneficial; it's just that it's hard to study due to the lengthy time periods required to do it justice and the individual differences among athletes.

For instance, when it comes to maximizing muscular strength, the research clearly indicates an advantage for periodizing training. But periodization currently doesn't appear to be mandatory for maximizing muscular hypertrophy. This is probably because most of the lifters tested pushed themselves to get stronger during the training period and therefore engaged in progressive overload, which is a form of linearity and is a central facet of periodization. In other words, they were periodizing their training despite being considered "non-periodized" because it didn't adhere to a predetermined plan.

As of 2019, there is zero research examining different forms of periodization on glute growth. So the main point I want you to remember is that all forms of periodization work as long as you factor in all of the program design variables and incorporate the principles inherent in the periodization strategies previously outlined. The secret is knowing which system to use and which variable to modify based on the situation. This is where periodization gets tricky, because you have to not only take into consideration individual differences and training goals but also understand how to switch things up from cycle to cycle or phase to phase.

GLUTE LAB TRAINING PHASES

If you're a beginner or you're simply someone who wants a well-rounded program with a glute training emphasis that factors in all of the aforementioned program design variables and principles of periodization, then the training plans offered later in this part of the book are a good place to start. But if you're a coach or someone who is interested in creating your own training plan based on your goals, experience, and preferences, then you need to take a systems-based approach to periodization by not only taking into account all of the strategies and variables previously covered but also understanding how to structure different phases of training.

For instance, unless someone needs to work on a specific lift or focus on developing a specific area of the body, I prefer to switch up the program every month for variety. For example, here's how I program for my online programming platform, Booty by Bret:

For the first month, I might implement a well-rounded plan where you train three days a week: the first day you prioritize squats, the second day you prioritize hip thrusts, and the third day you prioritize deadlifts. The next month, I might choose a squat specialization plan, and the month after that, perhaps a hip thrust specialization plan, meaning that you hip thrust first on all three days and program the squat and deadlift on only one training day per week after you've hip thrusted. For example, if you're following a hip thrust daily undulated periodization (DUP) plan—which is when you perform a certain lift multiple times a week with varying set and rep schemes—your program might look something like this (I have structured the sets and reps in the intermediate program this way):

HIP THRUST DUP

DAY 1		
SET	REPETITIONS	LOAD
1	10	~75%
2	10	~75%
3	10	~75%
4	AMRAP	~75%

DAY 2		
SET	REPETITIONS	LOAD
1	6	~85%
2	6	~85%
3	6	~85%
4	6	~85%
5	AMRAP	~85%

DAY 3		
SET	REPETITIONS	LOAD
1	15	~65%
2	15	~65%
3	AMRAP	~65%

If I'm putting a client through a hip thrust DUP program, I might keep them on it for up to six weeks and try to get them to increase each week using progressive overload (mainly reps or load in this scenario). The month (or phase) after that, I might do a deadlift specialization plan, and then the next month, a single-leg-focused plan.

The plan I choose largely depends—like everything—on the athlete's goals, but this is a universal blueprint that I've found to be very effective at building strength and developing the glutes. With my Booty by Bret plan, I almost always alter the training focus every four weeks in the following order: well-rounded to squat to hip thrust to deadlift to single leg and then back around. You're always squatting, deadlifting, hip thrusting, lunging, and doing abduction work, but the exercise selection, order, and volume are biased to emphasize one lift or category. I also include an upper-body exercise to focus on each month. Research shows that it's difficult to build strength but easy to maintain it. For this reason, greatly emphasizing one lift while putting other lifts on the back burner makes a lot of sense. In fact, I think it's the best possible way to build total body strength and maximum muscle over the long run. Here's what it looks like:

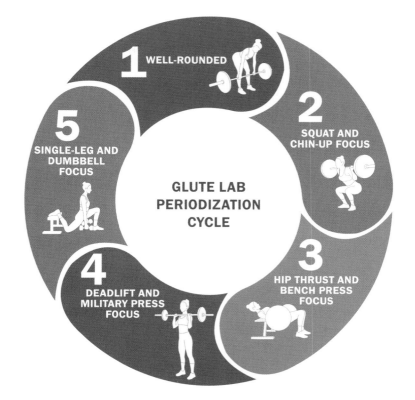

I realize that this type of periodization isn't all that common because it switches the focus instead of keeping the exercises the same and simply manipulating volume and intensity (actually load and effort in this case, but the mainstream term is intensity, which I don't like because it can mean either load or effort and is therefore ambiguous). But it is a superior form of planning in my opinion because it 1) keeps things interesting from a psychological standpoint, 2) naturally helps prevent overuse injuries, and 3) allows for well-rounded lower-body strength development and the full development of the upper and lower gluteus maximus subdivisions. But notice that the monthly focuses aren't haphazard; they're carefully planned. For example, after a squat month, you'll be eager to switch to hip thrusts because your knees may need a period of unloading, and after a deadlift month, your back may need a period of unloading, hence the single-leg-focused month that follows.

Now, do you really need to change up your workout every four weeks? Definitely not. Theoretically, you could do the same thing for years on end and see great results. But you will probably develop overuse injuries unless you really know what you're doing and you tolerate the lifts you perform well. More importantly, you will likely get so bored that you might stop enjoying your training. And when you don't enjoy your training, you're more prone to quit lifting altogether. The goal is to keep lifting and stay strong for life.

For these reasons, switching it up is important, but again, you can and should keep things similar. Each new phase shouldn't be radically different from the previous one, with totally different exercises, splits, and techniques. I like the "same but different" philosophy whereby you're always doing hip thrusts, squats, deadlifts, lunges, back extensions, kickbacks, and abduction work, but you do them in different order, choose unique variations, and tinker with the set and rep schemes and tempos to maximize your results by staving off overuse injuries, sparking new gains in the lifts and muscles you're focusing on, preventing habituation, and staying excited about your training.

It's also important to consider fluctuation of training stress. Many lifters go to the gym 52 weeks a year and attempt to push it to the limit every session. These types often fizzle out and end up injuring themselves or getting run into the ground. You can't go all out every session or even every week, for that matter.

As I mentioned, I like four-week training cycles, but you could just as well do three-, six-, or eight-week cycles and see great results. The first week of each cycle is a deload/introductory week. This is where you get a good feel for the new exercises, practice your technique, and figure out what loads to use for the following week. You can still get in a good workout, but you're not going to failure on anything, and you're definitely not going for any personal records. Think of this week as a 7 out of 10 in terms of overall effort. During the second week, you up the ante and go at an 8 out of 10 in terms of effort, still focusing hard on good form. For the third week, you ramp it up again and aim for a 9 out of 10 in terms of effort. Then, for week 4, you go all out (10 out of 10) and strive to hit some critical PRs. During this last week, you can let your form slide very slightly (think 10 percent degradation at a maximum) in order to crush some PRs. After the fourth week, you should feel a bit beat up and drained and should look forward to the upcoming deload/introductory week for the next phase. It looks like this:

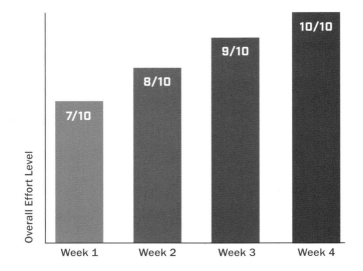

This is just one way to go about things, but it's certainly more effective than going at a 10 out of 10 every week and constantly being hurt, sick, or exhausted. This is how I want you to carry out the programs in Chapter 18.

The programs offered in this book (and the ones featured in my online training platform, Booty by Bret) adhere to the principles and general guidelines covered in this chapter. By following these programs, you can be sure that all of the program design variables have been carefully considered and periodized intelligently. It's my hope that I've provided you with the essential tools you need to construct your own training plan, but I also want to emphasize that sketching out a concrete month-by-month periodized training plan—though beneficial—is not a mandatory practice, especially for knowledgeable and experienced self-trained athletes.

When I initially stumbled across research showing how easy it is to maintain strength, I had a hard time believing it. But then I began experimenting in the gym (I've posted many of these experiments on my blog) and found it to be true.

The fact is, gaining strength is hard, especially after you've been lifting properly for a couple of years, but maintaining strength is easy. Because your physique is highly influenced by your relative total body strength, it makes sense to take advantage of the maintenance phenomenon and prioritize one or two lifts at a time.

In other words, don't try to build your squat, deadlift, hip thrust, lunge, bench press, incline press, military press, dip, chin-up, and row strength all at the same time. Instead, pick one or two lifts and focus on them by performing them (or similar variations) first in your workouts with more volume. Do less volume for the lifts that are on maintenance mode, and know that they'll get prioritized down the road.

Think of the aforementioned 10 lifts as balls that you're trying to juggle. Each ball corresponds to a main lift, which collectively represents your total body strength. In the beginning, you can juggle all of them because the balls are small, meaning that you're still learning the movements and probably not lifting too heavy. But as you gain strength and start lifting heavier loads, each ball gets bigger. Now you're trying to juggle larger and larger balls, which is difficult to manage. At a certain point, you can't juggle all of them simultaneously, and your gains plateau. So, rather than try to juggle all of the big lifts, focus on juggling two for an entire month while performing a couple of sets a week of the other lifts because, again, it's easy to maintain strength. After a month, rotate them and specialize in two different lifts for a month while the others are in maintenance mode. If you do this in a strategic, sequential fashion, you will experience better results and continue to gain strength and improve your physique.

This is what I do in my Booty by Bret program, and it works incredibly well. This method of periodization has the side benefit of building a balanced physique that is not hampered by overuse injuries. I could have achieved much better results had I understood this and developed this system 20 years ago. Now go build them balls!

TRAINING INTUITIVELY

Many people wonder whether it's absolutely necessary to plan out different training phases. The answer is, not necessarily. If you have vast experience and good instincts, you can train intuitively—deciding what you want to do on any given day based on how you feel and what you want to work—and see results that are just as good as long as you have some sort of structure (for example, you're following the Rule of Thirds) and utilize a progressive approach. In fact, for people with 10-plus years of lifting experience who read, train intelligently, and experiment in their training, pure intuitive training is probably the best way to exercise. But this same system would be detrimental to the average beginner. No matter how you plan your training, you must always listen to your body and make adjustments on the fly. But you have to earn the right to abandon a formal plan and "just wing it" in the gym.

In the next chapter, I outline various training splits, which you can use as templates to guide your training routines. Whether you're training intuitively or designing a periodized program, the training splits complement the Rule of Thirds by providing structure and organization to your workouts and training phases.

16

Training Splits

In the early days of powerlifting and bodybuilding, it was common to train the whole body during a training session. Strongmen from the classic era performed full-body workouts, and even old-school bodybuilders like Arnold Schwarzenegger started off with programs such as the "Golden Six Workout," which consisted of back squats, bench presses, chin-ups, overhead presses, curls, and sit-ups, three times per week.

Over time, though, bodybuilders and powerlifters rationalized that they might see better gains if they split up their workouts. Powerlifters began training their lower and upper bodies separately or focusing on one main lift per day with a couple of accessory lifts added in, and bodybuilders started splitting up their workouts based on muscles and body parts. Passionate and sometimes uncivil arguments over which is the most effective training strategy take place to this day. Is it better to train the full body or to split it up based on pushing and pulling muscles or body regions and muscle groups?

The truth is, they all work, and they're all awesome. But you have to learn how to make them work for you, as each one requires unique training strategies and styles. While almost all modern bodybuilders adhere to body part split training, most personal trainers prescribe full-body training.

There isn't much research on this topic, either. My colleague Brad Schoenfeld and I conducted a study and found full-body training to be slightly superior to body part split training for muscular gains, but all of the participants had previously been doing body part splits, so it could have been the novelty factor at play. At any rate, I believe everyone can benefit from experimenting with all of the various training styles and philosophies.

If you're new to training, I recommend following one or more of the 12-week programs offered in Chapter 18. Doing so will expose you to all of the main movement patterns and some of the basic periodization strategies. After you gain some experience and feel comfortable with the movements, you can experiment with the different training splits covered in this chapter. As you will see, I provide a one-week program template for each training split, which you can repeat for one month. And you still follow the same protocol previously outlined in that you start with a deload, or easy, week and progressively ramp up the effort and load each week, with the fourth week being the hardest.

Experimenting with the different training splits will give you a better understanding of what you like and don't like. Perhaps you like full-body training, or maybe you prefer to switch things up. The point is, you will never know what you like or how to train intuitively if you don't experiment with different training strategies. The training splits are there to give you options and to help you pick out the strategies that work best for you. To quote the late Bruce Lee, "Absorb what is useful, discard what is not, and add what is uniquely your own."

TRAINING SPLIT PROTOCOLS

There are several training split protocols that you can follow for strength and physique training.

BODY PART SPLIT

The body part split, widely used by bodybuilders, involves arranging training days based on body parts: for example, a chest/triceps day, a back/biceps day, a leg/glute day, a shoulder day, and an arm day. Most bodybuilders train frequently throughout the week, but some prefer to train just three or four times per week. In that case, you can pair pecs and lats on day 1, quads and glutes on day 2, delts and arms on day 3, and hams and glutes on day 4, as in Example 1 below. If you're really trying to build your glutes while adhering to a body part split plan, I suggest training five or six days per week and hitting your glutes three times on different days—one day pairing glutes with quads, one day pairing glutes with hams, and one day training the glutes on their own (see Example 2 on the next page).

Example 1: Body Part Split with Glute Focus: 4-Day Option with Two Leg Days

DAY 1: PECS AND LATS	
Bench Press	3x5
Wide-Grip Pull-Down	3x8
Dumbbell Incline Press	3x8
Chest-Supported Row	3x8
Dip	2x AMRAP
Inverted Row	2x AMRAP
Cable Crossover	2x12
Straight-Arm Pull-Down	2x12

DAY 2: QUADS AND GLUTES	
Back Squat	3x5
Leg Press	3x8
Dumbbell Walking Lunge	2x16
Barbell Hip Thrust	3x10
Leg Extension	2x20
Seated Hip Abduction	2x20

DAY 3: DELTS AND ARMS	
Military Press	3x5
Dumbbell Upright Row	2x8
Lateral Raise	2x10
Prone Rear Delt Raise	2x12
Chin-up	2x5
Hammer Curl	2x10
Close-Grip Bench Press	2x5
Rope Triceps Extension	2x10

DAY 4: HAMS AND GLUTES	
Deadlift	3x5
Dumbbell Back Extension	3x12
Lying Leg Curl	2x20
Seated Leg Curl	2x20
Frog Pump	2x50
Extra-Range Side-Lying Hip Abduction	2x30

Example 2: Body Part Split with Glute Focus: 5-Day Option with 3 Leg Days

DAY 1: GLUTES	
Barbell Hip Thrust	3x8
Glute Kickback Machine	3x10
Bodyweight Back Extension	3x20
Cable Standing Hip Abduction	3x10
Seated Hip Abduction Machine	3x20

DAY 2: CHEST/SHOULDERS/TRICEPS	
Barbell Incline Press	3x6
Barbell Military Press	3x8
Push-up	3x AMRAP
Dumbbell Lateral Raise	3x12
Rope Triceps Extension	3x10

DAY 3: QUADS AND GLUTES	
Front Squat	3x6
Leg Press	3x10
Dumbbell Walking Lunge	3x8
Leg Extension	3x10
Crunch	2x20
Hanging Leg Raise	2x10

DAY 4: BACK/REAR DELTS/BICEPS	
Chin-up	3x6
Chest-Supported Row	3x8
One-Arm Row	3x10
Prone Rear Delt Raise	3x10
Easy Bar Curl	3x10

DAY 5: HAMS AND GLUTES	
Conventional Deadlift	3x6
Weighted Back Extension	3x10
Stability Ball	3x8
Lying Leg Curl	3x10
Calf Raise Machine	2x10
Seated Calf Raise Machine	2x20

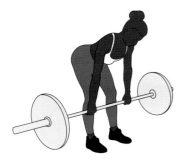

UPPER/LOWER SPLIT

This split is popular among strength coaches and powerlifters. It involves splitting up your training days between upper-body and lower-body muscles. Most lifters adhering to this plan train four days per week, with two lower-body sessions and two upper-body sessions. In my survey involving more than 13,000 participants, I learned that this was the most popular form of training with my followers, which was surprising.

Upper/Lower: 4-Day Full-Body Template

DAY 1: UPPER BODY	
Bench Press	3x5
Chin-up	3x5
Dip	3x8
Inverted Row	3x AMRAP
Lateral Raise	3x10

DAY 2: LOWER BODY	
Back Squat	3x5
Single-Leg Deadlift	3x8
Barbell Hip Thrust	3x10
Dumbbell Walking Lunge	3x8
Side-Lying Hip Raise	3x10

DAY 3: UPPER BODY		DAY 4: LOWER BODY	
Close-Grip Bench Press	3x5	Deadlift	3x3
Pull-up	3x AMRAP	Front Squat	3x5
Military Press	3x8	Glute Ham Raise	3x12
Chest-Supported Row	3x12	Dumbbell Back Extension	3x20
Prone Rear Delt Raise	3x10	Seated Hip Abduction Machine	3x20

What Type of Training Split Do You Typically Perform?

Answered: 13,675
Skipped: 39

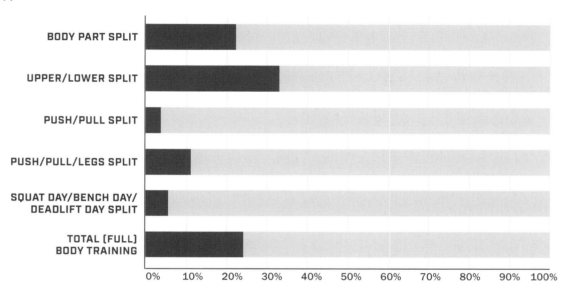

PUSH/PULL SPLIT

This type of program, used mostly by athletes and powerlifters, involves splitting up your training days between pushing exercises for the upper and lower body and pulling exercises for the upper and lower body. Most lifters adhering to this plan train four days per week, with two push sessions and two pull sessions.

Push/Pull: 4-Day Full-Body Template

DAY 1: PUSH		DAY 2: PULL	
Back Squat	3x5	Single-Leg Deadlift	3x8
Bench Press	3x5	Wide-Grip Pull-Down	3x8
Barbell Hip Thrust	3x8	Dumbbell Back Extension	3x15
Military Press	3x8	Seated Row	3x15
Banded Seated Hip Abduction	2x50	Cable Lateral Raise	2x10

Push/Pull: 4-Day Full-Body Template *(continued)*

DAY 3: PUSH	
Front Squat	3x5
Close-Grip Bench Press	3x5
Barbell Hip Thrust	3x12
Handle Push-up	3x AMRAP
Cable Standing Hip Abduction	2x12

DAY 4: PULL	
Deadlift	3x5
Chin-up	3x AMRAP
Glute Ham Raise	3x12
Inverted Row	3x AMRAP
Seated Face Pull	2x15

S/B/DL/HYP SPLIT

This is another popular split among powerlifters. One day focuses on squats, one day on bench presses, one day on deadlifts, and a final day on hypertrophy for the entire body. Obviously, you perform additional exercises on the S, B, and DL days. (See page 276 for another powerlifting training template with a glute training emphasis that utilizes this training split.)

S/B/DL/HYP: 4-Day Full-Body Template

DAY 1: SQUAT	
Back Squat	3x5
Walking Lunge	2x16
Pendulum Reverse Hyper	3x10
Single-Leg Romanian Deadlift	2x16
Lateral Band Walk	3x20

DAY 2: BENCH	
Bench Press	4x3
Close-Grip Bench Press	2x8
Chest-Supported Row	3x12
One-Arm Row	2x12

DAY 3: DEADLIFT	
Deadlift	3x3
Rack Pull	2x3
Front Squat	3x5
Barbell Hip Thrust	3x8
Monster Walk	3x20

DAY 4: HYPERTROPHY	
Weighted Push-up	5x10
Inverted Row	5x10
Pendulum Reverse Hyper	5x10
Glute Ham Raise	5x10
YTWL	2x10

TOTAL BODY (FULL BODY)

This style of training has achieved greater popularity in the past decade and is my personal favorite. Total body means you're hitting all of your muscles in a single session, not splitting up workouts. Most lifters who adhere to total-body training (TBT) perform three weekly workouts.

Total Body: 3-Day Template

DAY 1: MEDIUM	
Front Squat	3x8
Dumbbell Incline Press	3x8
Romanian Deadlift	3x8
Seated Row	3x8
Single-Leg Hip Thrust	3x8
Banded Side-Lying Clam	3x12

DAY 2: LIGHT	
Knee-Banded Hip Thrust	2x15
Dumbbell Overhead Press	2x15
Dumbbell Reverse Lunge	2x15
Supinated Pull-Down	2x15
Dumbbell Back Extension	2x15
Lateral Raise	2x15

DAY 3: HEAVY	
Sumo Deadlift	4x3
Close-Grip Bench Press	4x3
Pause Back Squat	4x3
Negative Chin-up	4x3
Pause Barbell Hip Thrust	4x3
Banded Standing Hip Abduction	3x12

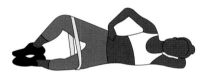

COMPOUND/BRO

This form of total-body training alternates between days involving heavier compound movements that are more taxing on the body and days involving lighter compound and single-joint movements that tend to be easier on the body. For example, you could perform three typical full-body workouts per week with two "bro" workouts (focusing on the mind-muscle connection and getting a muscle pump) sandwiched in between. Another example would be to perform a push day, a pull day, a bro day, and a total-body day.

Compound/Bro: 4-Day Template

DAY 1: PUSH	
High-Bar Back Squat	3x5
Close-Grip Bench Press	3x5
Leg Press	3x10
Military Press	3x10
Knee-Banded Glute Bridge	3x20

DAY 2: PULL	
Single-Leg Deadlift	3x8
Chin-up	3x AMRAP
Back Extension	3x30
Inverted Row	3x AMRAP
Nordic Ham Curl	3x3

Compound/Bro: 4-Day Template *(continued)*

DAY 3: BRO	
Lateral Raise	4x15
Rear Delt Raise	3x12
Dumbbell Curl	3x10
Cable Triceps Extension	3x10
Hammer Curl	2x10
Frog Pump	4x50
Banded Seated Hip Abduction	2x30

DAY 4: TOTAL BODY	
Barbell Hip Thrust Pyramid	10/8/6/15
Incline Press	3x8
Supinated Pull-Down	3x8
Dumbbell Walking Lunge	2x20
Push-up	2x AMRAP
One-Arm Row	2x10
Glute Ham Raise	2x15

THE COMPOUND/BRO SYSTEM

Many of you are like me—borderline addicted to the weight room. You'd probably see better results if you took more rest days or split up your workouts, but you love lifting and working your entire body at once. Several years ago, I developed the compound/bro system for the gym addict who still wants to see good results.

Here's what you're going to do: on days 1, 3, and 5 (for example, Monday, Wednesday, and Friday), perform compound lifts with low to moderate rep ranges (1 to 10 reps) and more rest time between sets (3 minutes). On days 2 and 4 and possibly on day 6 (for example, Tuesday and Thursday, with Saturday being optional), perform more targeted, isolated movements with moderate to high rep ranges (10 to 30 reps) and shorter rest times (1 to 2 minutes).

I provide fairly comprehensive lists in the chart on the next page, but obviously there are other movements you can perform. The main goal is to work your entire body every session but to alternate between taxing (compound lifts) and non-taxing workouts (isolated movements).

Effort is another important consideration. Push yourself harder on the compound days and leave more reps in the tank on the bro days. On the bro days, you're looking to feel the burn and get a pump, but you're not going to failure or trying to utilize progressive overload. Use the mind-muscle connection with strict form.

If you push yourself too hard on the bro days or get too sore, the following day's workout will be compromised, preventing you from getting stronger and gaining muscle. It takes a couple of weeks to really get the hang of this system, as you'll learn the best exercises for you and exactly how hard to push yourself so that you're still fresh the following day.

When I was doing compound/bro, I performed frog pumps, extra-range side-lying hip abductions, lying leg curls, cable lateral raises, prone rear delt raises, and face pulls. I'd get a nice glute and delt pump and still crush some heavy weights the following day. Full-body training is very demanding, and most people screw it up by doing too much. This system allows you to make gains while satisfying your daily urges to lift.

THE COMPOUND/BRO
SYSTEM

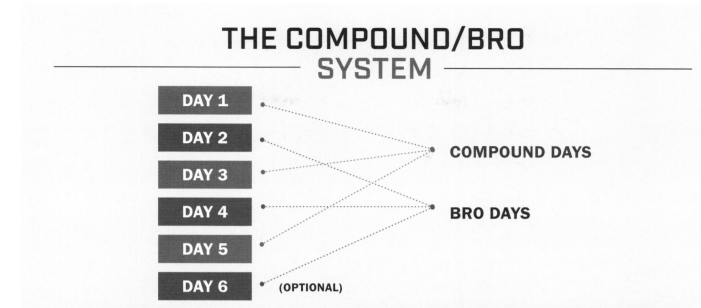

COMPOUND DAYS: Pick 4 exercises and do 3–4 sets of each		BRO DAYS: Pick 6 exercises and do 2–3 sets of each	
VARIATIONS OF:		**VARIATIONS OF:**	
Barbell Squat	Military Press	Bodyweight Frog Pump	Bodyweight Reverse Hyper
Barbell Deadlift	Bench Press	Bodyweight Curtsy Lunge	Cable Kickback
Barbell Hip Trust	Chin-up	Glute Ham Raise/Nordic	Abduction/Adduction Work
Barbell Glute Bridge	Pull-Down	Knee-Banded Glute Bridge	Leg Curl/Leg Extension
Leg Press	Incline Press	Bodyweight Step-up	Peck Deck/Fly/Crossover
Loaded Split Squat	Push-up	Light Goblet Squat	Pullover
Loaded Step-up	Dip	Light Kettlebell Deadlift	Straight-Arm Pull-Down
Barbell Good Morning	Row	Dumbbell Single-Leg RDL	Face Pull
		Kettlebell Swing	Rear Delt Raise
		Sled Push	Lateral Raise
		Banded Hip Thrust	Front Raise
		Cable Pull-Through	Curl
		Bodyweight Back Extension	Triceps Extension

You can follow any of these training templates and see good results. Each split has its own inherent strengths and weaknesses. For example, body part splits allow you to hit all of the angles, but training frequency is usually compromised. Total-body training is the most metabolically demanding, but you can't always fit in all of the exercises you love. I prefer total-body workouts (which technically aren't a split) because they allow for more frequent glute training and more variety as long as you treat the program like a glute specialization routine, which I do. In fact, the three programs included in Chapter 18 are all total-body training programs.

Again, you have to assess your goals and—equally important—consider what you enjoy. No system is perfect. I switch things up throughout the year and try to incorporate several different splits. When I perform total-body routines, I miss my delt day. When I perform split routines, I miss feeling like I hit everything in each workout. As long as you're performing adequate volume, following the Rule of Thirds, and training your glutes at least twice per week, you can essentially choose the split you like best and see great results.

Glute Training for Sports, CrossFit, Bodybuilding, and Powerlifting

If you follow my glute training system, there's a good chance that you will achieve your ideal physique while improving your athletic abilities. However, there are a ton of different ways to train your body. If glute training isn't your main jam, that's okay. Whether you're an athlete, you play sports, or you prefer other strength training modalities, like CrossFit, bodybuilding, or powerlifting, you can still train your glutes specifically without compromising your training. In fact, your athletic abilities, strength, and physique might improve because you're implementing glute-dominant movements that build and strengthen your glutes in a new and unique way.

GLUTE TRAINING FOR SPORTS AND PERFORMANCE (ATHLETES)

If you train your glutes, your strength and sports performance are very likely to improve. I've recognized this across the board with the athletes I work with, and we're noticing it at the Glute Lab with a variety of athletes from different sports. Even women who are purely interested in physique training tell me how much better and stronger they feel when playing sports or enjoying activities outside the gym.

However, when you're training for performance, you do things differently than when you're training for hypertrophy. If you're training purely for glute gains, you can focus on adding a lot more volume in the form of banded burnouts and high-repetition exercises. Also, you can and should train to failure or very close to it. For sports performance, you want the rep speeds to stay relatively fast, so you don't want to perform too many grinding, slow reps. This is why clusters and velocity-based training are popular in athletic weight rooms. So, instead of performing banded burnouts and training to fatigue and muscle failure, you use a variety of loads and keep the rep speeds explosive to better mimic the actions of sport (in most cases).

It's also important to train from different vectors—horizontal, vertical, and lateral/rotary (see Chapter 10 for a complete description of each vector)—and mix heavy, moderate, and light loads along with explosive training like Olympic lifts, jump squats, sled work, and of course sprints, agility drills, plyometrics, and ballistics.

In other words, you want to get strong and powerful from every vector or direction that you use in your sport—forward and backward, up and down, side to side, and rotating. And you have to work these directions against resistance to produce force across the athletic spectrum. In scientific terms, you want to shift your entire force-velocity curve rightward/upward so you're producing more force at every level of velocity and more velocity at every level of force required.

In the graph below, notice that you can pick any point on the Y-axis (force) and trace it rightward, or pick any point on the X-axis (velocity) and trace it upward, and find that the After Training value has increased compared to the Before Training value. You're now more forceful at any velocity and faster with any load.

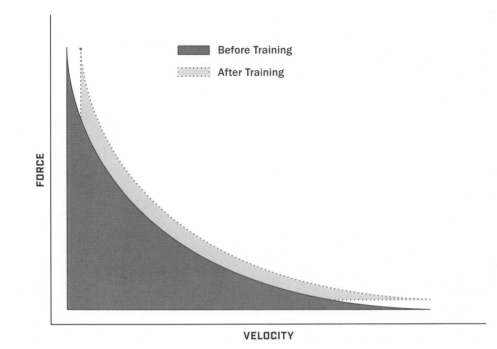

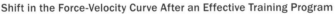

Shift in the Force-Velocity Curve After an Effective Training Program

Finally, you should prioritize heavy and explosive training in the gym. If you're a track athlete or you play sports, then speed training is a critical component—you need to be sprinting and doing plyometrics. And you need to perform your speed and explosive work first in the training session while you're fresh. If you have the simultaneous goal of building bigger, stronger glutes, then you should add glute-specific work as well. But you should also prioritize your hamstrings, as they're likely the most important sprinting muscles (the glutes are probably second), and perform Nordic ham curls, which can help prevent hamstring strain injuries.

However, if you're trying to sprint and perform plyometrics with the intention of building a better butt, please don't waste your time. These explosive actions are simply too rapid to grow meaningful amounts of muscle, because not enough cross-bridges can form to generate maximal tension in the glutes. Sprinters do indeed have huge glutes, but this has more to do with their genetics and resistance training than their activities on the track.

Athletes train in a variety of ways, but most of them stick to full-body training protocols. On the following page, I provide a sample program that combines explosive training with heavy lifting, which is necessary for most athletes. It assumes that the athlete trains three times per week and lifts after completing any sprint, plyometric, agility, and med ball work.

You might remember that I said to do 16 hard sets for glutes, but if you're an athlete, you can do more because the power exercises (the first two exercises on each day) are not as draining, you're not training to failure on high reps, and some additional low-demand accessories are needed (hip flexion and abs). This program isn't too demanding as long as it's the off-season.

DAY 1	
Hex Bar Jump Squat	4x3
Heavy Kettlebell Swing	3x8
Back Squat	3x6
Barbell Hip Thrust	3x6
Close-Grip Bench Press	3x6
Chest-Supported Row	3x8
Cable Hip Flexion	2x10
Ab Wheel Rollout	2x10
Side Plank	2x 30 sec

DAY 2	
Heavy Sled Push	3x 20 meters
Explosive 45-Degree Hyper	3x8
Dumbbell Bulgarian Split Squat	3x8
Block Pull	3x6
Incline Press	3x8
Weighted Chin-up	3x3
Nordic Ham Curl	3x3
Pallof Press	2x10
Hollow Body Hold	2x 20 sec

DAY 3	
Jumping Lunge	3x6 (3 jumps per leg)
One-Arm Power Snatch	3x5
Back Squat	3x6
Barbell Hip Thrust Pyramid	10/8/6/20
Close-Grip Bench Press	3x6
Dumbbell Bent-Over Row	3x8
Ankle Weight Standing Hip Flexion	2x12
RKC Plank	2x 20 sec
Farmer's Walk	2x 20 meters

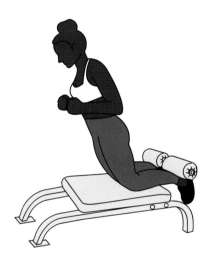

As you can see, this program builds and strengthens the glutes so that they can produce incredible amounts of force and power in sports. It has two explosive lifts per day (for example, the jumping lunge), along with a knee-dominant exercise (back squat), a hip-dominant exercise (hip thrust), an upper-body push (close-grip bench press), an upper-body pull (chin-up), and some accessories sprinkled in, such as multidirectional core stability (for example, the Pallof press), hip flexion (cable hip flexion), and/or eccentric hamstring work (Nordic ham curl). If you prefer Olympic lifts (such as power cleans), you can substitute those for the explosive lifts listed above.

There's no single best answer to this question. It depends on the sport and position. As I mentioned, for most sports it's important to train the entire body. Obviously, I'm biased toward the hip thrust, and I think every athlete can benefit from performing hip thrust, squat, and deadlift movement patterns. But—and this is crucial—you also need to focus on your entire body by emphasizing movements that are specific to your sport and target your weak areas.

In almost every case, the best way to improve your performance in your sport is to do the actions involved in your sport. This is the rule of specificity. At the most basic level, it means that if your sport is fighting, then the best exercise is fight training. If your sport is swimming, then you need to swim. Everything else you do is supplemental, and careful consideration should be given when programming strength and conditioning. If what you are doing in the weight room is not making you better at your sport or preventing injuries, then it's probably a waste of time.

What's more, which exercises are the best is subject to the individual, meaning it's different for everyone. For example, let's say all you've done is squats your whole life; you've never deadlifted or performed a lot of hinging patterns. In such a scenario (as unlikely as it may be), deadlifting will give you the most bang for your buck because you will see a lot of gains from performing this new movement pattern, which also happens to translate to your sport. It's the same with the hip thrust. If all you've done is squat and deadlift and you've never performed glute-dominant movements like the hip thrust, then you are likely to see huge gains from performing thrust movement patterns because you've relied so heavily on your quads and hamstrings until now. How you perform the exercises is important, too. For sports, you generally should avoid training to failure, keep the reps explosive, and experiment with cluster sets and velocity-based training.

In addition, a lot of recent research indicates that you get the most benefits from performing exercises with a specific load tailored to your individual force-velocity profile. Very strong athletes who are force dominant benefit more from performing exercises explosively with lighter loads, whereas very speedy athletes who are velocity dominant benefit more from performing exercises with heavier loads. More research needs to be conducted to determine which exercises improve each particular skill and action best and for how long this method should be practiced. For example, should athletes stick to their ideal loads for a month, a year, or a lifetime, and at what point should they incorporate more variety in loading?

I wish I could give you a blanket prescription that is ideal for all sports and all athletes, but the reality is that you have to figure out your weaknesses, select the best exercises to round out those weaknesses, and—most importantly—design a program that is specifically tailored to you and your sport and position. Although more and more strength coaches are coming around to glute training, I believe glute-dominant movement patterns are the missing link in a lot of athletes' strength training programs.

GLUTE TRAINING FOR CROSSFIT

CrossFit is undeniably one of the biggest trends in fitness, and it has profoundly influenced the way people train. CrossFit methods have been shown in the research and around the world to lead to incredible physiological improvements and, in terms of safety, have a similar injury rate as other popular training systems, like bodybuilding and powerlifting. Nevertheless, I believe CrossFit could be even better with some slight improvements in programming.

One of the central tenets of CrossFit is that the CrossFit approach is the best way to achieve elite physical results. The problem is that few CrossFit workouts of the day (WODs) include specific gluteus maximus exercises such as hip thrusts, barbell glute bridges, and horizontal back extensions. While they do tend to include squat and hip hinge variations, Olympic lifts, sled pushes, and American-style kettlebell swings, those exercises just aren't the same.

Here's another problem: Following the standard CrossFit template is unlikely to lead to optimal improvements in your ability to generate force and power horizontally. And you need to be able to generate force and power horizontally when sprinting (an activity commonly programmed in CrossFit WODs) or when pushing opponents out of the way during sport. My research indicates that hip thrusts are better for developing maximum horizontal pushing force than back squats.

What's more, CrossFit leaves ample glute strength and muscle mass increases on the table. Glute strength is very helpful for accelerating and moving in all directions, including vertical, horizontal, diagonal, side-to-side, and rotational vectors. Finally, there's a psychological edge that is achieved when glute development is at an all-time high, which I think would be warmly welcomed by CrossFitters worldwide. When your glutes are swole, you know it, and it builds confidence.

It's worth noting that CrossFit is doing a lot of things right when it comes to glute development. The great thing about CrossFit is that you perform a lot of squatting and hip hinging patterns, which, as you know, develop strong glutes, but mainly in flexed positions. To improve glute development, CrossFitters simply need to add glute-dominant thrust and bridging patterns as well as abduction exercises to their training programs. In addition to creating bigger, stronger glutes, these movements might help alleviate some of the hyperextension-based back pain that squatting and hinging movements tend to trigger. I've worked with a lot of CrossFitters, and I've found that when we add more thrust, bridge, and abduction work, their back pain tends to resolve itself—not just because it increases their glute strength but also because it encourages posterior pelvic tilt at end-range hip extension, which teaches them to not anterior pelvic tilt as they lock out.

The best part is that you can perform glute-dominant movements—specifically the glute bridge and hip thrust—safely at high intensity because these movements are very stable and smooth. In other words, you're less likely to get hurt when performing a hip thrust or glute bridge while fatigued as compared to a deadlift or squat variation.

From a physique training perspective, adding glute-dominant exercises to CrossFit also helps grow the glutes. Some of the women who come to me from CrossFit complain that their quads and hamstrings have taken over, which makes sense because they're performing a ton of quad- and hamstring-dominant movements. Now, some might argue that they don't care so much about their physique—all they care about is function. Well, having strong glutes and a well-balanced frame will make you more functional. If you're in less pain, you're more functional. And if you have a well-balanced frame and you are performing movements from every conceivable movement pattern and vector, again, you're more functional.

If you're a CrossFitter or you're working with someone who trains in CrossFit, it's important to realize that adding glute-specific movements will not negatively affect performance in CrossFit workouts as long as you program correctly. Glute-specific movements are likely to make you stronger, faster, and more resilient, but you can't go crazy with volume. You just need to add a few sets of glute-dominant and abduction movements to your strength sessions (which typically precede the WODs) and workouts. Or you can do your normal CrossFit training but add two glute-focused WODs per week. Here are a couple of examples:

GLUTE TRAINING CROSSFIT WOD TEMPLATES

EXAMPLE 1	
3 rounds of the following:	
Barbell Glute Bridge	12 reps
Rounded Back Extension	20 reps
Knee-Banded Hip Abduction	10 reps w/ 3-sec pause

EXAMPLE 2	
3 rounds of the following:	
Barbell Hip Thrust	8–12 reps
Frog Pump or Knee-Banded Glute Bridge	50 reps
Extra-Range Side-Lying Hip Abduction	20 reps

GLUTE TRAINING FOR BODYBUILDERS

All bodybuilders have their own unique routine, but the vast majority adhere to body part splits. Let's consider the lifter who prefers body part split training but is severely lacking in gluteal development. This lifter might benefit from straying from the norm and training the lower body three times per week and the upper body two or three times per week—for example, glutes on day 1 (Monday), chest/shoulders/triceps on day 2 (Tuesday), quads and glutes on day 3 (Wednesday), back/rear delts/biceps on day 4 (Thursday), and hams and glutes on day 5 (Friday). This way, the glutes are hit effectively on all three lower-body days. Let's assume that this lifter trains at a typical commercial gym. A productive glute training week might look something like this:

DAY 1: GLUTES	
Barbell Glute Bridge	3x12
Cable Kickback	3x15
Reverse Hyper	3x30
Lateral Band Walk	3x20
Banded Seated Hip Abduction	3x30

DAY 2: CHEST/SHOULDERS/TRICEPS	
Dumbbell Incline Press	3x8
Seated Shoulder Press	3x12
Push-up	3x AMRAP
Cable Lateral Raise	3x12
V-Bar Triceps Extension	3x12

DAY 3: QUADS AND GLUTES	
Back Squat	3x8
Hack Squat	3x12
Smith Machine Reverse Lunge	3x12
Leg Extension	3x20
Crunch	2x20
Side Crunch	2x20
Hanging Leg Raise	2x10

DAY 4: BACK/REAR DELTS/BICEPS	
Lat Pull-Down	3x8
Seated Row	3x12
Inverted Row	3x AMRAP
Reverse Pec Deck	3x12
Alternating Dumbbell Curl	3x12

DAY 5: HAMS AND GLUTES	
Romanian Deadlift	3x8
Single-Leg Back Extension	3x12
Valslide Leg Curl	3x12
Seated Leg Curl	3x20
Calf Raise Machine	2x10
Seated Calf Raise Machine	2x20

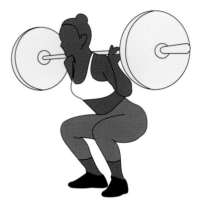

As you can see, this program hammers the glutes three times during the week. Day 1 involves high amounts of tension and metabolic stress for the glutes, day 3 involves moderate amounts of tension and high amounts of muscle damage for the glutes, and day 5 involves moderate amounts of tension and metabolic stress for the glutes. Moreover, the upper and lower glutes are hit hard, especially on day 1.

This lifter could attain even greater volume with the glutes by performing low-load glute activation exercises (see page 152 for examples) during the dynamic warm-up on each lower-body day and tacking additional hip thrusts and lateral band work onto the end of the day 3 and day 5 leg sessions. Of course, shoulders or arms could be taken out of the day 2 and day 4 sessions and added onto a separate day 6 (Saturday) session.

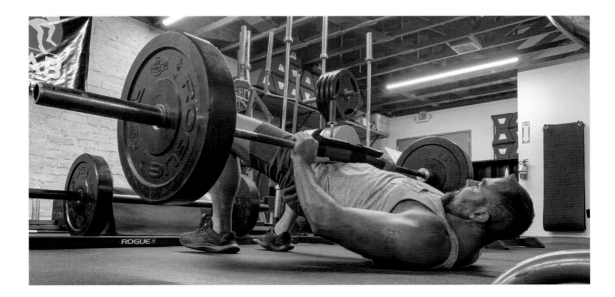

WHAT ABOUT YOGA, SPIN, AND PILATES?

I'm a big proponent of different training modalities as long as you enjoy them and they're not causing you harm. Granted, I have my opinions. I believe some people are misguided, especially when it comes to physique training goals. For example, if you want to put on muscle mass and all you're doing is yoga and spin class, you're not going to get the desired result. Moreover, if you're engaging in these activities as a way of "toning" your body, you are misguided.

The strength and conditioning industry has been trying to dispel the toning myth for several decades. Realize that there's no special neuromuscular adaptation for toning. You're doing things that cause muscles to grow efficiently, inefficiently, or not at all.

For example, let's say a dude wanted nice pecs. The best strategy would be to train them progressively twice a week with a variety of compound and isolation movements. Another good strategy would be to do a bunch of bodyweight push-ups and dips several days a week. A poor strategy would be to perform yoga or Tae Bo, thinking that it will grow pecs. The same goes for the glutes. Train using bodybuilding methods or train like a strength/power athlete, but don't train like a distance runner.

The toning myth began as a result of marketing efforts preying on the fears of women who saw images of bodybuilders and didn't want to become overly bulky. But here's the problem: If you're one of the lucky individuals who have the genetics to grow serious muscle, you could probably do just one 40-minute full-body workout a week and achieve your desired physique. But if you are a part of the vast majority, the only chance you'll have of achieving your desired physique is through resistance training. And if you have a goal, you should choose the most effective route.

For instance, if your main goal in life was to make $2,000 per week, you'd be foolish if you chose a job that paid $30 an hour over a job that paid $100 an hour. Same goes for physique training—resistance training will get you to your goal in a fraction of the time.

Please don't misinterpret what I'm saying here. I love all forms of exercise, and I encourage people to engage in physical activities that they enjoy. Yoga and Pilates are awesome, and they're great for overall health. Just know that resistance training is the single best activity you can do for aesthetic goals, and you can gain the same amount of muscle performing high or low reps as long as you push your sets hard.

In short, if you enjoy yoga and spin class and the way they make you feel, then you should do them. But if your goal is to grow your glutes, you still need to do the training that I'm recommending—unless you are part of the 0.1 percent who have amazing glute genetics.

The key, therefore, is to measure your goals against the activities you enjoy and find a balance. Of course, you will say that I'm biased, which I certainly am, but I believe everyone can benefit from glute training, regardless of which style of training they prefer.

Understand that doing these things—yoga, spin, Pilates, and so on—is not going to help your glutes substantially. If these training systems helped with glute growth, I'd be prescribing and recommending them. What's more, doing too much exercise is counterproductive. If you like doing yoga, spin, or whatever, by all means do it. Just make sure you're not overdoing it. And make sure you prioritize your strength workouts. That is, do your strength workouts first, making sure that you're well fed, well rested, and well motivated, and then do whatever else you enjoy afterward or on off-days.

GLUTE TRAINING FOR POWERLIFTERS

Powerlifters, especially those who plan on competing, need to focus on the three primary lifts: the squat, bench press, and deadlift. When it comes to program design, these are the lifts to prioritize first in your training. Your accessory work—which a lot of powerlifters do—is where you can hit glute-dominant exercises such as the hip thrust and abduction work. This is how powerlifters have always done it: main lifts and then accessory exercises.

Powerlifters have welcomed good mornings, Bulgarian split squats, 45-degree hypers, reverse hypers, pull-throughs, glute ham raises, sled work, and swings. And a lot of powerlifters have opened their minds to using bands and resistance bands (such as a Glute Loop) during their warm-ups. My only advice to powerlifters is to remain open-minded to hip thrusts, glute bridges, pendulum quadruped hip extensions (done underneath the reverse hyper), and rounded back extensions (done off the glute ham developer) because these movements improve strength and function for the squat and deadlift.

There are many effective ways to train for powerlifting strength. For the sake of simplicity, consider the powerlifter who has a squat day on day 1 (Monday), a bench day on day 2 (Wednesday), a deadlift day on day 3 (Thursday), and a hypertrophy day on day 4 (Saturday). Sticking to squats and deadlifts alone can build glutes, especially in men, but let's say this lifter isn't satisfied with their level of gluteal development. A program like this could work quite well:

DAY 1: SQUAT	
Back Squat	5x5
Barbell Hip Thrust or Barbell Glute Bridge	3x10
Barbell Back Extension or Pendulum Reverse Hyper	3x10

DAY 2: BENCH	
Bench Press	5x5
Military Press or Close-Grip Bench Press	3x10
Chest-Supported Row or Seated Row	3x10

DAY 3: DEADLIFT	
Conventional Deadlift or Sumo Deadlift	5x5
Dumbbell Front Squat or Dumbbell Bulgarian Split Squat	3x10
Single-Leg Hip Thrust or Pendulum Quadruped Hip Extension	3x12

DAY 4: HYPERTROPHY	
Lat Pull-Down	2x10
Dumbbell Bench Press	2x10
Inverted Row	2x10
Lateral Raise	2x10
Hammer Curl	2x10
Cable Triceps Extension	2x10
Prone Rear Delt Raise	2x10
Lateral Band Walk	2x20
Frog Pump	2x50

As in the case with the program for bodybuilders, the glutes are hit three times per week in this sample powerlifting plan. Saturday's session pumps some extra blood into the upper and lower glutes without interfering with recovery for Monday's squat session. To get extra volume for the glutes, this lifter can perform glute activation exercises during the dynamic warm-up on Monday and Thursday.

CHAPTER 18

Glute Training Programs

Following a program is great for several reasons. It helps you stay consistent, ensures that you perform intelligently structured workouts (assuming you're following a program that aligns with your goals and experience), exposes you to exercises that you might otherwise never do, and helps pave the way for training intuitively or designing your own programs down the road.

In this chapter, I provide three 12-week full-body programs with an emphasis on glute training, which take you from beginner to intermediate to advanced. In short, each program builds on the previous one by introducing more complex exercise variations. If you're new to strength training, start with the Novice Program and work your way sequentially through the Intermediate and Advanced Programs. If you're experienced, you can start with either the Intermediate or the Advanced Program.

The program you choose might also depend on the equipment available to you. For instance, if you want to train at home and you have minimal equipment—even if you're advanced—you can follow the Novice Program and still get great results. However, you will have to modify the program by performing more challenging exercise variations and pushing yourself hard on your sets. (More on this shortly.)

The three programs are aimed at giving you a solid foundation by integrating most of the methods, training strategies, and exercises covered in this book. Once you finish the programs, you can take a crack at designing your own programs by using the training splits as a template or consider one of the many program options offered in my store, which include personalized programming and my online training platform, Booty by Bret.

It's important to point out that each program has a customizable component built into each workout. At the end of each training session, you are allocated 10 free minutes to work on whatever you want (more on this on page 281). This is important because everyone has something unique that they want to focus on, which might not be included in the program. Whether it is a certain body part that you want to develop or an exercise that you really enjoy, you have the ability to customize the training to your preferences. So don't look at the program and assume that it isn't for you just because it is missing one of your favorite exercises. You can add it in at the end of your workout. If you believe the program will work and there is an element of freedom to do what you want, you are more likely to stay consistent, your confidence will increase, and you will get better results.

You will learn more about how to follow, customize, and get the most from the 12-week sample programs over the following pages, so I highly recommend you read through the FAQ before you get started.

PROGRAM GUIDE FAQ

When you start following a prewritten program, it's natural to have questions. In the coming pages, I answer the most frequently asked questions that people ask me when I design a program for them, and from people who follow my online Booty by Bret program. These are the questions I'm sure will come up when you follow the 12-week programs offered later in the chapter.

Most of the material covered here is distilled from the previous section. Consider it as both a guide to following the 12-week programs and a recap to the methods and instructions echoed throughout this book.

SHOULD I FOLLOW THE PROGRAM EXACTLY AS IT IS WRITTEN?

Each program is meant to be followed in sequence, meaning you should progress sequentially through all 12 weeks and then advance to the next program. However, you can and should replace exercises that are not well tolerated with exercises that are. So, if squatting hurts your knees, perhaps substitute a step-up or another quad-dominant exercise. It's also important to push your sets to get the most from the workouts. For example, you should increase the load or reps on the first couple of exercises each day throughout the month, as these tend to be the bigger movements that work more overall muscle. To accomplish this, perform more reps with the same load or use heavier loads for the same number of reps. However, don't try to set PRs on every exercise every week. Toward the ends of the workouts, strive for quality over quantity; you don't have to set PRs to highly activate the muscles and produce an adaptive stimulus.

THE WORKOUTS ARE TOO EASY. AM I TOO ADVANCED FOR THEM?

Most people don't know how to push themselves hard in the gym and never come close to reaching their full potential. If you think the workouts are too easy, chances are you're not pushing your sets with sufficient effort.

I made this mistake early on in my training when I first experimented with HIT, which involves performing one all-out set of each exercise to failure. My body and mind were conditioned to perform multiple sets and multiple exercises for one muscle. I never thought that just one exercise (or one set, for that matter) was enough to make strength and muscle gains, which is how a lot of other people feel. Now, I'm not suggesting that you perform just one set to failure of each exercise, although this may benefit you depending on your physiology. What I am suggesting is that you don't need to do 5 sets of each exercise. When you're used to doing 5 sets, anything less feels like a step in the wrong direction because you're conditioned to do more work. In your mind, you need many sets, often with multiple exercises for one muscle or movement pattern, to feel like you got a good workout. But that is not the case. When you push your sets close to or to muscle failure, you don't need to perform as much volume. In fact, doing less volume and putting in more effort is just as effective at building strength and muscle, with the added benefit of reducing training time and possibly decreasing your chances of developing overuse injuries and burnout.

Here's the deal: it takes time to push yourself to failure, because you don't know what going to failure feels like until you've done it for several weeks or even months. Once you develop the skill and the conditioning, you will realize that doing less and pushing yourself harder actually yields better results.

I'M USED TO DOING MUCH MORE VOLUME. HOW WILL I MAKE PROGRESS WITH THESE PROGRAMS?

As I've said, many lifters, especially female lifters, do too much volume. Research has confirmed that there's a "sweet spot" of volume, with too little or too much being suboptimal for muscular adaptations. It's a common misconception that the more you exercise, the better results you'll see. But this is not the case. In my experience, the sweet spot for most lifters is 12 to 20 sets per day, but obviously, many factors interact to determine this amount of volume, including exercise selection, load, effort, frequency, fitness level, age, and especially genetics. At any rate, I have been very successful as a personal trainer by avoiding crazy high-volume regimens and instead focusing on moderate-volume protocols with the goal of gaining strength and setting PRs over time. Many of my clients see immediate, rapid progress when they start training with me and cut back on the number of exercises and sets. So trust the programs as they are written, and most importantly, concentrate on form, put in the effort, and load your sets accordingly.

HOW SHOULD I WARM UP?

The programs don't include a warm-up, so it's up to you to get your body prepped for the exercise session. I outline a sample warm-up routine on page 152, which should serve you well when following any of the 12-week programs, but I want to emphasize that warm-ups are highly individualized. Some lifters require just 5 minutes of movement, while others might require or prefer 45 minutes. Most of my clients do something similar to what is covered on page 152, or do one or more of the following: lunges, goblet squats, back extensions, dumbbell stiff-leg deadlifts, high knees, rectus femoris stretches, leg swings, lateral band walks, and sometimes some foam rolling, which takes around 5 minutes.

If it's early in the day and it's cold, you might require a longer warm-up than if it's later in the day and it's warm. And on some days, you might need more or less time depending on how you feel. If you're stiff and tight, you might need to do some light dynamic stretching, whereas if you feel loose, you might just need a few light warm-ups before you start adding load. That said, it's always a good idea to do some form of general warm-up, like dynamic stretching (see page 154), before you jump into your specific warm-up sets.

Remember, a warm-up is exactly as the name implies: you're just getting warmed up. Many people make the mistake of turning the warm-up into an exercise circuit. You can use the movements you're going to perform as a guide. For example, if you're squatting for your main lift, it makes sense to perform a warm-up set of light squats or a similar movement pattern that works the same muscle groups. However, how much you decide to do depends on how you feel on that particular day, the exercises you're performing, the order of the exercises within the session, your strength and fitness level, the set and rep scheme you're following, and your individual physiology.

For instance, when I'm warming up for heavy squats as the first exercise of the day, I take quite a while to get into it. I may hit 2 sets of 10 bodyweight squats and then do 135 pounds for 3 reps, then 225 pounds for 2 reps, then 275 pounds for 1 rep, then 365 pounds for 1 rep, and then I'm ready to start my set.

For deadlifts, I might perform 3 sets of 10 bodyweight squats prior to pulling and then go straight to 315 pounds for 1 to 3 reps, then 405 pounds for 1 rep, then 495 pounds for 1 rep, and then I'm ready to go.

For hip thrusts, I perform a couple of sets of 10 bodyweight squats and then jump into 315 pounds for 3 reps, then 495 pounds for 1 rep, and then I start my set.

Let's say I'm performing heavy squats, deadlifts, and hip thrusts all in the same workout. I do the squat warm-up I mentioned above and then do my squat sets. But then I'm primed and warm, so I'll do only 1 warm-up set for deadlifts with 405 pounds for 1 rep. After my deadlifts, I can go right into my hip thrust sets without doing any specific warm-up sets.

When it comes to upper-body warm-ups, I follow a similar protocol. That is, I tailor my warm-up to the exercise and how I'm feeling. For example, I never need any warm-up sets when I'm performing rows. For chin-ups, I do a couple of sets of lat pull-downs and then hang from the pull-up bar prior to performing my sets. For bench presses, I take more time warming up. I press just the bar for 5 reps, then 135 pounds for 5 reps, then 225 pounds for 2 to 3 reps, then 275 pounds for 1 rep, then I'm ready to start my set. For "smaller" lifts performed later in the workout, I don't do any warm-up sets because I'm already warm, so I jump right into my work sets.

I hope this gives you some insight into how individualized warming up can be. I encourage you to develop your own warm-up protocol that suits your body and how you are feeling on that particular day.

ARE THESE PROGRAMS PERIODIZED? HOW DO I PROPERLY DELOAD ON YOUR PROGRAMS?

The programs offered in this book are strategic and methodical. The first week of each four-week phase is a deload week. This doesn't mean you take the week off; it means you don't push that hard and focus on practicing the lifts and figuring out what loads you will use for the following week. In general, your deload weeks will be around 60 to 70 percent as hard as the last week in the program. For week 1, think 60 to 70 percent; week 2, think 70 to 80 percent; week 3, think 80 to 90 percent; and week 4, think 90 to 100 percent effort.

How is this done, specifically? Well, you don't have to overthink it. On week 1, don't go as close to failure on your sets. This doesn't mean you can't do anything hard; it just means you should use common sense and ease into the training phase.

Deadlifts drain you more than any lift, so definitely don't do anything hard on deadlifts on week 1. Squats and hip thrusts and bench and chin-ups aren't quite as hard, so you can push those a bit harder, but still not to failure. Single-joint lifts like lateral raises, curls, and lateral band walks don't take much out of you, so you can go hard on these exercises.

Then, on week 2, you can do a more typical workout, but without going to failure on anything. On week 3, go to failure and up your effort, but leave some room in the tank. On week 4, crush it and go for PRs. Please do not write off deloads as "wimpy." Too many lifters fail to be strategic in their training, fail to utilize self-control, and never end up seeing results. Deloads accomplish several key things: they allow hormones and neurotransmitters to normalize, they give the body time to repair nagging little injuries, and they provide a psychological reprieve, all while you practice your technique and prepare your muscles for future gains.

I WANT MORE VOLUME FOR A CERTAIN BODY PART.
CAN I ADD IN SOME ADDITIONAL STUFF?

Nobody likes following a program with zero freedom. Not only that, but everyone has different areas or exercises they want to spend extra time working. For this reason, I always include 10 minutes of optional training at the end of a workout. For example, let's say you feel you could use some more delt work in your program. After you complete the programmed workout, you might perform a couple of sets of lateral raises, front raises, and rear delt raises. Or perhaps you want to get in some extra core work because you really enjoy blasting your abs. This is what the 10 minutes of free time is designed to accomplish; it allows you to home in on a specific body part or focus on an exercise that you love that might be missing from the program.

However, there are a few important considerations. The first is not to exceed the 10-minute window, which adds up to 40 minutes of extra exercise per week. I keep it limited to 10 minutes because the majority of women I train would be happy doing four additional hours of exercise, even when I tell them it is counterproductive. And if I were to tell you to pick one or two exercises instead of giving you a time limit, you might spend 30 minutes on those extra exercises. So whatever exercise option you decide to do, make sure you stay within that 10-minute window, as that limit will prevent you from doing too much and hampering your recovery.

The second is to avoid the big compound lifts and high-intensity interval training, which work more than one muscle group and can be taxing on the body. Instead, focus on isolation exercises that don't beat you up too badly, such as leg extensions, leg curls, calf raises, crunches, biceps curls, delt raises, triceps extensions, and so on. For example, if you want more leg work, you could do three supersets of leg extension and leg curls, which would take around 10 minutes.

The third is not to do additional heavy glute exercises, like barbell hip thrusts, barbell glute bridges, or back squats. The programs already emphasize the glutes, so the 10 minutes is really for working other areas of your body that you feel need more attention. You can, however, do a glute burnout, which I address next.

Lastly, I want to emphasize that the 10 minutes of extra work is optional. Some of my clients who really push the envelope with their effort don't use their 10 free minutes because they're getting enough stimulus from the programmed workout. So don't feel obligated to use it if you feel like you're getting enough work from the program.

CAN I ADD A GLUTE BURNOUT AFTER THE TRAINING SESSION?

If you want to add a 3-minute burnout, it falls into the 10-minute window. Let's say you want to do some extra core work (or focus on another body part) and then blast your glutes. In this scenario, make sure that the ab workout doesn't exceed 7 minutes and the glute burnout doesn't exceed 3 minutes. It's also important to stick with bodyweight and banded glute exercises like glute bridges, lateral band walks, and pulse squats. To learn more about how to construct a glute burnout, flip back to page 213.

YOU DON'T PROGRAM MUCH AB WORK. CAN I ADD SOME?

This is true. The abs are incorporated in many of the exercises I prescribe in the programs. Abdominal definition has much more to do with getting lean than developing big abdominal muscles. However, you will develop stronger and more muscular abs if you train them directly, so if that is your goal, definitely add ab exercises in the 10 minutes of optional time at the ends of some of your training sessions. I recommend performing 2 sets of two different ab exercises twice per week. It doesn't take a lot of volume since they're getting hit during the regular workouts.

CAN I ADD A BURNOUT SET AFTER MY BIG LIFTS?

Let's say a program calls for 3 sets of 6 reps for back squats. Say you do 155 pounds for 6 reps on all 3 sets. After you finish, you may want to lower the weight to 95 pounds and "burn out" for reps. This is tricky. On the one hand, it'll give you a better workout on the spot. You'll fatigue your muscles and feel the burn. However, take a step back and consider the entire week of training. If you are squatting 3 times per week, adding extra sets of squats will prevent you from recovering for the following session.

Always look at the big picture when making training decisions and veering from the plan. It is vital to modify the program from time to time, but you should be more cautious when adding to the program than when subtracting from the program.

CAN I THROW EXTRA WORKOUTS INTO YOUR PROGRAM?

In general, no. Definitely don't do any additional big lifts like squats, deadlifts, bench presses, chin-ups, military presses, or even heavier hip thrusts. But if you want to throw in some extra glute work, you could pull it off as long as you don't do anything crazy. For example, you could certainly add in a session once or twice per week consisting of a few sets of bridges, frog pumps, or lateral band walks. That wouldn't detract from the following day's training session. Always consider your next training sessions and make sure you're recovered for them. You won't make progress if you don't gain strength, and you won't gain strength if you aren't recovered from your workouts.

IS IT OKAY IF I DO SOME YOGA OR ADDITIONAL CONDITIONING WORK ON THE SIDE?

As I discussed on page 274, I support and encourage you to do the things you enjoy. However, you also have to consider your goal. If you want to build bigger, stronger glutes, then you have to consider whether doing anything extra will negatively impact your training sessions later in the week. If it won't, then go ahead and add it in. There are different types of yoga, with some being more hardcore than others, so try to stick to the relaxing kind instead of intense yoga. And I prefer walking over HIIT and intense conditioning work, as the latter can be a bit taxing and take away from your workouts. Maybe you find that you can do incline treadmill, cycling, kettlebell swings, or sled pushes without getting sore or fatigued, but hiking, stair climbing, plyos, and sprinting kick your butt and prevent you from making strength gains. In short, continue to do the things you enjoy, but listen to your body and don't do anything that might disrupt your strength training sessions or move you further away from your physique goals.

HOW MUCH CARDIO SHOULD I DO?

If you like doing cardio, you can and should add some in. But just like yoga and other conditioning work, cardio can interfere with your training sessions. Whether or not endurance training interferes with strength training is debated in the research, but it's safe to say that you'll never be your best at running marathons and your strongest at the same time.

Obviously, there's a point at which the body cannot become the best it can be at one thing if you're giving it mixed signals by telling it to be good at two opposing things. So don't go crazy on the cardio. Do "relaxing" cardio sessions where you're not striving for records and pushing it too hard. Jogging interferes with muscular adaptations more than cycling and walking. If you don't like cardio and are active in your daily life, don't feel compelled to do much of it at all. Your heart will be healthy from all of the walking and non-exercise activity thermogenesis (NEAT—such as cleaning the house and running errands) and lifting. Instead of doing cardio, you may have to daily step count goals, such as 10,000 steps a day.

I prefer for you to limit your cardio to three 30-minute sessions per week, but sometimes you may want to go for a big hike or compete in something. When that happens, adjust your training program accordingly. For example, don't go for a deadlift PR the day after performing a 12-mile obstacle race—it won't happen!

If you're wondering whether you should do cardio for weight loss, flip back to page 219, where I discuss this in more detail.

IS IT OKAY IF I EXERCISE EVERY DAY?

This is tricky. Yes, we should all move daily for health purposes. Most of the population is too sedentary and falling far short on exercise for optimal health. However, many of you (the ones who are following the programs in this book) are on the opposite end of the spectrum. When you strive for PRs and train the way we do, it's a different kind of training than is recommended by health and fitness organizations.

Walking, jogging, general cardio, circuit training, and lifting weights the way most people do aren't too intense. These activities can and should be carried out every day if there's no progressive component. However, progressive resistance training and HIIT are stressful to the system, and they can easily throw off your physiology if you don't take days off from exercising and periodize your training (we do this with our deload and progressive system).

I can't tell you how many bikini competitors I've worked with who have unhealthy relationships with exercise (and food, for that matter). They're obsessed with training and feel guilty and anxious to the point where they cannot take a day off. This is unfortunate, as the body needs days off to recover.

When you lift heavy, you create microlesions in the muscles as well as microdamage to tendons, ligaments, and fascia. You also tax your brain. Psychologically speaking, how many lifting sessions per year can you truly get fully aroused for? Definitely not 365. Probably more like 52. This implies that many of your sessions will be middle of the road, some will feel great, and others will outright suck. That's the way the body works. But you mustn't throw your body out of whack in terms of hormonal milieu if you want to reach your full potential. You want to do what's optimal for your physiology, not what your brain has fooled you into doing.

Have self-control and stick to a strategy. You'll see better results if you take at least one day off per week from exercising altogether. Many people see great results when they lift heavy just 2 to

4 days per week. The programs included in this book contain four training days per week simply because it's the number of days that most people want to train, and it works well for the masses. If you prefer a different training frequency, consider using the principles and guidelines covered in Parts 3 and 4 to design your own training plan.

HOW LONG SHOULD I REST BETWEEN SETS?

Rest for 2 to 3 minutes with "big" lifts such as squats, deadlifts, bench presses, chin-ups, and hip thrusts. When going for a big PR, you may even want to rest for more than 3 minutes. When performing "medium" lifts like rows, push-ups, and back extensions, rest for 2 minutes between sets. "Small" lifts like curls, triceps extensions, lateral raises, and lateral band walks may require only 1 minute of rest. But don't feel the need to use a stopwatch and be super strict with rest times; research has shown that going by feel leads to the best results. If you listen to your body, you'll know when you're recovered and ready for the next set. To learn more about rest periods and sets, flip back to page 181.

WHAT TEMPO SHOULD I UTILIZE?

To reiterate, *tempo* refers to the cadence you use when lifting. Sometimes you'll see things like 4/1/2/0, which means to lower the weight for a count of 4, pause for a second, lift the weight for a count of 2, then repeat with no pause between reps. Don't think about tempo when you lift; it just throws you off. The only time I want you to pay attention to tempo is when you're performing pause reps or accentuated eccentrics. In that case, I'll spell it out for you and tell you what to do. In all other cases, just lift. Don't be super slow with your reps; you want an explosive concentric contraction and a controlled eccentric contraction. You always want to control the weight and lift in a smooth manner. Some exercises have more range of motion and will therefore take longer to carry out than others.

IS IT OKAY IF I SUPERSET THE WORKOUT OR PERFORM IT AS A CIRCUIT?

Sometimes it's okay to superset (see page 213). This means that you do an exercise and then immediately move into the next exercise and then rest. Sometimes it speeds up the workout without interfering with performance. Just make sure that if you do superset, you pick noncompeting exercises. For example, squats and bench presses are okay to superset, or hip thrusts and rows. But you wouldn't want to do this for deadlifts and chins since both use the lats a lot, or for military presses and dips since both utilize the triceps.

I do not recommend making the workout into a circuit (performing one exercise after another with minimal rest). To effectively build muscle and have productive sets, you need to rest between sets, and you need to get comfortable with resting (know that it's important in order to see results). Sometimes it's okay to do a glute training circuit as a separate workout, but not for the prescribed main workouts contained within the programs.

WHAT ABOUT A COOL-DOWN?

If you like performing a cool-down activity like stretching or walking, then go ahead and do it. But it's not necessary. Your body will cool down just fine when you stop training.

I DIDN'T SET ANY PRS THIS MONTH, AND I AM VERY FRUSTRATED. DOES THIS MEAN THE PROGRAM ISN'T WORKING?

No, it does not. It's a normal phenomenon with adaptation. The body works in waves. Progress is never, ever linear—not for strength, not for weight loss, not for fat loss, and not for muscle growth. Get comfortable with stagnation periods and know that they are a normal part of training.

I DON'T FEEL A CERTAIN EXERCISE WORKING. SHOULD I SUBSTITUTE SOMETHING ELSE OR KEEP AT IT?

Well, some exercises you may not "feel" in any one area. For example, I don't really know where I "feel" deadlifts the most; they're just hard all over. Moreover, I feel squats mostly in my quads, and when I hip thrust heavy, I feel my quads and hams almost as much as my glutes. Yet I still perform all of these because I know that getting stronger at the big lifts makes me more muscular. That said, never stick with an exercise just because you think you have to. If something doesn't feel right, then nix it. Maybe you can come back to it later, or maybe you never do. No exercise is mandatory to perform for results. There are plenty of great exercises to go around. When you ditch an exercise, do something in its place that works similar muscles and/or involves a similar pattern.

HOW DO I PERFORM A CERTAIN EXERCISE YOU PRESCRIBE?

In the next section, I provide detailed descriptions for all of the glute training exercises. For upper-body movements, which are not covered in this book, visit glutelabbook.com to see a short video demonstration of each exercise. If you're new to training, I highly recommend working with an experienced coach, or progressing sequentially through the programs offered in this book. As you will see, I start out with just bodyweight movements and then add more challenging variations over the following weeks.

I'LL BE TRAVELING DURING THE MONTH. WHAT SHOULD I DO?

First, enjoy your trip. Don't stress out about your workouts. It is easy to maintain strength and even easier to maintain muscle. Try to stay active and walk a lot. This will prevent you from gaining weight, as most people eat more when away from home (the assumption here is that you're not trying to gain weight, of course). If you can get to a gym, great. Do as much of the prescribed workout as possible, and make substitutions when needed.

If you can't access a gym, do bodyweight workouts consisting of squats, push-ups, Bulgarian split squats, lunges, frog pumps, single-leg hip thrusts, frog reverse hypers, side-lying hip raises, and extra-range side-lying hip abduction. If you have someone who can hold onto your ankles, do Nordic ham curls and back extensions. You can also do partner rows if the other person is strong enough to hold you up. If you have mini bands, do various lateral banded glute exercises.

Ideally, you'll be able to make it into the gym at least one day per week. This will allow you to maintain your strength and coordination on the lifts. You can do quick 20-minute bodyweight workouts 3 to 5 days per week to keep your muscles primed. If you want to just enjoy your trip and avoid exercise altogether, try to have this week come right after a very hard week of training (ideally the fourth week of the training phase); this is known as *functional overreaching*. In this case, you're purposely/strategically overdoing it, knowing that you'll have some time off for the body to repair.

To learn more about what you can do on vacation, check out page 240.

HOW MUCH SHOULD I PROGRESS EACH WEEK?

It is impossible to say. It depends on your gender, age, current strength and fitness levels, and genetics, as well as the exercise in question. What I can tell you is that you won't be able to continuously increase by 10 pounds per week, and you won't be able to continuously increase most lifts by 5 pounds per month. This would equate to 60 pounds over a year. You might make this kind of progress on big lifts like squats, deadlifts, and hip thrusts for your first year or two of training, but it won't continue indefinitely. If so, you'd be Superman within a decade. You also won't get 1 more rep each week with the same weight, and you won't be able to get 1 more rep per month on most lifts.

Consider chin-ups. Doing 10 chin-ups is a difficult feat, and it's one that many people never achieve—even lifters who have been training for years. The rate of improvement is lackluster with chin-ups, but with hip thrusts, it's not so bad. You could easily start out with 135 pounds for 10 reps and end up getting 30 reps within a few months of training, but eventually you'll hit a plateau. To learn how to overcome plateaus, flip back to page 234.

When following the programs offered in this book (or any program, for that matter), try to bump things up gradually over time—5 more pounds here, another rep there. If you're doing 3 sets of an exercise, consider your 3-set total or your 3-set volume load. For example, let's say you're doing squats, and you perform 135 pounds for 3 sets of 5 reps in week 2 of your program. Maybe in week 3, you hit 135 pounds for 6 reps, then 5, and then 5 again. You should be proud of this achievement, as you have set a PR. Then, in week 4, maybe you end up hitting 135 pounds for 3 sets of 6 reps. If so, this is a big improvement. These little progressions accumulate over time and lead to big changes in strength and physique.

YOU DON'T WRITE DOWN PERCENTAGES OF 1RM TO USE. HOW DO I KNOW HOW MUCH TO LIFT?

If you're a strength training researcher or a savvy personal trainer, you'll notice that the number of reps people can get with a certain percentage of 1RM varies considerably. For example, I just had 12 women do max reps on hip thrusts with 50 percent of their 1RM. The range was 16 to 29, meaning that one subject got 16 reps and another got 29 reps with the same relative load. With 80 percent of 1RM on certain lifts, some subjects can get 5 reps, while others can get 10 reps. If I had prescribed 3 sets of 6 reps with 80 percent of 1RM, the first subject wouldn't have come close, while the other would have found it too easy. For this reason, I avoid prescribing percentages. Simply establish a baseline and then bump things up little by little.

For instance, let's say you underestimate your loading. In this scenario, you should try to do more reps on your last set (assuming you do an AMRAP set), and then, in the following week, you should bump up the load. If you overestimate your loading, you will end up falling short of the total reps, so cut back a bit on the load on the following week.

DO I NEED TO FOLLOW THE SET AND REP SCHEMES EXACTLY AS WRITTEN?

The short answer is no. You won't always nail the prescribed rep schemes exactly as written. Think of them as recommendations to calculate your working weight and then try to get close.

For example, let's say a workout calls for 3 sets of 8 reps. There are three protocols you can implement to carry out your sets.

The first protocol is to do the same loading on each set (I refer to this as *straight sets*), which gives you two options. Option one is to start with a working weight that you can do for only 8 reps. In this situation, you go to muscle failure on all of your sets. So you will hit 8 reps to muscle failure on your first set, and then you may get only 5 reps and then 4 reps on your second and third sets. With this option, you will never have a nice, neat set and rep scheme because the load is the same, and you can't get as many reps with the second and third sets due to fatigue. Option two is to pick a working weight that you can do for 10 to 12 reps. In this situation, your first two sets are easier, and only your last set is to muscle failure. In this case, you may indeed end up getting 3 sets of 8 reps.

The second protocol is to adjust your working weight so that every set is to failure. These are known as *descending sets* because you have to reduce the load with every set. For instance, say the program calls for 3 sets of 8 reps of back squats, and you want to push every set to muscle failure. If your max 8-rep back squat is 155 pounds, then that is your load for your first set. In order to get 8 reps with your second and third sets, however, you have to lower the load. So your second set might be 145 pounds, and your third set might be 135 pounds.

The third protocol is to increase the load with each set, which is the opposite of descending sets and hence is referred to *ascending sets*. Keeping with the same example, if the program calls for 3 sets of 8 back squats and your max 8-rep back squat is 155 pounds, then you might perform 135 pounds on your first set, 145 pounds on your second set, and 155 pounds on your third set. In this situation, only your third set is to failure.

When it comes to choosing the protocol, it depends on the exercise, how you are feeling that day, and where you are at in your training cycle. If you want to push yourself in your workout, choose the same weight and go to failure on every set. If you're feeling beat up or you're building yourself up, then perhaps you push only your third set to failure. The point is this: if the program calls for 3 sets of 8 reps, you don't have to do exactly that. As long as you're going to failure on at least one of your sets, then you are following the program recommendations and getting enough stimulus to improve strength and grow muscle.

SET AND REP LOADING OPTIONS	
Straight sets (all sets to failure)	155x8, 155x5, 155x4
Straight sets (last set to failure)	140x8, 140x8, 140x8
Descending sets (all sets to failure)	155x8, 145x8, 135x8
Ascending sets (last set to failure)	135x8, 145x8, 155x8

WHAT IF I CAN DO MORE REPS ON MY LAST SET? SHOULD I STICK TO THE PROGRAM OR REP OUT TO FAILURE?

I alluded to this in a previous question. This is called an AMRAP (as many reps as possible) set, and it's a double-edged sword. On the one hand, it will ensure that you go to failure and go all-out, thereby theoretically recruiting all of the available motor units in the muscle. However, training to failure has been shown to be lackluster in the literature, meaning that you do not have to carry out all of your sets until you fail in order to see great results. What's worse, if you train a lift or muscle frequently, an AMRAP set could fatigue you to the point where you're not recovered by the time you perform the exercise again. In this case, it would prevent you from having a stellar workout, and a PR would be unachievable.

SHOULD I ALWAYS GO TO FAILURE?

Absolutely not. Remember the Rule of Thirds (covered on page 198): about a third of your sets should be taken to failure, about a third of your sets should be 1 to 2 reps shy of failure, and the remaining third should be nowhere close to failure.

ON WHICH DAYS SHOULD I SCHEDULE MY WORKOUTS?

This depends on your training frequency and logistics. The programs offered in this book include four workout sessions per week, so make sure you split up the days so that you're not training four straight days in a row. I like to train on Monday, Tuesday, Thursday, and Friday and then relax and enjoy my weekends. Other people prefer to have a couple of days off during the week and hammer it hard over the weekend. If you drink alcohol on weekends, I don't recommend training the day after a big night out. Remember, you want to set PRs here and there, and this won't happen if you're hungover. Monday, Tuesday, Thursday, and Saturday would work, as would many other combinations that spread out the training days evenly.

Strategize your training schedule if possible. For example, if I'm going to deadlift, I like to have a day off beforehand so that I'm fresh and recovered.

HOW LONG SHOULD EACH SESSION LAST?

This depends on the number of exercises you perform, the types of exercises you perform, the loads you use, your personal preference regarding rest times between sets, how long it takes you to warm up, and the number of warm-up sets you do. In general, your workouts should take between 50 and 90 minutes (including the 10 minutes of optional exercise).

I FEEL STIFF AND REALLY SORE. SHOULD I TAKE THE DAY OFF, MODIFY THE WORKOUT, OR JUST PUSH THROUGH IT?

I cover training around discomfort, soreness, and injuries extensively on pages 223 and 226, which I encourage you to read. As a recap, always err on the side of caution. When in doubt, take the day off. Hindsight is always 20/20. Almost every time I've hurt myself in training, my body was trying to tell me something, but I was too stubborn to listen. Learn from my mistakes by paying close attention to the signals your body is sending you. Many times, you can warm up and end up feeling much better and ready to go, but don't lie to yourself and think you feel great when you really don't. Your body should feel good most of the time, not beat to smithereens. Always know that you can and should modify training sessions depending on how you feel. Never push through "bad" pain. You intuitively know when something is somewhat normal and when something is off. Sometimes I warm up and still feel like crap, and I end up just doing some light sets for glutes or delts or whatever and then call it a day.

The goal is to keep the goal the goal. If you hurt yourself, your new goal will be to rehabilitate and get back to baseline.

WHAT SHOULD I DO IF I MISS A DAY OF TRAINING?

First, don't sweat it! It happens. If you miss a training session due to being busy and overwhelmed, you could skip the session completely without making any further adjustments. But a slightly better strategy would be to combine your following sessions. Maybe I shouldn't use the word *combine* here, as you'll definitely need to subtract some things. But consider the big lifts: squats, bench, deadlifts, chin-ups, and hip thrusts. You want to do these at least once per week, assuming they are included in the program (not everyone can or should do all of these lifts). So, if you miss Monday and that's the day you were scheduled to squat, then maybe squat in your next training session, but nix an exercise that's less important.

If you know in advance that you're going to miss a session, you can make adjustments ahead of time. Let's say you know you're going to miss a Friday, and the deadlift is the main exercise on that day. In this case, just do deadlifts on Wednesday but omit any other hip hinging work prescribed for that day. For example, you wouldn't also do any dumbbell 45-degree hypers or stiff-leg deadlifts. The deadlift is the most important exercise of the three, so it gets prioritized. Here's another example. Let's say you were scheduled to perform 15 total sets on Monday, Wednesday, and Friday, and you miss Monday's session. On Wednesday and Friday, after making adjustments, maybe you end up doing 18 total sets to make up for some of what you missed on Monday. You will have performed 36 total sets for the week, not 45 as originally planned. Don't try to get all 45 sets in on Wednesday and Friday, as this would be a recipe for overtraining. If, however, you take a day off because you're beat down and overly fatigued, then just take the day off and try to have a couple of easy sessions before merging back into the swing of things full bore.

Now, if you miss an entire week of training because you're on a business trip or on vacation, you can just start the program where you left off. And if you get injured or you really fall off the wagon and miss a few weeks of training, you might consider easing back into the program by starting from the beginning.

WHAT CAN I DO ON NON-TRAINING DAYS TO FEEL PRODUCTIVE?

A decade ago, I felt like I should always be doing something for my recovery: hot tub, contrast showers, sauna, cold plunges, massages, foam rolling, light stretching, active recovery, and so on.

When you train progressively, you don't need more exercise on off-days; you need rest. Don't consider doing "active recovery." Life will give you plenty of active recovery when you walk and move around and do chores and have sex (if you're lucky). Many of the recovery modalities are overrated, and you should never feel guilty for failing to stretch or foam roll. These things can be considered icing on the cake, and they should be done in moderation. These modalities mostly work on the nervous system; they aren't changing your tissue like you think. (To learn more about recovery protocols, flip back to page 151.)

You know what else needs recovery? Your brain. Lifting weights progressively is stressful. Don't underestimate this fact. The majority of the time, the best thing you can do on your days off is sleep more and do something you enjoy. Being in a good state of mind throughout the week is good for the muscles and good for the body. So take a nap, watch that show you've been wanting to watch, go see a movie, dive into that book you've been wanting to read, or hang out with that friend or family member you've been missing. Not many people talk about this in S&C, but it is important.

WHAT IF I WANT TO TRAIN ONLY MY GLUTES AND NOT MY FULL BODY?

Just eliminate the upper-body exercises and you are good to go.

NOVICE PROGRAM

Throughout the entire novice program, days 1 and 3 and days 2 and 4 are repeated to give you more practice with each movement pattern. Although this training strategy isn't as exciting as having a new workout each day of the week, it's better for your development, as motor patterning requires practice and repetition. I want you to ingrain solid movement patterns from the get-go, which will pay dividends in the years to come. With bodyweight training, you progress by performing more reps and by graduating to more advanced variations, which you will do from one phase to the next. If you purchased this book with the hope of diving right into the training but you don't currently have a gym membership or access to equipment, your wish is granted.

The first four weeks involve solely bodyweight exercises. This gives you a chance to get more accustomed to bodyweight loading, which forms the base for most foundational movements. It also gives you some time to obtain a gym membership or purchase some items such as a Glute Loop, dumbbells, a bench, a set of rings, and a chin-up bar (which you'll need to complete the entire 12-week plan).

The second four weeks build on the first phase, include slightly more advanced variations, and incorporate some basic equipment. Remember, with single-leg exercises, always begin with the weaker leg and then match reps with the stronger leg.

The final four weeks take things up a notch and incorporate some additional basic equipment. Your coordination will be much better at this point, and you'll be ready to take on more advanced exercises. To reiterate, the first week of each phase is dedicated to learning the movements, and the remaining three weeks are performed more aggressively with the primary goal of achieving progressive overload.

I have some additional advice for this program that is very important to your success. I want you to consider the prescribed set and rep schemes as general targets, knowing that you will necessarily stray from them as you gain strength and push yourself to set personal records. For example, let's say you hit 3 sets of 20 bodyweight box squats one week. The next week, you might aim for 3 sets of 22 reps, then 3 sets of 25 reps the following week. In addition, you may or may not be able to perform full-range bodyweight push-ups and chin-ups by week 9. If you can, great. But if you can't, this is not uncommon. Just do the best you can. Continue to perform eccentric push-ups and chin-ups, but try to "do more" over time by lowering yourself in a more controlled manner. Or purchase a long band and perform band-assisted push-ups and chin-ups. The bottom line is that you can always perform the right variation for your level of fitness, and you can always work progressively to improve your strength.

PROGRAM REQUIREMENTS

The first eight weeks of this program are just body weight, so you don't need any equipment to perform the first two phases. For the third phase (weeks 9 to 12), however, you will need dumbbells and a resistance band. I recommend using two light dumbbells with which you feel comfortable bench pressing and deadlifting and one heavier dumbbell that you can use for hip thrusting and goblet squatting. For the resistance band, you can purchase a Glute Loop on my website, or you can find many other options online.

When it comes to sizes, the vast majority of lifters prefer the S/M Regular Glute Loop. If you have very large thighs or prefer long strides and wide sumo stances, you might prefer the L/XL Regular Glute Loop. Strong and Extra-Strong Glute Loop options are available for more advanced lifters. That said, some people like the S/M for thrust and bridge patterns and the L/XL for squat and quadruped movement patterns, so you might consider getting both. Finally, you also might consider purchasing a 41-inch resistance band (also referred to as a *long band*) for band-assisted pull-up and chin-ups.

WEEKS 1–4

DAYS 1 AND 3	
Bodyweight Feet-Elevated Glute Bridge	3x20 (elevate feet onto couch)
Bodyweight Torso-Elevated Push-up	3x10
Bodyweight Parallel Box Squat	3x20 (sit onto a low table)
Bodyweight Inverted Row	3x10 (use two chairs)
Bodyweight Side-Lying Clam	3x20
Bodyweight Side Plank	2x 20 sec

DAYS 2 AND 4	
Bodyweight Glute Bridge	3x20
Bodyweight Knee Push-up	3x10
Bodyweight Medium Step-up	3x10 each leg (use a chair)
Bodyweight Bent-Over YTWL	3x10
Bodyweight Side-Lying Hip Abduction	3x20
Bodyweight Plank	2x 40 sec

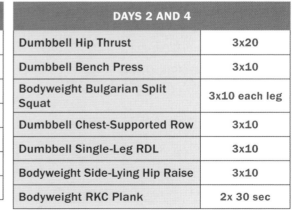

WEEKS 5–8

DAYS 1 AND 3	
Bodyweight Knee-Banded Glute Bridge	3x20
Bodyweight Eccentric Push-up	3x5 (4-sec lowering phase)
Goblet Parallel Box Squat	3x20
Bodyweight Eccentric Chin-up	3x3 (4-sec lowering phase)
Banded Seated Hip Abduction	3x30
Bodyweight Side Plank	2x 40 sec

DAYS 2 AND 4	
Bodyweight Hip Thrust	3x20
Dumbbell Standing Shoulder Press	3x10
Bodyweight Reverse Lunge	3x10 each leg
Dumbbell One-Arm Row	3x10
Bodyweight Extra-Range Side-Lying Hip Abduction	3x20
Bodyweight RKC Plank	2x 20 sec

WEEKS 9–12

DAYS 1 AND 3	
Single-Leg Hip Thrust	3x10
Bodyweight Push-up	3x3
Goblet Deep Squat	3x20
Bodyweight Chin-up	3x1
Dumbbell Romanian Deadlift	3x10
Banded Seated Hip Abduction	3x30
Bodyweight Side Plank	2x 1 min

DAYS 2 AND 4	
Dumbbell Hip Thrust	3x20
Dumbbell Bench Press	3x10
Bodyweight Bulgarian Split Squat	3x10 each leg
Dumbbell Chest-Supported Row	3x10
Dumbbell Single-Leg RDL	3x10
Bodyweight Side-Lying Hip Raise	3x10
Bodyweight RKC Plank	2x 30 sec

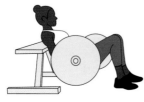

INTERMEDIATE PROGRAM

By now, you'll have gotten accustomed to the main movements. You've been pressing, pulling, bridging/thrusting, squatting/lunging, hinging, and abducting. Now it's time to crank up the dial and begin performing the movements with greater loading. You need to get friendly with the barbell throughout these 12 weeks. Unlike during the novice program, you will perform four different workouts in each week of the intermediate program.

Each phase includes all of the main movement patterns, but the first four weeks focus on the hip thrust and military press, the second four weeks focus on the squat and chin-up, and the last four weeks focus on the deadlift and bench press. Note that this is the Glute Lab periodization strategy that I discussed on page 256, where you switch the focus from month to month, and it is the same format that I use in my Booty by Bret online training platform (except I also include a well-rounded month and a single-leg month in the rotation).

Now, if you're like me, you're definitely going to look ahead and glance at the advanced program. You might even be tempted to jump right into it, even if you don't belong there, just because you think you'll see quicker results. Don't do it. Although the advanced program contains a lot of fancy methods, advanced routines aren't necessarily better than basic routines (as discussed in detail on page 216). Strong and fit lifters will definitely love the advanced program because of the novelty factor, but getting stronger during the intermediate program is paramount.

Think of the intermediate program as your home base program that you'll stick to most of the time. For example, let's say you want to train indefinitely using the guidelines you learned in this book. You perform the novice, intermediate, and advanced programs back to back to back and are 36 weeks in. At this point, you might want to joint Booty by Bret or experiment with some of the other training splits or strategies mentioned in this section. Eventually, however, you'll want to work your way back to the intermediate and advanced programs; just make sure to modify them by swapping out exercises from the same category (see pages 123 to 129 for categories) and adjust some of the set and rep schemes to your fitness level.

When you get to this point in your training, I want you to perform two cycles of intermediate-style programming for every cycle of advanced-style programming. The intermediate program is your meat and potatoes, whereas the advanced program is your dessert.

PROGRAM REQUIREMENTS

To carry out the intermediate program, you will need the following equipment:

- Barbell and plates
- Glute Loop
- Adjustable bench
- Squat rack/stands
- Chin-up bar
- Rings
- Dumbbells
- 45-degree hyper
- Cable column

WEEKS 1–4

DAY 1	
Barbell Hip Thrust Pyramid	1x10, 1x8, 1x6, 1x15
Military Press Pyramid	1x10, 1x8, 1x6, 1x15
Back Squat	3x6
Chin-up	3x AMRAP
Gliding Leg Curl	3x10
Lateral Band Walk	2x20

DAY 2	
Knee-Banded Bodyweight Glute Bridge	3x30
Push-up	3x AMRAP
Dumbbell Stiff-Leg Deadlift	3x10
Seated Row	3x12
Bodyweight High Step-up	3x10
Banded Fire Hydrant	2x12

DAY 3	
Knee-Banded Constant Tension Barbell Hip Thrust	3x20
Military Press	3x6
Pause Front Squat	3x5 (1-sec pause)
Underhand Grip Lat Pull-Down	3x10
Dumbbell 45-Degree Hyper	3x12
Banded Standing Hip Abduction	2x20

DAY 4	
Pause Barbell Hip Thrust	3x5 (3-sec pause)
Seated Dumbbell Overhead Press	3x12
Between Bench Dumbbell Squat	3x20
Inverted Row	3x AMRAP
Good Morning	3x8
Monster Walk	3x20

WEEKS 5–8

DAY 1	
Back Squat	3x5
Chin-up	3x AMRAP
Single-Leg Foot-Elevated Hip Thrust	3x10
Incline Press	3x8
Banded Frog Pump	2x30

DAY 2	
Dumbbell Deficit Reverse Lunge	3x30
Eccentric-Neutral Grip Pull-up	3x5 (3-sec lowering phase)
Romanian Deadlift	3x10
Push-up	3x AMRAP
Knee-Banded Hip Abduction	2x30

DAY 3	
Goblet Squat	3x10
Eccentric Chin-up	3x5 (3-sec lowering phase)
Barbell Glute Bridge	3x12
Eccentric-Accentuated Push Press	3x6 (4-sec lowering phase)
Frog Reverse Hyper	2x20

DAY 4	
Front Squat	3x6
Neutral Grip Pull-up	3x AMRAP
Semi-Sumo Deadlift	3x6
Pause Close-Grip Bench Press	3x10 (1-sec pause)
Cable Standing Hip Abduction	2x12

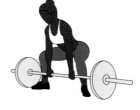

DAY 1	
Deadlift	3x5
Pause Bench Press	3x5 (1-sec pause)
Dumbbell Bulgarian Split Squat	3x8
One-Arm Row	3x10
Extra-Range Side-Lying Hip Abduction	2x20

DAY 2	
Low-Bar Parallel Box Squat	3x8
Dumbbell Bench Press	3x10
Pause Dumbbell 45-Degree Hyper	3x8 (3-sec pause)
Chin-up	3x AMRAP
Banded Cha-Cha	2x20

DAY 3	
Dynamic Effort Deadlift	3x5
Bench Press	3x8
Deadstop Foot-Elevated Single-Leg Hip Thrust	3x8
Dumbbell Bent-Over Row	3x10
Banded Supine Abduction	2x20

DAY 4	
Rest Pause Barbell Hip Thrust	3x10 (6, 2, 1, 1)
Handle Push-up	3x AMRAP (off dumbbells)
Dumbbell Squat	3x8
Wide-Grip Lat Pull-Down	3x10
Spread-Eagle Reverse Hyper	2x20

ADVANCED PROGRAM

You've completed the novice program, you've finished the intermediate program, and now you're ready for the advanced program. Here you do the same movement patterns but with heavier loading and more challenging schemes. This program contains the majority of advanced methods covered in Chapter 13 with alterations in tempo and includes machines and other equipment commonly found in commercial gyms.

If you're a seasoned lifter, you'll undoubtedly love this program due to the novelty factor alone. You will incorporate some new techniques like dropsets, pre-exhaustion, clusters, supersets, and ladders. This type of training plan can be very effective in short spurts, but basic progressive overload using straight sets and pyramids on the big lifts—although not fancy or sexy—will always lay the foundation for a strong, muscular physique. So don't look at the advanced program as being better than the intermediate program. Instead, think of them as complementary and synergistic.

Down the road, you can always revisit the advanced program while swapping some exercises from the glute exercise categories and augmenting the set and rep schemes. Your first time through, you should stick to the routines as listed. In time, through studying this book and experimenting in the gym, you'll become the expert when it comes to your body, and you'll be able to effectively write your own training programs.

PROGRAM REQUIREMENTS

You'll need access to a commercial gym for this program.

WEEKS 1–4

DAY 1	
Barbell Hip Thrust Dropset	2x10/10/10
Military Press	3x10
Dumbbell Curtsy Lunge	3x10
Inverted Row	3x10
American Deadlift	3x10
Banded Pallof Press	2x10

DAY 2	
Trap Bar Deadlift	3x6
Close-Grip Bench Press	3x4
Cable Kneeling Kickback	3x12
Wide-Grip Lat Pull-Down	3x10
Ring-Supported Pistol	3x10
Superset: RKC Plank/ Kettlebell Swing	3x 20 sec/ 20

DAY 3	
Pre-Exhaustion Nordic Ham Curl/Leg Extension	3x8/20
Reset Knee-Banded Barbell Hip Thrust	3x10
Bench Press	3x6
Lunge Isohold	2x 30 sec
Chest-Supported Row	3x8
Standing Glute Squeeze	3x10 (5 sec on, 3 sec off)

DAY 4	
Back Squat	5x3
Incline Press	3x8
1¼ Barbell Hip Thrust	3x8
Chin-up	3x8
Bodyweight Glute-Dominant Back Extension	3x30
Sled Push	3x 20 meters

WEEKS 5–8

DAY 1	
Conventional Deadlift	3x10
Standing Single-Arm Dumbbell Overhead Press	3x8
Enhanced-Eccentric Barbell Single-Leg Hip Thrust	3x6 (2 legs up, 1 leg down)
Single-Arm Pull-Down	3x8
1¼ Heel-Elevated Goblet Squat	3x8
Cuff/Dip Belt Cable Hip Rotation	2x10

DAY 2	
Barbell Hip Thrust	5x5
Pause Bench Press	5x3 (3-sec pause)
Cable Pull-Through	3x20
Chin-up	3x AMRAP
Dumbbell Deficit Curtsy Lunge	3x12
Banded Standing Hip Abduction	2x20

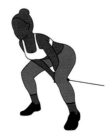

DAY 3	
Cluster Deadlift 5 reps with 70% 1RM EMOM	5 mins
Dumbbell Incline Press	3x8
Banded Kneeling Hip Thrust	3x20
Dumbbell One-Arm Row	3x12
Goblet Squat Pulse	2x30
Banded 45-Degree Kickback	3x20

DAY 4	
Pause Front Squat	3x5 (1-sec pause)
Military Press	3x6
Braced Single-Leg RDL	3x10
Narrow Neutral Grip Pull-Down	3x10
Pause Barbell Hip Thrust	3x5 (3-sec pause)
Knee-Banded Glute Bridge/Supine Abduction Ladder	12/11/10/...3/2/1

WEEKS 9–12

DAY 1	
Banded Hip Thrust	3x20
Bench Press	3x3
Stiff-Leg Deadlift	3x8
Weighted-Eccentric Chin-up	3x3
Dumbbell Between-Bench Squat	3x20
Banded Standing Hip External Rotation	2x12

DAY 2	
Double-Banded Hip Thrust	3x10
Feet-Elevated Push-up	3x AMRAP
Pistol Squat	3x AMRAP
Eccentric-Accentuated Chin-up	3x3 (lowering phase as slow as possible)
Prisoner Single-Leg 45-Degree Hyper	3x10
Extra-Range Side-Lying Hip Raise	3x10

DAY 3	
Triple-Banded Hip Thrust	3x8
Pause Bench Press	3x6 (3-sec pause)
Nordic Ham Curl	3x6
Feet-Elevated Inverted Row	3x AMRAP
Lateral Raise	3x10
Superset: Cable Kickback/ Hip Abduction	3x12/12

DAY 4	
Barbell Hip Thrust	5x5
Arnold Press	3x10
Back Squat	3x10
T-Bar Row	3x10
Dumbbell Glute-Dominant Back Extension	3x12
Burnout	3 mins nonstop Knee-Banded Glute Bridges/ Abductions

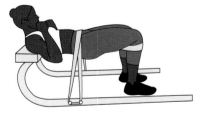

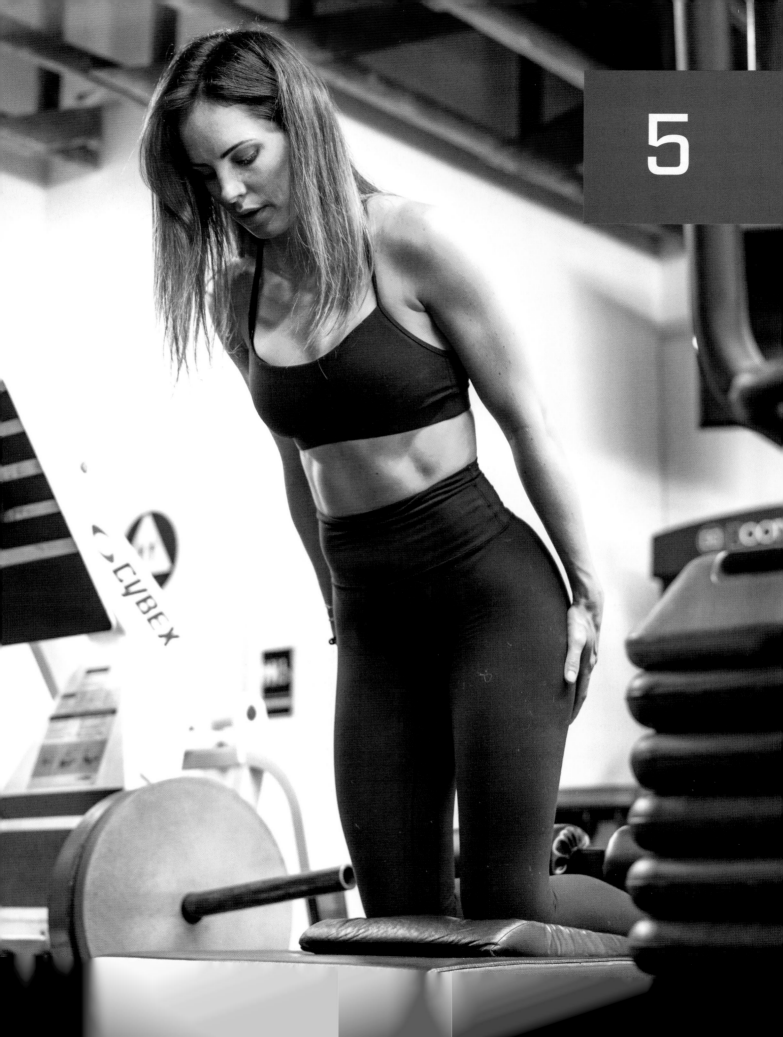

EXERCISES

To make the techniques in this part of the book easy to navigate, I've organized them into three chapters: Glute-Dominant Exercises, Quad-Dominant Exercises, and Hamstring-Dominant Exercises.

As you will recall from Chapter 10, there are several ways to categorize hip extension exercises. The most accurate and comprehensive method is to look at the position of the body relative to the line of resistance (load vector—see page 116) and knee action (the knees stay bent as in a hip thrust, the knees stay straight as in a back extension, the knees move slightly as in a stiff-leg deadlift, the knees flex as in a glute ham raise, or the knees extend through a full range of motion as in a squat).

Although looking at the load vector and knee action tells you why certain exercises work your glutes better than others and how to target a specific muscle region based on the position and load, it's difficult to organize techniques into broad categories using such methods. For this reason, I've organized this part based on the dominant muscle group working during the exercise. For example, hip thrust and glute bridge variations are considered glute dominant because they primarily work the glutes. Squat and lunge variations are considered quad dominant because they primarily work the quads. And deadlift and other hip hinge variations are considered hamstring (ham) dominant because they primarily work the hamstrings. Now, it's important to point out that the dominant muscle is not the only muscle active during the movement. Other muscles (referred to as *synergists*) play a crucial role. Your quads and hamstrings, for instance, are highly active during a hip thrust even though it is considered a glute-dominant exercise. And your glutes are active during squat and hip hinge movements even though they are considered quad- and hamstring-dominant exercises, respectively. In short, all hip extension exercises work the glutes to varying degrees.

I'll recap how each category works the glutes in a unique way in the coming pages. For now, just understand that organizing techniques based on the dominant muscle is a simple way to lump movements into broad, general categories.

However, I want to emphasize that this is not a perfect system of classification. There is a continuum in that some exercises fall into two categories depending on the knee action, body position, and how the exercise is performed. For instance, a high-bar full squat performed with the heels elevated and torso upright works the quads more (knee dominant), whereas a low-bar parallel back squat performed with a marked forward torso lean works the hamstrings more (hip dominant). But both fall into the quad-dominant category because they are squat variations. The same applies to stiff-leg deadlifts versus trap bar deadlifts: the former is hip dominant while the latter is knee dominant. To browse the exercises based on the movement and muscle region you want to work, refer to the Glute Exercise Categories chart on pages 124 and 125.

HIP- AND KNEE-DOMINANT CONTINUUM

DEADLIFT

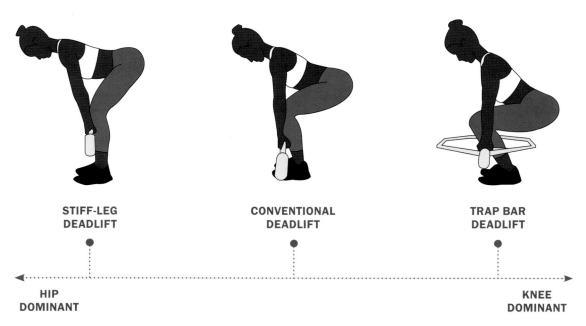

Another reason why organizing exercises into these three main categories is not sufficient is that there are different types of movements (glute bridge, hip thrust, and abduction exercises), as well as double- and single-leg variations of each movement. Put simply, there are a ton of exercises and variations of each movement that fit within the framework of the dominant muscle categories.

To further separate and distinguish the exercise variations, I also classify exercises based on the movement pattern. For example, the glute-dominant exercises include these movement patterns: hip thrusts, glute bridges, kickbacks, upright hip thrusts, quadruped hip extensions, abduction, and external rotation. Each of these movement patterns represents a section within the glute-dominant chapter. And the same is true for the quad- and hamstring-dominant chapters.

GLUTE DOMINANT	QUAD DOMINANT	HAMSTRING DOMINANT
Hip Thrusts	Squats	Deadlifts
Glute Bridges	Split Squats	Good Mornings
Quadruped Hip Extensions	Step-ups	Back Extensions
Kickbacks	Single-Leg Squats	Reverse Hypers
Upright Hip Thrusts	Sled Drags	Swings
Hip Abduction Exercises	*Knee Extensions	Straight-Leg Bridges
Hip External Rotation Exercises		Knee Flexion Exercises
Posterior Pelvic Tilt		

*Knee extensions are not covered in this book because they can be performed only on a knee extension machine. However, they fall into the quad-dominant category and should be considered an effective accessory exercise for isolating and developing the quads.

To categorize the exercise variations—that is, the different ways to perform the same exercise—I look at four things:

- Limb number (or stance)
- Range of motion
- Load position (where the weight is placed on the body)
- Equipment

As I will describe in more detail in the coming pages, you're still performing the same movement pattern, but by changing your stance, range of motion, load position, or equipment, you're performing a slightly different variation of the exercise.

LIMB NUMBER

For glute training purposes, *limb number* refers to double-leg (bilateral), single-leg (unilateral), and B-stance variations.

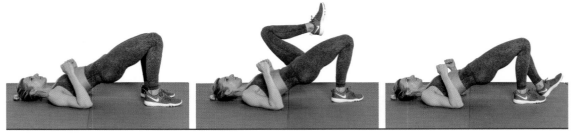

DOUBLE LEG   SINGLE LEG   B-STANCE

RANGE OF MOTION

You can also alter an exercise by changing the range of motion (ROM). For example, you can perform a glute bridge with your feet on the ground or elevated on a box, or you can perform a stiff-leg deadlift or a deficit stiff-leg deadlift (which increases ROM).

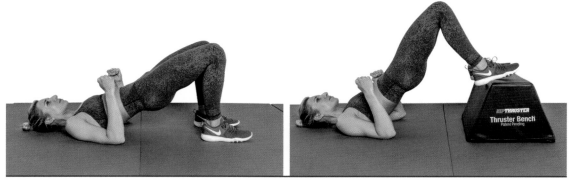

GLUTE BRIDGE

FEET-ELEVATED GLUTE BRIDGE

LOAD POSITION

Load position refers to the position of the weight on your body. For example, you can perform squats with the load positioned on your upper back (high- or low-bar back squat), in the crooks of your arms (Zercher squat), or hanging from your hips (belt squat).

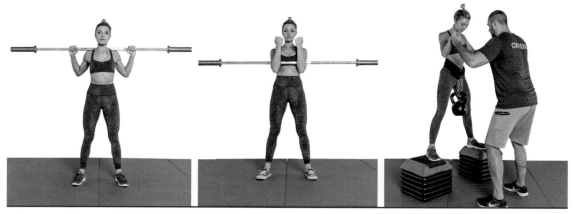

BARBELL BACK SQUAT

ZERCHER SQUAT

BELT SQUAT

EQUIPMENT

You can also create unique exercise variations from the same movement pattern by using different equipment. For example, you can perform a front-loaded squat with a barbell or dumbbell, each of which offers a unique stimulus. In this part of the book, you will learn how to create variations using all of the different kinds of equipment, including free weights, bands, and machines.

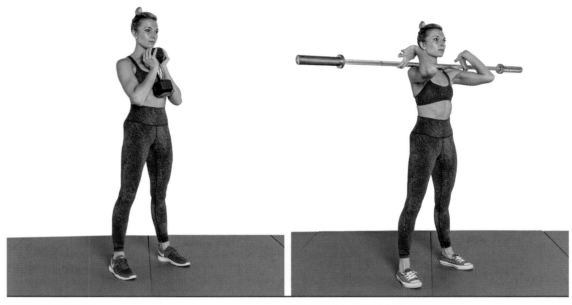

GOBLET SQUAT   BARBELL FRONT SQUAT

As you can see, you have a lot of options. To get the most out of this part of the book, I strongly encourage you to read the chapter and section introductions—specifically the "Guidelines and Cues," which apply to all of the exercise variations. From there, you can learn why each variation is different, what it is good for, and how to perform it correctly.

I know that the sheer volume of techniques can be overwhelming. As I've said before, at any point you can turn back to Chapter 18, pick a program to follow, and then browse the technique sections based on the movements you want to perform on any given day or workout. But, for the best results, it's important to experiment with different techniques to figure out which exercises and variations work best for you. This is why it's so important to have a broad arsenal of techniques at your disposal: so you can pick the variations that best suit your situation, goals, and anatomy.

BUYING EQUIPMENT

I'm hesitant to offer specific equipment recommendations because everyone has different preferences when it comes to brands and suppliers. What's more, some people are more economical and like to seek out the best deal, while others just want the best piece of equipment money can buy, regardless of price. For instance, you can find most of the equipment listed here on Amazon.com, on Craigslist, at secondhand stores, or at most local sports stores at an inexpensive price, but you risk buying faulty or cheap equipment. Personally (and I'm not saying you need to do this), I prefer spending a little extra money and getting something that is durable and highly rated.

Below are my favorite websites where you can buy the equipment recommended for each phase. In my opinion, these websites sell the best strength training equipment and weightlifting gear.

- Bretcontreras.store, EliteFTS.com, Performbetter.com, Roguefitness.com, Sorinex.com

Glute-Dominant Exercises

When it comes to exercises that target and develop the glutes, glute-dominant movements reign supreme. The exercises featured in this chapter are considered glute dominant because there is constant tension on your glutes throughout the entire range of the movement. The constant tension not only maximizes muscle contraction in the glutes but also prevents blood from escaping the muscle, producing a burn and pump. In addition to feeling your glutes swell, the burn is associated with metabolic stress, which is thought to further aid in the development of muscle.

Conversely, when you squat or deadlift, there are moments when your glutes are highly active and on tension and moments when they are not. So the glutes get a break where blood is pumped out of the muscle, which prevents the buildup of metabolites (molecular by-products of fatiguing muscles) and swelling. If you've ever wondered why you don't get a glute pump when you squat or deadlift, this is the reason. I'm not trying to scare you away from squats and deadlifts; these movement patterns are critical to glute development, function, and performance. But if your goal is to grow and strengthen your glutes, it's best to prioritize the glute-dominant exercises covered in this chapter.

STRUCTURE AND ORGANIZATION

This chapter is broken into eight main sections—hip thrusts, glute bridges, quadruped hip extensions, kickbacks, upright hip thrusts, hip abduction exercises, hip external rotation exercises, and posterior pelvic tilt exercises. The hip thrust, glute bridge, and quadruped hip extension exercises are all the same in that your back is flat and your knees stay bent during the movement. The kickback exercises are not considered a hip thrust movement pattern because you have to straighten your legs to perform the movement, but they're still glute-dominant exercises because they work the heck out of your glutes.

The hip thrust ranks highest because your shoulders are elevated, allowing you to move your hips through an increased range of motion. The glute bridge shares the same movement pattern, but your shoulders are on the ground, which reduces hip range of motion. The quadruped and kickback movements are easy to learn and can be done anywhere, making them great for activation drills and building muscle through high repetitions. The upright hip thrust techniques are essentially standing and kneeling hip thrust variations. They are not as good as the hip thrust, but they're great to mix in for variety. Hip abduction exercises are great for burnouts and developing the upper glutes. And hip external rotation exercises are essential for athletes, especially those who play rotational sports like baseball and tennis. Finally, posterior pelvic tilt exercises are considered diagnostic or assessment drills aimed at developing proper pelvic tilt action and maximal glute contractions.

GLUTE-DOMINANT EXERCISES

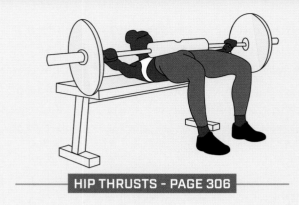

HIP THRUSTS - PAGE 306

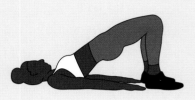

GLUTE BRIDGES - PAGE 340

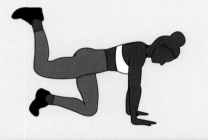

QUADRUPED HIP EXTENSIONS - PAGE 357

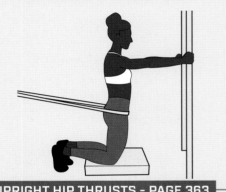

UPRIGHT HIP THRUSTS - PAGE 363

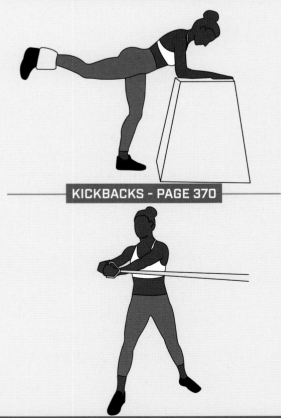

KICKBACKS - PAGE 370

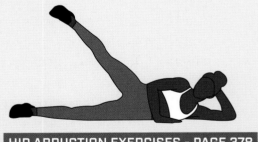

HIP ABDUCTION EXERCISES - PAGE 378

HIP EXTERNAL ROTATION EXERCISES - PAGE 397

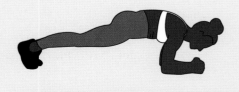

POSTERIOR PELVIC TILT - PAGE 401

Hip Thrusts

It's hard to believe that just 13 years ago, the hip thrust didn't exist. If you wanted to train your glutes with a loaded exercise, you had no other choice but to squat, deadlift, or lunge. Today, a wide range of people regularly use the hip thrust in a variety of settings—from top-level physique athletes, bodybuilders, powerlifters, and professional sports teams to celebrities and generalist exercise enthusiasts. It's not a stretch to say that the hip thrust is one of the fastest growing exercises in the fitness industry.

What has led to the success of the hip thrust? Naturally, my ego wants to take all of the credit, but that's not the real reason. Though I played a big role in promoting the exercise initially, the rapid growth and popularity stem from the results. The majority of the before-and-after photos that people send me are transformations credited solely to the hip thrust. These people didn't change anything in their training other than to add the hip thrust, and their physique improved.

Although the transformations do a lot to validate the exercise, there is much more to the hip thrust than improving physique. For starters—as I discussed in the introduction—the hip thrust is a movement pattern for the glutes that you can load with considerable weight. This has a couple of advantages:

- It's conducive to progressive overload due to the stability, short learning curve, and ability to hoist serious weight.
- Lifting heavy helps increase tension in the muscle, which, as you learned in Part 2, is a mechanism for muscle growth and strength development (see page 80).

Second, the ability to load the exercise with weight allows you to create strength goals that clearly measure progress. Having something tangible to work toward—say, hip thrusting 225 pounds for a set of 10 reps—helps you stay on track and be consistent with your training. Conversely, training simply to look good or working toward aesthetic goals is difficult to measure. It's subjective to the person judging the physique. And if you're judging yourself, you're probably comparing yourself to others and not being fair. This can derail your training and crush your motivation. So, even if you're training to improve your physique, it's important to create strength goals so that you can track your progress. Numbers don't lie, but your eyes might, and usually not to your advantage.

Third, the hip thrust is easy to perform. With both feet on the ground and your back braced against a bench, you have three points of contact, making the movement very stable and safe. Generally, the more stable the movement, the safer it is and the easier it is to learn and execute. This means you can take a beginner who is not proficient at squats or deadlifts, which require more coordination and are typically more challenging to learn, and give them a simple, safe, and effective glute and leg workout.

In addition to having a short learning curve, the added stability of the hip thrust allows for maximal glute activation. More specifically, your knees stay bent through the entire range of motion, which inhibits your hamstrings and prevents them from firing optimally. Your brain will allow you to contract the muscle, but not maximally, because it knows it's not the right muscle for the job. So, when your knees are bent, your central nervous system will call upon the glutes to get the job done. This is why the hip thrust movement patterns are considered glute dominant because you're deemphasizing the hamstrings so that the glutes can do the lion's share of the work. To put it another way, when your knees stay bent and you extend your hips, your glutes contract more than when your knees stay straight, as in a stiff-leg deadlift or back extension, or when they bend and straighten, as in a squat or cable pull-through.

Another reason why the hip thrust is so effective for building the glutes is that it stresses end-range hip extension, which is the zone of maximum glute activation. The gluteus maximus activates the most when it's in a shortened position. And the glutes are shortened markedly at the top of the hip thrust as you lock out or fully extend your hips.

Lastly, the hip thrust position allows you to move your hips through a full range of motion. Elevating your back against a bench creates more of a bend in your hips (hip flexion) in the bottom or start position. To reach the top or finish position, you have to raise your hips through a larger range of motion compared to the glute bridge. This larger range of motion and the tension maintained in the bottom position are what make the hip thrust a great glute exercise.

10 REASONS TO HIP THRUST

I've already explained why the hip thrust is great for glute development. Here, I provide a more succinct but comprehensive list of the top ten reasons why the hip thrust rocks:

1. It places constant tension on the glutes.
2. It moves the hips through a large range of motion.
3. There is high tension in the peak glute activation position (at end-range hip extension).
4. The bent-knee position reduces hamstring contribution and increases gluteal contribution.
5. The stable position and simple technique make it easy to learn and execute.
6. It is well suited for all body types, unlike other popular lifts.
7. It allows for heavy lifting, so a variety of loads and set and rep schemes can be utilized.
8. It is the safest heavy lower-body exercise and is easy on the lower back if performed correctly.
9. It is well suited for building confidence in women and beginners due to the high loads that can be used.
10. It is a versatile exercise that can be performed using a variety of stances, loads, and equipment.

GUIDELINES AND CUES

BARBELL HIP THRUST

Keep your head forward and tuck your chin

Reach full hip extension, posteriorly tilt your pelvis, and contract your glutes maximally

Position the bar just above your pubic bone in the lower abdominal region. Use a pad and make sure it is centered on the bar and the bar is centered on your hips.

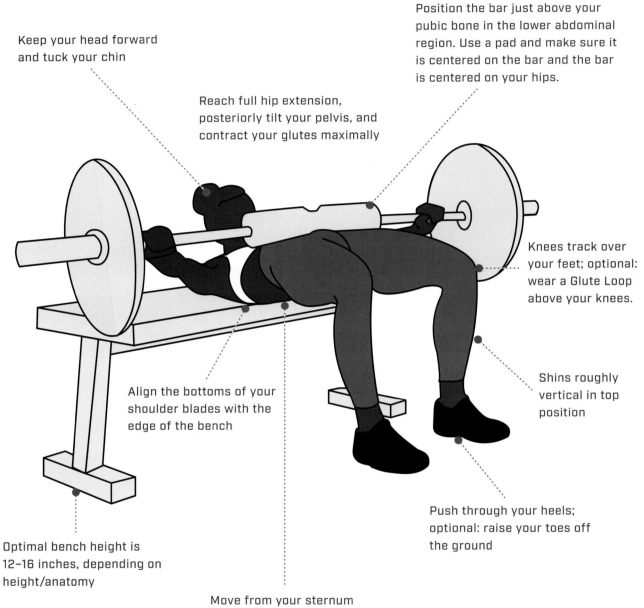

Knees track over your feet; optional: wear a Glute Loop above your knees.

Align the bottoms of your shoulder blades with the edge of the bench

Shins roughly vertical in top position

Optimal bench height is 12–16 inches, depending on height/anatomy

Move from your sternum down and think about keeping your ribs down

Push through your heels; optional: raise your toes off the ground

As you will soon learn—or you may already know—there are several ways to hip thrust based on your body position and the equipment you use. For instance, you can perform a barbell hip thrust, a bodyweight hip thrust with both feet elevated, or a single-leg hip thrust with a dumbbell (to mention a few options). Later in this section, I cover all of the variations in detail. But first, I want to address some important guidelines and cues that apply to every variation. Consider what is covered here as a universal blueprint for achieving perfect hip thrust technique.

BENCH HEIGHT: ALIGN THE BOTTOMS OF YOUR SHOULDER BLADES WITH THE FRONT OF THE BENCH

What makes the hip thrust unique is that your shoulders are elevated off the ground. The general rule is to position your back against a bench so that the bottoms of your shoulder blades are in line with the top edge of the bench.

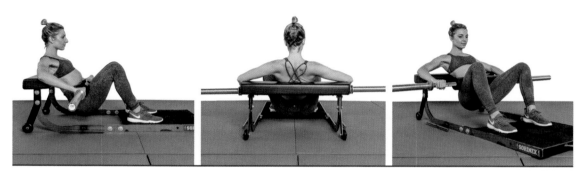

Aligning the top edge of the bench just below the shoulder blades is the optimal setup for most people.

To set up, you need a Hip Thruster, a bench, or an aerobic step with risers. The Hip Thruster is designed for the hip thrust movement pattern, but I realize that most people don't have access to one, which is not a problem. Virtually every gym has benches and aerobic steps. The key is to find a setup that works for you.

The ideal bench (or step) height is around 14 inches (35.5 cm). If you're tall, you may want to experiment with a 15- to 16-inch bench. If you're smaller—say, 5-foot-2 or shorter—or if you have relatively long legs and a short torso, you might need to lower it to 12 inches. If your gym has only taller benches, you can still hip thrust, but you may have to elevate your feet as well so that your shoulders, hips, and knees line up in the top position. If the bench is too high, you might feel the movement more in your quads than in your glutes. If the bench is too low, you might bend from your back instead of from your hips.

Depending on your height, the height of the bench, and whether or not you have a pad under your butt, your butt may touch down to the pad or the ground or it will hang in midair, with the latter being the most common.

Below I describe four hip thrust setups. First is the optimal setup with a Hip Thruster bench. Next, I show you how to set up on a flat or adjustable bench or an aerobic step with risers. If you're wondering how to set up with a barbell, I cover those variations later in the section. For now, I want you to focus on getting into the right start position.

Hip Thruster

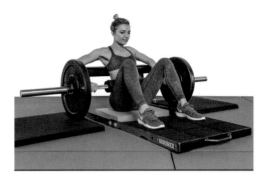

The Hip Thruster is about 14 inches in height (it's 16 inches tall with a 2-inch-tall mat). If the bench is too high and the edge of the bench hits above your shoulder blades, try sitting on a balance pad as shown in the photo. This will elevate your butt a couple of inches, positioning your back right where it needs to be. It's rare that 14 inches is too short—I'm 6-foot-4 and it's fine for me—but if it's too low for you, using a taller bench is your best option.

Flat Bench

Most benches are 16 inches or taller, which is too high for most people. Even elevating your butt off the ground by sitting on a pad is still too high, so most people set their stance and hover above the ground. If you're performing a barbell hip thrust, you may need to employ a different setup—see page 334. It's also imperative to secure the bench so that it doesn't slide backward or tip over. There are several ways to do so. The safest option and the one I recommend is to shove the bench against a wall or power rack. You can also place heavy dumbbells against the bench or have someone sit on it or push against it from behind, but these methods are not as safe or effective.

Adjustable Bench

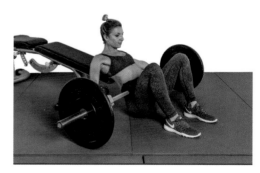

An adjustable bench with a decline setting is another popular option. The advantages are that you can adjust the height of the bench to your body, it's relatively stable, the downward-sloping angle might feel good on your back, and most commercial gyms carry this piece of equipment.

Aerobic Step

An aerobic step with risers is a good option because you can adjust the height to suit your body. It is also stable as long as the risers are on a rubber surface, which is common in most gyms. Even so, I recommend placing the step against a wall for added safety. Many people love the way the curved edge of the aerobic step feels on their back, but most find it necessary to drape a yoga mat or towel over the edge to protect their back, as shown in the photos. The most common setup is to use five risers per side (which makes the step the same height as the Hip Thruster). Shorter individuals can use four risers per side and taller individuals six per side.

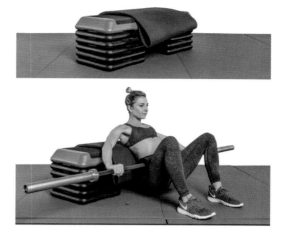

AMERICAN HIP THRUST

You perform the American hip thrust with your back higher on the bench (with the edge of the bench centered on your midback instead of your mid-upper back), which positions your feet a little closer to your butt. This variation leads to higher hamstring activation and less quad activation as compared to the traditional hip thrust, and it naturally positions your head so that you are looking forward, which creates more pelvic action. I typically prescribe this variation for people who feel hip thrusts in their back. So, if your back hurts, you have a history of lower back pain, or you feel too much tension in your back when you hip thrust, try the American variation and see if you prefer it.

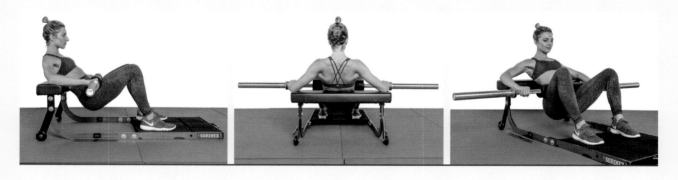

FOOT DISTANCE: GET YOUR SHINS ROUGHLY VERTICAL

Now that you know where to position your back, the next step is to figure out where to position your feet. Getting into the top position of the hip thrust by aligning your shoulders, hips, and knees is a good way to determine proper foot distance. You may need to set up in front of a mirror, film yourself from the side, or have a friend check your position to ensure proper alignment.

To begin, position your back against the bench, aligning the top edge of the bench just below your shoulder blades. Next, extend your hips so that your torso is roughly parallel to the ground. From here, adjust your feet until your shins are roughly vertical. Consider this your starting point. As you practice the movement, adjust your feet forward and backward while paying close attention to how your glutes activate. You might find that you prefer a slightly longer stance with your knees behind your shins or a slightly shorter stance with your knees in front of your shins. In general, the farther away your feet are, the more you will feel your hamstrings, and the shorter your stance, the more you will feel your quads.

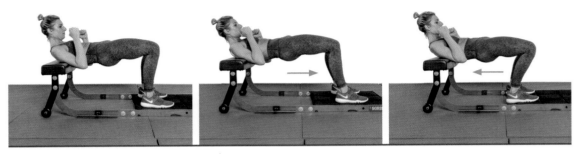

SHINS ROUGHLY VERTICAL   LONG STANCE   SHORT STANCE

STANCE AND FOOT PRESSURE: PUSH THROUGH YOUR HEELS

Once you've determined the proper foot distance, the next step is to experiment with foot flare and stance width. I like to position my feet roughly shoulder width apart and fairly straight, with my knees flared outward, because this setup gives me the most glute activation. But I've trained a lot of people who like a narrow stance with straight feet and some who like their feet wide and turned out. So experiment and use the stance that feels best to you. You may feel that one stance hits your glutes much harder than the others (this is the stance you want to prioritize), or you may feel your glutes working similarly in all styles. If you fall into the latter category, choose the stance that feels the most comfortable.

Though foot position might vary from person to person, the cue for initiating the movement is the same for everyone—push through your heels. Pushing through the balls of your feet shifts tension to your quads and often to your hamstrings, which is not the purpose of this exercise.

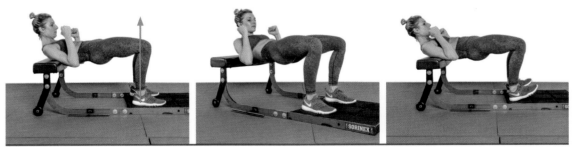

FEET FLAT HEEL DRIVE   RAISE TOES OFF THE GROUND

You can either keep your feet flat or raise your toes off the ground via ankle dorsiflexion. Employ the option that feels more comfortable and yields higher glute activation.

KNEE POSITION: PUSH YOUR KNEES OUT

Pushing your knees out as you extend your hips not only increases glute activation but also puts your knees in the optimal position. Whether you're thrusting, squatting, lunging, or deadlifting, you usually want your knees to track over your middle toes.

Allowing your knees to cave inward from the bottom position not only reduces tension in your glutes but also places strain on your knee joints. However, if your knees come in a bit at the top of the movement, this isn't necessarily a problem; it may just be a natural movement for your particular hip joint and glute attachment anatomy.

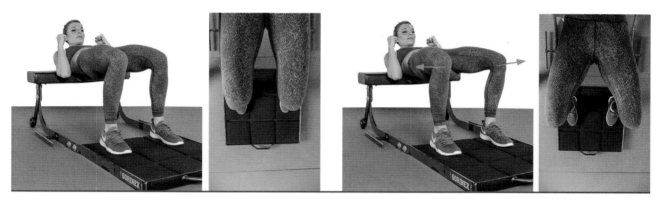

Push your knees out while keeping your feet flush with the ground as you extend and lower your hips.

HIP POSITION: REACH FULL HIP EXTENSION

Full hip extension is the zone in which you achieve peak glute activation. Again, the goal is to get your shoulders, hips, and knees in line. Think about squeezing your glutes to reach full hip extension and pausing for a moment at the top. This one-second pause increases time under tension and ensures proper tempo and control throughout the movement. Don't skimp on range of motion just to perform more reps. If you can't reach full hip extension, end the set and start again fresh.

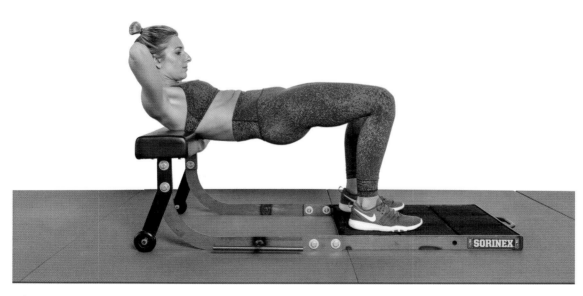

When you reach full hip extension, your knees, hips, and shoulders should be roughly in line.

SPINAL MECHANICS: MOVE FROM YOUR STERNUM DOWN

When I started teaching the hip thrust exercise, I didn't give any cues to help with spinal-pelvic posture, which caused some people to develop lower back pain. To remedy this problem, I developed the American hip thrust and began experimenting with different spinal-pelvic strategies. I realized that the majority of people get the most glute activation with a low occurrence of lower back pain when they hinge at the lower scapulae region and maintain a forward head position. I used cues like "head forward" and "ribs down" to encourage this action.

Though these cues work well, some of my clients still experience lower back pain when they hinge or rock back and forth over the bench. So more recently, I've been utilizing another cue: "move from your sternum down." This cue encourages more pelvic action—specifically, posterior pelvic tilt in the top position—reduces erector activation, helps people feel their glutes more during the exercise, and prevents lower back pain and discomfort. Though this cue seems to work well for the majority of people, you should experiment with the spinal-pelvic strategies outlined on pages 317 to 319 and employ the option that works best for you.

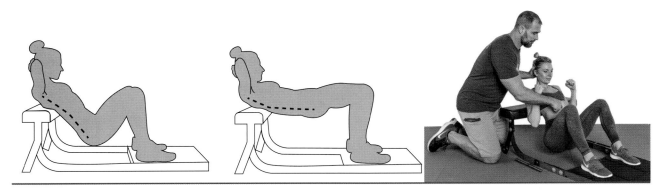

To posterior pelvic tilt, move from your sternum down. You can also think about keeping your ribcage down as you extend your hips.

HEAD POSITION: TUCK YOUR CHIN

A forward head position not only puts your body in proper alignment but also helps keep tension on your glutes and away from your spinal erectors and hamstrings. Here's how it works.

OPTION 1: HEAD FORWARD/CHIN TUCKED

At the bottom of the hip thrust, look straight ahead. As you elevate your hips, maintain your forward gaze, which will cause your neck to flex forward during the movement. You can also think about tucking your chin to your chest as you extend your hips.

Although I've never heard of anyone getting hurt by tucking their chin, some people say that neck flexion is harmful and will cause injury. But your neck is unloaded, so there is no real cause for concern. However, if it doesn't feel right to you, then keep your head and neck neutral throughout the entire range of motion. As you can see in the photos, you look up at the top of the hip thrust. Unless this causes you pain during or after the exercise, it is not wrong; it's just a variation. Maybe 1 in 10 of my clients prefer this method.

OPTION 2: HEAD AND NECK NEUTRAL

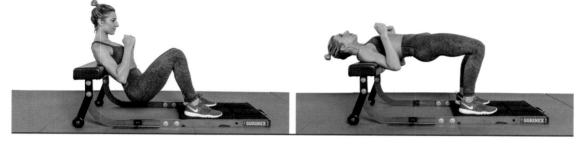

Focus your gaze forward. As you elevate your hips, keep your head and spine neutral.

BRACING: BRACE YOUR CORE

Bracing increases spinal stability, prevents hyperextension, and allows for better performance. It's simple: at the bottom of the movement, take a deep breath and then "lock it down" by tightening your abs, obliques, and diaphragm muscles.

EVOLUTION OF THE HIP THRUST MACHINES

Just as the hip thrust has evolved over the last decade, so too has the equipment. It started with the Skorcher, then came the Hip Thruster, and now there are even more options, such as the Booty Builder, Glute Builder, and Nautilus Glute Drive.

To be clear, all you need to hip thrust is a stable bench. So don't think you need to go out and spend thousands of dollars just to get your thrust on. However, these machines are specifically designed for hip thrusting, which makes the setup and execution much easier.

I don't want to try to sell you on any of this equipment because—again—it is not required to hip thrust. But there are pros and cons to each machine, and it might be helpful to know what those are in case you want to buy one for your home gym, or the commercial gym at which you train has one or more of these models.

SKORCHER

The Skorcher is still one of my favorite hip thrusting machines because it is comfortable, it allows for the most hip range of motion, and the handles provide additional stability, which make double- and single-leg hip thrusts feel incredible. The problem is that you can add resistance only in the form of a band, and it's not designed for barbells. So you're limited in what you can do.

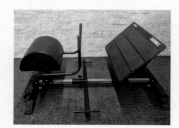

HIP THRUSTER

The Hip Thruster is probably the least cool compared to the newer models, but it is the most affordable and takes up the least space, and you can use it to perform a wide range of glute exercises, from barbell and banded hip thrusts to abduction exercises, Bulgarian split squats, and banded deadlifts. The one caveat is that the barbell hip thrust can be cumbersome to set up: ideally, you need to roll the weights onto an elevated surface to get your hips in place. But again, the versatility, size, and price make the Hip Thruster the best option for home gyms and most fitness facilities.

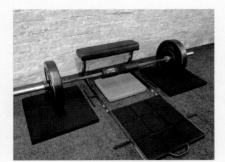

BOOTY BUILDER

The Booty Builder is the most expensive but also the smoothest. To perform the hip thrust movement, you buckle the strap around your waist and adjust the weight by moving the pin up or down the weight stack, making the Booty Builder the most convenient machine for loading. You can also use bands and perform cable kneeling hip thrusts. But this machine is expensive, takes up a lot of space, and isn't as versatile, meaning that it is designed primarily for hip thrusting.

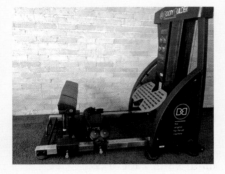

GLUTE BUILDER

The Glute Builder is the Swiss Army knife of hip thrust machines. You can do all of the exercises that you can on the Hip Thruster, plus quadruped and reverse hyper variations, which are unique to this machine. In addition, the Glute Builder has a barbell rack, which makes setting up and loading easier to manage. It falls in the middle in terms of cost and size.

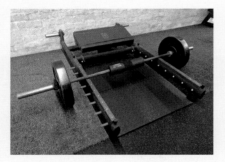

NAUTILUS GLUTE DRIVE

The Glute Drive is easy to load, and the ergonomics help you maintain good form. Nautilus did a great job of making it look like it belongs in a commercial gym. However, the setup is not for everyone. Some people feel the exercise too much in their quads, and many complain about the pad digging into their hips. But the execution is smooth and super safe, making this a great piece of equipment. Like the other machines, it's heavy and a bit more expensive, and it can take up quite a bit of space if you add the plate storage.

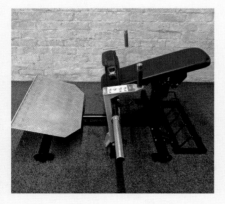

At my Glute Lab gym, we have all of these hip thrust machines, and they are all valuable for different reasons. What's interesting is that there isn't a clear favorite among the people who train there.

SPINAL-PELVIC STRATEGIES

When it comes to performing the hip thrust correctly, there is no one-size-fits-all approach. The majority of people can follow the hip thrust guidelines and cues and they're good to go, while others might need to experiment with different strategies to get the desired result: to maximize glute activation without causing damage to the body.

The spinal-pelvic strategies outlined in this section—that is, the positions of your spine and pelvis—give you options. There are pros and cons to each strategy, and they are different for everyone. For example, you might find that slightly hyperextending your spine as you elevate your hips fires your glutes optimally. If you don't feel pain or wear-and-tear on your body, then perhaps that is the right technique for you. As with all of the variations I offer, I suggest that you experiment with the different strategies and choose the one that best suits your unique body type and movement mechanics.

NEUTRAL SPINE

Perhaps the most universal and widely taught spinal strategy is to keep your spine and pelvis neutral—head, ribcage, and hips in line. This is my least favorite option because your head tilts back at full hip extension, which in my experience almost always leads to spinal hyperextension at the end of the set. You see lifters who use this technique arching their chests as they rep to failure. But a lot of coaches teach the neutral spine, so it's important to include here.

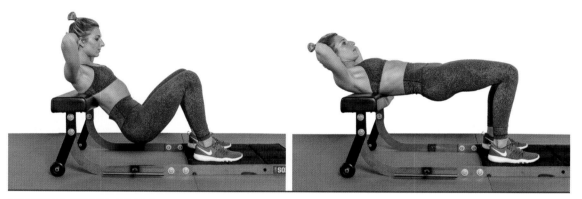

NEUTRAL SPINE: BOTTOM POSITION   NEUTRAL SPINE: TOP POSITION

NEUTRAL SPINE IN THE BOTTOM POSITION, POSTERIOR PELVIC TILT IN THE TOP POSITION

Another option is to keep a neutral spine and pelvis in the bottom position and then tuck your chin and allow your pelvis to tilt backward slightly as you reach the top position, or full hip extension. Sure, there is a little bit of spinal flexion when you reach the top, but squeezing your glutes causes it. With your glutes squeezed, your lower back is braced and protected, and it shuts your erectors off so there's markedly less compressive loading, which also safeguards your spine. What's more, you achieve maximal glute activation, which is the primary purpose of the exercise. But you don't want maximum posterior pelvic tilt; just tilt slightly with your ribcage down (keeping a forward gaze and head and neck position usually accomplishes this). This is the strategy I recommend for people who are susceptible to lower back pain.

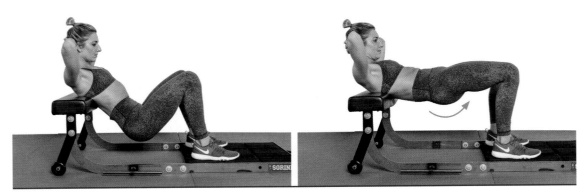

NEUTRAL SPINE: BOTTOM POSITION   POSTERIOR PELVIC TILT: TOP POSITION

POSTERIOR PELVIC TILT IN THE TOP AND BOTTOM POSITION

You can also stay locked in a posterior pelvic tilt throughout the entire range of the movement. So you crunch your abs slightly, tuck your chin so your gaze changes from downward to forward during the motion, bring your ribcage down at the bottom of the movement—keeping your back slightly rounded—and maintain that position as you elevate your hips into the top position. Although this strategy works for some of my clients, it's not my favorite.

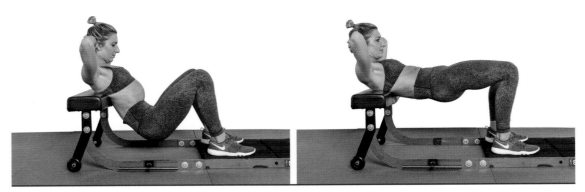

POSTERIOR PELVIC TILT: BOTTOM POSITION   POSTERIOR PELVIC TILT: TOP POSITION

ANTERIOR PELVIC TILT IN THE BOTTOM POSITION, POSTERIOR PELVIC TILT IN THE TOP POSITION

This spinal-pelvic strategy is my favorite and is probably the most popular. I hip thrust this way, and most of my clients do, too. In the bottom position, you're in slight spinal extension and anterior pelvic tilt, and then at the top, you reverse it into a little bit of spinal flexion and posterior pelvic tilt.

Most people tolerate this strategy well. According to the research, people can lift more weight with this method because their hips are strongest in deep hip flexion, and anterior pelvic tilt mimics hip flexion (just like posterior pelvic tilt mimics hip hyperextension). So it helps you get more weight off the ground, but you'll still need to finish it off by locking out your hips using the power of your glutes. To achieve this type of form, think chest up at the bottom of the movement and ribs down at the top. You can also think about moving from your sternum down.

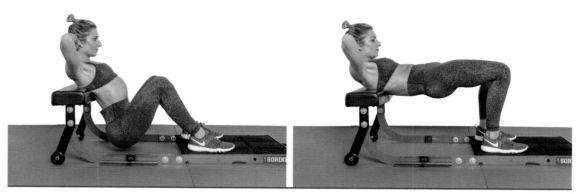

ANTERIOR PELVIC TILT: BOTTOM POSITION   **POSTERIOR PELVIC TILT: TOP POSITION**

FAULTS AND CORRECTIONS

If you follow the guidelines covered earlier in the section, you will avoid many of the most common hip thrust faults. However, it's important to understand why certain faults are suboptimal and how to correct them. Equally important, you need to know how to adjust your stance or position to get the most glute activation possible, as well as how to train around and avoid pain while hip thrusting.

FAULT: SPINAL HYPEREXTENSION

Excessive spinal hyperextension, or overarching your lower back, shifts tension from your glutes to your lower back muscles. It commonly occurs when you try to extend your hips with an anterior pelvic tilt, where the front of your pelvis drops downward and the rear of your pelvis rises upward. People often commit this fault when they try to lift more weight than their glutes can support. For instance, instead of using their glutes to finish the movement, they drop their pelvis and arch their back in an attempt to lock out their hips. This can happen due to weak glutes or simply poor mechanics or technique.

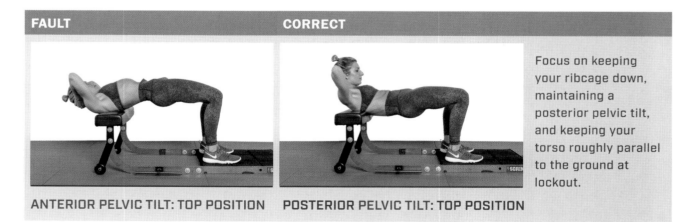

FAULT	CORRECT	

Focus on keeping your ribcage down, maintaining a posterior pelvic tilt, and keeping your torso roughly parallel to the ground at lockout.

ANTERIOR PELVIC TILT: TOP POSITION   **POSTERIOR PELVIC TILT: TOP POSITION**

FAULT: SLIDING UP AND DOWN THE BENCH

If you set up too low or high on the bench, you tend to slide up and down during the movement. This can shift tension away from your glutes to your quads.

CORRECTION:
Position your back against the bench so that the bottoms of your shoulder blades are lined up with the edge of the bench and maintain that position as you perform the movement.

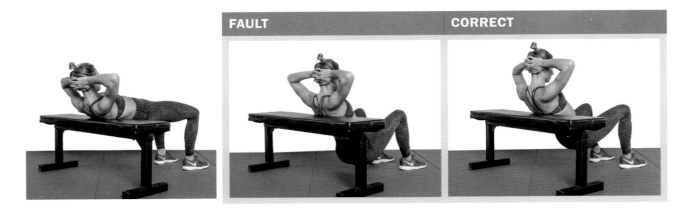

FAULT   CORRECT

FAULT: INSUFFICIENT HIP EXTENSION

Failing to lock out your hips typically happens when you try to lift too much weight or do too many reps. It's important to reach full hip extension with each repetition because this is the zone in which you get the most glute activation.

CORRECTION:
Reduce the load and focus on squeezing your glutes with a one-second pause with your hips in full extension. Again, your shoulders, back, and knees should be in line with your torso and parallel to the ground. Stop the set when you can no longer achieve a full range of motion.

FAULT: "FEELING IT" TOO MUCH IN YOUR QUADS

If you feel too much tension in your quads or you don't feel enough tension in your glutes, try one or more of the following corrections.

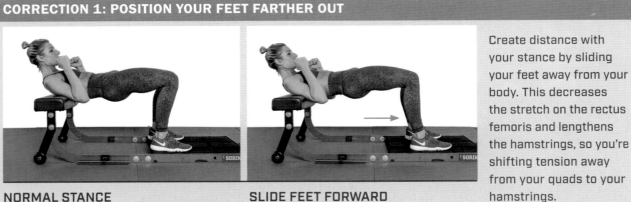

CORRECTION 1: POSITION YOUR FEET FARTHER OUT

NORMAL STANCE   SLIDE FEET FORWARD

Create distance with your stance by sliding your feet away from your body. This decreases the stretch on the rectus femoris and lengthens the hamstrings, so you're shifting tension away from your quads to your hamstrings.

CORRECTION 2: ADD A MINI BAND OR RESISTANCE BAND AROUND YOUR KNEES

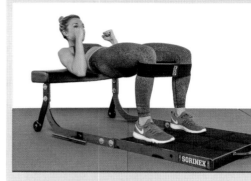

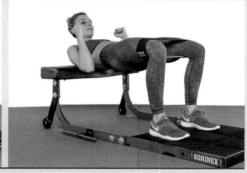

Add a mini band or resistance band (Glute Loop) either below or above your knees. This doesn't take tension out of your quads but rather adds tension to your glutes.

GLUTE LOOP BELOW KNEES

GLUTE LOOP ABOVE KNEES

CORRECTION 3: DRIVE THROUGH YOUR HEELS

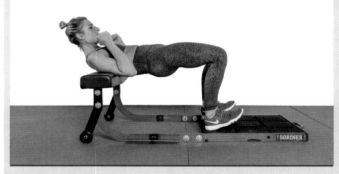

Focus on driving through your heels. You can elevate your toes by dorsiflexing your ankles to encourage this action.

DORSIFLEXION

CORRECTION 4: USE A SHORTER BENCH

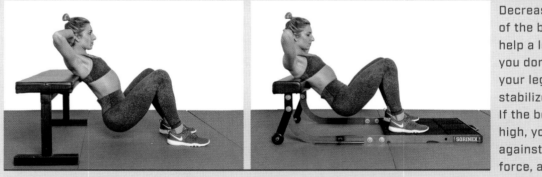

Decreasing the height of the bench can help a lot because you don't have to use your legs as much to stabilize your body. If the bench is too high, you have to push against it with more force, adding tension to your quads.

BENCH (HIGHER)

HIP THRUSTER (LOWER)

CORRECTION 5: LOOK UP WITH HIP HYPEREXTENSION

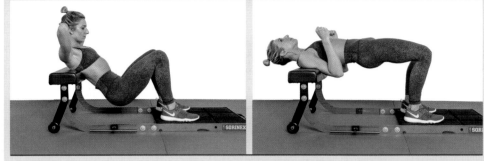

NEUTRAL

LOOK UP W/ HYPEREXTENSION

For some people, looking up increases glute activation. Probably 1 in 5 to 10 clients I train finds success with this technique. It's usually someone who is prone to feeling their quads too much when they hip thrust.

CORRECTION 6: PERFORM THE AMERICAN HIP THRUST

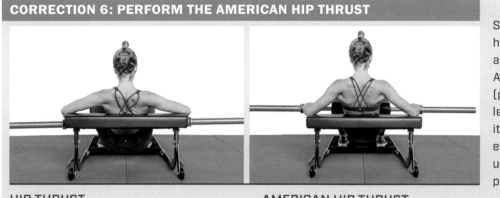

HIP THRUST

AMERICAN HIP THRUST

Sliding your back higher up the bench and performing the American hip thrust (page 311) shortens the lever length and makes it more of a pelvic tilting exercise because your upper torso is naturally positioned forward.

FAULT: "FEELING IT" TOO MUCH IN YOUR HAMSTRINGS

If you feel your hamstrings overworking during the hip thrust, you essentially reverse the "too much quads" corrections.

CORRECTION 1: POSITION YOUR FEET CLOSER TO YOUR HIPS

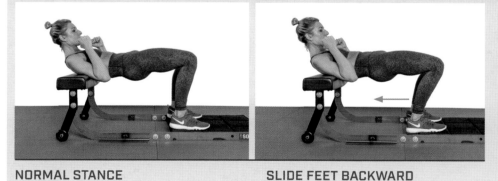

NORMAL STANCE

SLIDE FEET BACKWARD

Slide your feet closer to your body. This shifts tension from your hamstrings to your quads, which increases the perception of glute activation for some people.

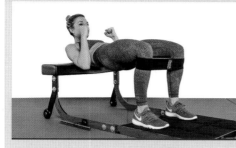
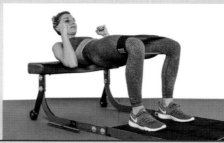

GLUTE LOOP BELOW KNEES　　GLUTE LOOP ABOVE KNEES

Adding a mini band around your knees—again—places more tension on your glutes.

CORRECTION 3: PUSH THROUGH YOUR WHOLE FOOT

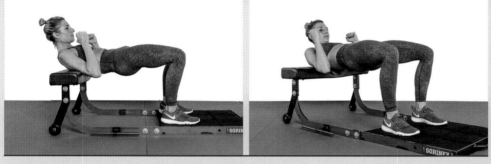

WHOLE FOOT

Instead of pushing through your heels, focus on driving through your whole foot, including the toes. (Obviously, you would not dorsiflex your ankles or raise your toes off the ground here.)

CORRECTION 4: USE A TALLER BENCH

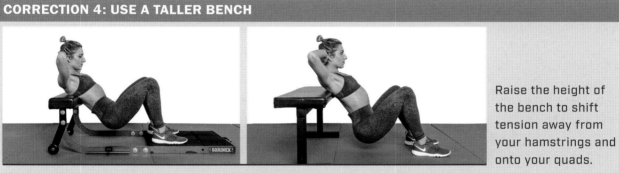

HIP THRUSTER　　BENCH

Raise the height of the bench to shift tension away from your hamstrings and onto your quads.

CORRECTION 5: LOOK FORWARD WITH POSTERIOR PELVIC TILT

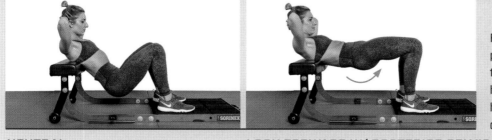

NEUTRAL　　LOOK FORWARD W/ POSTERIOR PELVIC TILT

For the majority of people, especially those who tend to feel hip thrusts in their hamstrings, this is the optimal technique.

5

EXERCISES

TRAINING AROUND PAIN

Lower Back Pain

Lower back pain almost always stems from hyperextending the spine with an anterior pelvic tilt in the top position. In most cases, simply keeping your spine neutral or maintaining a slight posterior pelvic tilt will correct the issue. Learn to look forward, keep your ribs down, and tuck your chin at the top of the thrust.

SIJ Pain

Sacroiliac joint (SIJ) pain is tricky because the exercises used to strengthen the glutes—like the hip thrust and glute bridge, which theoretically should help prevent SIJ pain—are often the same exercises that can exacerbate it. This is another scenario in which you have to listen to the signals your body is sending you. If hip thrusting lights it up, consider backing off for a couple weeks. When you return to training, stay out of the painful ranges and progress slowly. Over time, strengthening your glutes should improve persistent SIJ pain, but it's a delicate balance of training your glutes without pushing too hard.

Knee Pain

Most knee pain stemming from hip thrusts is not due to movement errors (not even knee caving), but rather is a by-product of high quad activation. The solution is to employ variety and reduce the number of heavy barbell hip thrusts you perform. You can opt for barbell glute bridges or B-stance hip thrusts, for example. To reduce quad tension, you can reduce the load, elevate your feet, adjust your stance, place a resistance band around your knees, or employ a glute bridge variation.

Neck Pain

Typically, hip thrust–related neck pain stems from having a weak neck. What most people don't realize is that tucking your chin or focusing your gaze forward when hip thrusting is difficult. It's not that it's straining your neck; it's that holding your neck in that position is fatiguing. So a lot of the pain is actually sore muscle, not pain stemming from bad mechanics. If you notice that your neck gets fatigued every time you hip thrust, you might want to consider doing some neck strengthening exercises. However, if tucking your chin causes acute pain, which it does for some people, try looking up and tilting your head back or keeping it neutral. Staying pain-free is priority number one, and you can still work your glutes just fine.

Upper Back Scrapes

Upper back scrapes are almost always due to insufficient bench padding. If you're trying to hip thrust off a plyometric box or other hard surface, you will scrape and bruise your back. It's like trying to barbell hip thrust without a bar pad; it's not recommended. Obviously, using a bench with adequate padding is ideal and will solve this problem. If you don't have a bench, you can add your own padding in the form of a yoga mat or balance pad.

Wrist Pain

Wrist pain is more common with barbell glute bridges due to the downward angle of your body at the top of the movement. But it occurs with the hip thrust every once in a while. In both cases, pain is a result of hyperextending your wrists. The solution is simple: maintain a neutral wrist position.

Hip Pain

In almost every case, hip pain results from not using a bar pad and not setting up correctly.

HIP THRUST SAFETY

To ensure that you come out of your hip thrusting experience unharmed, you must heed several safety considerations:

- Make sure that the bench is stable and secure. An unstable bench is dangerous, especially when lifting a lot of weight. If it tilts or slides backward, you risk injury. You can secure your bench by positioning it against a wall or power rack.

- To protect your upper back, make sure that the bench you are using has enough padding.

- To protect your pelvis when performing barbell hip thrust variations, use a squat sponge or other thick bar padding, such as a yoga mat.

- Lower back discomfort is the most common complaint associated with the hip thrust. Although it is important to experiment with the spinal-pelvic strategies outlined on pages 317 to 319, most people find that keeping their chin tucked and ribs down prevents lower back pain.

- Have a dedicated area for hip thrusts with all of the right equipment and accessories. This applies specifically to coaches who work at or own a gym and to people who have home gyms. In addition to ensuring safety, having a station dedicated to hip thrusting makes it easier to perform the exercise. In other words, if you have to organize all of the equipment every time you want to hip thrust, you are less likely to do it. Even worse, you're more likely to do it suboptimally due to all of the steps required to set up the equipment.

HIP THRUST CATEGORIES

There are five hip thrust categories based on foot position. Here I describe each bodyweight variation. Later in the section, I show you how to add resistance and load within each category by using different equipment.

When it comes to selecting a hip thrust variation, you have to take a lot of factors into account: your goals, your access to equipment, and how you feel that day. These categories give you options. If you're just starting out and you want to learn how to hip thrust, or you want to lift a lot of weight, stick with the double-leg hip thrust techniques. If you don't have any weights on hand, the single-leg variations may be the best choices. If you want to shift tension away from your quads to your hamstrings, you can implement the elevated variations.

DOUBLE-LEG (BILATERAL) HIP THRUST

This variation is the easiest to perform, is ideal for lifting heavy weight, and gets the highest glute activation. Both feet are in contact with the ground, and your back is braced against the bench. With multiple points of contact, the lift is very stable and safe.

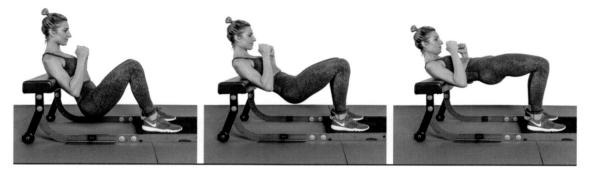

First, make sure your bench is secure and won't slide backward. Seated on the floor, position your upper back against the bench. With the bottoms of your shoulder blades lined up with the front of the bench, assume your hip thrust stance. If you're performing the movement with just body weight, curl your arms, dig your triceps into the bench, and make fists with your hands. Next, drive through your heels, push your knees outward, and thrust your hips upward while squeezing your glutes. Think about using your glutes to push your hips upward so the movement occurs at your hips, not your spine. As you reach full hip extension, focus on squeezing your glutes maximally for one second. Keeping your back and elbows pinned against the bench, lower into the bottom position with control before beginning your next repetition.

SINGLE-LEG (UNILATERAL) HIP THRUST

This variation is bit more challenging because you have only one point of contact on the ground, meaning that you have to stabilize your body on one leg. This category of hip thrust is great because you can get a good workout with low weight and repetitions. You get slightly less glute activation compared to the double-leg variation, but the single-leg hip thrust is still a great exercise to include in your program.

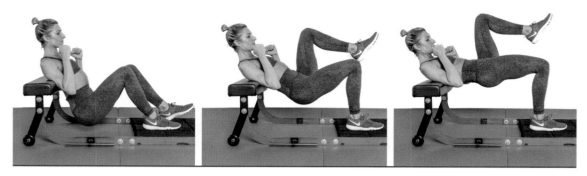

Set up exactly as you would when performing a double-leg hip thrust: make sure your bench is secure and won't slide backward, position your upper back against the bench, curl your arms, dig your triceps into the bench, and make fists with your hands (or put your arms in a T position). With the bottoms of your shoulder blades lined up with the front of the bench, assume your hip thrust stance, positioning your feet together along your center line. Next, lift one leg by pulling your knee toward your chest. Note: You can keep your leg bent as shown, or straighten it—whichever you prefer. To perform the movement, drive through your heel, raise your hips until they are roughly in line with your grounded knee and shoulders, and squeeze your glute as you reach the top position.

B-STANCE HIP THRUST

The B-stance hip thrust variation is essentially a cross between the single- and double-leg variations. Instead of raising your leg off the floor, you keep your foot on the ground slightly in front of your other leg, which provides balance and stability. This requires less coordination, making it slightly easier to perform. The key is to use your extended leg only for balance and stability. Your rear foot (the one that is closer to your body) should produce around 70 percent of the force, while your extended leg produces about 30 percent of the force when you extend your hips. I suspect that as you lift more weight—say, when performing a heavy barbell B-stance hip thrust—you will inevitably use your extended leg more to counterbalance the weight, which defeats the purpose of trying to load mostly one leg. So, as with the single-leg hip thrust, it's better to keep the load light.

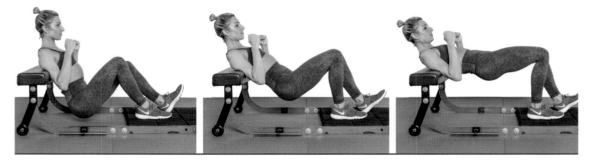

Position the bottoms of your shoulder blades along the front of a secured bench and assume your hip thrust stance. Next, straighten one leg, placing your heel just in front of your other foot and keeping the toes of the extended leg in the air. To execute the movement, drive through the heel of the foot that is closer to your body and raise your hips. Realize that your extended leg is there only to provide balance and stability. In other words, don't actively push your extended leg into the floor as you extend your hips.

The frog pump, which I cover on page 348, is a popular glute exercise that you typically perform with your back on the ground. However, you can elevate your shoulders or your feet to increase hip range of motion. If you elevate your shoulders, you create a hip thrust movement pattern—hence the name frog thrust. I don't prescribe the frog thrust as often as other hip thrust variations because you can't load the movement with a lot of weight, and some people feel their quads more in this particular stance. Consider the frog thrust variations accessory exercises that you can throw in from time to time for variety. I recommend a smaller bench (the Thruster Bench in the photos is 12 inches tall) and using lighter loads with high reps.

HIP-BANDED FROG THRUST   **BARBELL FROG THRUST**   **DUMBBELL FROG THRUST**

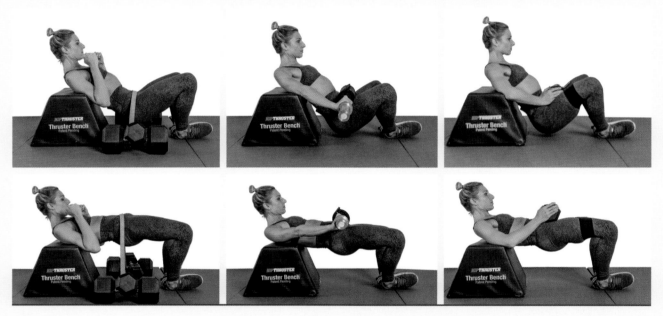

FEET-ELEVATED HIP THRUST

Elevating your feet on a box, step, chair, or bench can almost double your hip range of motion. It also increases hamstring activation and decreases quad activation. This variation is great if your quads are smoked from a workout, you want to shift tension away from your quads, or you want to increase the range of motion for the exercise. It is best performed with just body weight or using light dumbbells and bands.

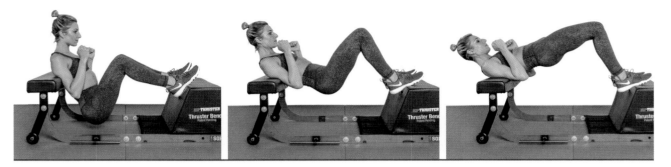

Set up in your hip thrust start position with a box secured where your toes would normally be if you were performing a hip thrust with your feet on the floor. You can either place the centers of your feet on the edge of the box, which tends to work the glutes more, or place both heels on top of the box with your toes pointed toward the ceiling, which tends to work the hamstrings more. Adjust the box backward or forward as needed so that your knee angle is slightly greater than 90 degrees in the bottom position. To perform the movement, push your hips toward the ceiling, driving through your heels or the centers of your feet until you reach lockout. Think about squeezing your glutes for one second as you reach full hip extension.

FOOT-ELEVATED HIP THRUST

Like the feet-elevated hip thrust, this single-leg variation increases hip range of motion and shifts tension to your hamstrings. However, it's more challenging due to the increased stabilization demands. For best results, it's best to keep the weight light and focus on your form (the mind-muscle connection).

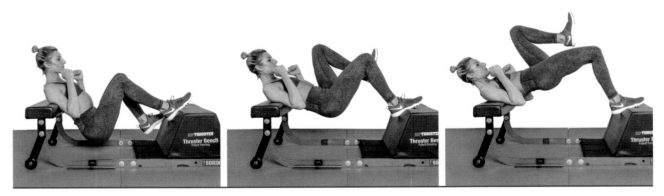

Set up in front of a bench or plyometric box with another box in front of you. The front edge of the box should be where your feet would normally rest on the ground. You can either place the centers of your feet on the edge of the box to work your glutes more or place both heels on top of the box with your toes pointed toward the ceiling to work your hamstrings more. Next, position your feet together along your center line, then lift one leg by pulling your knee toward your chest. Note: You can keep your leg bent, as shown, or straighten it—whichever you prefer. With the bottoms of your shoulder blades lined up with the front of the bench, drive your elbows back, push through your heel, and extend your hips. Squeeze your glute as you reach the top position, then lower yourself back into the bottom position with control.

LOADING AND EQUIPMENT VARIATIONS

You can create variations within the five hip thrust categories by adding a dumbbell, band, or barbell. Just as the technique variations provide a slightly different exercise stimulus, each piece of equipment adds a different element to the hip thrust technique.

While it's not required to have all of the accessories and equipment listed, it will make your hip thrusting experience better and—equally important—will give you options. For instance, you might hip thrust three days a week, but on one of those days you use a barbell and on the other two days you use a band or dumbbell.

KNEE-BANDED VARIATIONS

A resistance band (Glute Loop) is my favorite tool for increasing gluteal tension with the hip thrust. When you add a band either above or below your knees, you have to drive your knees outward to resist the inward pressure of the band, which increases glute activation—specifically upper glute activation.

KNEE-BANDED HIP THRUST

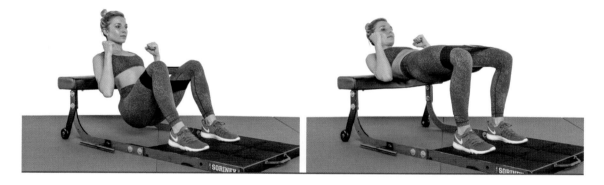

FEET-ELEVATED KNEE-BANDED HIP THRUST

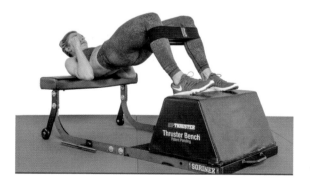

To perform the double-leg knee-banded bodyweight variations, simply position the band above or below your knees, assume a comfortable stance, and then drive your knees into the band. Maintaining outward knee pressure, extend your hips, squeezing your glutes as you reach full hip extension. As you lower your hips back to the ground, continue to drive your knees outward against the band.

SINGLE-LEG KNEE-BANDED HIP THRUST

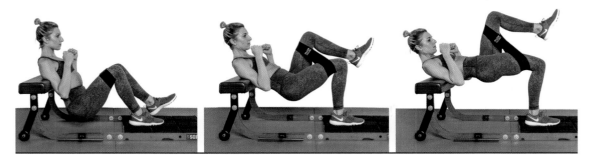

You can also use a band to add resistance to the single-leg hip thrust. To perform this variation, position the band above your knees, then raise one leg to put a stretch into the band and create resistance. The higher you raise your leg, the more stretch you put into the band and the more resistance you create. The key is to keep the same stretch in the band as you raise and lower your hips through a full range of motion; it's the separation of the band that causes the increased glute activity.

It's important to mention that you can use a band in combination with the dumbbell, barbell, and hip-banded variations. Sometimes when you add load to the hip thrust, you feel more tension in your quads and hamstrings. It's not that your glutes are not activating; they're actually activating to a higher degree—it's just that the extra load is causing the other muscles in your legs to work harder. If this happens, you can add a resistance band to increase glute activation when using the dumbbell, barbell, or hip band. The benefit of using the band with other forms of resistance is you don't have to use as much weight or perform as many reps to get a good pump and burn. However, if you're going for a one-rep max or want to increase the number of reps you can perform, then it's best not to use the band.

KNEE-BANDED DUMBBELL HIP THRUST

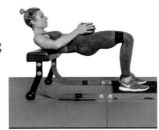

DUMBBELL VARIATIONS

The dumbbell should be the first stop for beginners when adding load to the hip thrust. Start light and work your way up. Once you feel comfortable with the movement, try the barbell variation. In general, I recommend the dumbbell hip thrust for higher reps and glute burnouts. To perform the dumbbell hip thrust variations correctly, be sure to center it directly over your hips and keep it positioned over your pelvis as you raise and lower your hips. You may need to roll the dumbbell forward slightly as you elevate your hips and roll it backward as you lower your hips to keep the weight centered over your pelvis. If you're performing a double-leg hip thrust, grip the outsides of the dumbbell. If you're performing a single-leg hip thrust, position the handle over your hip flexor on the same side as your grounded leg.

5

EXERCISES

331

DUMBBELL HIP THRUST

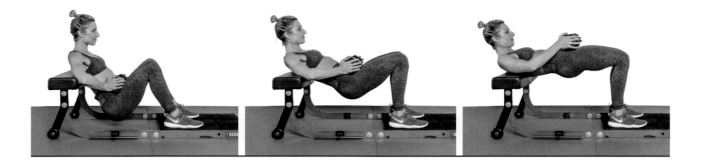

FEET-ELEVATED DUMBBELL HIP THRUST

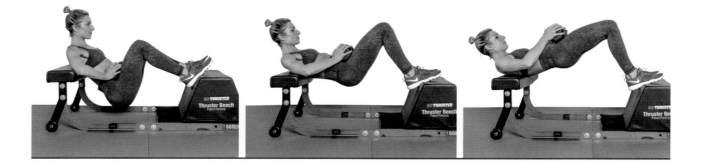

SINGLE-LEG DUMBBELL HIP THRUST

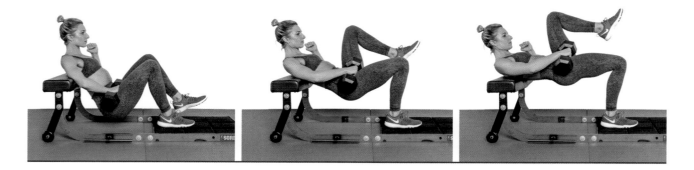

B-STANCE DUMBBELL HIP THRUST

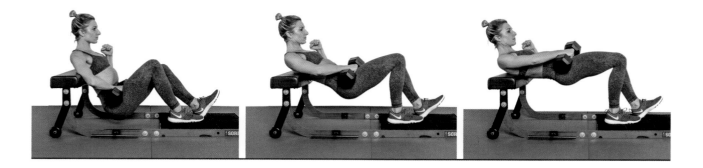

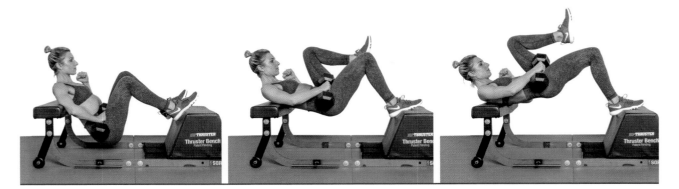

BARBELL VARIATIONS

The barbell hip thrust is a great way to challenge your strength and add load to the hip thrust movement. Depending on your height and the height of your bench, there are a few different setups. If you don't have the ideal setup—like a bench set to 14 inches or what feels right for your height—then getting the barbell into position can be a bit awkward at first. But once you get the hang of it—and assuming you have the right equipment—it's no more challenging than taking a barbell out of a rack to back squat.

Barbell Placement

The ideal bar position for the barbell hip thrust is just above your pubic bone in the lower abdominal region. I recommend a squat sponge, Hampton bar pad, or balance pad. If you don't have access to any of these, you can use a folded yoga mat, but it doesn't work as well. If the bar still hurts your hips, you may have to double up on the padding by using a combination of materials.

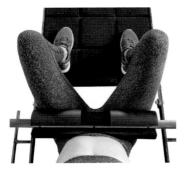

Another important aspect of barbell placement is to make sure that the pad is centered on the bar and that the bar is centered on your hips.

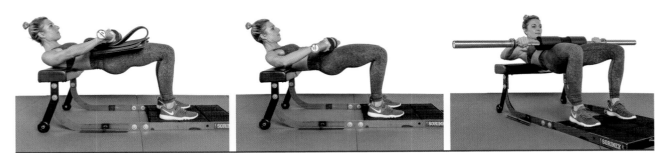

DOUBLE PAD:
SQUAT SPONGE + YOGA MAT

SINGLE PAD: THRUSTER
SPONGE OR SQUAT SPONGE

Over-Under Setup

The over-under setup is the most common way to get the barbell into position. The first step is to align the bottoms of your shoulder blades with the front of the bench. Then, from a seated position, you reach forward and roll the barbell over your legs until it is positioned across your hips. If the bench is too high, you can sit on a balance pad to put your back in the ideal position. However, elevating your hips might make it a struggle to roll the barbell over your thighs. To get the barbell into the correct position, pull the barbell onto two rubber mats (1.5-inch-thick mats are ideal in this scenario) or use specialized weight plates (Thruster Plates). If you don't have access to either mats or plates, you might need to lift the bar slightly and then slide your feet into the correct position. To exit, simply sit down and push the barbell over your legs.

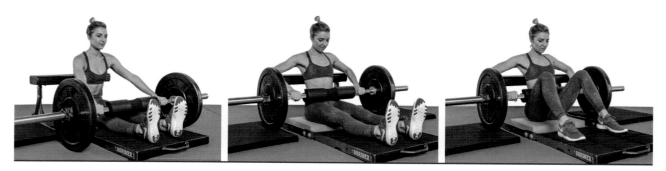

If you don't have specialized weight plates (Thruster Plates), which are rare in most commercial gyms, you can pull the barbell onto bumper plates or 1.5-inch-thick mats. Again, this is necessary for people who have big quads and need to elevate the bar so they can get into a good hip thrust position.

Down-Up Setup (Tall Bench Option 1)

Until the Hip Thruster machine becomes a staple in commercial gyms, a flat, stable utility bench is the most widely available option. The key—and this is crucial—is to secure the bench against a wall or power rack to prevent it from sliding around or tilting backward. Hip thrusting on a bench that is not secure is a recipe for disaster.

Although a lot of benches will work just fine, many are too tall for this exercise. If you can't find a bench of a suitable height, you may have to use your arms and bridge your hips to get your back into the right position before executing the lift.

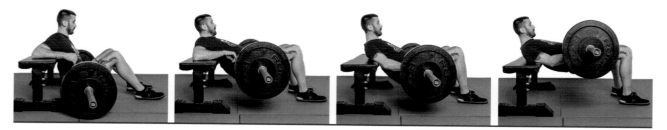

Roll the barbell over your legs and hips. Next, place your forearms over the bench and move your feet toward your butt. Pushing off the ground and driving your forearms into the bench, elevate your hips and slide your back into position with the lower shoulder blades resting against the bench. Keeping your hips elevated, form your grip on the bar. Make whatever adjustments necessary and you're ready to thrust.

Up-Down Setup (Tall Bench Option 2)

If the down-up setup doesn't feel right, the up-down setup is a great alternative, especially for beginners. As with the down-up setup, you have to secure the bench against a wall and keep the load light. And "light" is probably much lighter than when performing the over-under or down-up setup because you have to deadlift the weight and then slowly lower yourself into position with the bar balanced on your hips. This option is mainly for people who don't have access to light bumper plates and are not strong enough to use 45-pound weight plates. In short, this is how you get the bar into place if you're using small plates or just the bar. Otherwise, rolling it over your legs using the over-under setup is the best option.

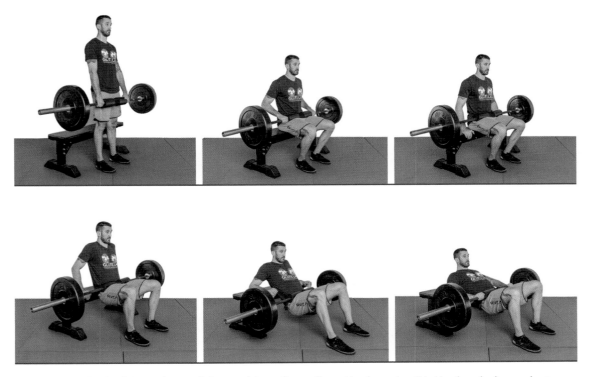

Deadlift the barbell into the upright position, then sit on the bench with the bar balanced on your hips. Place your hands on the bench. Using your arms and legs to support your weight and the barbell, slide your butt off the bench and lower yourself until the bottoms of your shoulder blades line up with the edge of the bench. Keeping your back in place, form your grip on the bar and adjust your feet to the appropriate distance. Now you're ready to thrust. When you're finished with your set, sit your butt to the ground and push the barbell over your legs.

Barbell Hip Thrust Execution

Once you have set up and have the barbell in place, form a wide grip on the bar, spacing your hands far enough apart that there is a slight bend in your elbows. Finding the right grip might take some adjusting. To lift the weight, you do several things at once: drive through your heels, push your knees outward, elevate your hips into the bar, and hinge at the bench while keeping a forward head position and moving mostly from the sternum down. Think about using your glutes to push the bar upward so that the movement occurs at your hips, not your spine. As you reach full hip extension, focus on squeezing your glutes maximally for one second. You may have to push on the bar to keep it centered over your hips. Keeping your back and elbows pinned against the bench, lower into the bottom position with control before beginning your next repetition.

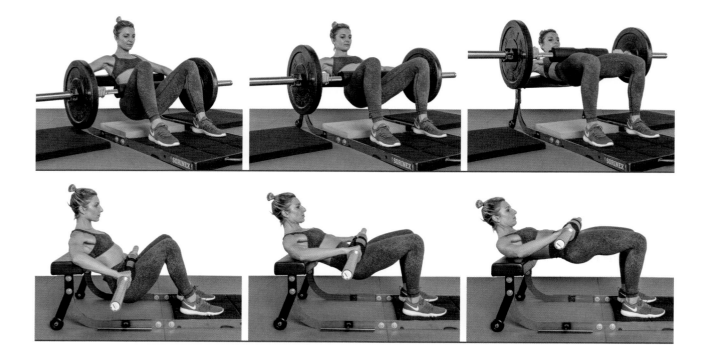

Barbell Plus Short Bands Hip Thrust

Adding short bands to the barbell emphasizes end-range hip extension, which is where most people are weak. Although the setup can be tricky, the lifting experience is amazing. The bar glides up and down, and you feel a ton of glute activation in the top position, more so than with just a barbell. There is an escalating loading curve, meaning that it is easier at the bottom and harder at the top as the bands stretch, so there is a gradual increase in load. Remember, variety is a great thing, especially when it comes to growing muscle.

To set up for this variation, hook a short band or mini-band around each end of the barbell. If you're using a Hip Thruster, you can hook the other ends of the bands around the pegs. If you're hip thrusting off a bench, you can hook the other ends around heavy dumbbells.

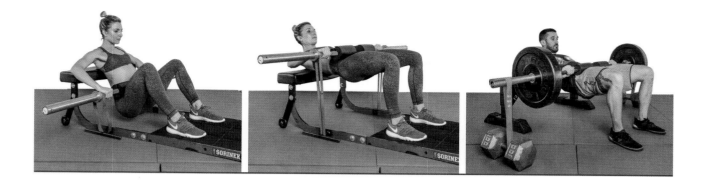

Single-Leg and B-Stance Barbell Hip Thrusts

You can also use a barbell when performing single-leg and B-stance hip thrusts. Again, these variations require more skill and coordination, so it's best to keep the weight light. As the weight increases, your form is likely to degrade, and you will have a harder time feeling your glutes work during the exercise. If you're performing the B-stance variation and you go too heavy, you will use your extended leg more to perform the movement, which defeats the purpose of the single-leg variation.

The setup and execution of the lift, however, are the same as for the double-leg barbell hip thrust variation. Sit on the ground with your legs straight, then either roll the barbell over your legs or use one of the other setup options. Next, make sure the pad is centered on the bar and that the bar is centered on your hips. From here, form a wide grip on the bar, slide your feet back, and assume your single-leg hip thrust stance—feet together and positioned along your center line. Keeping the barbell positioned over your hips, elevate one leg, then drive your heel into the ground as you raise your hips into the bar. If you're performing the B-stance variation, extend one leg just in front of your other leg and raise the toes of your extended leg off the ground. Again, you're not pushing off this leg, but rather using it for support and stability.

SINGLE-LEG BARBELL HIP THRUST

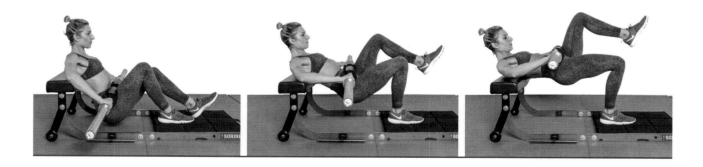

B-STANCE BARBELL HIP THRUST

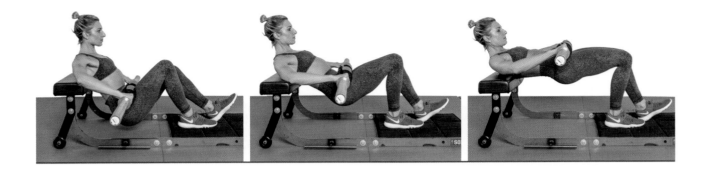

HIP-BANDED VARIATIONS

A hip band provides a unique stimulus to the hip thrust in that there is little resistance in the bottom position and maximum resistance in the top position. Conversely, a barbell weighs the same the whole way through. For example, if you're lifting 185 pounds, it's 185 pounds throughout the entire range of the movement. If you're using a band, on the other hand, it might be 15 pounds in the bottom position and 185 pounds in the top position. This means the exercise causes less muscle damage because there is not as much loading in the bottom position, where the muscles are stretched. However, you still get a ton of muscle tension and metabolic stress.

Hip-banded hip thrusts are great because they force you to focus on the lockout, which, as you know by now, is the zone in which you get the most glute activation. It's also the zone that people tend to skimp on, especially as the weight gets heavier. Just as people stop shy of parallel when they add load to the squat, people quit going as high in the hip thrust—stopping short of lockout—as the weight gets heavier. Adding a band helps prevent this tendency by strengthening the lockout position.

For the best results, keep the band positioned over your hips. You may need to hook your thumbs around the sides to keep the band in place and prevent it from flipping backward on you as you thrust.

You have a few different options for securing the band. If you have a Hip Thruster, the band attachments allow for an easy setup. You can also hook the bands around the feet of a power rack or Smith machine or around crisscrossed heavy dumbbells.

HIP-BANDED HIP THRUST

SINGLE-LEG HIP-BANDED HIP THRUST

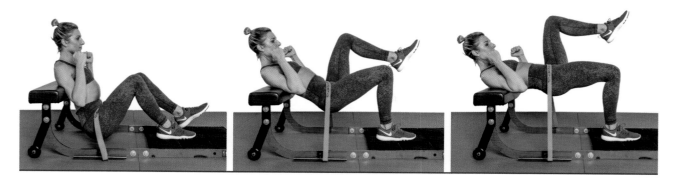

ARE MACHINES USEFUL FOR GLUTE DEVELOPMENT AND ATHLETICISM, OR SHOULD I STICK TO FREE WEIGHTS?

Free weights may have a slight edge, but machines are also great for glute development. In some scenarios, machines have the advantage. Personally, I use both in my training. If your goal is to build the nicest glutes possible, then you should implement all of the exercises that work for you—whether they involve machines or free weights.

We know that unstable surface training isn't ideal for building explosive power. Stability is important for maximizing prime mover muscle activation and force production. Machines are, in fact, the most stable options for resistance training, so they can be well suited for athleticism if they train athletic movement patterns. Think of lever machines that are plate loaded instead of single-joint machines like leg extension and leg curl machines. But free weights have some instability to them, which might be beneficial because it better coordinates the stabilizing muscles.

The bottom line is, you shouldn't avoid machines because you perceive them as being not functional. If you are prone to injury or you get beat up by the barbell counterparts, machines will give you better results over the long run because you're not getting injured. For instance, a lot of people prefer Smith machine hip thrusts over barbell hip thrusts because it's easier to get set up and they feel more stable when performing the movement. If you fall into this category, don't feel like you have to perform barbell hip thrusts. You can stick with Smith machine barbell hip thrusts and see great results.

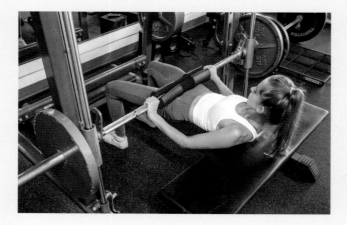

If you're using a vertical Smith machine, you can set up in either direction. If you're using an angled Smith machine like the one in the photo, on the other hand, you have to position the bench so that the bar moves away from your hips as you rise upward.

Glute Bridges

When glute bridge techniques first popped up on my radar back in the early 2000s, I didn't pay them much attention. They were great glute activation exercises, but I had to perform a ton of reps to get a good glute workout. This was when I thought you had to lift super heavy in order to grow muscle. For that reason, I mainly stuck to barbell glute bridges. But once I realized that performing high reps is just as effective for growing muscle as lifting heavy weights, I saw the glute bridge variations in a whole new light. I started using these techniques more and more in my programs with great results. Then I started experimenting and coming up with new variations, such as frog pumps, and realized even more benefits.

Now I consider glute bridge techniques foundational to my glute training system for several reasons. For starters, they are easy to perform. With your back flat on the ground and your knees bent, all you have to do is extend your hips. In this sense, the glute bridge serves as a foundation for the more challenging hip thrust variations. For example, I might start someone out with the bodyweight glute bridge and then, depending on their strength and form, increase the difficulty by introducing more challenging glute bridge variations. If they continue to show proficiency, I can progress them to the hip thrust variations, which are more challenging due to the increased hip range of motion (but are more effective for that same reason).

Second, glute bridges are excellent low-load activation exercises, meaning that they prep your glutes for more strenuous lifts like the back squat and deadlift. Just as trying to bake a cake without preheating the oven will produce poor results, jumping into a heavy lift without warming up the dominant muscle group can compromise performance. Utilizing glute bridge techniques is particularly important for people who have allowed their glutes to atrophy due to lack of activity. If your muscles are not activated throughout the course of the day—for example, you sit for half of the day and don't regularly perform glute-specific exercises—they tend to weaken. It's safe to assume that your glutes are not activating, causing them to atrophy. Performing glute activation techniques like the glute bridge not only improves your brain's ability to fire the glutes but also primes them to fire optimally when you perform more complex movements that involve the glutes.

Third, you can use glute bridges to build muscle by performing high repetitions or lifting heavy. Because there are more techniques that cater to high reps and only a few that can be done with significant weight (such as the barbell glute bridge and double dumbbell glute bridge), the majority of muscle-building glute bridge techniques are done with light weight and fall into the 20- to 60-rep range. But it's different for everyone. The key is to focus on quality over quantity.

If you're just starting out, 20 bodyweight glute bridges might be challenging for you. In that case, sticking with the bodyweight glute bridge and then progressing sequentially through the variations in this section is a great idea. Just remember, the goal is to feel your glutes working during the movement. If it's too easy and you're not focusing on glute activation, you might not feel your glutes working much. This is typical for people who can perform 50 bodyweight glute bridges without struggle. If you or someone you coach falls into this category, add resistance in the form of a band, dumbbell, or barbell and focus on control, not speed or load. If you go too fast or too heavy, your form will deteriorate. If you feel tension in your back, quads, or hamstrings, you may need to slow down the movement or change the setup or variation.

Lastly, the glute bridge techniques activate the glutes maximally without overloading the quads. For example, performing a hip thrust increases the range of motion by elevating your shoulders off the ground, but it also increases quad activation. This doesn't necessarily take away from the hip thrust; it just means that you have to activate your quads to a higher degree when performing the movement. Glute bridges, on the other hand, have less quad activation due to the angle of your body (going from level to inclined) and the lack of a bench to push into for stability. So, if you want to decrease quad activation—either because your quads are sore from a workout or you want to shift tension away from the area—glute bridges might be a better option for you.

Although I didn't give glute bridges the attention they deserved early on in my personal training career, I have spent a lot of time since developing new techniques and variations to grow and maximize their effectiveness, all of which you will learn about in this section. I use these variations in my own training and extensively with my clients.

GUIDELINES AND CUES

GLUTE BRIDGE

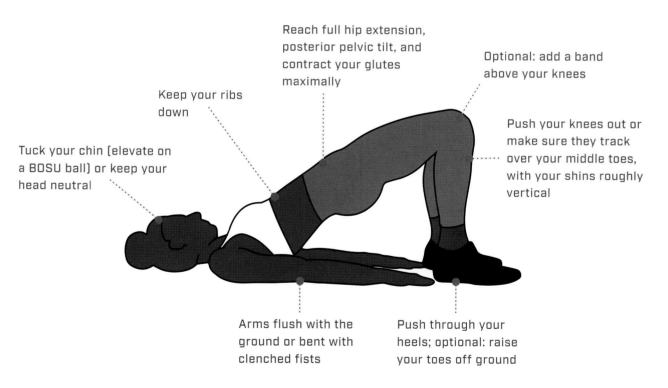

Reach full hip extension, posterior pelvic tilt, and contract your glutes maximally

Optional: add a band above your knees

Keep your ribs down

Push your knees out or make sure they track over your middle toes, with your shins roughly vertical

Tuck your chin (elevate on a BOSU ball) or keep your head neutral

Arms flush with the ground or bent with clenched fists

Push through your heels; optional: raise your toes off ground

FROG PUMP

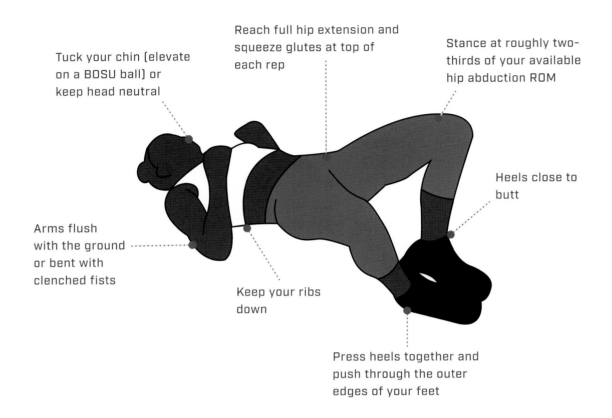

Tuck your chin (elevate on a BOSU ball) or keep head neutral

Reach full hip extension and squeeze glutes at top of each rep

Stance at roughly two-thirds of your available hip abduction ROM

Heels close to butt

Arms flush with the ground or bent with clenched fists

Keep your ribs down

Press heels together and push through the outer edges of your feet

In the following pages, I teach the universal principles of glute bridging, which you can apply to every glute bridge variation. In short, if you go through these steps, you'll have the foundation you need to master the glute bridge exercises.

SETUP: HIPS, SHOULDERS, AND KNEES IN LINE

Although you can make specific adjustments to your head, foot, and arm position, the top of the movement should look roughly the same for most people—that is, your hips, shoulders, and knees should be aligned. This helps you determine how far to position your feet from your body.

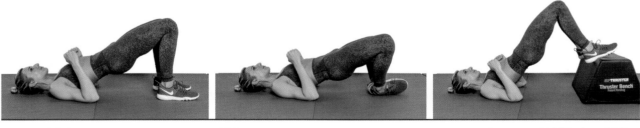

GLUTE BRIDGE   FROG PUMP   FEET-ELEVATED GLUTE BRIDGE

Notice that the hips, shoulders, and knees are in roughly a straight line. This is the optimal position for most people.

ASSUME A STANCE THAT ALLOWS FOR MAXIMUM GLUTE ACTIVATION

Simply getting into the top position is a great way to determine where to position your feet in relation to your hips. As with the hip thrust, if you feel the glute bridge too much in your quads, try sliding your feet away from your body. If you feel it too much in your hamstrings, try bringing your feet closer to your body.

You can also experiment with stance width and foot flare. Some prefer to assume a narrow stance and keep their feet straight, while others prefer a wider stance with their feet turned out. Your stance width and the degree to which you flare your feet depend largely on your hip anatomy and personal preference. Some of my clients prefer a very wide stance with their feet turned out, and a couple over the years have preferred a narrow stance with their feet turned slightly inward. Neither of these positions is ideal for me; I prefer a medium stance with my knees out, which brings me to my next point. You can choose to flare your knees out more or less depending on the above-mentioned variables. Play around with different stances and adopt the position that feels best to you.

DRIVE THROUGH YOUR HEELS

Once you determine your ideal stance, you can play around with driving through your heels with your feet flush with the ground or with your toes elevated. Many people like to keep their feet flush with the ground, but some feel the exercise more in their glutes when they elevate their toes. The common assumption is that keeping your feet flat shifts tension to your quads and lifting your toes shifts tension to your hamstrings, but this is not always the case. Many people feel it more in their hamstrings when they push through their toes. Nevertheless, if you feel a lot of tension in your quads when your feet are flat, try positioning just your heels on the ground— or on top of the box if you're performing the feet-elevated variation—and see if you get more glute activation.

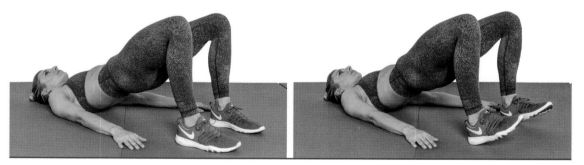

FEET-FLAT STANCE   TOES-ELEVATED STANCE

ARMS FLUSH WITH THE GROUND OR BENT WITH CLENCHED FISTS

Two arm positions are commonly used for glute bridge techniques. The first is to position your arms at your sides with your palms flush with the ground. The second is to bend your arms and clench your fists. Play around with both and choose the option that feels more comfortable.

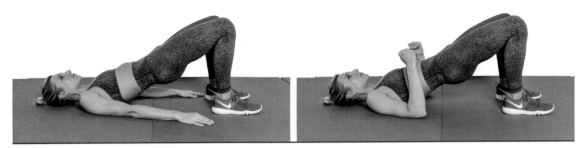

ARMS STRAIGHT   ARMS BENT

HEAD POSITION: CHIN TUCKED OR HEAD NEUTRAL

When it comes to head position, you can lay your head flat on the ground, raise it off the ground using your neck muscles, or prop it up on a BOSU ball, yoga block, or balance pad. Again, this is a matter of personal preference.

In my experience, elevating your head by tucking your chin has a couple of advantages. The first is that it keeps your ribcage down and helps prevent your back from overarching. So, if you feel tension in your back instead of your glutes, then the chin tuck is a good option. The second advantage is that it prevents you from sliding backward. Positioning the BOSU ball or whatever you're using against something sturdy like a wall will prevent you from sliding across the floor as you perform the movement, which can be a problem when glute bridging on a hard, slick surface. As your feet slide away from your body, tension shifts to your hamstrings. More than anything, it's annoying to have to adjust your stance constantly. Bridging on a yoga mat or with your shoulders pinned in place by a bench straddle or a partner's feet will also solve this problem.

4 OPTIONS TO PREVENT SLIDING

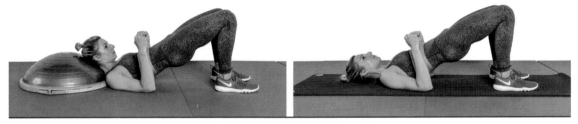

BOSU BALL   YOGA MAT

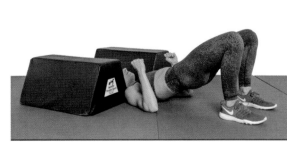

DUAL THRUSTER BENCH STRADDLE

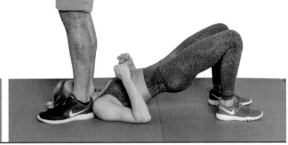

PARTNER-ASSISTED STRADDLE

FAULTS AND CORRECTIONS

FAULT: SPINAL HYPEREXTENSION

This fault occurs when you hyperextend through your lower back as you extend your hips into the top position. The problem is your back muscles will fire hard for no good reason. You want hip extension (and some hip hyperextension), not spinal hyperextension. If you overarch, you'll feel tension in your spinal erectors and not as much in your glutes. Not only will your spinal erectors fatigue, but you may unnecessarily develop hyperextension-related lower back pain.

The tendency is to extend your hips maximally, but if you're flexible, you can actually extend your hips past your knee and shoulder line. This extra extension doesn't always happen at your hips, though; it could be happening at your spine. Most people have around 10 degrees of hip hyperextension mobility when their knees are bent, but the range in humans is vast—from 0 to 50 degrees or more! Therefore, it's important to keep your spine relatively neutral during the bridge and make sure that any hyperextension comes at the hip joint, not the spine.

This fault is especially problematic if you're performing the barbell glute bridge variation because your torso is angled downward at the top of the movement and you have to use your hands to keep the bar from sliding down your body. If you're bridging a lot of weight—say, 315 pounds—and you hyperextend, you are putting an insane amount of stress not only on your lower back but also on your wrists, which are helping to support the barbell.

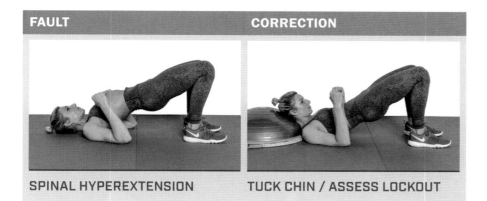

FAULT	CORRECTION
SPINAL HYPEREXTENSION	TUCK CHIN / ASSESS LOCKOUT

CORRECTION:
Tucking your chin by propping your head on a BOSU ball or other implement will help keep your ribcage down, preventing hyperextension through your lower back and keeping your spine stable. You should also assess your lockout position by filming yourself from the side. Make sure that the extension stops when your hips run out of range of motion. This is fairly easy to spot since your back will bow upward and your ribs will flare away from your pelvis.

FAULT: PUSHING THROUGH THE TOES

Positioning your feet too close to your body or pushing through the balls of your feet shifts tension away from your glutes and into your quads or even your hamstrings.

CORRECTION:
Try raising your toes off the ground (ankle dorsiflexion) and focus on driving through your heels.

GLUTE BRIDGE CATEGORIES

There are two ways to create variations for the glute bridge techniques. The first is to modify your position, which I outline in this section, and the second is based on the equipment you use, which I outline next.

All of the glute bridge positions are similar in that your back is on the ground and your legs stay bent. The variations are created by changing your stance—either double leg, single leg, B-stance, or frog pump—or by positioning your feet on the ground or an elevated surface.

As with the hip thrust, each variation has certain benefits and caters to certain goals and body types. Just as it's important to experiment with all of the techniques to see what works best for you, all of the variations are important because they provide slightly different stimuli. For example, if you're trying to maximize muscle tension, you might perform the bilateral barbell glute bridge, or perhaps you will find that the single-leg or frog pump variations fire your glutes more.

The exercise category you select might also be circumstantial. If you're traveling and you don't have access to weights, you might choose the single-leg glute bridge variation or elevate your feet off the ground.

For the best results, experiment with the different exercise categories with just your body weight.

GLUTE BRIDGE

With both feet positioned on the ground, this variation is stable, allowing you to lift heavier weight to create greater muscle tension. The added stability also means that it is easy to perform. In other words, it doesn't require a lot of coordination because you have multiple points of contact, making it a great regression for the hip thrust.

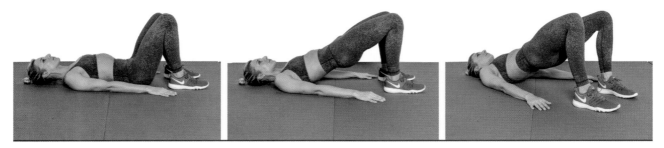

Lie on your back and assume a comfortable stance. Drive through your heels and raise your hips as high as you can without arching your lower back. Squeeze your glutes as you reach the top of the movement. Lower your hips all the way to the ground (or at least until the plates touch the ground) in order to maximize range of motion during the movement.

SINGLE-LEG GLUTE BRIDGE

This variation is typically more challenging because you have to stabilize your body with one leg. What's great about the unilateral variations is they can be done anywhere, and bodyweight resistance alone can provide an amazing glute workout.

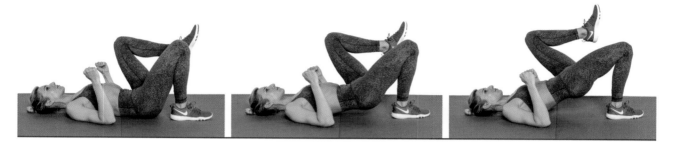

Lying on your back, get your arms into position—either down at your sides with your palms flat on the ground or bent with clenched fists, as shown here. Position your feet together along your center line and then elevate one leg. Note: You can bend or straighten your nonworking leg. Choose the option that gives you better mechanics and glute activation. Next, drive through your heel and raise your hips until they are roughly in line with your grounded knee and shoulders.

B-STANCE GLUTE BRIDGE

The B-stance variation is essentially a single-leg glute bridge, but instead of raising your leg off the floor, you keep your foot on the ground slightly in front of your opposite foot and elevate the toes. This provides a little more stability, making this variation slightly easier to perform. Think of the B-stance variation as a cross between the single- and double-leg glute bridge. You're not actively pushing off your extended leg, but rather using it to stay balanced. Imagine that 70 percent of your weight is on your working leg and 30 percent is on your other leg.

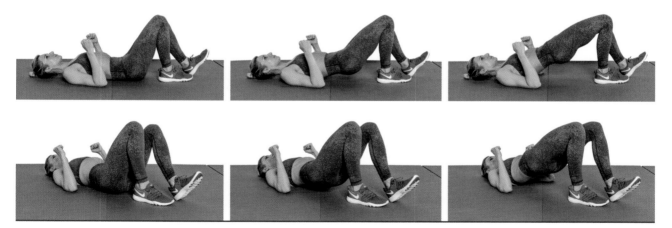

Lie on your back and assume a comfortable stance, positioning your feet together along your center line. Next, move one leg forward, placing your heel just in front of your other foot. To execute the movement, drive through the heel of the foot that is closer to your body and raise your hips. Remember that your extended leg is there only to provide balance and stability.

FROG PUMP

The frog pump variation is different from the others in that the bottoms of your feet are touching—specifically your heels. This provides a different stimulus, which for many people elicits more glute activation than the traditional glute bridge due to the inherent hip abduction and external rotation associated with setting the feet in the frog/butterfly position.

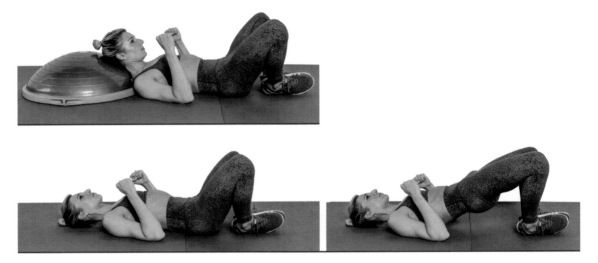

Lie on your back and position your heels together. When it comes to stance distance and knee angle, there's a sweet spot: you don't want your feet too far from your body or too close, and you don't want your knees touching the ground or straight up in the air. I recommend positioning your head on a BOSU ball to keep your chin tucked. To perform the movement, keep your knees and feet in the same position, drive through your heels (or the outsides of your heels), and elevate your hips, squeezing your glutes as you reach the top position.

GLUTE MARCH

The glute march is a cross between a double- and single-leg glute bridge. As you can see in the photos, you perform a double-leg glute bridge, hold the top position, and then raise one leg at a time. At Glute Lab we use the glute march as a warm-up drill and as a regression for the single-leg glute bridge (2 sets of 10 reps with each leg or 20 single-leg marches). Say you're good at double-leg glute bridges but not quite ready for the single-leg variation. In this situation, you can use the glute march to develop your single-leg glute bridge technique and coordination. You can also employ the two up, one down method by performing the double-leg glute bridge and then lowering with a single leg, switching legs after each bridge.

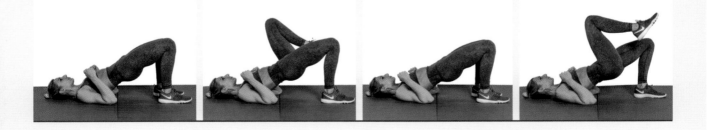

FEET-ELEVATED GLUTE BRIDGE

To perform this technique, position both feet (or both heels) on an elevated surface, such as a box, step, chair, or bench. This shifts tension to your hamstrings, increases hip range of motion, and decreases quad activation. If you want to shift tension away from your quads or increase tension in your hamstrings, this is a great variation to implement.

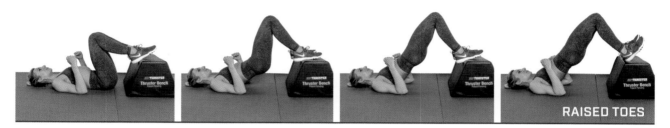

Lie on your back in front of a plyometric box or bench. You can either place the centers of your feet on the edge of the box or place both heels on top of the box with your toes pointed toward the ceiling. Slide backward or forward so that your knee angle will be at around 90 degrees at the top of the movement. Push your hips toward the ceiling, driving through your heels or the centers of your feet, until a straight line runs from the middle of your back through your knees. Think about squeezing your glutes for one second as you reach full hip extension.

SINGLE-LEG FOOT-ELEVATED GLUTE BRIDGE

If single-leg glute bridges from the ground are challenging for you, then these are slightly more difficult due to the increased range of motion and stabilization demands. Like double-leg feet-elevated glute bridges, this variation shifts tension from your quads to your hamstrings.

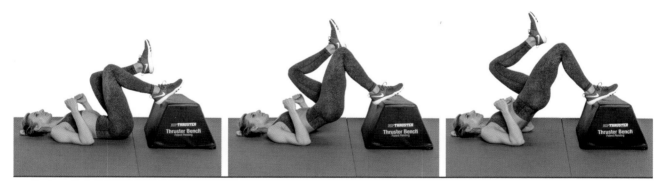

Lie on your back in front of a plyometric box or bench. You can either place the centers of your feet on the edge of the box or place both heels on top of the box with your toes pointed toward the ceiling. Slide backward or forward so that your knee angle is slightly greater than 90 degrees. With your feet together and positioned on your center line, elevate one leg. Note: You can keep your leg bent, as shown, or straighten it. Choose the option that gives you better mechanics and glute activation. Next, drive through your heel or the center of your foot and raise your hips until you reach full hip extension. Lower yourself with control.

LOADING AND EQUIPMENT VARIATIONS

The glute bridge equipment options are basically the same as the hip thrust equipment options. You can use a resistance band (Glute Loop or mini band), dumbbell, barbell, or hip band. The descriptions for the knee band, dumbbell, and barbell are strikingly similar to those for the hip thrust because the glute bridge and hip thrust share a similar movement pattern.

KNEE-BANDED VARIATIONS

Adding a resistance band to the glute bridge puts double duty on your glutes, meaning they have to work twice as hard to carry out the movement. With the band around your knees pulling your knees inward, you have to use your glutes not only to extend your hips but also to drive your knees out to resist the band, creating a deeper, quicker burn.

You can place the band above or below your knees. In my experience, positioning it above the knees fires the glutes more, but it's different for a lot of people. Like all variations, choose the one that gives you more glute activation. It's also important to note that the band position you prefer may differ from one glute exercise to the next, so keep this in mind when performing knee-banded squat or hip abduction variations.

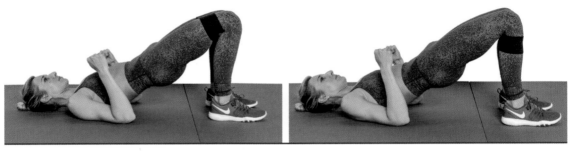

BAND ABOVE KNEES   BAND BELOW KNEES

Knee-Banded Bodyweight Variations

To perform the knee-banded variations, position the resistance band above or below your knees, assume a comfortable stance, and then drive your knees outward into the band. Maintaining outward knee tension, extend your hips, squeezing your glutes as you reach full hip extension. As you lower your hips to the ground, continue driving your knees outward against the band.

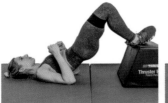 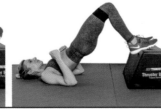 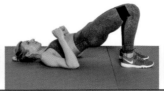 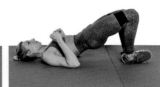

FEET-ELEVATED KNEE-BANDED FROG PUMP

FEET-ELEVATED KNEE-BANDED GLUTE BRIDGE

KNEE-BANDED GLUTE BRIDGE

KNEE-BANDED FROG PUMP

Single-Leg Knee-Banded Variations

You can also use a resistance band for single-leg variations. As shown in the photos, you use your top leg to control the resistance. In other words, the higher you raise your leg, the more stretch you put into the band. And the more stretch you put into the band, the harder you have to work to extend your hips. So, by simply separating your legs, you're adding resistance to the hip extension movement. The key is to keep the same stretch in the band as you raise and lower your hips through a full range of motion.

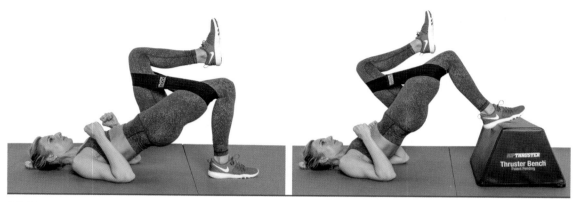

SINGLE-LEG KNEE-BANDED GLUTE BRIDGE   SINGLE-LEG FOOT-ELEVATED
KNEE-BANDED GLUTE BRIDGE

Knee-Banded Dumbbell/Barbell Variations

You can also use a band in combination with the dumbbell or barbell variations. The benefit of using a band with a dumbbell or barbell is that you don't have to use as much weight or perform as many reps to get a good pump and burn.

However, the resistance band works more upper glute max than lower glute max. Theoretically, it could limit the total number of reps you can do, which would provide an inferior stimulus to the lower glute max. A recent paper showed that it didn't negatively impact total rep performance, but I don't believe that to be the case across the board for all of the exercises. (The study looked at squats.)

Using a resistance band is always a great idea if you want to get more upper-glute activation, but if you're going for a barbell glute bridge one-rep max or you want to increase the number of reps you can do to tie in the lower glute max, then you may want to train without a band from time to time.

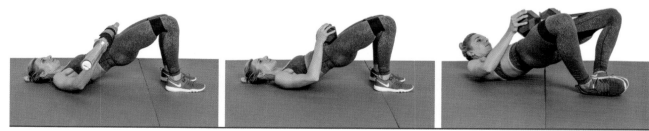

KNEE-BANDED BARBELL   KNEE-BANDED DUMBBELL   KNEE-BANDED DUMBBELL
GLUTE BRIDGE   GLUTE BRIDGE   FROG PUMP

DUMBBELL VARIATIONS

The best way to challenge your glutes while bridging is to add resistance to your hips. This can be done using a dumbbell or barbell. A dumbbell is smaller, lighter, and easier to handle, making it a good progression for the barbell glute bridge. For this reason, I typically start people out with the dumbbell glute bridge before progressing to the barbell variation. This is not to say that the dumbbell is reserved only for beginners, however. I use dumbbells all the time in my own training and with my clients. If the bodyweight glute bridge is too easy and you don't feel it in your glutes until you hit rep 50, then place a dumbbell on your hips and see how you feel.

The idea is to perform high reps but with more resistance. You should feel the burn at rep 20 (or sooner), and you should use enough weight that you can't do more than 60 reps. If you can do more than that, consider using a heavier weight or implementing frog pumps, which are the only technique we commonly do up to 100 reps of due to the short hip range of motion.

Single Dumbbell Variations

To perform the dumbbell glute bridge variations, position a dumbbell directly over your hips. You may have to tinker to find the right placement. With your hands gripping the outside of the dumbbell, drive through your heels, push your knees out, and extend your hips upward into the dumbbell. As you elevate your hips, use your hands to roll the dumbbell forward slightly, keeping it centered over your pelvis. Squeeze your glutes as you reach the top of the movement. As you lower your hips to the ground, keep the dumbbell positioned over your hips by rolling it backward slightly.

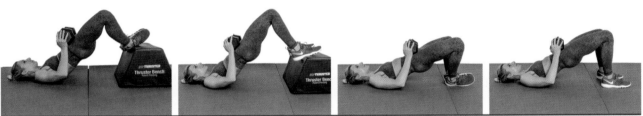

FEET-ELEVATED
DUMBBELL
FROG PUMP

FEET-ELEVATED
DUMBBELL
GLUTE BRIDGE

DUMBBELL
FROG PUMP

DUMBBELL
GLUTE BRIDGE

Double Dumbbell Variations

As an alternative, you can use two dumbbells when executing the glute bridge and frog pump. This is a great option if you don't have access to heavy dumbbells. For example, say you like to dumbbell glute bridge with 80 pounds, but the gym you're training at doesn't have heavy dumbbells (a common occurrence in most hotel fitness centers). In this scenario, you could use two 40-pound dumbbells.

Although the double dumbbell variations are great when you don't have access to heavy single dumbbells, using two dumbbells can present some problems: some people find it uncomfortable, it's hard to stabilize as you move, and it can be tricky to get the dumbbells in place, especially if they are heavy.

For this reason, I recommend the double dumbbell variations for the glute bridge and frog pump because you're not moving through a large hip range of motion, making it easier to hold the dumbbells in place as you execute the movement. As you can see in the photos, you want to position the dumbbells on each hip, over your hip flexor muscles.

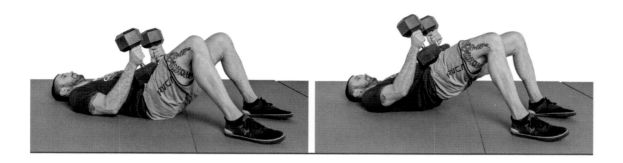

Single-Leg Dumbbell Variation

To perform the single-leg dumbbell variation, place your feet together along your center line and place a dumbbell on the same side as your grounded leg. Position the dumbbell over your right hip and bend your opposite arm with your fist clenched. With the dumbbell in place, elevate your opposite leg. You can bend your knee, as shown, or reach for the ceiling by straightening your leg. Using your arm to keep the dumbbell positioned over your hip, drive through your heel and extend your hip. Squeeze your glute as you reach the top position and dig your opposite elbow into the ground for stability.

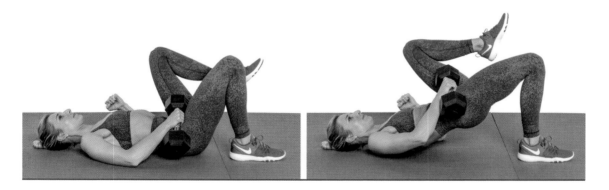

BARBELL VARIATIONS

People often ask me which is better for building big, strong glutes—the barbell glute bridge or the barbell hip thrust. As I've said, the hip thrust is the best booty builder due to the increased hip range of motion, but your body can take a heavier load (assuming equal practice with both lifts) with the barbell glute bridge, which might increase glute activation. For this reason, it's smart to incorporate both into your program. In other words, prioritize the hip thrust, and every once in a while, go from the floor and bridge as heavy as possible in the desired rep range.

To perform the barbell techniques safely, you will need to protect your pelvis with a folded towel, a yoga mat, or, even better, a squat sponge. Otherwise, the bar will dig into your hips, compromising your mechanics and limiting the amount of weight you can lift. Position the barbell directly over your hips, right above your pubic bone, but play around with the exact placement. There is a sweet spot for everyone, and it will take some tinkering to find yours. The key is that it doesn't hurt. If you position the barbell so that it is pushing straight down on your hips, which is ideal, but it is painful because it's digging into your pelvis, then the lesser of two evils is to adjust the barbell position or double up on the padding (for example, a yoga mat and a squat sponge). Remember, your glutes will not fire maximally if the exercise hurts.

Another useful barbell glute bridge tip is to use smaller 25-pound plates instead of the bigger 45-pound plates. The former are lower to the ground, meaning that there is no gap between your hips and the barbell at the bottom of the movement. If you're using bigger plates, there may be an inch or two where there is no connection, so you have to elevate your hips in order to make contact with the bar. Using smaller plates removes this gap, and you have tension on your hips from the beginning of the movement, which creates resistance through a larger range of motion.

Forming a grip on the barbell depends on torso and arm length, but the general rule is to secure a comfortable grip with a slight bend in your elbows, as shown in the photos.

Barbell Glute Bridge

To perform the barbell glute bridge, sit on the ground with your legs straight and then either roll the barbell over your legs or have a spotter place the bar over your hips. Make sure the bar pad is centered on the bar and that the bar is centered on your hips. From there, form a wide grip on the bar, spacing your hands far enough apart that there is a slight bend in your elbows. It might take some adjusting to find the right grip. Once you have your grip, slide your feet back and assume your glute bridge stance. Keeping the barbell positioned over your hips, drive your heels into the ground and thrust your hips into the bar. As you raise your hips, use your arms to push on the barbell to keep it in place. Squeeze your glutes as you reach full hip extension. As you lower your hips to the ground, continue pushing on the barbell with your arms to keep it centered over your hips.

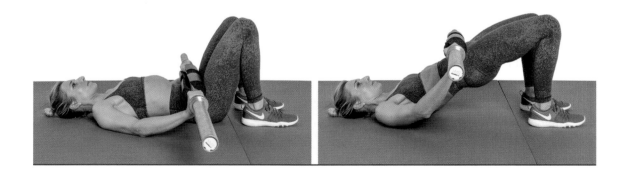

Frog Stance Barbell Glute Bridge

In general, the more skill and coordination an exercise requires, the less effective it is at activating the glutes. The single-leg barbell glute bridge has a considerable balance requirement, which makes it hard to perform rhythmic reps. For this reason, I don't perform or prescribe single-leg barbell glute bridges often. It still works the glutes, but not to the same degree as the other variations. Instead I prefer the frog stance barbell glute bridge. Keep the load light and stick with higher rep ranges. As with the barbell glute bridge, I recommend using smaller plates, 25 pounds or less, so you don't have to elevate your hips into the bar to close the gap.

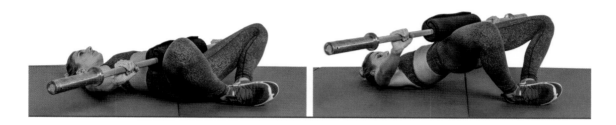

HIP-BANDED VARIATIONS

The hip-banded variations are used primarily for hip thrusts, but you can also perform them with the glute bridge and frog pump. As I discussed in the hip thrust section, the band provides a unique exercise stimulus because there is less resistance in the bottom position and more resistance in the top position. This is a great option if you want to avoid muscle soreness and emphasize metabolic stress. Like most banded variations, I typically reserve these for the end of a workout in the form of a high-repetition burnout.

To get the most out of hip-banded glute bridges, it's best to perform them on a bench. If you attempt hip-banded glute bridges from the ground, it's difficult to get enough tension in the band. But using a bench takes the slack out of the band, and there is tension right from the start.

The problem is getting set up. The execution of the exercise looks great on Instagram, but what you don't often see is how difficult it is to get into the right position.

To perform the technique properly, you need to position a bench in the middle of a power rack, hook the band around the legs of the bench, and then slide underneath the band, positioning it directly over your hips. Because there is tension on the band, the sliding underneath part is awkward. Once you get the band around your hips, you assume your glute bridge stance and elevate your hips into the band, squeezing your glutes as you reach full hip extension.

Lastly, there are a couple of tips that will improve your hip-banded glute bridge experience. The first is to have a training partner help you hook the band around your hips while you're on the bench. The second is to use a wide bench with stiff padding.

If you don't have access to a power rack, you can hook the band around heavy dumbbells. In this scenario, I recommend using a lighter band and going for higher reps. You can also elevate your feet on a short bench or box and perform feet-elevated glute bridges or frog pumps.

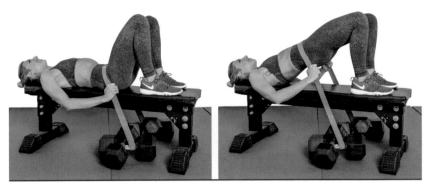

HIP-BANDED GLUTE BRIDGE OFF BENCH

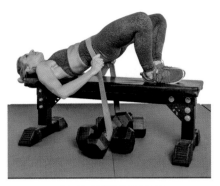

HIP-BANDED FROG PUMP
OFF BENCH

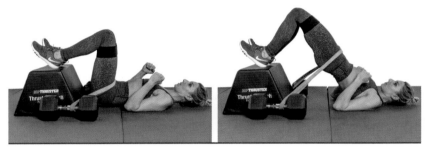

FEET-ELEVATED HIP-BANDED GLUTE BRIDGE

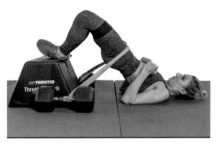

FEET-ELEVATED HIP-BANDED
FROG PUMP

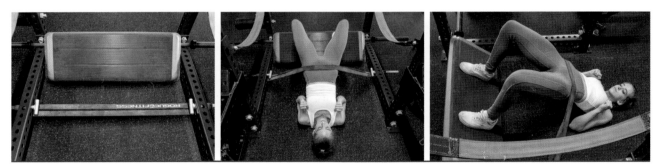

POWER RACK SETUP

3 Quadruped Hip Extensions

Quadruped hip extensions are among the easiest glute-building movements you can perform. But don't let the simplicity of these movements mislead you. When people think an exercise is "easy," they sometimes assume it's not functional, or if it targets only one muscle, they view it as a throwaway movement.

As I've said, you should learn how to perform compound movements, and compound movements should comprise the majority of training for most people. But—and this is important—you also need isolation exercises that target particular muscle groups. What if you want to target your glutes without working other muscles? Or suppose you have an imbalance and you need to target one side of your body. Or perhaps you want to warm up or activate your glutes for more strenuous exercise. These are all good reasons to have a glute isolation movement like the quadruped hip extension in your exercise toolbox.

Consider the techniques outlined in this section as precision glute exercises. About 10 studies have tested glute activation with the quadruped exercises, and in every one it was sky-high. This means the quadruped techniques are great for targeting the glutes but also can build muscle if a strong mind-muscle connection and additional load are utilized. Yet most strength trainers label these techniques as wimpy because they're easy, they primarily target the glutes, and they are not movements that can be loaded with a lot of resistance. I think the quadruped hip extension is a good glute-building exercise for these exact reasons, but you need to learn how to progress it, which I show you how to do in the following pages.

Although you can load the quadruped movement pattern using a band, dumbbell, or ankle weight, it is generally considered a bodyweight exercise. For this reason, the quadruped variations are typically used for warm-ups, for high-repetition burnouts, or to create a mind-muscle connection. Say I'm training a new client who is having trouble feeling their glutes during movement. I'll put the client in the quadruped position and have them perform some bodyweight repetitions. Right away, they feel their glutes activate. In addition to prepping the glutes for more strenuous exercise, the quadruped position creates a mind-glute connection, meaning that the client now knows what it's like to fully activate the glutes. This is useful for a couple of reasons.

First, there are people out there who don't know what it feels like to fully activate their glutes. Either they're sedentary and not using their glutes, or they're so used to relying on their quads and hamstrings that their mind-body connection with the glutes is poor. In both cases, the quadruped hip extension helps reestablish that connection and increases the brain's output to the glute muscles.

Second, you can carry that feeling over to other glute-dominant movements, like the glute bridge and hip thrust. Suppose you feel your quads and hamstrings working too much during the glute bridge and hip thrust. Simply performing a few bodyweight quadruped hip extensions will help you connect what you should be feeling when you activate your glutes while thrusting. You can then use this sensation as a guide while you adjust your position and experiment with glute bridge and hip thrust variations to find the ones that give you the most glute activation.

To summarize, the quadruped hip extension variations are easy to perform, are great for activating your glutes, and can be used to build muscle if you use load and go close to failure. I call them penalty-free volume exercises because they don't add much to total-body stress and don't beat up your joints; they just add volume to your glute workout without compromising your recovery.

Quadruped hip extensions, reverse hypers, cable kickbacks—all of these exercises fall into the penalty-free volume exercise category. In general, I program them in the middle of a workout at least once a week (for example, 3 sets of 20 reps) for variety. You're not trying to set PRs; you're just trying to get a good burn and glute pump.

GUIDELINES AND CUES

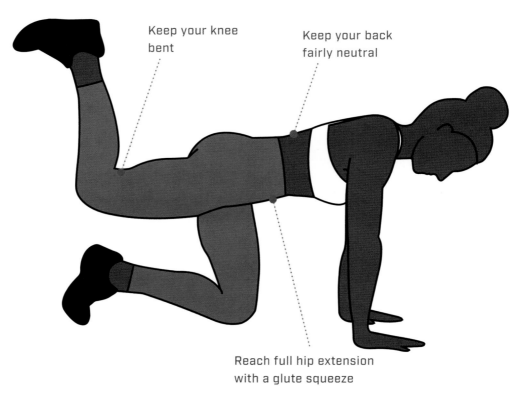

Keep your knee bent

Keep your back fairly neutral

Reach full hip extension with a glute squeeze

Because the quadruped movement is so easy to perform, there are only a few things you need to consider when executing the movement.

SETUP: POSITION KNEES UNDER HIPS AND HANDS UNDER SHOULDERS

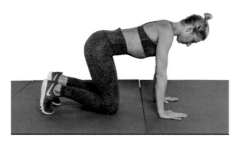

Getting into position is as simple as getting on your hands and knees. Typically, I don't have to cue people to get into the right position. They tend to put their hands and feet in the right place or automatically adopt a position that feels right. If you're looking for a place to start, position your knees directly underneath your hips and place your hands a little bit out in front of you, slightly outside shoulder width. Perform a couple of reps and adjust your position to ensure pain-free movement and maximal glute activation.

SPINAL MECHANICS: STAY IN THE NEUTRAL ZONE

Although the goal is to keep your spine neutral and your back flat, you might arch a little bit as you kick your leg rearward. This is perfectly acceptable for most people. If you don't feel any lower back pain or too much tension in your erectors, then a little bit of arching or anterior pelvic tilt at the top of the movement is fine. As with all exercises, the idea is to keep your back in your neutral zone.

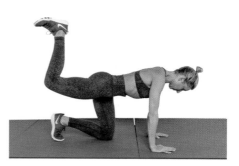

KNEE PATH

To perform the quadruped hip extension, you kick your leg back while keeping your knee bent at roughly a 90-degree angle. Some people flare the knee outward a little bit, and that's fine. This is primarily due to hip anatomy and the action of the glute engaging and acting on the hip. I don't try to correct it, because a little abduction and external rotation might be ideal.

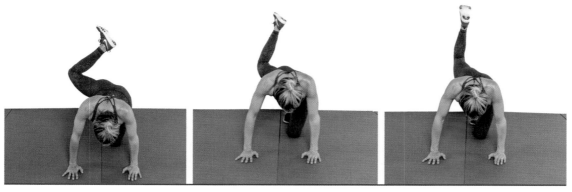

KNEE FLARE   SLIGHT KNEE FLARE   STRAIGHT BACK

FAULTS AND CORRECTIONS

FAULT: SPINAL HYPEREXTENSION

Not a lot can go wrong with the quadruped hip extension movement. The only thing that tends to happen is an overly dramatic arch. There is an acceptable range, which I've already covered; anything outside this range puts unnecessary stress and tension on the lower back.

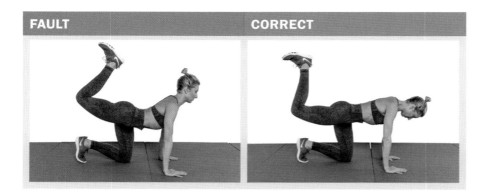

FAULT   CORRECT

CORRECTION 1:

The easiest way to correct this fault is to lower the elevation of your leg—that is, don't kick your leg as high. Hyperextension happens at end range, so simply lowering your leg slightly and remaining conscientious of your position should keep you in an acceptable range. Make sure to squeeze the glute of your working leg and consciously strive to keep your back fairly flat.

CORRECTION 2:

If you're having trouble staying in the neutral zone, try positioning a bench underneath your belly. The bench will help cue you not to hyperextend as you kick your leg back.

QUADRUPED HIP EXTENSION VARIATIONS

There are two ways to perform the quadruped hip extension exercise: from the ground in a horizontal position or on a bench in an incline position.

HORIZONTAL QUADRUPED HIP EXTENSIONS

Horizontal refers to the position of your body in relation to the ground. Variations performed from this position are easy and can be done anywhere. They're more difficult to load with weight, but you can add resistance in the form of a band, making them great for warm-ups and burnouts.

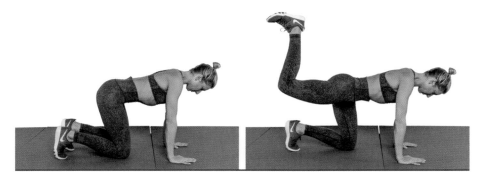

Get down on all fours with your knees underneath your hips and your hands underneath your shoulders. Keeping your back flat and your knee bent, extend your leg backward until you reach full hip extension. Make sure to squeeze your glute and hold the finish position for a one-second pause. Your leg may abduct (move laterally) as you reach full hip extension, which is fine. Again, the degree of abduction largely depends on your hip anatomy.

Knee-Banded Quadruped Hip Extension

Adding a band is a great way to add resistance to the quadruped hip extension. Like all banded variations, it's easier at the bottom and gets increasingly more difficult as you reach the top of the movement.

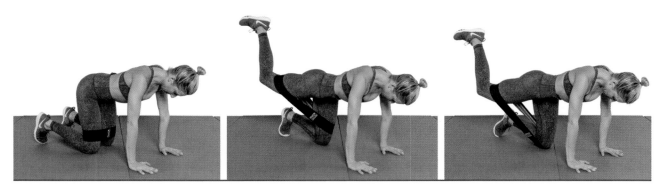

Position the band above your knees, then kick your leg back while keeping your knee bent or slightly bent. If you want to increase the resistance or you're using a larger or more elastic band, pin the loop underneath your grounded knee (opposite your working leg), as shown in the third photo above.

Ankle Weight Variation

An ankle weight is another great way to load the quadruped hip extension. You can position the weight around your ankle or just below your knee.

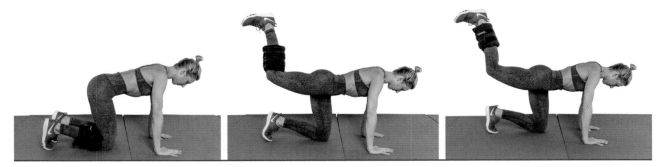

Wrap the weight just below your knee or around your ankle and set up in the quadruped position. Then simply kick your leg back—keeping your knee bent—and squeeze your glute as you reach full hip extension.

Reverse Hyper (Pendulum Quadruped Hip Extension Variation)

My absolute favorite way to load the quadruped hip extension is to kick upward into the pendulum underneath a reverse hyper machine—specifically an old-school reverse hyper from Westside. Though the ankle weight and knee-banded variations are good, you can add only so much weight, and the resistance can feel awkward. Not the case with the reverse hyper. In addition to providing constant, smooth tension throughout the entire range of motion, you have the option to load the movement with significant weight. However, I recommend keeping the load light, sticking with moderate to high reps, and focusing on the mind-muscle connection.

The problem is, very few gyms have a reverse hyper. To make matters even more challenging, you're not using the machine as it's intended, which makes the setup a bit tricky. Instead of pulling the weight with your feet as you would when performing an actual reverse hyper on top of the unit, you position yourself underneath the machine and kick upward into the weight sleeve, as shown in the photos on the following page.

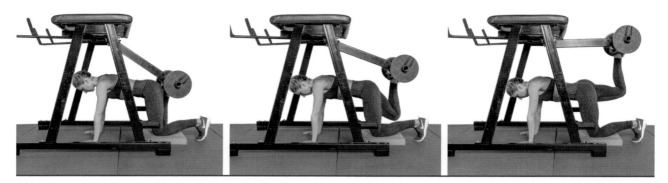

Get into the quadruped position underneath the reverse hyper machine with your butt positioned below the pendulum. I recommend kneeling on a yoga mat or balance pad to protect your knees. From here, position the arch of your foot over the weight sleeve, kick your foot back slightly—pushing the pendulum rearward—and then scoot back until the shin of your extended leg is roughly vertical. Now push straight upward by driving your foot skyward into the weight sleeve. Make sure to control the downward motion so you don't slam your knee on the ground. (This is why it's important not to go too heavy.)

INCLINE QUADRUPED HIP EXTENSION

For this variation, you need an incline bench. The bench changes the angle of your body to make it more conducive to utilizing resistance. You can perform incline variations using a dumbbell or ankle weight behind your knee. If you try to perform the dumbbell variation from the ground, the weight will roll down your hamstrings, compromising the mechanics of the exercise.

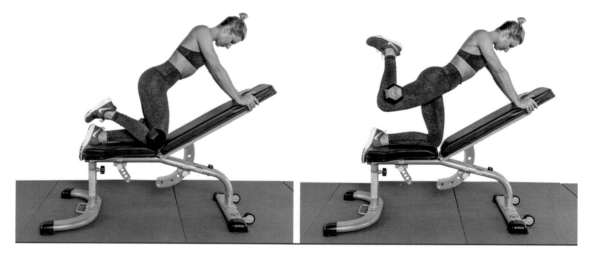

Set the bench at about a 45-degree incline. Place one knee on the seat and allow the other knee to hang off to the side. Position a dumbbell in the crook of your knee and keep your leg bent. To stabilize your upper body, grip the outsides of the bench. Keeping your back flat, bring your free knee past your hip (this is the start position), then extend your leg backward until you reach full hip extension. Again, squeeze your glutes and hold the finish position for at least one second. Perform controlled, rhythmic reps to prevent the dumbbell from sloshing around.

4 Upright Hip Thrusts

If I polled all of my clients and asked them to name their favorite glute exercise, I would get a wide range of answers. Some love the conventional hip thrust. Others prefer an upright hip thrust variation like a pull-through), which is interesting because I don't like this movement at all—not because it is a bad glute builder but because I much prefer the conventional hip thrust.

The fitness industry tends to value standing exercises more than supine exercises, so this might be why many people gravitate toward the upright hip thrust. Although the upright hip thrust is an effective glute exercise, it has limitations. You can't use a lot of load, and the more resistance you add—like a thick band, or a big stack for the cable upright hip thrust—the more balance it requires. And the more balance and stabilization an exercise requires, the less glute activation you get.

At the end of the day, we all need variety, and mixing things up is exactly what the upright hip thrust techniques are good for. If they happen to be your favorite glute exercises, I recommend performing them once or twice a week near the beginning or middle of your workouts.

GUIDELINES AND CUES

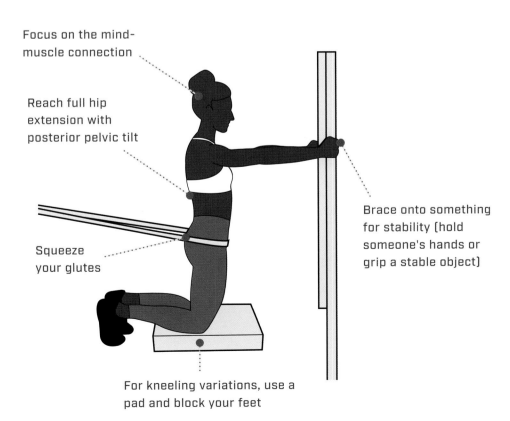

Focus on the mind-muscle connection

Reach full hip extension with posterior pelvic tilt

Squeeze your glutes

Brace onto something for stability (hold someone's hands or grip a stable object)

For kneeling variations, use a pad and block your feet

The upright hip thrust encompasses two exercise categories: the hip-belted upright hip thrust, which employs a dip belt, and the pull-through, which utilizes a triceps rope. These exercises share the same movement pattern and work the same muscles but are performed slightly differently based on the equipment being used.

In the photos, you'll notice that the pull-through requires you to pull the weight between your legs, while the hip-belted upright hip thrust centers the resistance around your hips, which more closely resembles a conventional hip thrust. You can perform both exercises either standing or kneeling.

Whether you're performing the hip-belted variation or the pull-through, standing or kneeling, the general setup and execution are the same.

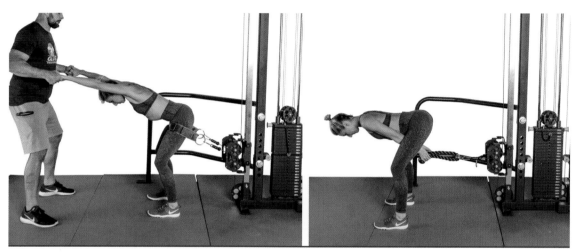

STANDING UPRIGHT HIP THRUST   STANDING PULL-THROUGH

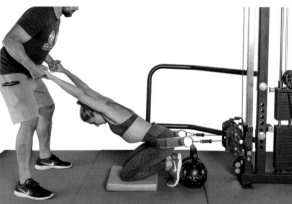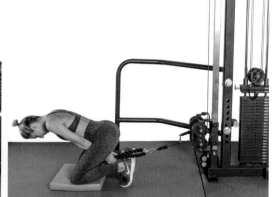

KNEELING UPRIGHT HIP THRUST   KNEELING PULL-THROUGH

START POSITION: SIT YOUR HIPS BACK

Before you experiment with the two variations, it's important to understand how to get your body in the right position. As you can see in the photos, you want to tilt your torso forward and—this is key—sit your hips back. Think of it like performing a Romanian deadlift (see pages 514 and 515). Your back is flat, your hips are back, there is a slight bend in your knees, and your shins are nearly vertical (if performing the standing variation). When you do it correctly, you will feel tension in your hips and a stretch in your glutes. This is your start position.

FOCUS ON THE MIND-MUSCLE CONNECTION

As I said, the upright hip thrust techniques are not very stable, meaning that the more resistance you apply to the movement, the less balance you have. More specifically, the resistance at your hips pulls your body backward. To counter the backward pull and remain balanced, you have to tilt your torso and lean forward.

But again, the more resistance or weight you try to pull, the harder it is to stay balanced, which can reduce glute activation. So, rather than try to pull a lot of weight or progressively overload the resistance, it's better to keep the weight light and focus on the mind-muscle connection—that is, concentrate on getting the most glute contraction possible with every rep.

Like every exercise, there is a happy medium when it comes to loading. If you don't have enough resistance, you will have to perform a ton of reps to get meaningful work done, and if there is too much resistance, you will be off-balance and won't get as much glute activation. It's worth repeating when it comes to the upright hip thrust: don't focus on lifting as much weight as possible, but rather on getting as much tension in your glutes as you can with each rep. This will take some tinkering. Experiment with different stances (kneeling and standing), equipment variations (band, cable, triceps rope, and dip belt), and load and rep schemes, and stick with the variation and resistance level that work your glutes the most.

GRIP SOMETHING STABLE (HIP-BELTED UPRIGHT HIP THRUST VARIATIONS)

If you're performing the hip-belted upright hip thrust, you can add more resistance because your hands are free, which allows you to grab onto a friend's hands, a squat rack, or any kind of stable pole. Upright hip thrusts are much more effective when you have something to grab onto for stability, so I hope you can figure something out. But even performing them in this manner has its drawbacks. Often, lifters use their arms to pull their hips forward instead of using the power of their glutes. In short, use your grip to maintain balance, not to extend your hips and move your torso into an upright position.

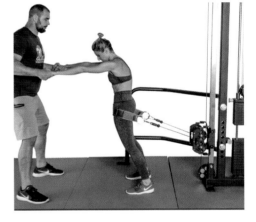

BLOCK AND SPREAD YOUR KNEES (KNEELING UPRIGHT HIP THRUST VARIATION)

For the kneeling upright hip thrust, you need padding for your knees and two heavy kettlebells to block your feet. The padding protects your knees from the hard ground while the kettlebells prevent you from sliding backward as you extend your hips.

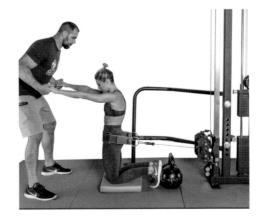

FAULTS AND CORRECTIONS

If you've read some of the other technique sections, you know that you can avoid many faults simply by following the guidelines and cues and technique descriptions. This is especially true with the upright hip thrust variations, which are challenging to set up and execute.

The most common faults associated with the upright hip thrust are positioning the cable or belt too high or too low, using too much resistance, and tilting the torso forward without sitting the hips back. To prevent and correct these faults, experiment to find the best cable or belt height, keep the load light, and focus on sitting your hips back as you tilt your torso forward.

BANDED VARIATIONS

Using a band is another way to add resistance to the upright hip thrust. It's not quite as effective as the cable column because there is little resistance in the start position, so you don't work your glutes as much while they are stretched. You get tension only as you reach full hip extension. You can play around with the band tension and the distance from the object used to tether the band, but you're limited by logistics unless you have a partner. For example, say you do these in a power rack; you put the bands around the rear uprights and have to hold onto the front uprights for support. But in this situation, you can't adjust your position or move farther away to increase the tension because you're holding onto the front uprights. So it's better to hold a partner's hands. Pause reps are ideal with these—anywhere from 1 to 3 seconds. You can perform both kneeling and standing variations.

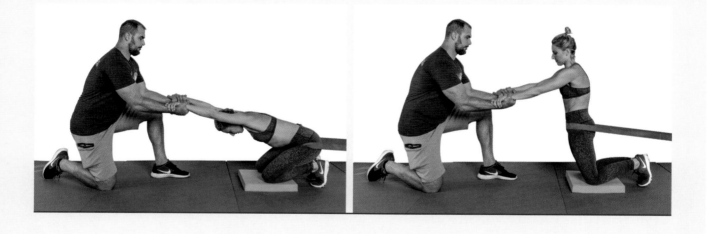

UPRIGHT HIP THRUST VARIATIONS

You can perform upright hip thrusts using a dip belt (hip-belted upright hip thrust) or a rope handle (pull-through). And you can perform them from either a standing or a kneeling position.

STANDING UPRIGHT HIP THRUST

This variation is the easiest to perform because you're standing, which for many people is a more stable position than kneeling. If you can, hold onto a squat rack or someone's hands as you extend your hips for added balance and stability. If you don't have a partner or something to grab, keep the weight light and focus on higher reps. You also need to lean forward considerably to counter the backward pull on your hips, especially as you get stronger and use heavier weight. A dip or strongman belt (we use the Spud, Inc. brand in the Glute Lab gym) is ideal for performing this variation. If you're using a dip belt, remember to remove the long chain attached to the belt so that you can stay close to the cable column.

Some people prefer to place a band or loop around their knees and try to spread their legs as they sit back to increase glute tension during this variation. If you don't feel your glutes working and you feel it more in your hamstrings, experiment with the kneeling variation.

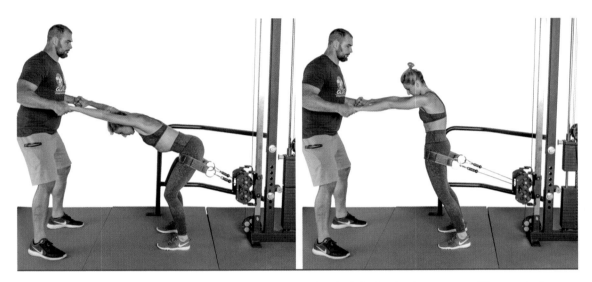

Position the band or cable just below or at roughly hip height in the bottom position and place a dip belt or strongman belt around your waist, centered over your hips (just above your pubic bone). From there, walk forward and get into your start position. Once the belt is in place, create tension so that there is resistance in the start position. With your feet positioned at roughly shoulder width, your hips back, and your torso tilted forward (the heavier you go, the more you'll lean), drive your hips into the belt, squeezing your glutes as you reach full hip extension. If you're holding onto something—say, your trainer's hands or a squat rack—use your grip only to maintain balance and counteract the need to lean forward excessively. In short, don't use your arms to pull yourself into the upright position. Once you reach full hip extension, think about dropping your torso downward and exaggerate sitting your hips back. I tell my clients to "shut the door with your butt" to emphasize sitting the hips back, which seems to click.

KNEELING UPRIGHT HIP THRUST

The kneeling upright hip thrust is the closest approximation of the conventional barbell hip thrust. It's a little more challenging to set up, but a lot of people prefer it to the standing variation because they feel their glutes working more. Like supine hip thrusts, your knees stay bent, which reduces the role of your hamstrings and shifts more tension to your glutes. The problem is that you need additional equipment. To protect your knees, you need adequate padding (two balance pads are ideal), and some people need to block their feet to keep them from sliding backward. To accomplish this, position two heavy kettlebells behind your feet. If you don't have a belt or training partner, then it might be better to perform the pull-through variations with a triceps rope.

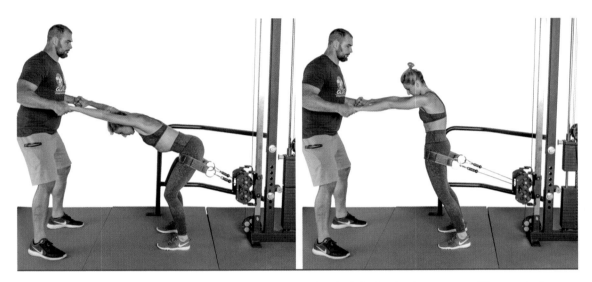

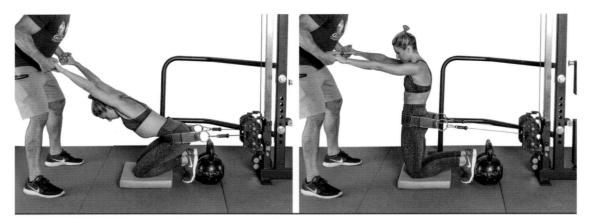

Find adequate padding for your knees, such as two balance pads or ab mats or a folded yoga mat. Position the belt around your hips, just above your pubic bone. Walk forward, putting tension into the cable. Kneel on the pads, then sit your hips back. You can spread your knees and position your heels together in a frog/butterfly-like setup—many people feel it more in their glutes when they adopt this stance. With your torso forward and your back flat, drive your hips into the belt using the power of your glutes to extend your hips forward. As your torso rises, use your hands to maintain balance or, if you don't have something to grip, shift your weight forward slightly to achieve an upright position. Your upper back will round as you extend your hips if you tilt your pelvis properly.

STANDING PULL-THROUGH

For the standing pull-through variation, you grip a triceps rope or band between your legs. You can use other handles, but a triceps rope is best due to the knobs at the end, which help keep your grip in place. This is a great option if you don't have a partner or the proper equipment to perform the hip-belted upright hip thrust variation or if you simply prefer the pull-through.

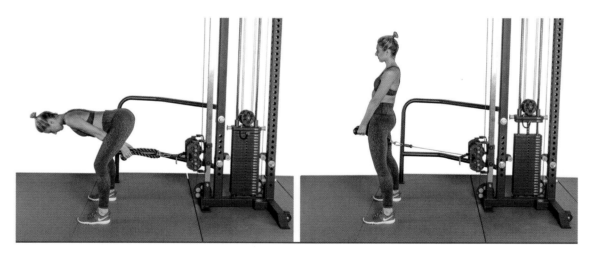

Form your grip on the triceps rope so that your thumbs are forward and your palms are facing each other. Take slack out of the cable by walking forward and assume your stance—most people position their feet at about shoulder width. Next, sit your hips back and allow your torso to tilt forward. Try to keep your back flat and your shins vertical. From here, drive your hips forward into your forearms, squeezing your glutes as you extend your hips. Don't try to pull on the rope with your arms; instead, use the power of your glutes to push your hips forward. To maximize glute tension, it's helpful to keep your chin tucked or head down and posterior pelvic tilt as you stand upright, just as you do at the top of a back extension or hip thrust.

KNEELING PULL-THROUGH

The kneeling pull-through is a great option if you feel the standing pull-through too much in your hamstrings. Like the hip-belted kneeling upright hip thrust counterpart, your knees stay bent, which shortens your hamstrings, putting even more emphasis on your glutes. But the setup is a bit awkward in that you need padding for your knees and something to block your feet to keep them from sliding backward, and the cable path is odd and seems too close to the ground.

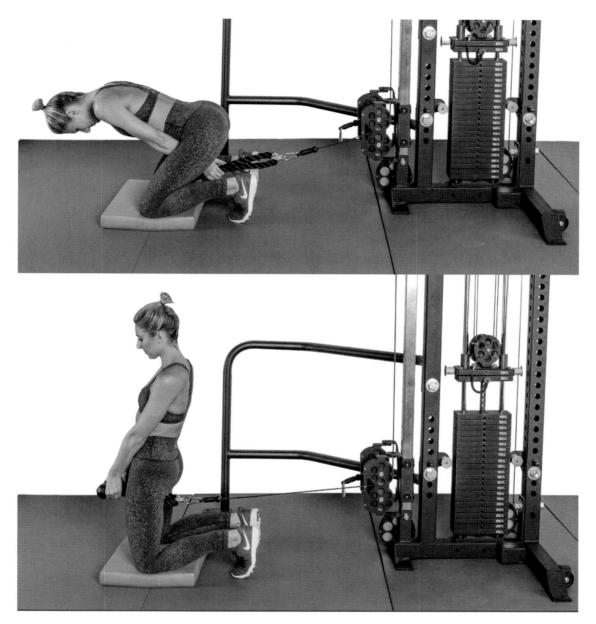

As with the hip-belted kneeling variation, position two balance pads or ab mats or a folded yoga mat (or some other form of padding) where you plan to place your knees. With adequate tension in the cable, form your grip on the triceps rope so that your thumbs are forward and your palms are facing each other. Next, kneel on the pads, sit your hips back, tilt your torso forward, and allow the cable to pull your hands underneath your hips. Using the power of your glutes, drive your hips into your forearms and extend your hips—keeping your chin tucked with a slight posterior pelvic tilt. Your upper back will round as you extend your hips if you tilt your pelvis properly. Again, don't pull on the rope; just keep your grip tight and your back flat as you drive your hips forward.

Kickbacks

The kickback movement pattern includes standing and kneeling kickbacks, both of which fall into the category of penalty-free glute exercises, meaning that they don't make you too sore or put a ton of stress on your body. These techniques are great in a variety of scenarios.

The first is establishing or strengthening the mind-muscle connection with the glutes, which I often refer to as the mind-glute connection. Kickbacks are helpful for warming up the hips with low reps (not to failure) at the beginning of a workout to prime the glutes for the main lift.

The second way to use kickbacks is in the middle of a workout. As with the other glute accessory exercises—like the quadruped and pull-through variations—kickback techniques are great for adding a little extra volume to your workout. For example, I might program 3 sets of 20 reps between a hip thrust or deadlift (primary lift) and an abduction exercise (workout finisher) to get in a little extra glute work.

GUIDELINES AND CUES

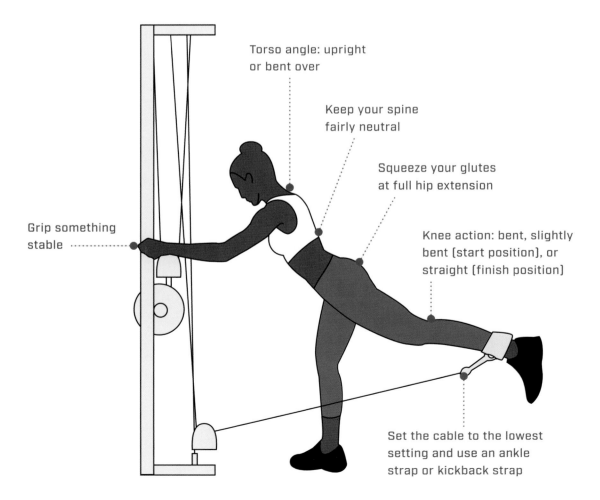

Torso angle: upright or bent over

Keep your spine fairly neutral

Squeeze your glutes at full hip extension

Grip something stable

Knee action: bent, slightly bent (start position), or straight (finish position)

Set the cable to the lowest setting and use an ankle strap or kickback strap

Kickbacks are fairly easy to perform, and you can do them from a standing or quadruped position. Below are four general guidelines that will help you get the most out of the kickback exercise variations.

SPINAL MECHANICS: KEEP YOUR SPINE IN THE NEUTRAL ZONE

When you kick your leg back, the tendency is to arch your back slightly. A little bit of hyperextension is fine and is probably necessary to maximize glute activation. However, too much extension will shift tension to your lower back, which is not ideal. There's a zone in which you get good glute activation with just a little bit of back and hamstring activation. In short, avoid excessively hyperextending your hips and keep the weight and repetitions manageable. As you get closer to muscle fatigue and failure, make sure you're still feeling tension in your glutes. The moment you start to feel the exercise more in your back and hamstrings than in your glutes, stop the set.

GRIP SOMETHING STABLE (STANDING VARIATIONS)

When performing the standing variations, it's ideal to grip something stable. As you kick your leg back, you have to shift your weight onto your grounded leg to maintain balance. In addition to making the movement more stable and easier to perform, gripping something allows you to counterbalance your weight and maintain a vertical torso. This creates a smooth line of action when kicking your leg back and translates to higher glute activation and better movement mechanics. Most cable machines have arms for this exact purpose. If you're performing a banded variation, position a tall box or set up in front of a wall, pole, or squat rack so you have something to grip.

KNEE ACTION: KNEE CAN STAY SLIGHTLY BENT OR STRAIGHT

There's a lot of variance with the kickback exercises; it depends on the person and the equipment being used. For example, your leg can stay slightly bent or straight—neither is wrong. Or you can move from bent knee to extended knee as you kick rearward. You may find that you prefer one option over all others, or you might apply different knee action to particular variations.

GLUTE SQUEEZE: FOCUS ON THE MIND-MUSCLE CONNECTION

Squeezing your glutes for one second is a universal rule that you can apply to all glute-dominant movements, but it's especially important to emphasize with the kickback. As with the quadruped hip extension, you get only a brief spike in glute activation. Squeezing your glutes for one second increases time under tension and helps you make a mind-glute connection. Moreover, you can't load the kickback with a lot of weight without compromising your form, so keep the resistance light and perform very slow, controlled reps.

FAULTS AND CORRECTIONS

FAULT: SPINAL HYPEREXTENSION (TOO MUCH BACK AND HAMSTRINGS)

When it comes to performing kickback exercises—especially the standing variations—it's important to take time to set up properly. Most faults occur when people rush into the movement without trying to dial in the nuances first. The most common fault is to hyperextend through the lumbar spine, which increases the tension in your back and hamstrings. If you feel the exercise working your back and hamstrings, there are a couple of easy solutions.

CORRECTION 1:
Reduce the resistance or number of repetitions and focus on squeezing your glutes as you reach full hip extension.

CORRECTION 2:
Don't kick back as far or as high. Stop when you feel your hips running out of range of motion and resist the temptation to swing your leg higher, which typically leads to lower-back arching and anterior pelvic tilt.

KICKBACK CATEGORIES

You can perform the kickback techniques while standing or on all fours (quadruped position).

STANDING KICKBACKS

For the standing variations, you can keep your leg straight, slightly bent, or bent in the start position, and you can either remain upright or tilt your torso forward. Remaining upright represents a true horizontal vector or line of resistance, while tilting creates a blended vector, or angled line of resistance relative to the body, which creates higher levels of glute activation at the bottom of the movement when you are in a flexed position. Experiment with both and choose the one that works your glutes more. In my experience, the bent-over and knee-bent-to-extended variations tend to be the most popular and effective because you can get more tension through a broader range of motion. *Note:* You can add load in the form of a cable, band, or ankle weight for moderate to high reps.

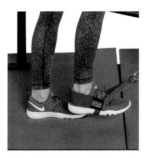

Cable Kickback

A cable column is my favorite tool for performing standing kickbacks because there is constant tension on the glutes. To perform cable kickbacks correctly, the line of resistance should be low on your ankle, over your Achilles tendon. Position the cable at the bottom and use an ankle strap. You can hack the exercise by using a handle, but it might change your mechanics. At Glute Lab, we also use a special strap designed for kickbacks that wraps around your shoe.

KNEE FLEXED

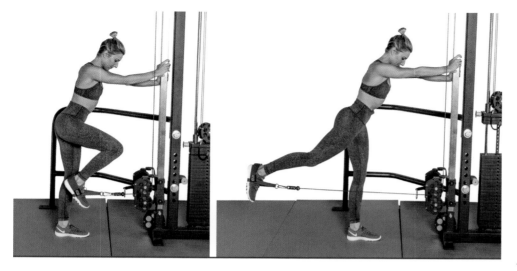

KNEE STRAIGHT/SLIGHTLY BENT

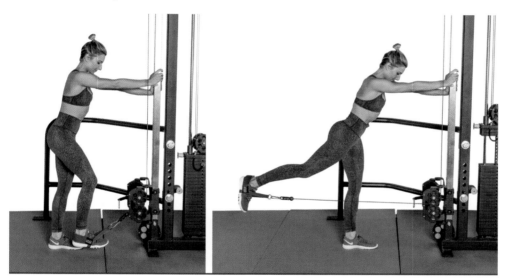

BENT OVER

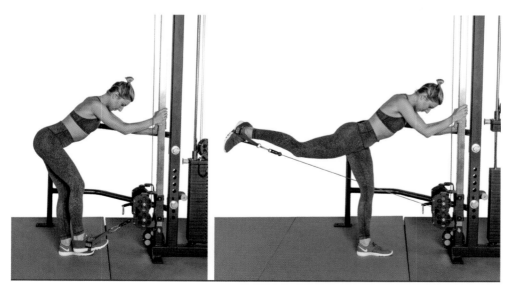

Set the cable column so it lines up with your instep. (This is the lowest setting on most cable column machines.) If the cable column doesn't drop low enough for you, stand on a step. Hook the strap around your Achilles tendon. With your strapped foot lifted off the ground and positioned just in front of your body, lean forward slightly (or remain upright) and hold onto something stable to maintain balance. Kick your leg straight back, squeezing your glutes as you extend your leg and reach full hip extension. Note: You can start with your leg bent, semi-straight, or straight, but you always straighten or almost straighten your leg as you reach full hip extension.

Ankle Weight Kickback

If you don't have a set of ankle weights at home, I highly recommend that you buy a pair. Ankle weights are inexpensive, and using one is the easiest way to load the kickback movement.

When using an ankle weight for standing kickbacks, it's important to control the kickback throughout the entire range of the movement. In other words, you don't want to use the momentum created by the weight to transition into your next rep. Instead, pause at the start and finish position to keep steady tension on your glutes. It's also important to bend over and support your weight on a tall box or bench or brace against a wall. This increases the range of motion and provides stability and balance.

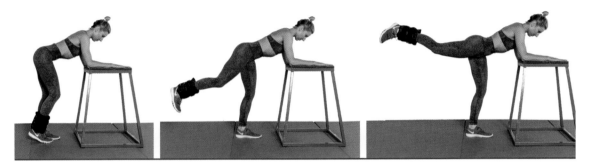

With the ankle weight in place, lean forward (or remain upright) and place your hands against a wall or box or grip something stable, like a plyometric box. Next, shift your weight onto your grounded leg and lift your opposite foot off the floor slightly. Kick your leg straight back while maintaining a fairly neutral spine and squeeze your glute as you reach full hip extension.

Banded Kickback

Like the ankle weight variation, the banded variation is a great option if you don't have access to a cable column. The key is to keep the resistance light so you don't struggle to kick your leg back. You can also use a resistance band (Glute Loop) and wrap it just above your knees. Banded kickbacks are great for performing sets with high reps of 20 to 30. Like all of the kickback variations, focus on squeezing your glute for one second at end range.

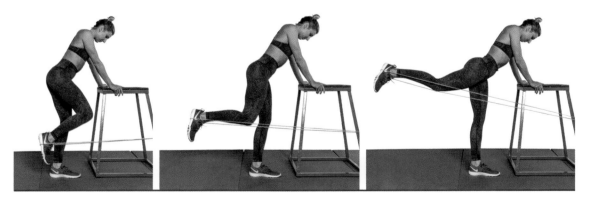

Set the band to the height of your instep or just below your knee and grip something stable, like a plyometric box. For straight-leg kickbacks, hook the band around the back of your ankle. For bent-leg kickbacks (see photos above), hook the band around the arch of your foot. Then simply kick your leg back until you reach full hip extension.

QUADRUPED KICKBACKS

The quadruped kickback variations share the same technique cues and loading options as the standing variations. They work your glutes in a similar way but are easier to perform because you have multiple points of contact, making these movements a lot more stable compared to their standing counterparts.

Bird Dog

The bird dog is a classic glute exercise that ties in the shoulders and upper back. The bodyweight bird dog is generally used as a warm-up exercise, while the loaded (ankle weight and dumbbell) variation is an accessory glute exercise that you can place in the middle or at the end of your workout. In most situations, 2 sets of 10 to 15 reps on each leg/side is a good starting point.

BODYWEIGHT BIRD DOG

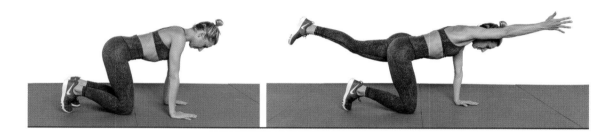

ANKLE WEIGHT + DUMBBELL BIRD DOG

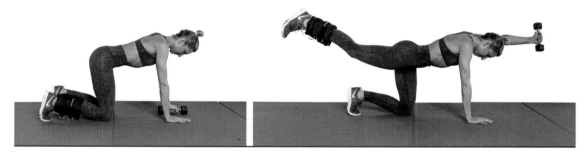

As with the quadruped hip extension exercises, the idea is to position your hands underneath your shoulders and your knees underneath your hips. From here, kick your leg straight back while simultaneously extending your opposite arm. Raising your opposite arm not only counterbalances your weight but also ties in the muscles of your core and upper back. Try to keep your back flat and get your extended leg and arm horizontal. A little bit of hip hyperextension is okay as long as you feel tension in your glutes and not in your lower back.

Cable Quadruped Kickback

Again, a cable column provides constant resistance and allows for a smooth and rhythmic tempo; it's the most effective way to load the kickback movement pattern.

KNEE BENT

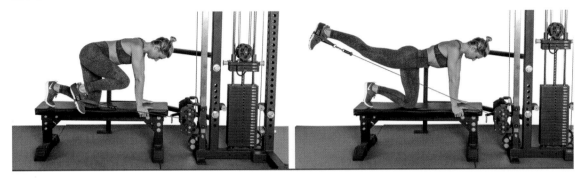

KNEE STRAIGHT/SLIGHTLY BENT

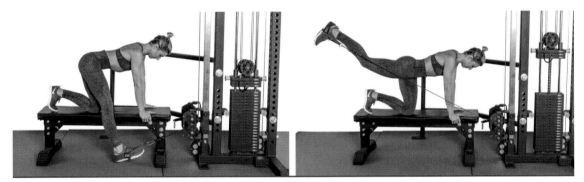

Place a bench in front of the cable column, position the cable to the lowest setting, and—depending on the strap you are using—hook it either around your Achilles tendon or the heel/arch of your foot. You can start with your leg bent, semi-straight, or straight. If your leg is bent, kick it straight back as you extend your knee. If your leg is straight, slowly swing it back until you reach full hip extension. (You might feel your hamstrings working more with this variation.) With both variations, squeeze your glute as you reach full hip extension.

Banded Quadruped Kickback

Like the standing banded kickback, the banded quadruped kickback is a good option when you don't have access to a cable column. To reiterate, keep the resistance light to ensure a smooth tempo.

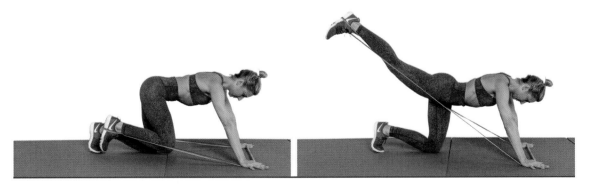

Get down on all fours, then hook a small band around the arch of your foot and around both of your thumbs. Pinning the band in place underneath your palms, kick your leg back at an upward angle.

Ankle Weight Quadruped Kickback

The ankle weight quadruped kickback is similar to its standing counterpart in that you pause at the start and finish position. Pausing not only helps you maintain constant tension but also keeps you from swinging your leg and using the momentum of the weight to transition into your next rep.

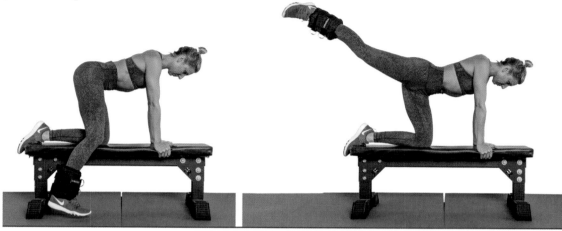

Wrap the ankle weight around your ankle/lower shin and set up in the quadruped position on a bench. Allow your weighted leg to hang off the bench, then slowly kick your leg back—keeping your knee slightly bent or straight—and squeeze your glute as you reach full hip extension.

Pendulum Quadruped Kickback

A final kickback option is to perform donkey kicks underneath a reverse hyper. Yes, reverse hypers are rare in gyms, but if you have access to one, give this variation a try. It is similar to the pendulum quadruped hip extension, with two slight differences. First, you shift your body forward relative to the machine. Second, you kick back instead of up, which allows you to extend your knee instead of keeping it bent.

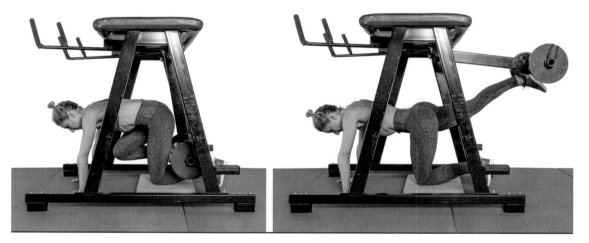

Get into the quadruped position underneath the reverse hyper. I recommend kneeling on a yoga mat, balance pad, or some other kind of thick padding to protect your knees. From here, position the arch of your foot against the loading pin and scoot back so that your working leg is in full hip and knee flexion. Then simply kick your leg straight back and slightly upward.

Hip Abduction Exercises

When it comes to glute growth, I'd venture to guess that about 85 percent of your gains will come from hip extension exercises, like hip thrusts, glute bridges, squats, deadlifts, and lunges. The other 15 percent will come from abduction exercises, which primarily target the upper glutes.

I noticed this early on in the bikini competitors I train. The ones who did abduction exercises had much better upper-glute development than their peers. So, if you want to build a glute shelf (where your upper glutes protrude from your hips), you should emphasize and perform the exercises outlined in this section.

The best part is, hip abduction exercises don't typically beat you up or leave you overly sore, so you can get in a good workout without taxing your body. The one drawback is that they are difficult to load. You typically have to use a band, cable, or hip abduction machine to create resistance. For this reason, I often place abduction work at the end of a training session and focus on high repetitions and burnouts—performing several exercises in sequence to fatigue the region.

GUIDELINES AND CUES

To get the most out of the hip abduction exercises, you need to keep a few guidelines in mind.

REST BETWEEN LEGS/SIDES

There are some hip abduction movements that seem to be performed with one leg, such as fire hydrants, side-lying hip abduction, and cable standing hip abduction, but they actually hit both legs at the same time. For these variations, it's important to take a break after working one side. For example, if you perform the fire hydrant exercise, do one leg and then rest for 30 to 60 seconds before working the other leg. Think about it like this: one leg is moving dynamically while the other leg is stabilizing. Both glutes get worked during abduction movements, even though it appears that one leg is doing all of the work. So, if you start working the other side immediately, you might not be able to match the reps on the opposite side due to fatigue. This is the case with all single-leg hip abduction exercises.

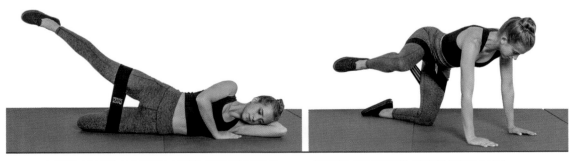

SIDE-LYING KNEE-BANDED HIP ABDUCTION   KNEE-BANDED FIRE HYDRANT

ROLL ONTO THE LATERAL EDGES OF YOUR FEET

This guideline applies to transverse plane exercises like the hip hinge knee-banded hip abduction and seated banded hip abduction variations. Rolling onto the lateral (outside) edges of your feet helps you get a little more range of motion and increases the tension. In fact, it's important not to skimp on range of motion and focus on maximizing the full potential of the movement with every rep, regardless of the variation you're performing.

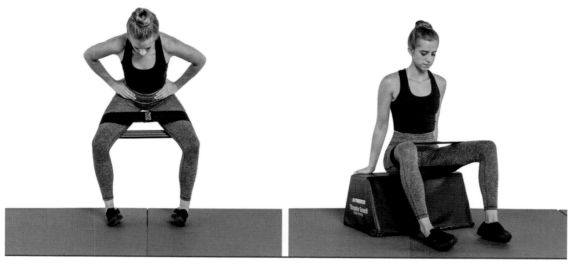

HIP HINGE KNEE-BANDED HIP ABDUCTION   SEATED KNEE-BANDED HIP ABDUCTION

KEEP YOUR FEET STRAIGHT OR TURNED SLIGHTLY INWARD AND PUSH YOUR KNEES OUT

This guideline applies to frontal plane hip abduction exercises, specifically lateral band walks. To get the most from these exercises, position your feet straight or turn them slightly inward, drive your knees outward into the band, and keep your hips even. In other words, don't allow your knees to cave inward, turn your feet out excessively, or laterally tilt your pelvis as you step. With lateral band walks, you want to push laterally through your grounded leg rather than reach laterally with your stepping leg. This cue may seem unimportant, but your intention affects glute activation and mechanics.

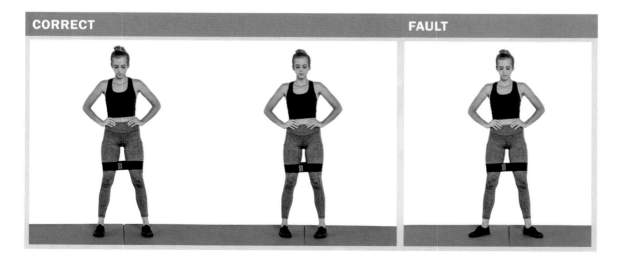

CORRECT   FAULT

FAULTS AND CORRECTIONS

Hip abduction exercises are fairly easy to perform due to the limited range of motion and light resistance. However, the characteristics that make these techniques easy can create complacency when it comes to form, which is never a good thing. For instance, people sometimes perform lateral band walks or seated hip abduction exercises with poor posture or skimp on range of motion as the set goes on.

To prevent these faults, think about looking athletic, maintaining good posture (avoid slouching), and express the full range of motion with every repetition. You also want to remain symmetrical. A lot of people point their feet in different directions, which indicates that they are not taking the exercises seriously. Just because the techniques are easy doesn't mean that you should let your form go by the wayside or brush them off as worthless. Keep the right intent and don't devalue the movement just because you're not moving a ton of weight.

HIP ABDUCTION CATEGORIES

The hip abduction exercises can be divided into two categories based on body position: frontal plane and transverse plane. The former encompasses abduction exercises with the hips extended, and the latter encompasses abduction exercises with the hips flexed.

FRONTAL PLANE HIP ABDUCTION

As you may recall from Chapter 10, frontal plane hip abduction captures lateral movement in either a standing or a side-lying position. This includes lateral band walks, standing hip abduction, and side-lying hip abduction variations. Remember, these are the only exercises that completely target the upper gluteus maximus and gluteus medius. If you're interested in developing your upper glutes, employ exercises from this category in the form of high reps and burnouts at the ends of your workouts.

Lateral Band Walk

To perform the lateral band walk, position a resistance band or mini band above or below your knees. You can either walk along one side or move back and forth, switching between legs. The key is to drive laterally into the ground with your grounded leg while stepping with your opposite leg.

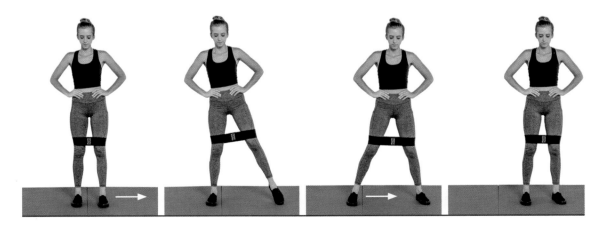

X-Band Walk

You can also wrap a long band around the outsides of your feet and under the arches of your feet and then cross it in front of your body. This is called an X-band walk, and it's a great variation to throw in from time to time for variety.

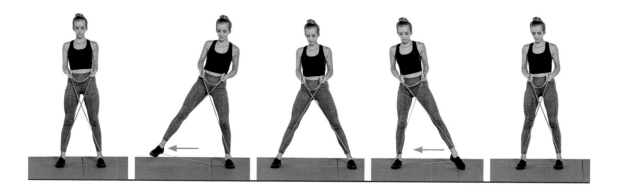

Monster Walk

The monster walk is similar to the lateral band walk, but instead of walking from side to side, you walk forward or backward. You can either walk straight forward and back with a wide stance—keeping constant tension on the band—or zigzag back and forth in a diagonal fashion.

WIDE-STANCE MONSTER WALK

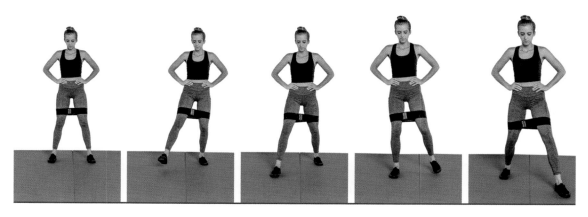

ZIGZAG MONSTER WALK

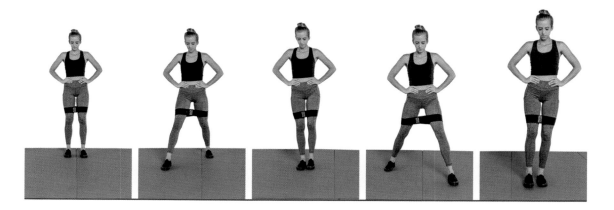

Standing Hip Abduction

Although you can perform standing hip abduction out in the open, it's better to grip a pole or balance against a wall for stability. To perform the movement, shift your weight onto one leg, internally rotate your opposite leg, bring it slightly in front of or next to your grounded foot, and then abduct or move your leg laterally out to the side until you reach the end of your range.

You can perform bodyweight standing hip abductions or add resistance in the form of a band, ankle weight, weight plate, or cable column. The cable column is the smoothest and my favorite variation. To execute this variation, set the cable height to the lowest setting and wrap the strap around your ankle. Again, you will need to hold onto the legs or center column to maintain balance. The ankle weight variation is great because it utilizes constant resistance on the hips and can be done anywhere. However, you have to keep the weight light to avoid heaving or using the momentum of the swing to assist in the movement. You can also use a resistance band or long band, which is good for warm-ups and burnouts. The key is to keep the resistance light so you don't struggle to abduct your leg.

STANDING HIP ABDUCTION

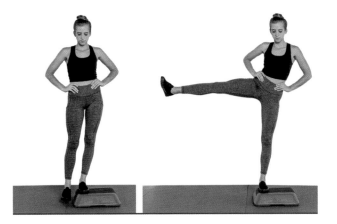

STANDING ANKLE WEIGHT HIP ABDUCTION

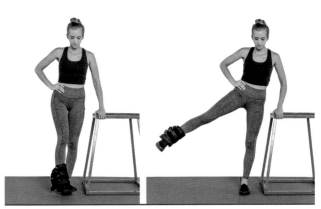

STANDING CABLE HIP ABDUCTION

STANDING KNEE-BANDED HIP ABDUCTION

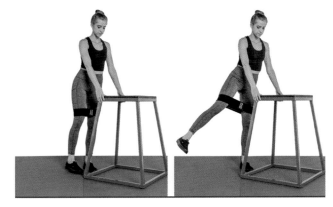

STANDING BAND ABDUCTION   **WEIGHT PLATE STANDING HIP ABDUCTION**

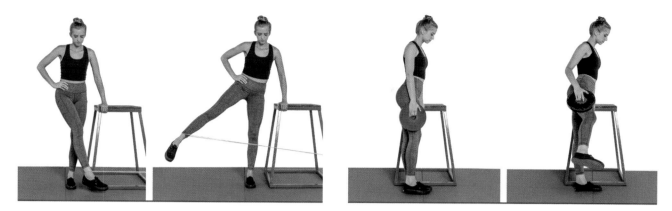

Side-Lying Hip Abduction

To set up for side-lying hip abduction, lie on your side with your shoulder and elbow on the floor. You can bend your bottom leg or keep it straight—whichever you prefer. To execute the movement, internally rotate your top leg and bring it just in front of your bottom leg. Keeping that leg internally rotated, abduct your leg by raising it straight up until you run out of range of motion. Bring your foot all the way down to the ground to complete the repetition.

You can add resistance to this movement by using a resistance band, such as a Glute Loop or mini band, or an ankle weight or weight plate. If you use a band, you have to reverse the movement in midair to maintain tension in the band. You lose a little range of motion, but it's great for creating a burn. An ankle weight creates more constant tension on the glutes and allows you to perform the full range of motion, which is ideal. To increase the range of motion, you can perform the extra-range side-lying hip abduction by planking on your knee and elbow or lying on a flat or incline bench.

SIDE-LYING HIP ABDUCTION

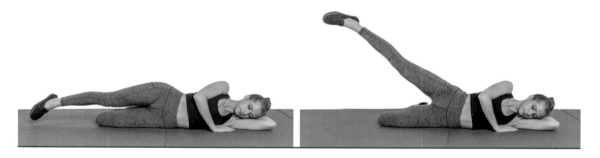

KNEE-BANDED SIDE-LYING HIP ABDUCTION

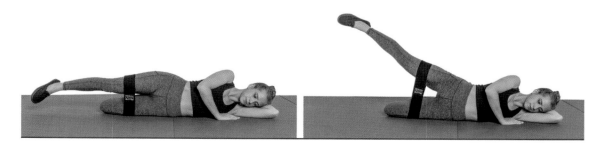

ANKLE WEIGHT SIDE-LYING HIP ABDUCTION

WEIGHT PLATE SIDE-LYING HIP ABDUCTION

PLANK EXTRA-RANGE SIDE-LYING HIP ABDUCTION

EXTRA-RANGE SIDE-LYING HIP ABDUCTION OFF BENCH

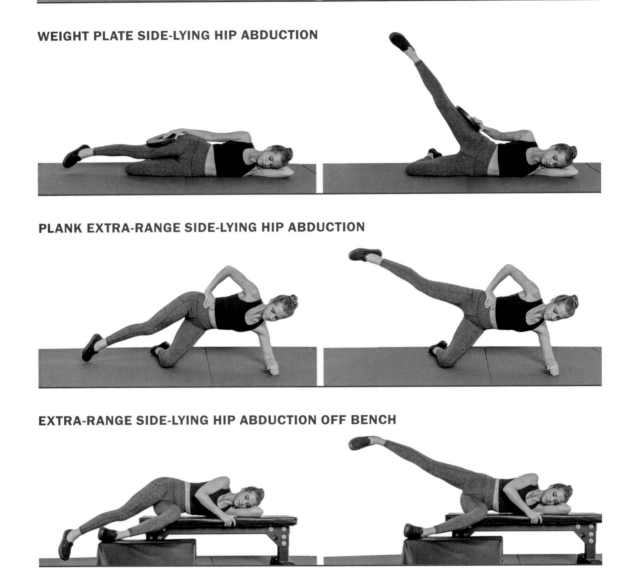

ANKLE WEIGHT EXTRA-RANGE SIDE-LYING HIP ABDUCTION OFF BENCH

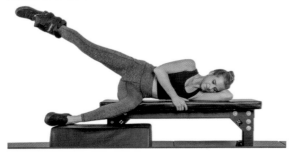

45-DEGREE SIDE-LYING HIP ABDUCTION (BACK)

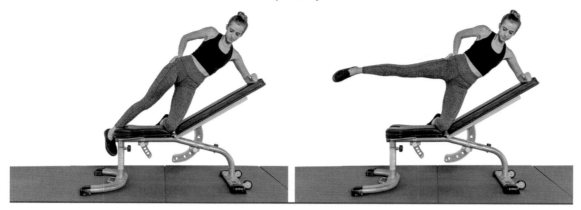

45-DEGREE SIDE-LYING HIP ABDUCTION (FRONT)

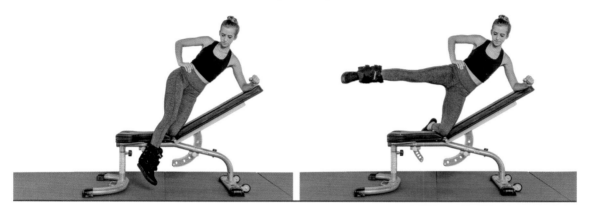

Top Glute Bridge Abduction

This technique works your glutes in two ways: you're holding the top position of the glute bridge in hip extension and then abducting your knees. In this sense, you're making your glutes pull double duty, meaning that they contract to maintain the top position and then contract more as you drive your knees outward into the band. In scientific terms, you're using your glutes to carry out simultaneous hip extension and hip abduction torque. In addition to increasing glute activation, abducting ties in your upper glutes, producing a potent glute burn. You can create burnouts with this exercise by performing a set number of glute bridges and then immediately performing a set number of top glute bridge abductions. To execute this variation, position a band above or below your knees, lie on the ground, and get into the glute bridge position. From here, simply extend your hips and then drive your knees out laterally into the band as far as you can while keeping your hips locked out.

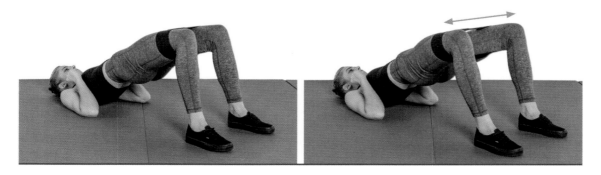

Top Hip Thrust Abduction

Top hip thrust abduction shares all of the same characteristics and technique as top glute bridge abduction. The only difference is that your shoulders are elevated off the floor. Again, you can combine the hip thrust with abduction to create burnouts—for example, you can perform 12 banded hip thrusts and then 12 top hip thrust abductions. You could also do a ladder burnout with a descending rep pattern or stick with traditional sets and reps.

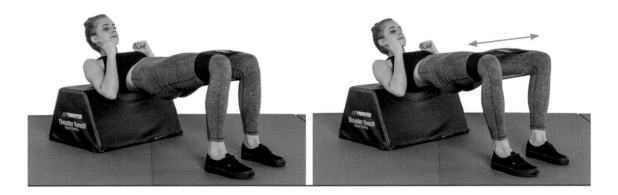

TRANSVERSE PLANE HIP ABDUCTION

Whenever you bend over or flex your hips and then move your leg(s) laterally, you're working transverse plane hip abduction movements. These exercises primarily work the upper glutes but also tie in the lower glutes. They include exercises like side-lying clams, squat walks, and seated and hip hinge hip abduction exercises. Like frontal plane hip abduction exercises, you can perform high reps in the form of burnouts toward the end of your training session or low reps as a low-load activation warm-up at the beginning of a workout.

Squat Lateral Walk

Squat walks are similar to lateral band walks in that you're stepping from side to side with a resistance band above or below your knees. But instead of remaining upright, you lower into a squat, which ties in more of your lower glutes. To execute the movement, wrap the band below or above your knees, lower into a squat, and then step laterally by driving into the ground and away with your grounded leg while reaching with your opposite leg. Be sure to take a wide step so that you put a full stretch into the band.

You can also perform sumo squat walks by adopting a wider stance. You can't take as wide of a step, but there is more tension on your glutes for the duration of the exercise. As with the other lateral band walk variations, you can either walk along a line and then switch after a given number of steps or stay in one area by switching back and forth between legs.

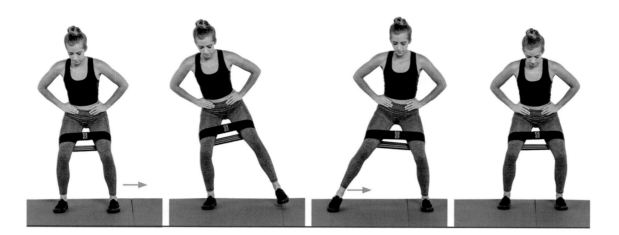

Squat Monster Walk

You can also perform squat walks in a forward and backward direction. This variation works your glutes through a broader range of motion because you're altering between hip flexion and extension with each step. However, a lot of people don't get the same level of glute pump or burn when stepping forward and backward as they do when stepping from side to side.

As with the monster walk, there are two ways to step: you can adopt a wide stance and keep the stretch in the band as you step straight forward or backward, or you can zigzag by bringing your foot toward your center line and then back out again with each step. Similarly, you can walk for a set distance or number of steps or take two steps forward and two steps back to stay in the same area.

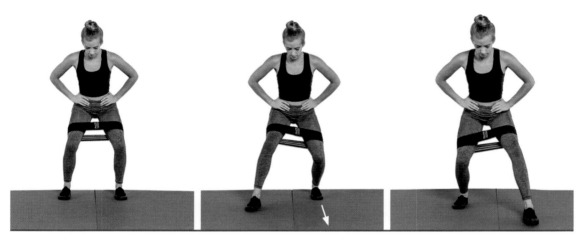

Banded Cha-Cha

We came up with this exercise at Glute Lab. We called it the banded cha-cha because we thought it resembled the cha-cha dance. We later learned that it looks nothing like the dance, which tells you how much we know about dancing. Nevertheless, the name stuck. The best way to set up is to grasp a plyometric box, the uprights of a power rack, or anything stable that you can grip. Place a resistance band above your knees, position your feet together along your center line, sit your hips back—keeping your shins roughly vertical—and then shift the majority of your weight onto one leg. Next, drive your non-loaded leg back at a 45-degree angle. You will feel this exercise uniquely in both legs. The grounded leg holds an isometric squat position while the moving leg performs hip abduction with slight hip extension. We typically prescribe 2 or 3 sets of 20 to 30 reps. Perform all reps with one leg, rest, and then repeat with your other leg.

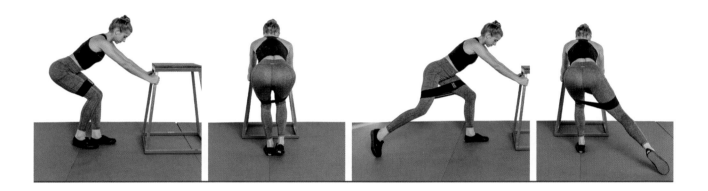

Side-Lying Transverse Hip Abduction

Some people have a hard time with normal side-lying hip abduction due to their hip anatomy and muscle architecture. They have to fight hard to stay in the frontal plane—that is, to keep their top leg over their bottom leg as they perform the movement. These people generally like the transverse plane side-lying hip abduction variation, which emphasizes bringing the top leg in front of the bottom leg. In short, the exercise works similar muscles and shares the same setup as the frontal plane variation, but the execution is different in that your top leg is in slight hip flexion as you lower and raise your leg.

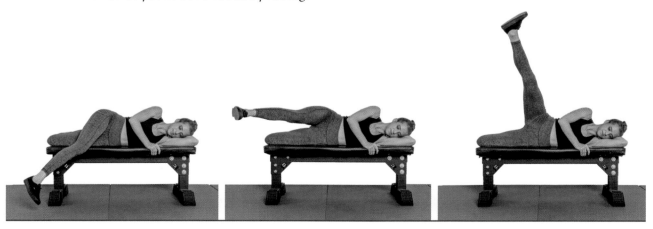

Side-Lying Clam

The setup for the side-lying clam is similar to side-lying hip abduction in that you lie on your side with your shoulder or elbow on the floor. But instead of keeping your leg straight, you bend both legs and flex your hips, creating roughly a 45-degree angle between your knees and your hips. To perform the movement, crisscross the arches of your feet (see the bottom-right photo below) and then raise or abduct your top leg.

You can add resistance in the form of a band by positioning it above your knees or by holding a weight plate over your thigh. To perform these variations, come up onto your bottom elbow and raise your top leg while keeping your feet together. Your hips should reach full extension as you open your legs.

SIDE-LYING CLAM

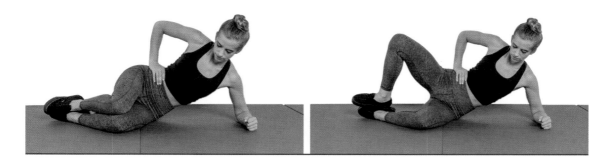

KNEE-BANDED SIDE-LYING CLAM

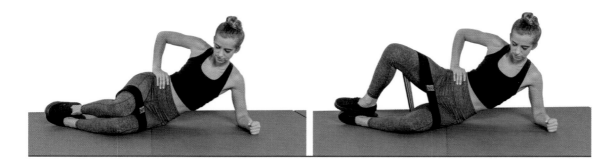

WEIGHT PLATE SIDE-LYING CLAM

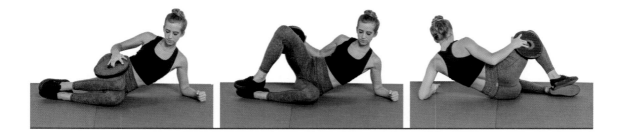

Side-Lying Hip Raise

The side-lying hip raise is an advanced hip abduction exercise that is similar to a clam but ties in your bottom leg and extends your hips. Begin in the side-lying position on your elbow with your hips and knees bent. Pushing through your grounded knee, raise your body upward. Abduct both hips at the same time while driving the hips forward. Aim to achieve maximum hip separation at the top of the movement. As you descend, sink back into your bottom hip. To make the exercise even more challenging, elevate your grounded knee on a balance pad to increase the range of motion, or position a band above your knees.

SIDE-LYING HIP RAISE

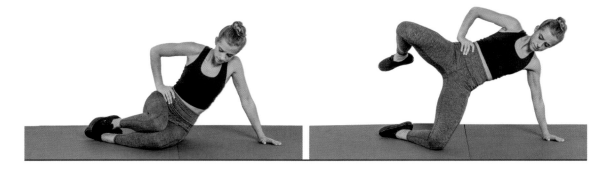

EXTRA-RANGE SIDE-LYING HIP RAISE

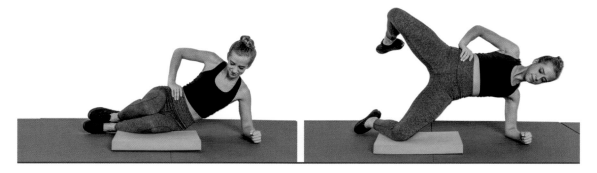

KNEE-BANDED SIDE-LYING HIP RAISE

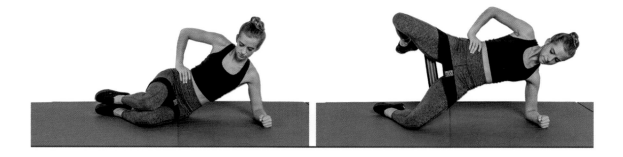

Fire Hydrant

The fire hydrant is a classic quadruped glute exercise that can be done with body weight, a resistance band, or an ankle weight. Whether you're doing just body weight or adding resistance, the key is to maintain a neutral spine (don't flex or extend) and remain in an athletic quadruped stance as you abduct with your free leg. Some people mistakenly twist their body to raise the leg higher, which is unnecessary.

If you want to get more range of motion from the exercise, shift your hips to one side—sinking your weight into one hip—and then come back to center as you abduct or raise your opposite leg. What's great about this extra-range variation is that it works your grounded leg almost as much as your top leg. For the knee-banded variation, you can position the band just above your knees or slip it underneath the knee of your grounded leg to pin it in place (possible only if you're using a stretchy band). For the ankle weight variation shown on the next page, you can position the weight around your ankle or your knee.

FIRE HYDRANT

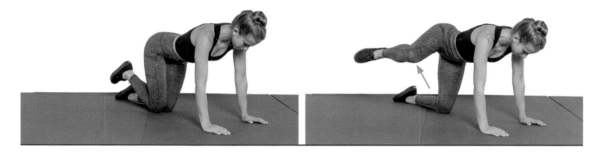

EXTRA-RANGE FIRE HYDRANT

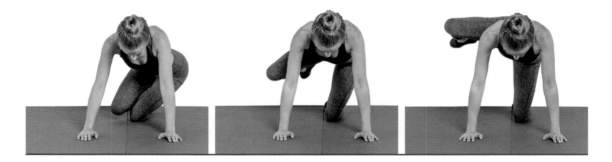

KNEE-BANDED FIRE HYDRANT

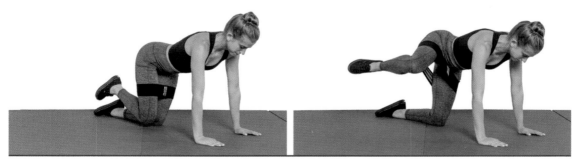

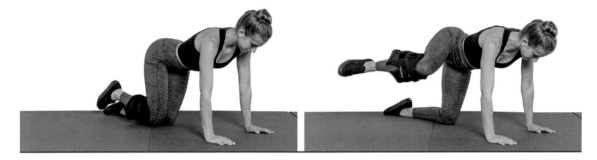

Knee-Banded Standing Hip Hinge Abduction

You can perform dual hip abduction from a standing, seated, or supine position. All of the variations require you to position a resistance band, such as a mini band or Glute Loop, either above or below your knees. To perform the standing variation, assume a comfortable stance—most people prefer to position their feet shoulder width apart (you need enough tension in the band to prevent it from sliding down your legs)—tilt your torso forward, sink your hips back, and keep your shins roughly vertical as if you were setting up for a Romanian deadlift. With your back flat and your torso positioned at roughly a 45-degree angle, drive your knees outward into the band until you reach the end of your range of motion or you can't stretch the band any farther. Strive to hit this range with each rep. You can also roll onto the outsides of your feet to get a little more range of motion.

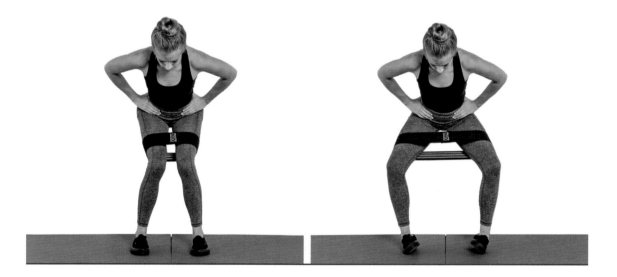

Knee-Banded Seated and Supine Hip Abduction

To perform the seated and supine variations, sit on the edge of a box, chair, or bench or on the ground with roughly a 90-degree bend in your knees. With the band wrapped either above or below your knees, drive your knees outward maximally into the band, just as you would when performing the hip hinge variations. You can perform the seated variations from different torso angles. If you're seated, you can lean back slightly, sit straight up, lean forward slightly, or lean really far forward. If you're supine, you can sit upright using your hands, lean back by resting on your elbows, or lie flat on your back. You might find that a certain angle fires your glutes more than the others, and that might be the angle you use most often. However, I typically have my clients break up their sets by performing a certain number of repetitions from each of three torso angles to ensure that they fully hit their glutes. There are three strategies for abducting your legs. You can

- Roll onto the edges of your feet to get a little more range of motion
- Perform these with a deliberately wide stance so that your knees are in valgus (caved inward) at the onset of the exercise and move to a neutral position at lockout
- Slide your feet outward maximally using Valslides or Gliding Discs

BACKWARD LEAN SEATED HIP ABDUCTION

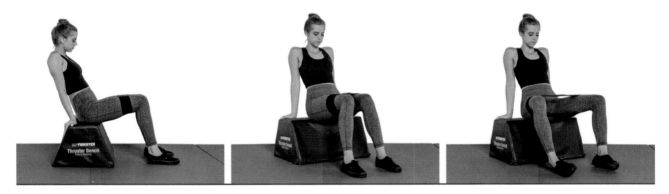

UPRIGHT SEATED HIP ABDUCTION

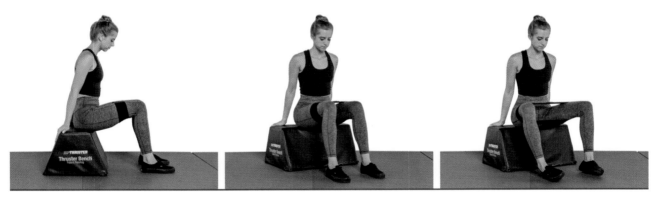

FORWARD LEAN SEATED HIP ABDUCTION

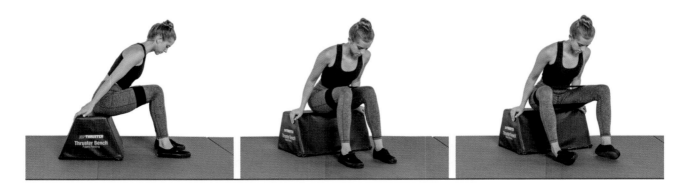

VALGUS SEATED HIP ABDUCTION

SLIDING SEATED HIP ABDUCTION

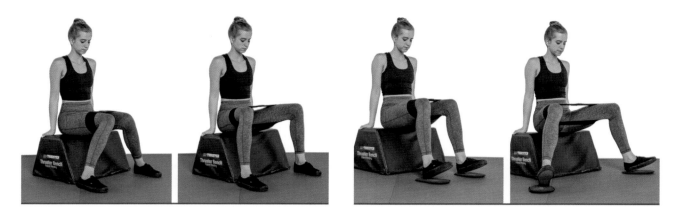

SUPINE FROM HANDS HIP ABDUCTION

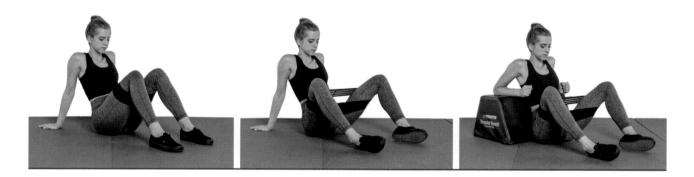

SUPINE FROM ELBOWS HIP ABDUCTION

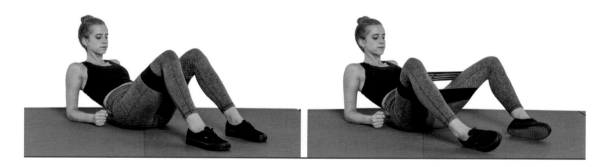

SUPINE HIP ABDUCTION

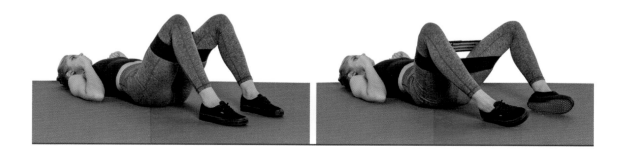

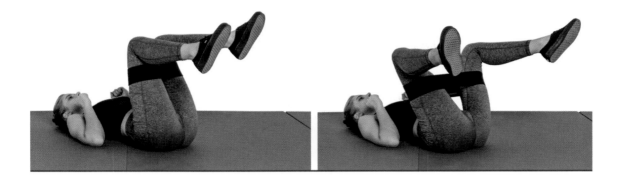

LOADING AND EQUIPMENT VARIATIONS

When it comes to loading the hip abduction movement pattern, I recommend two excellent pieces of equipment: the seated hip abduction machine and the Gluteator.

SEATED HIP ABDUCTION MACHINE

The seated hip abduction machine is a client favorite at my gym. The good news is that most commercial training facilities have this machine, making it a great option for people with gym memberships.

As with most hip abduction exercises, seated hip abduction machine work is generally done at the end of a training session with high reps (20 reps or higher), and the focus revolves around getting a good pump and burn.

When it comes to training methods, I employ several strategies. The first relates to torso angle. For example, you can perform seated hip abductions by leaning back, remaining upright (this can be done seated or hovering in a squat), or leaning forward. Each torso angle strengthens and targets different subdivisions. While all of them work both the upper and the lower glutes, leaning back emphasizes the upper glutes, while leaning forward brings the lower glutes more into play. Hitting all three torso positions ensures that the glutes are hit from all angles. A sample set and rep scheme might look like this: 1 set of 10 to 20 reps with the same weight at each of the three torso angles, for a total of 3 sets. Perform the same number of reps at each torso angle.

You can also perform dropsets, such as 2 sets of 3 dropsets. For example, to complete a set, you perform 10 reps at a heavy weight, immediately lower the weight (move the pin one or two places up the weight stack), perform another 10 reps, lower the weight again, and then, without pausing, perform the last 10 reps.

Manual resistance is another method I use with my clients to enhance the eccentric phase, otherwise referred to as *enhanced eccentric reps*. I assist with the concentric portion and then push to add resistance on the eccentric phase.

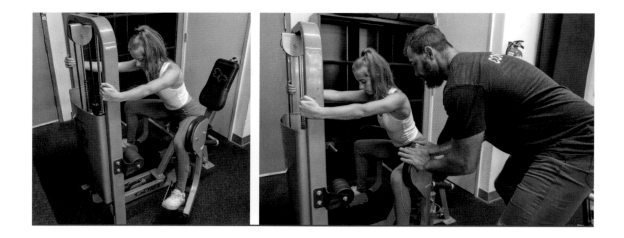

GLUTEATOR

I make sure to equip the Glute Lab with the absolute best glute training equipment. One of my favorite machines is the Gluteator from Dynavec Resistance Systems, which combines hip extension and hip abduction. This machine is easy to load, feels smooth, and produces a crazy glute burn. The first time I used it, I did 3 sets of 20 reps with two 45-pound plates on each side. I had to get out of the seat and stand up between sets 2 and 3 because my glutes were burning so badly.

As glute training becomes more and more popular, new innovations and better equipment are hitting the market. My hope is that the Gluteator and various hip thrust machines will become staples in all commercial gyms.

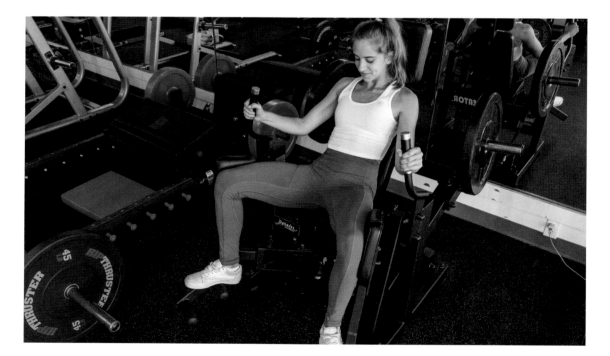

Hip External Rotation Exercises

Eighteen years ago, at age 24, I got together with my friends for a softball game. I went five for five with five home runs. One of them cleared the fence by probably 150 feet. My friends and I were amazed, as I hadn't been that good of an athlete in high school. So what had changed? Well, I'd been lifting heavy weights and had gotten much stronger.

Rotational power fascinates me. During the steroid era in baseball, guys were knocking balls out of the park like it was nothing. Muscle mass and strength seem to be very good for bat-swinging power.

The same isn't always true for sprinting and jumping power; they can be beneficial or detrimental depending on the athlete and the sport.

I got better at hitting home runs from doing squats, deadlifts, bench presses, chin-ups, and probably even heavy ab work. But power development is usually better achieved with explosive movements—for example, with various med ball throws—and of course by practicing the sport.

I've always wondered if rotational weight room exercises would increase rotational power. In theory, they would, but not much research has been done on the subject. Nevertheless, hip external rotation exercises are great to sprinkle into your glute training program. In addition to developing the upper and lower glutes, hip external rotation (and abduction) exercises are essential for athletes, especially those who play rotational sports like baseball, tennis, and martial arts. When you rotate, you're combining all three actions controlled by the glutes: hip extension, hip abduction, and hip external rotation. For example, say you're swinging a bat to hit a baseball. You start in slight hip flexion. As you transition to swing, you move into hip extension; shift forward, which is hip abduction; and twist, which is hip external rotation.

My point is that hip external rotation exercises integrate the entire body, and you'll feel them in your obliques and especially in the glute max of your rear leg. The glute max is the most powerful hip external rotator, but many athletes struggle with this exercise in the beginning. I've measured the glute activation of the standing cable hip external rotation movement, and it reaches maximum capacity. I don't think it's a great glute builder because of the limited range of motion, but in my opinion, athletes should train all three primary roles of the glutes (hip extension, hip abduction, and hip external rotation).

GUIDELINES AND CUES

Hip external rotation exercises mimic a swinging and throwing motion in that you assume an athletic stance and rotate your body using the power of your hips. This is actually a lot more difficult than it sounds, which is why I don't typically teach it to my physique clients. However, as I said, it's worth doing, especially if you play sports. To help you get the most from these exercises, I want to address one important guideline, which applies to both techniques.

When executing the hip external rotation exercises—whether you're performing the cable or the banded variation—the idea is to keep tension in your glutes throughout the full range of motion, which is best achieved by controlling the rotation and extending your arms away from your body as you rotate. In other words, keep the rotation slow and steady and reach away with the cable or band as you twist. If you rotate too much and allow the cable or band to wrap around your body, you will lose glute tension.

CUFF/DIP BELT CABLE HIP ROTATION

The cable and band hip external rotation exercises are the most popular hip rotation exercises. But, as I've said, they are difficult to learn and teach. More recently, I've been implementing a new technique that utilizes a cuff or dip belt and cable column. (You can also use a light band.) As you can see in the photos, you wrap the cuff, belt, or band below your knee, brace onto a box or the arm of the cable column, raise your knee to hip level, and then abduct and externally rotate your leg. Although the traditional hip rotations are still effective—and you should try to master them, especially if you're a coach or someone who plays sports—this is a much easier variation to learn. Granted, you're not rotating your body as much, which is specific to sport, but you can effectively target the gluteal muscles that are responsible for producing rotation. You also feel your glutes working a lot more compared to the traditional hip external rotation exercises. If you're interested only in developing your glutes and the other variations are too difficult, you can stick with this variation and get great results. If you play sports, I recommend implementing all of the techniques covered in this section.

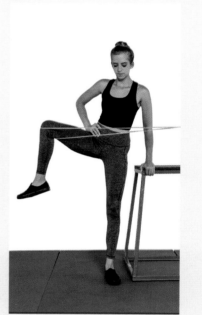

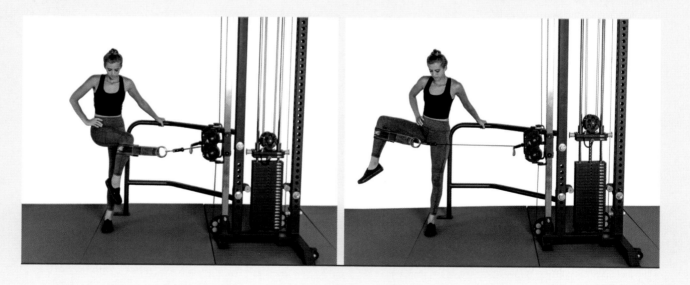

HIP EXTERNAL ROTATION VARIATIONS

Only a couple of hip external rotation exercises are worth doing, and they are difficult to execute. If your primary goal is to build bigger glutes, then you don't need to worry too much about performing these exercises. If done properly, they do lead to high levels of glute activation, but they are not as valuable for glute growth as they are for function and performance. If you play sports or you want to improve your rotational ability, then programming a few sets at the end of your workout is definitely a good idea. In fact, there's a study that showed around 70 percent of glute force can be transferred into hip external rotation due to the diagonal orientation of the glute fibers. To maximize and develop rotational power, you need to know how to use your glute as a hip external rotator, which is a skill that these exercises help develop.

CABLE HIP EXTERNAL ROTATION

Hip external rotation exercises can be done using a resistance band, a rope handle on a cable column, a Cook bar, or a Rip Trainer, which is essentially a bar with a band attached to the end. My preference is a cable column with a Cook bar (you could also use a rope handle) because it offers a smooth line of action and there is constant tension throughout the entire range of the movement, which makes it easier to control the rotation.

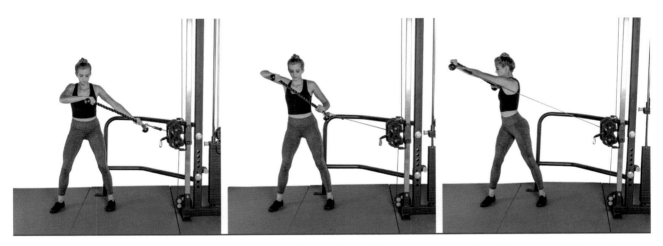

Position the cable low or around hip level. If that doesn't feel right, experiment with different heights until you find the setup that feels best. Grip both ends of the bar, step away from the cable column, and assume an athletic stance. Next, you do several things at once: pivot on your rear foot, rotate your hips, and extend your rear arm in an upward diagonal angle across your body. More specifically, as your rear arm passes your center line, you reach outward so that your arm is fully extended. There should be a little distance between the cable and your body. To complete the rep, momentarily pause in the finish position, then slowly rotate with control back to the start position. This is a difficult exercise to learn from reading, so have your coach walk you through it, or consider filming yourself and comparing your form to what is shown in the photos.

RIP TRAINER/BAND HIP EXTERNAL ROTATION

These variations using a Rip Trainer or a band are not as smooth because the tension increases as you reach end range, making it harder to control the rotation and potentially creating a jerkier motion. For this reason, I much prefer the cable version. That said, the Rip and band variations are good options if you don't have access to a cable machine. The setup and execution are exactly the same as for the cable variation.

RIP TRAINER HIP EXTERNAL ROTATION

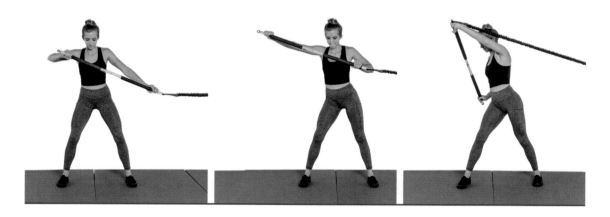

BAND HIP EXTERNAL ROTATION

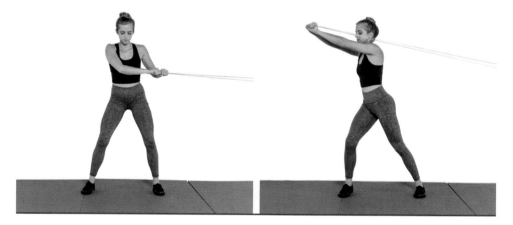

Posterior Pelvic Tilt

When it comes to activating your glutes, you need to be able to create and maintain tension in a wide range of movements and in any position—whether you're seated, standing, hip hinging, or squatting. You could be playing Twister, and when someone says, "Turn on your glutes," you should be able to fire them instantly. But not everyone can.

In fact, about one in four new clients I work with has a hard time activating or tensing their glutes when their hips are in full or nearly full hip extension while their legs are straight (but not while bent), which—as you know—is the zone in which you get the highest glute activation.

In addition to not developing their glutes properly, these people have a hard time locking out their hips when performing deadlifts or back extensions or even keeping their glutes tensed in a plank or push-up position. Realizing that poor glute activation was the root of the problem, I devised a simple solution. I call it the posterior pelvic tilt (PPT) activation test, which is a simple progression of exercises to test glute activation and help people develop the mind-glute connection.

PPT ACTIVATION TEST

Personal trainers don't get a ton of time with clients. Most trainers see their clients for only one to three hours a week if they're lucky. This doesn't leave a lot of time to run clients through their workouts while simultaneously dialing in their technique, let alone experiment with different exercise variations to tease out weaknesses and provide corrections. This is where the PPT activation test comes into play.

Say I'm working with a new client or someone who has a hard time firing their glutes. Rather than put them through a ton of complex movements, I start by teaching them how to posterior pelvic tilt because it's a position that creates a ton of tension in the glutes. I do so using four different techniques: the standing glute squeeze, the RKC plank with the toes on the ground, the RKC plank from the knees, and the PPT hip thrust.

Depending on where the client falls on the glute activation spectrum, I have them perform one or more of the PPT activation exercises for homework. This allows them to work on developing glute tension while they are at home so that we can focus on getting a good workout while I have them in the gym.

For example, I might have a client do planks twice a day on their own, starting with a 10- to 20-second hold. My goal is to build them up until they can perform a 1-minute RKC plank while maintaining tension in their glutes the entire time.

Someone who has developed a mind-muscle connection with their glutes (also referred to as the mind-glute connection) or who has been training for a long time can typically hold a plank or standing glute squeeze for a minute without much struggle. But a lot of beginners can't keep tension on their glutes, and their glutes shut off or flutter after about 5 seconds. Hypothetically, an advanced athlete could keep the glutes activated in a plank at above 80 percent of maximum capacity for the entire minute, whereas a beginner might be able to keep the glutes activated at only 40 percent of maximum capacity for that minute.

To build a client up to a 1-minute plank, I might start by programming 3 sets of 20 seconds and then increase the time and reduce the number of sets as they get stronger. I have beginners start with the short-lever RKC plank. Once they get good at that, I progress them to the standing glute squeeze, then the RKC plank, and lastly the PPT hip thrust.

Once the client can do a 1-minute plank and maintain solid glute tension the entire time, I don't need to assign homework anymore. In other words, the PPT activation test drops out of the program once they gain the muscle endurance and strength to perform a 1-minute plank. This achievement also demonstrates that they have developed the mind-glute connection—meaning they can fire their glutes on command—and eliminates many of the faults that stem from poor glute activation, such as not feeling tension in the glutes or being unable to lock out the hips properly. What's more, it can help with glute growth because it creates tension in the muscle. Granted, it's not as good as performing a loaded hip thrust, but for beginners, every little bit helps.

You can still use the exercises in the PPT activation test as a warm-up prior to strenuous exercise. The key is to do just enough to wake up the muscle and avoid going to fatigue. You can also use these exercises anytime you've been imprisoned in a chair for an extended period, such as after a long flight or car ride. You can use them in a burnout circuit as well—we throw in RKC planks at Glute Lab all the time, typically for 20-second holds. In short, using the PPT exercises to wake up the glutes might diminish or help prevent hip and lower back pain associated with poor hip extension mechanics (excessive anterior pelvic tilt).

GUIDELINES AND CUES

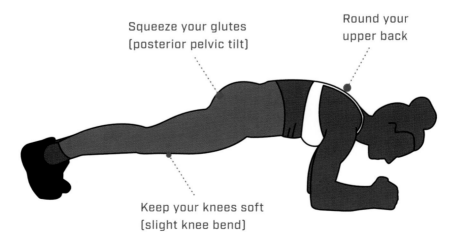

Squeeze your glutes
(posterior pelvic tilt)

Round your
upper back

Keep your knees soft
(slight knee bend)

All of the PPT activation exercises are similar in that you create tension in your glutes by rotating your pelvis rearward and then hold tension to develop the mind-glute connection. One particular cue will help you do exactly that.

In previous sections, you saw that tucking your chin and rounding your upper back encourages posterior pelvic tilt. For example, when you tuck your chin during a hip thrust or glute bridge, your pelvis naturally tilts rearward as you reach full hip extension, which for most people increases glute activation. The same is true when performing back extensions: tucking your chin and rounding your upper back reduces tension in your hamstrings and spinal erectors and increases tension in your glutes. We apply this same cue to the PPT activation exercises to encourage posterior pelvic tilt. Whether you're standing or planking, you want to round your upper back slightly, tuck your chin, and think about keeping your ribcage down.

FAULTS AND CORRECTIONS

The biggest problem people have with the PPT exercises is achieving high levels of glute activation on the first attempt. Again, this could be due to lack of activity, being new to glute training, or simply not having developed the mind-muscle connection with the glutes. But if you follow the progression I've outlined, your ability to contract your glutes will improve over time.

People fail either because they do not get into a good position or because they give up after a couple of attempts. You have to take these exercises seriously and concentrate if you want to see improvement. If you're a beginner, it might help to follow the PPT categories sequentially and work your way up to a minute by performing 3 sets of 20-second holds. Once you can hold the position for a minute, move on to the next exercise. When you can hold every position for a minute with what you perceive to be 80 percent of maximum glute activation, you no longer need to practice the sequence unless you're using it as a warm-up or to wake up your glutes after extended periods of inactivity or as part of a burnout.

PPT CATEGORIES

There are four categories of PPT activation exercises. As I said, it's important to work through these categories sequentially. Start with the short-lever RKC plank and then progress down the list to the RKC plank, standing glute squeeze, and PPT hip thrust as you gain proficiency—that is, you increase your ability to maintain near-maximal contraction in your glutes for at least a minute.

PPT SHORT-LEVER RKC PLANK

Of all the PPT activation exercises, this variation is the easiest to perform. In most cases, I start people off with the RKC plank, or even the standing glute squeeze, and then regress to the short-lever plank if they struggle to contract and maintain tension in their glutes. In other words, if you're having trouble posterior pelvic tilting and activating your glutes in an RKC plank or standing glute squeeze, then you should start here.

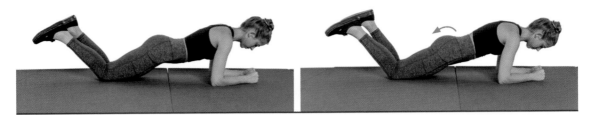

Get on your hands and knees in a quadruped position. Walk your hands out until you're in a push-up position—keeping your lower back flat—and then drop to your elbows, positioning your arms underneath your shoulders. To posterior pelvic tilt, round your upper back, tuck your chin, and then squeeze your glutes. You should feel your pelvis tilt rearward as you contract. To help facilitate this action, think about pulling your belly button toward your ribcage as you contract your glutes and then maintaining that tension for 20 seconds or longer.

PPT RKC PLANK

Traditionally, the RKC plank is an exercise for developing core stability and strength, but here you're using it as an activation drill to practice posterior pelvic tilting and help prime your glutes to contract harder and longer. As a result, it's important to differentiate the plank from the posterior pelvic tilt glute squeeze. If you're performing a normal plank, the goal is to keep your knees straight, but with the PPT RKC plank, you can have a slight bend in your knees and round your upper back to help increase posterior pelvic tilt and glute activation.

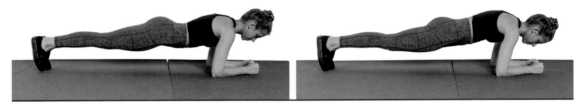

Get into the push-up position, then drop to your elbows. With your elbows positioned underneath your shoulders, round your upper back, tuck your chin, and then squeeze your glutes. Again, you can think about pulling your belly button toward your ribcage as you contract your glutes to emphasize the posterior pelvic tilt action.

STANDING GLUTE SQUEEZE

The standing glute squeeze is one of the best ways to test and measure glute activation, as well as highlight the role of the glutes. In fact, this is where I start the majority of people because you can feel the hip movements that your glutes control. When you have a strong glute squeeze, for example, you will feel your hips move into hip extension and your pelvis posterior pelvic tilt, and you will feel an outward external rotational force at your feet. But not everyone will feel it. If you don't feel your glutes activate, regress to the PPT RKC plank and short-lever RKC plank until you develop the strength to contract and maintain tension in your glutes.

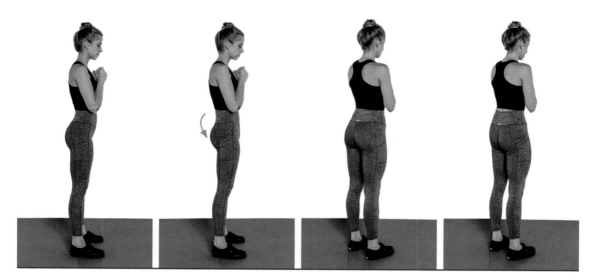

Find your preferred stance. The vast majority of people position their feet just outside shoulder width and turned slightly outward. However, you should experiment with wider and narrower stances and tinker with foot flare to determine the stance that allows you to achieve the highest level of glute activation. Once you find your ideal stance, bend your elbows, clench your fists, and then squeeze your glutes. Again, you should feel your hips extend and your pelvis tilt underneath your body with an outward force on your feet. You can add resistance by attaching a weight to a dip belt and challenge your ability to posterior pelvic tilt under load. To perform this variation, wrap the dip belt around your hips with the loop anchored over your butt and get into a neutral standing position. Then squeeze your glutes and posterior pelvic tilt. If done correctly, the weight will rise slightly. It's only a few inches of range of motion, but you can really feel your glutes moving the weight.

STANDING LOADED POSTERIOR PELVIC TILT

The standing loaded posterior pelvic tilt challenges your ability to posterior pelvic tilt under load. This exercise is good for glute hypertrophy, as well as strengthening PPT action and end-range hip extension. I recommend placing this exercise at the end of your workout and performing 2 or 3 sets of 10 reps of 5-second squeezes.

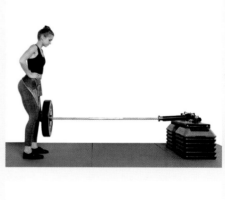

To set up for this exercise, elevate a landmine about 16 inches off the ground and load the other end of the bar. (You need a lot of weight to make this exercise effective.) Wrap a dip belt around your hips with the loop anchored over your butt, hook the chain around the bar sleeve, and then clip it in place using a barbell collar. Note: If the landmine is on the ground, the chain pulls the collar off the end of the bar, which keeps the weight plates in place. To execute this exercise, get into an upright position with a slight hip hinge, then squeeze your glutes and posterior pelvic tilt. If done correctly, the weight will rise slightly. It's only a few inches of range of motion, but you can really feel your glutes moving the weight. You can also use a dip belt with a Pit Shark and cable column.

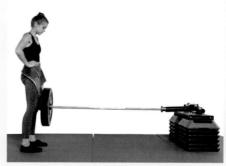

PPT HIP THRUST

Most people (myself included) feel the highest levels of glute activation in the lockout position of the hip thrust while posterior pelvic tilting. This is not the case for everyone, but it's worth testing and perhaps drilling if you don't feel your glutes activate when performing the full movement. You can also experiment with the spinal-pelvic hip thrust strategies outlined on pages 317 to 319. But for this exercise, you're isolating the top range of the movement—full hip extension with posterior pelvic tilt—as a way of testing and strengthening the mind-glute connection. You can either hold the position or move within the top 6-inch range. For example, one test is to hold the end-range position, while the other is to pulse (a short up-and-down movement using hip flexion and anterior pelvic tilt on the way down and hip extension and posterior pelvic tilt on the way up) within the top 6-inch range of motion. To increase glute activation, you can also add load in the form of a resistance band or dumbbell, but don't get carried away and use a barbell.

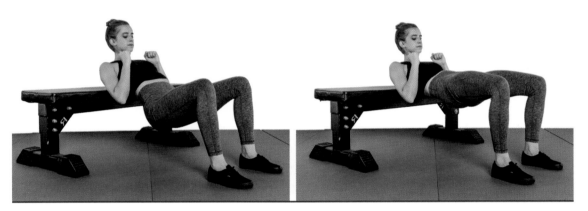

Get into the start position of the hip thrust by positioning the tops of your shoulder blades against a bench and then raising your hips, keeping your knees bent at a roughly 90-degree angle. Again, you're not moving through a full range of motion or dropping your hips; you're just holding the top position. In most cases, simply squeezing your glutes to hold the top position will cause you to posterior pelvic tilt. If this doesn't happen, drop your hips slightly and then focus on really squeezing your glutes. You should feel your pelvis rotate underneath your body. Like the plank variations, think about keeping your ribcage down, keeping your chin tucked, and pulling your belly button toward your ribcage. Once you get the posterior pelvic tilt down, the next step is to pulse within the top 6-inch range of motion.

Quad-Dominant Exercises

As I've said throughout this book, to fully develop your glutes and body, you need to perform a wide range of exercises and target your glutes from different angles and load vectors. In this chapter, I cover quad-dominant exercises, which, as you know, primarily target the quadriceps muscles. However, these lower-body exercises—which include squats, single-leg squats, split squats, step-ups, and sled pushes—do a lot more than develop bigger, stronger quads. Just as glute-dominant movements work more muscles than just your glutes, quad-dominant exercises do more than grow your legs. You're targeting your glutes in a unique way and growing muscle through different hypertrophy mechanisms.

For instance, instead of reaching peak muscle activation when the glutes are shortened, as in a hip thrust, peak glute activation is reached during quad-dominant movements when the glutes are stretched. This provides four distinct advantages for both glute growth and overall function.

First, when the glutes are fully lengthened while activated, muscle damage occurs, meaning that you experience tears and lesions at a microscopic level in the various components of your muscle cells. Though muscle damage is often overrated and can be counterproductive if you're overly sore, it seems to play a role in generating muscle growth. As I've said, you could probably get about 85 percent of your glute gains from glute-dominant exercises with the remaining 15 percent coming from quad- and hamstring-dominant exercises.

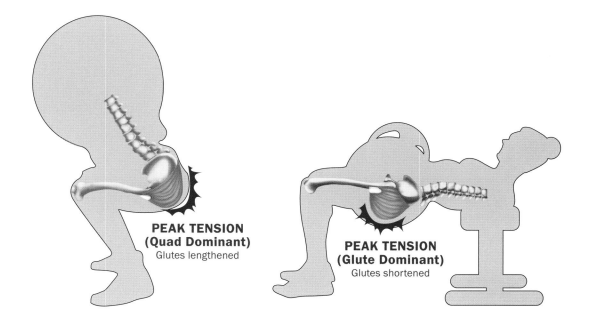

**PEAK TENSION
(Quad Dominant)**
Glutes lengthened

**PEAK TENSION
(Glute Dominant)**
Glutes shortened

Second, quad-dominant exercises such as squats, lunges, and step-ups target the lower subdivision of your gluteus maximus. Research comparing long to short muscle length training shows regional specific muscle growth, meaning that stretching the muscle under tension (quad- and hamstring-dominant exercises) targets regions that aren't recruited when you train only at short muscle lengths (glute-dominant exercises). To put this in simpler terms, you target different muscle fibers and work your glutes in a unique way, ensuring that these muscles develop maximally. So, if you have overdeveloped upper glutes or you simply want to focus on building the lower subdivision of your gluteus maximus—specifically near the attachment point, informally referred to as the butt crease region—then prioritizing quad-dominant movements in your training aligns perfectly with your goals.

The third advantage is that building your quads using the exercises in this chapter helps shape a leaner physique. The stronger you are at any given body weight, the leaner you'll be, which is why it's important not to omit big movements like squats and deadlifts that work a lot of muscles throughout the body.

Lastly, the majority of exercises in this chapter are considered functional movement patterns, meaning that they work muscles and mimic movements that are performed in daily life. Take the squat, for example. If you understand how to squat with good form, you can apply the mechanics to every action that involves the squat movement pattern, such as getting in and out of a chair. To be clear, I'm not saying you need to move with perfect form every time you get in and out of a chair, but if you understand the principles that govern good squatting, lunging, and step-up mechanics, you can use those same techniques to guide your movements outside the gym.

Although my main objective as a personal trainer is to help people reach their physique goals, I like to think that I do more than help people look good naked. I want to make my clients stronger, more resilient human beings. Because quad-dominant movements are buried in the actions of everyday life, I believe that teaching people how to perform the exercises in this chapter (and in the next chapter focused on hamstring-dominant movements) helps them carry out everyday movements with greater efficiency. So, even if your goals revolve primarily around building bigger, stronger glutes, it's important to experiment and integrate quad-dominant exercises into your training program.

STRUCTURE AND ORGANIZATION

In this chapter, I cover all of the quad-dominant exercises (also referred to as squat movement patterns), which I've broken into five sections: squats, split squats, step-ups, single-leg squats, and sled pushes. The squats section includes exercises such as the back squat and front squat, which, for most people, will serve as the primary lifts throughout the week. Split squats encompass all of the lunge variations, and Bulgarian split squats are great for targeting the lower glutes. Step-ups and single-leg squats are typically done in the middle of a workout as accessory exercises. And sled pushes are great for warming up, as a finisher to a workout, or as a tool to rebuild the glutes after an injury.

QUAD-DOMINANT EXERCISES

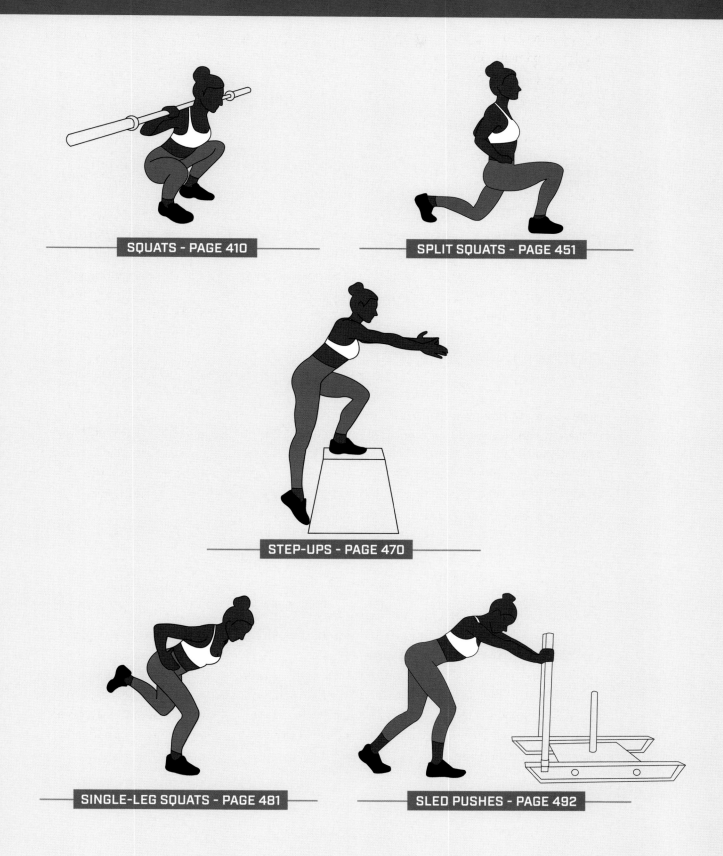

SQUATS - PAGE 410

SPLIT SQUATS - PAGE 451

STEP-UPS - PAGE 470

SINGLE-LEG SQUATS - PAGE 481

SLED PUSHES - PAGE 492

1

Squats

At one time, the squat was regarded as the king of all glute exercises. If you wanted to build bigger, stronger glutes, the prevailing advice was to "just squat." I've spent a great deal of time dispelling this mantra over the years, and I've highlighted some of the most salient points as to why "just squat" is terrible advice for anyone looking to maximize glute development. But that doesn't mean squats are bad. If maximum glute growth is your goal, you should prioritize glute-dominant movements, but you should also squat and perform squat variations, as well as hip hinge and deadlift variations.

In this section, I break down the types of squats and explain what each type it is good for, how to perform the movement correctly, and how to create exercise variations based on load position and equipment options. Consider this section the ultimate guide to mastering the squat movement pattern.

GUIDELINES AND CUES

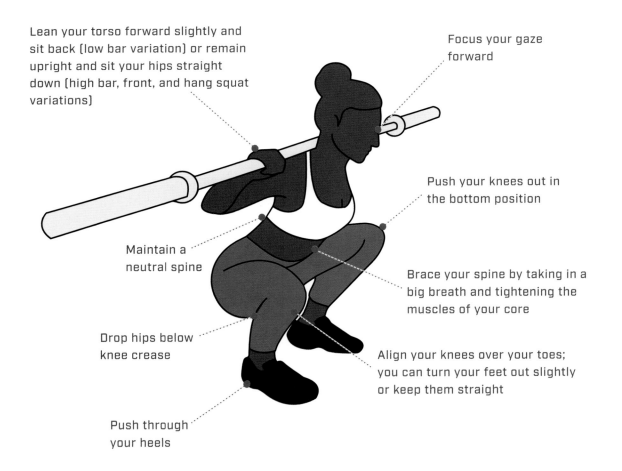

Lean your torso forward slightly and sit back (low bar variation) or remain upright and sit your hips straight down (high bar, front, and hang squat variations)

Focus your gaze forward

Push your knees out in the bottom position

Maintain a neutral spine

Brace your spine by taking in a big breath and tightening the muscles of your core

Drop hips below knee crease

Align your knees over your toes; you can turn your feet out slightly or keep them straight

Push through your heels

Squats are classified by stance, load position, and the equipment you're using. You can squat in a wide stance with a barbell on your back (known as a sumo back squat), in a narrow stance while holding a kettlebell or dumbbell in front of your chest (known as a goblet squat), or with your feet on a box and a weight hanging from your hips (known as a belt squat), to mention a few variations.

Before I delve into the different types of squats (front squat, back squat, hang squat, and so on), let's address some universal guidelines that apply to the squat movement pattern.

STANCE AND FOOT POSITION

Finding a stance that works with your unique anatomy and training goals is the first step to squatting correctly and getting the most from the exercise variations. The problem is that there is no one-size-fits-all squat stance, and you may have different stance preferences for different squats. For example, you might prefer a slightly wider stance with your feet straighter when low bar back squatting but a narrow stance with your feet turned out while front squatting. What's more, it's important to switch up your stance from time to time to stress your muscles in different ranges of motion and positions. (More on this shortly.)

Below, I provide a general overview of your stance options. Study the different foot positions, get a feel for the different stances, and see what works best for you as you progress through the other guidelines. As a general rule, you want to adopt a stance that feels good on your joints, doesn't cause you pain, expresses the full potential of your mobility, and allows you to maintain good form.

Feet Orientation

When it comes to the orientation of your feet, you can position them straight, turn them outward 45 degrees, or align them anywhere in between these two extremes. As with all exercises that have different stance options, you should do some experimenting to determine the right degree of foot flare for you. Some people like to keep their feet straight, some prefer a slight foot flare, and others like to turn their feet out a lot. Regardless of the stance you choose, both feet should be flared to the same degree. A lot of people make the mistake of adopting an asymmetrical stance by positioning one foot straight and turning the other out, which throws off their balance and technique. Always pay attention to the orientation of your feet and make sure you're setting up symmetrically—unless, of course, you have asymmetrical hips and you've determined through experimentation (and ideally through working with an experienced coach) that squatting feels better when each foot is uniquely aligned, but that is rare.

Stance Width

When it comes to stance width, you can stand with your feet positioned underneath your hips (narrow stance), shoulder width or just outside shoulder width (standard stance), or outside shoulder width apart (wide/sumo stance). In general, standing with your feet just outside shoulder width allows you to squat to full depth without compromising your strength, making it the most common and universal squat stance.

Adopting a wide stance enables you to lift heavier loads and is great if you want to squat only to parallel, making it the preferred stance for most powerlifters, especially those who use specialized training gear.

A narrower stance is often required if you want to squat to full depth or deeper than parallel, but everyone is different—some people can get deeper with a wider stance.

I recommend employing all three stances in your routine. Most people, myself included, squat primarily from a standard stance (just outside shoulder width), but I also squat from a wide/sumo stance for variety. Switching up your stances targets your glutes and stresses your muscles in slightly different ways, forcing your body to adapt in ways that potentially improve strength and grow muscle.

STANDARD STANCE

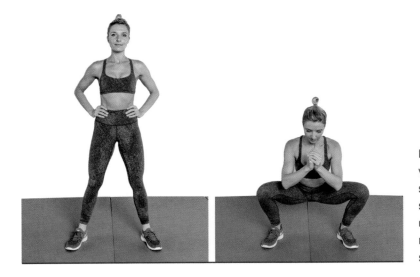

In general, standing with your feet just outside shoulder width allows you to squat to full depth without compromising your strength, making it the most universal squat stance.

SUMO (WIDE) STANCE

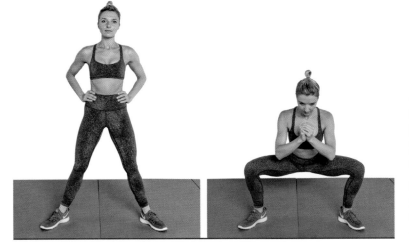

Adopting a wide, or sumo, stance allows you to lift heavier loads and is great if you want to squat only to parallel, making it the preferred stance for most powerlifters, especially those who use specialized training gear.

NARROW STANCE

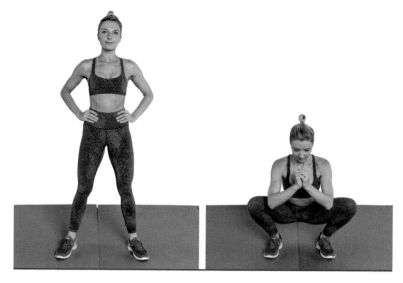

Some lifters prefer a narrow stance, likely due to hip anatomy and ankle mobility.

B-Stance

The B-stance is a hybrid between a single-leg and a double-leg exercise. You place around 70 percent of your weight on your front leg, with the remaining 30 percent on your back leg. Typically, I use the B-stance for the high-bar back squat, but you can use it for front squats, too. This stance is great for athletes because a staggered stance is common in most sports. If you have one side that is weaker than the other, you can also use the B-stance to home in on your weak side and create balance and symmetry.

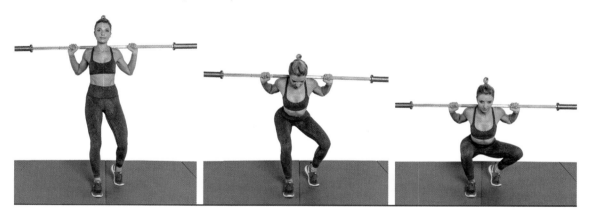

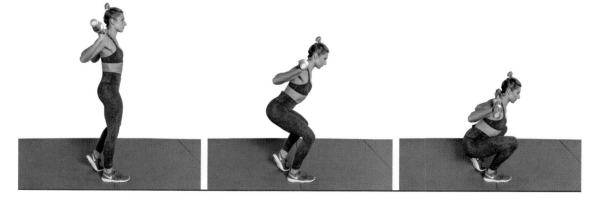

SPINAL POSITION: ARCH YOUR BACK, KEEP YOUR CHEST UP, AND KEEP YOUR SPINE IN THE NEUTRAL ZONE

As with most exercises, you want to keep your spine as neutral as possible throughout the entire range of the movement. In other words, the less spinal motion, the better. (To learn more about the importance of keeping your spine in a neutral zone, refer to page 139.) Many people break into spinal hyperextension or round forward. To prevent these faults, most trainers tell their clients to "arch your back" or "keep your chest up," which is another way of saying "don't round."

But you have to be careful when using these cues. They do work, especially when people are struggling out of the bottom position, but they can be misinterpreted. For example, some people hear the "chest up" or "arch your back" cue and hyperextend by creating an exaggerated bend in their lower back, which takes them outside the neutral zone. But this tendency is more common in individuals with hypermobile spines and can easily be avoided by stabilizing the spine properly.

Trainers also have to be careful with the "arch your back" cue because beginners might interpret it as rounding. I made that mistake early on in my personal training career. A client I was working with was doing box squats, and on her first rep, she rounded forward a little bit. So, on the next rep, I told her to arch more, and to my surprise she rounded even farther forward because she thought *arch* meant to round forward, which makes sense for a beginner who has never heard that cue before. If you think of an arch on a bridge, for example, then it is easy to see how someone might interpret arching as flexion, or rounding forward. It was a good lesson for me. As trainers, we have to realize that our clients might not know what we mean, so we need to be careful to explain and demonstrate proper spinal mechanics before we start shouting cues.

BRACING AND BREATHING: BRACE YOUR SPINE BEFORE YOU INITIATE THE MOVEMENT

To stabilize your spine and maintain a neutral spinal position, take a big breath into your belly and chest (around 70 percent of your maximum lung capacity) and then tighten your core (abs, obliques, erectors, and diaphragm muscles). If you're performing a one-rep max, you can hold your breath throughout the entire range of the movement and then breathe out once you reach the top position, or you can start to let out air as you rise out of the bottom position and pass the sticking region (the part of the lift where you slow down due to a mechanical disadvantage) and take a breath in once you complete the lift. More specifically, when you reach the top position, relax your diaphragm and let out the rest of your air. Keep your postural muscles on tension to maintain a neutral spine. Then rebrace by drawing in another breath and tightening the muscles of your trunk.

If you're performing a heavy set of 5 to 10 reps, you can still hold your breath on each rep to maximize spinal stability and strength, but you have to breathe in at the top position and rebrace before starting your next rep. If you're performing high repetitions—say, 10 or more—you can breathe rhythmically by inhaling during the lowering (eccentric) phase and exhaling during the rising (concentric) phase.

HEAD POSITION: FOCUS YOUR GAZE FORWARD

The same rule that applies to your spine also applies to your head position: you want your head and neck in the neutral zone. More specifically, don't look up or down.

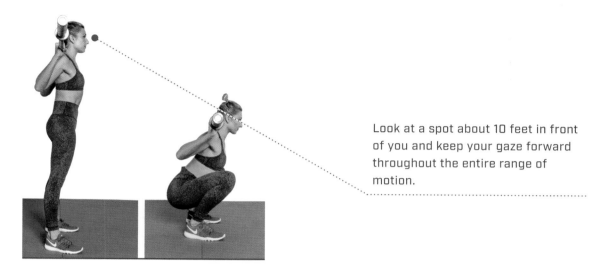

Look at a spot about 10 feet in front of you and keep your gaze forward throughout the entire range of motion.

KNEE POSITION: PUSH YOUR KNEES OUT

Driving your knees out helps you lower deeper into the squat and prevents your knees from collapsing inward, which is a mechanism for knee pain and other injuries. (See page 141 to learn more about the valgus knee fault error and how to correct it.)

Just as people can misinterpret the "chest up" and "arch your back" cues, a lot of people think that "knees out" means to take a wider stance. So I often say that "knees out" means not letting your knees cave inward, known as knee valgus. Another way to think about knee position is to keep your femurs (thighs) over your toes as you squat.

The "knees out" cue is particularly important as you rise out of the bottom of the squat. Hardly anyone caves on the way down; it's on the way up, right out of the hole, when you really need to focus on driving your knees out.

KNEE FLARE CONTINUUM

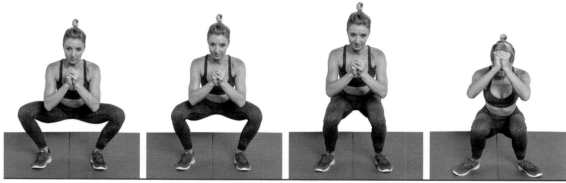

Depending on your mobility, you can flare your knees out past your feet or align your thighs over your toes. Driving your knees out in the bottom of the squat helps prevent knee valgus, which occurs when your knees cave inward.

FOOT PRESSURE: PUSH THROUGH YOUR HEELS

As you squat, think about keeping your weight evenly distributed over your heels. This places tension on your hips/glutes and keeps you balanced. You can also experiment with distributing your weight over your ankles or driving through your entire foot. Avoid driving through the balls of your feet, which would shift tension to your knees/quads and compromise your balance. Put simply, "push through your heels" means "don't come up onto the balls of your feet."

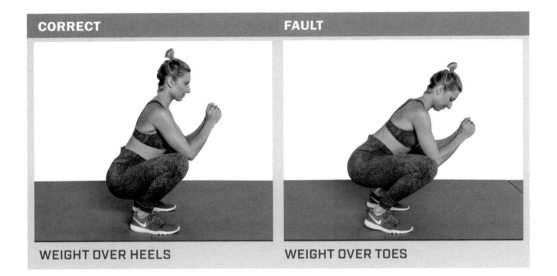

CORRECT — WEIGHT OVER HEELS

FAULT — WEIGHT OVER TOES

SQUAT DEPTH

To get the best results from squatting, you need to squat to parallel, sinking your hip crease just below the center of your knee joint. Depending on your anatomy and mobility, this may be as deep as you can squat. If you can maintain good form while squatting deeper, then a full-depth squat might be beneficial. I'm a big fan of deep squats as long as they are well tolerated, meaning that you can maintain good form and don't feel pain. Some individuals can perform only half squats properly, and this is fine; these lifters actually see better results because they get strong in their functional ranges without experiencing any discomfort.

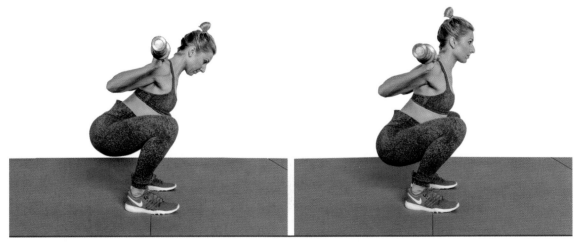

PARALLEL SQUAT

FULL-DEPTH SQUAT

TORSO LEAN

As you lower into the bottom of the squat, you need to lean your torso forward slightly. How far you lean depends on your hip and ankle mobility, hip anatomy, and anthropometry (limb length), but for most people, the lean shouldn't exceed 45 degrees. The only exception is if you have relatively long femurs and a short torso. As you learned in Chapter 5, people with long femurs and short torsos have a more pronounced forward lean when they squat, whereas people with short femurs and long torsos typically squat with a more upright posture.

The degree of your torso lean is also determined by the type of squat you're performing. People who squat only to parallel generally have more pronounced forward-leaning torsos, while people who perform full squats generally have more upright torsos.

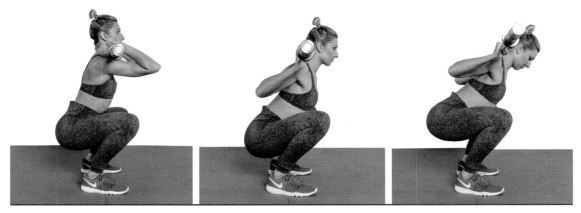

UPRIGHT SQUAT   SLIGHT LEAN SQUAT   FORWARD LEAN SQUAT

HIPS AND KNEES BREAK SIMULTANEOUSLY

As you lower into a squat, your hips and knees should break (bend) at the same time. Simply stated, you should have relatively even motion from your hips and knees as you initiate and lower into the squat. This is especially true for a parallel squat. Think about sitting your hips back as you lower your elevation and bend your knees. In a full squat, you initiate the downward movement by sinking your hips straight down between your thighs while flaring your knees outward at a 45-degree angle. The former type requires a deeper hip hinge, while the latter entails a more pronounced knee bend. In both versions, your hips and knees break simultaneously.

INITIATING PARALLEL SQUAT   **INITIATING FULL SQUAT**

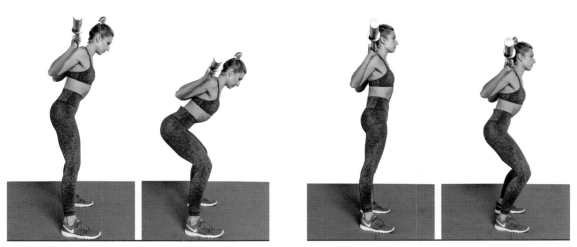

HIP AND KNEE DRIVE

Just as you want fairly even hip and knee motion as you lower into a squat, you want even motion at your hips and knees as you drive upward. Your torso angle should remain constant during the first half of the rising phase and then become more upright as you stand into the finish position.

PARALLEL SQUAT

FULL SQUAT

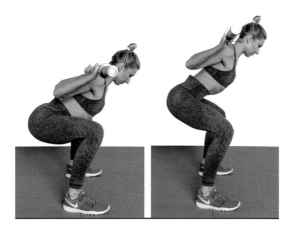

SQUEEZING YOUR GLUTES

Some people squeeze their glutes as they reach the top position to help lock out their hips and stabilize their spinal position. This is fine as long as you don't excessively push your hips forward and it doesn't throw off your technique. But don't do it as a strategy for increasing glute hypertrophy. Squeezing your glutes does increase glute activation, which is a good thing, but I highly doubt it will lead to greater glute gains, especially if you're already performing hip thrusts and back extensions.

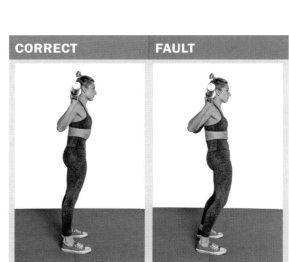

KEEP THE LOAD BALANCED OVER THE MIDDLE OF YOUR FEET

This cue applies mostly to barbell squat variations such as front, back, and Zercher squats. From a profile view, the barbell should bisect the middle of your foot. If the bar floats over your toes, it will place unnecessary pressure on your lower back. If the bar shifts backward toward your heels, it will throw you off-balance. The best way to check your form is to have someone film you or take photos of you from the side. From there, you can make the necessary adjustments.

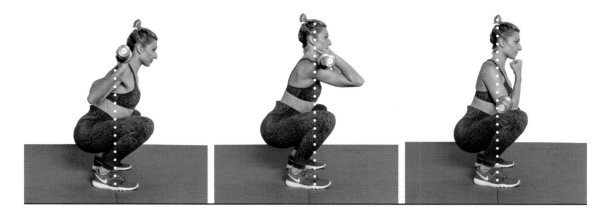

MASTER A ROUTINE

Squatting correctly is a serious skill. And like any skill, it's important to master a routine to ensure a successful outcome. Think of setting up for a squat like shooting a free-throw in basketball or putting in golf. Patterning a routine increases your chances of success.

Watch experienced lifters perform squats, and you will notice that every rep looks the same, meaning that they squat to the same depth with the same form every single time. When taking a barbell out of a rack, they move precisely and efficiently. Though squatting routines differ slightly from person to person, they are similar in that the lifter forms their grip symmetrically on the bar, unracks the weight, takes only a couple of steps back, assumes their stance, braces their spine, and then squats down and up with the same form.

Watch beginners squat, on the other hand, and you will notice that they squat to a different depth on every rep and that their form is all over the place. When they perform barbell lifts, they line up asymmetrically, take too many steps back, and then shimmy their hips and constantly adjust their stance in an attempt to get comfortable.

The point is, you want to develop a routine that sets you up to squat with optimal technique. Consider all of the squat guidelines previously covered and experiment to find the right sequence of movements. Once you find your ideal routine, practice squatting the same way over and over again until it becomes instinctual. The less you have to think about the individual steps, the better you will become at squatting and the stronger you will be. In short, once you master your routine, the easier it is to get in the zone and focus on the task at hand.

Many lifters are interested in squatting deeper—especially powerlifters. We all have unique skeletons, and the sizes and shapes of our bones highly influence our movement patterns. Often we can perform mobility drills and exercises to improve our joint range of motion, but other times our bones and ligaments limit us. Nevertheless, there are several strategies that can help you get deeper in a squat, and these strategies have sound biomechanical rationale supporting them.

If you train for aesthetics/physique purposes, then you should squat to the depth that suits your body best. For some people, this means a full squat, but for others, it means stopping just shy of parallel. If you compete in powerlifting, however, then you must descend at least to parallel—that is, your hip crease must sink deeper than the center of your knee joint.

If you're interested in increasing your squat depth, experiment with the following strategies and choose the methods that work well for you.

HIP MOBILITY DRILLS

In order to squat deep, you need to sink your hips deep, which requires hip mobility. I'm only scratching the surface with the techniques I offer here, so I encourage you to experiment with different mobility drills that might not be listed.

Dynamic means you're moving and performing repetitions or pulses. For example, when you pulse, you move into your end range, hold the position for one or two seconds, move just out of end range, and then repeat. For example, 3 sets of 10 repetitions on each side is a sample warm-up. Dynamic mobility drills will reduce stiffness, increase your overall joint range of motion, and help prepare you for more strenuous exercise without interfering with your strength.

Static means you're holding at end range for a set period of time, say 30 seconds or 1 minute per side. Static mobility drills also improve flexibility, but they interfere with strength, which is why they are done after a training session. For more hip stretches, flip back to page 154.

QUADRUPED STRETCH

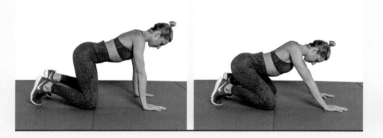

DEEP LUNGE STRETCH

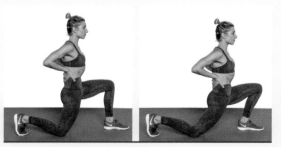

HIP EXTERNAL ROTATION STRETCH

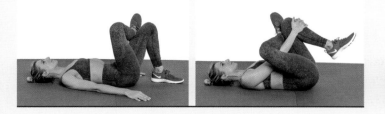

PIGEON POSE STRETCH

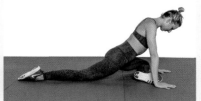

ANKLE MOBILITY DRILLS

Ankle mobility probably has the biggest impact on squat depth. As you lower into a squat, you need to maintain an upright torso, and your knees have to track forward over your ankles. Put simply, squatting deep requires good ankle dorsiflexion range of motion, which these drills will help improve. Just like the hip mobility drills, you can perform dynamic ankle mobility drills at the beginning of a workout and static calf stretches after the workout.

STANDING KNEE GLIDES

KNEELING KNEE GLIDES

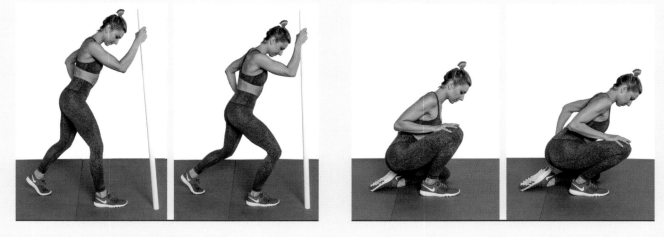

FRONT LOAD PLACEMENT

Positioning a load in front of your body helps you sink deeper into the squat because you have to maintain an upright torso position. Let's say your spine and femur form a 40-degree angle. If you're upright, this angle gets your hips deeper than if you're leaning forward.

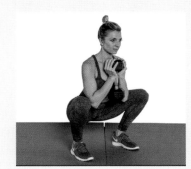

HIGH BAR PLACEMENT

Like the front squat variations, the high-bar back squat forces you to keep your torso more upright, which allows you to sink deeper into the squat. When you place the bar lower on your back, you have to lean your torso forward to maintain your balance, which prevents you from dropping your hips past parallel.

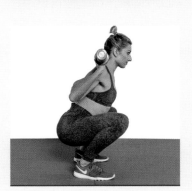

QUAD STRENGTHENING

When you squat with an upright torso, your quads have to work a lot harder to achieve full squat depth. So the stronger your quads, the easier it is to maintain an upright torso. You can strengthen your quads by squatting—specifically by doing front squats, goblet squats, and high-bar back squats—but also by doing Bulgarian split squats, leg presses, and leg extension exercises.

HEEL ELEVATION

Though ankle mobility drills may help improve ankle dorsiflexion, which in turn will improve squat depth, improving mobility can take a long time. What's more, some people may never get enough ankle dorsiflexion due to their anatomy, regardless of how much they stretch. Elevating your heels reduces the amount of ankle dorsiflexion required, allowing your knees to come forward and your hips to drop lower. There are several ways to do this: you can wear squat shoes with elevated heels, stand on a wedge, or place your heels on 5- or 10-pound plates. This is an immediate solution for most people, and it's one of my favorite deep squat hacks.

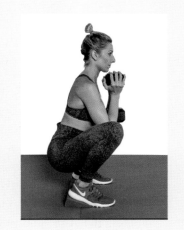

Now, some coaches say never to use heel lifts because they set you up for future problems, but I disagree. How does improving your ability to squat with good form create future problems? You stay more upright and it feels better. Olympic lifters wear shoes that elevate their heels, and these are people who squat three to five days per week.

Their rationale is, "You need to teach people how to squat without a heel lift and prescribe ankle mobility drills so they can build that mobility." But you can still work on improving your mobility while working on your squat. Elevating your heels gives you artificial ankle mobility, not only making it easier to squat upright but also allowing you to target your quads. And for people with really bad ankle mobility who want to squat to full depth, elevating the heels is a must. I've used this variation in my own training and with a lot of my clients with great success.

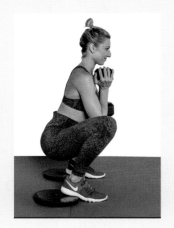

GLUTE ACTIVATION

When the glutes contract, they exert a rearward pull on the heads of the femurs. If your glutes are not firing optimally, your hip flexion range of motion may decrease slightly because the heads of your femurs are bumping into your acetabulums (hip sockets). Performing glute activation drills essentially wakes up your glutes and helps them fire optimally, which can help clear this impingement, allowing you sink a little deeper into the squat. I offer a few options below. For a more comprehensive list of glute activation drills and a sample warm-up, see page 152.

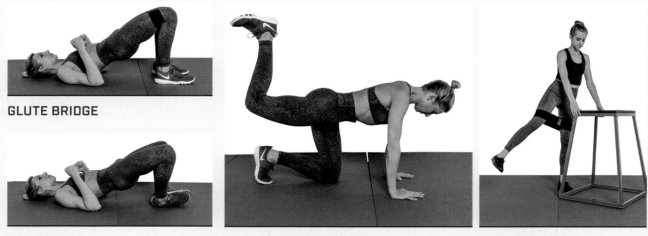

GLUTE BRIDGE

FROG PUMP

QUADRUPED HIP EXTENSION

HIP ABDUCTION

FAULTS AND CORRECTIONS

Squatting is a movement pattern that requires a lot of coordination. All of the muscles in your body have to work in concert to balance a vertical load as you move your hips, knees, and ankles through a full range of motion: you have to find your ideal stance, brace your spine and stay in your neutral zone, break at your hips and knees to initiate the movement, lean your torso forward but not too much, and push your knees out as you rise out of the bottom position. That's a lot of actions to coordinate. And things get a lot more challenging when you add weight and start experimenting with different load positions.

But here's the deal: you can prevent potentially harmful form-related errors simply by following the guidelines previously outlined and studying the individual technique descriptions covered later in the section. However, a few faults that apply to all of the squat exercise variations—butt wink, knee valgus, and early hip drive—are worth examining. If you can avoid these faults, you will not only get stronger in every variation but also significantly reduce your risk of getting injured or feeling pain while squatting.

FAULT: BUTT WINK

The term "butt wink" refers to a posterior pelvic tilt in the bottom of a squat. It's true that butt winking, or allowing the pelvis to rotate posteriorly (tilt backward), can cause lower back pain and injury, especially during a heavy squat. Depending on your hip anatomy, anthropometry, motor control, and mobility, you may butt wink early in the squat, later on as your hip crease drops below your knees (past parallel), or as you reach full depth.

But there is a little bit of wiggle room, or an acceptable butt-winking zone. This is where having a trained eye for the art of lifting is important. I can't give you a precise zone or tell you exactly how many degrees of winking is acceptable because it is different for everyone. You need to listen to your body and the signals it's sending. If you tend to butt wink a little bit and you never feel pain, then it might be fine. If you butt wink a lot and your lower back hurts every time you squat, then it's a problem. So you shouldn't be paranoid about butt winking, but you should be cognizant of your technique and try to err on the side of maintaining a neutral spine.

When your spine is neutral, you're set up optimally to withstand the compressive forces acting on your spine (think core muscle contractions and load). But when you posterior pelvic tilt or butt wink, you pull your lumbar spine into flexion. Now, you're not in the best position to handle these compressive forces, and you risk disc herniation and other lower back injuries.

To help you understand why the butt wink occurs, I'll address each of the variables that can contribute to this fault. You can also check out the video I posted on my YouTube channel titled "Squat Biomechanics and Butt Wink."

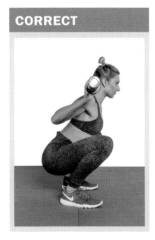

FAULT

CORRECT

Hip Anatomy

It should come as no surprise that the shape of your pelvis determines how deeply you can squat without butt winking. To put this in more technical terms, the way the head of your femur articulates within your hip socket governs how deeply you can squat. For example, say the head of your femur jams into the ridge of your acetabulum (hip socket) as you squat to parallel. In this scenario, it doesn't matter how mobile and flexible you are; there's nowhere for your femur to go. The only way to drop below parallel is to butt wink. That is, your pelvis has to rotate posteriorly to accommodate deeper ranges of hip flexion, causing your lumbar spine to round with it.

CORRECTION:

Squat only to ranges that feel comfortable and allow you to maintain good form. To accurately gauge how far to squat, use the box squat techniques on pages 428 to 430.

Motor Control

A lot of muscles are working in concert when you squat: glutes, hamstrings, quads, adductors, erectors, and abdominals, to mention a few. If you're an inexperienced squatter or you haven't learned how to squat correctly, then your muscles may not act in proper coordination. For example, the glutes can pull rearward on the heads of the femurs when activated, which keeps them centered properly in the socket. This is what I mean by motor control. If you're not moving with proper form—you're not stabilizing your spine, driving your knees out, activating your glutes, and so on—then that might contribute to excessive butt winking.

CORRECTION:

Follow the guidelines previously outlined, reduce the range of motion of your squat, and practice box and bodyweight squats before progressing to the more complex variations.

Mobility

The vast majority of people assume that the butt wink is caused by poor flexibility. For example, some say that when your hamstrings are tight, they pull on your pelvis, causing you to butt wink. While a lack of hip mobility—that is, the ability to move actively through a joint range of motion—certainly can cause the butt wink, this mobility restriction is not usually related to tight muscles. Now, I'm not saying that stretching can't help, because it can, but saying that your hamstrings, hip flexors, or adductors are the cause of your butt wink is inaccurate. Your hamstrings and rectus femoris don't lengthen (that much) as you lower into a squat, which would have to be the case for tight hamstrings and quads to be a limiting factor. And some of your hip flexors shorten as you descend, so that can't be it, either.

However, if your ankles are tight, meaning that you have limited ankle dorsiflexion range of motion, then your knees will be prevented from moving forward, which is necessary for staying balanced and centered in the squat. If you severely lack ankle dorsiflexion mobility, the only way to stay balanced and centered in a deep squat is to butt wink. In this situation, working on your ankle mobility can certainly improve and may even prevent your lower back from rounding into flexion, but there's only so much improvement to be made with various stretching techniques. Mobility is greatly influenced by skeletal anatomy, and not everyone can develop superior ankle dorsiflexion range of motion.

CORRECTION:

Work on your hip and ankle mobility. Another option is to elevate your heels by positioning your heels on plates or wearing squat shoes with elevated heels. See the sidebar on pages 420 to 423 for more options and to learn how to increase squat depth.

FAULT: EARLY HIP DRIVE

Early hip drive occurs when the hips shoot up out of the hole. Your knees extend rapidly while your hips remain at a similar angle, which causes you to essentially turn the squat into a good morning. The main cause of this fault is insufficient quad strength. If the quads can't do the job, the only way to get the bar up is to rely more on the hips. And the hips are stronger when the legs are straighter since they're in a position to better use the hamstrings for hip extension strength.

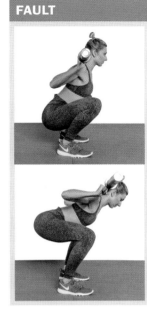

FAULT

Many squatting experts blame glute or back strength for early hip drive, but it's actually weak quads. It is true that you're carrying excessive knee extension out of the hole when you shoot your hips up, but the barbell won't move upward much because the hips don't extend; you're essentially dumping your torso forward and "stalling" until your hamstrings lengthen to a position where the hips can take over and carry out the lift. The problems with this technique are that 1) it's ugly, 2) it puts more pressure on your lower back, and 3) it turns a squat, which is a knee-dominant exercise, into a good morning, which is a hip-dominant exercise.

CORRECTION:
Strengthen your quads with front squats, high-bar squats, goblet squats, and leg extensions. Keep your form in check so that you never practice and ingrain the early hip drive. Eventually, your quad strength will catch up, and your go-to movement pattern for the squat will become more balanced, with your hips and knees extending in sync.

FAULT: KNEE VALGUS

Knee valgus (also referred to as *valgus collapse* or *medial knee displacement*) occurs when the knees cave inward. It's characterized by hip adduction, internal rotation, and ankle inversion. This fault is particularly problematic when landing from a jump, which is how people tear their ACLs or damage their knees. Serious injuries like these are not as common with the squat, but over time, excessive and consistent knee valgus puts unnecessary stress on the lateral aspect of the knee, which can eventually lead to knee pain. What's more, you're ingraining a movement pattern that might rear its ugly head when you're doing something more dynamic. In short, it's best to avoid the knee valgus fault when squatting.

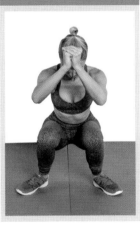

FAULT

If you're an advanced athlete, you might have a little wiggle room when it comes to this fault. For example, Olympic weightlifters sometimes catch weight in the bottom of a squat with their knees slightly caved in, but they immediately reclaim a good position by pushing their knees out. I call this a *valgus knee twitch* because the motion is subtle and looks athletic. When beginners do it, however, it doesn't look nearly as athletic. Strength coaches call it the *melting candle syndrome* because they cave everywhere; the back rounds, the knees cave inward, and the ankles collapse, and they rarely reclaim a good position.

This is one of those circumstances in which you need to learn the rules before you can break the rules. In the beginning, everyone should try to avoid the knee valgus fault. But once you become more advanced and you understand the pros and cons, you can decide whether to

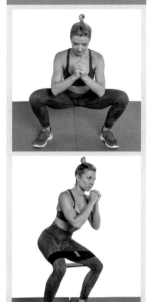

accept more risk. Sometimes lifters are willing to sacrifice their form to lift more weight, such as rounding the upper back in a deadlift or allowing a slight knee valgus in the bottom of a squat.

CORRECTION 1:

Knee valgus generally occurs as you drive out of the bottom position. One of the best strategies for correcting it is to film yourself squatting. I had a client who had horrible knee valgus, and I thought I would never be able to get her to break the pattern. I would tell her "knees out," but she just couldn't get it. So I started filming her head on, and to my surprise she enjoyed watching the videos. She started memorizing the association between a proper squat and a valgus squat. In a very short period, she had corrected her movement pattern and was squatting with great form—that is, she started driving her knees out as she descended and rose out of the bottom position.

CORRECTION 2:

If you struggle with knee valgus, try positioning a resistance band (such as a Glute Loop or mini band) above or below your knees. The inward resistance of the band forces you to drive your knees outward to counter the inward pressure, which is the action I'm referring to when I say, "knees out." If you're using a Glute Loop, I recommend the large/extra-large size to allow for more knees-out action.

SQUAT CATEGORIES AND VARIATIONS

There are many ways to squat: in a wide stance, in a narrow stance, in a B-stance (staggered stance), or to a box. You can also vary the exercise based on the equipment you're using and where you place the load on your body. For example, if the load is positioned on your back, it's considered a back squat. If the load is positioned on your delts, it's considered a front squat. And if you're holding the load in your arms/hands below your chest, it's considered a hang squat (this is a name I created to categorize this squat).

In the following pages, I explain the characteristics of each squat variation: what it's good for, who it's good for, and how to change it up with different equipment. Before you delve into the variations, though, I want to emphasize the importance of experimenting with *all* of the various types of squats, because different types might activate your glutes to different degrees.

Sure, all squat exercise variations are similar for glute activation, but some people get the highest activation from low-bar back squats, while others get more activation from front squats. And some report more glute activation with a sumo (wide) stance over a narrower stance and vice versa. So the squat variation that is best for glute development is the one where you feel your glutes activate the most and allows you to progressively overload safely and comfortably over time. If deep squats hurt your hips or lower back, then those are not the best for your glute development. If you tolerate back squats and box squats well, then stick with those variations. In short, choose the variations that feel best and then prioritize those in your training.

Load also plays a factor. I've trained a lot of people who report feeling higher levels of glute activation with submaximal loads—where they're not lifting as much weight as they can and not going to failure, but rather focusing on technique—compared to lifting ultra-heavy, probably because their form breaks down. I also believe that you get higher activation when the load is positioned closer to your center. For example, goblet squats tend to elicit high levels of glute activation because the load is generally light and centered on the body. You can also increase glute activation by performing knee-banded squat variations, which I cover on page 446.

Again, we all have different hip anatomy, anthropometry, and muscle architecture, and these factors dictate which squat variation is best for glute development. However, it's impossible to know the precise technique and loading that maximize glute gains, which is why it is important to use a shotgun approach. That is, you have to practice a variety of squats with a variety of loads and effort, and then, through experience and tinkering, you can find the variations that produce the best results—the ones that feel good, don't cause you discomfort, and align with your goals.

To help you understand the utility and application of each type of squat, the different loading and equipment options, and the proper way to set up and execute the exercises, I've divided the squat variations into six categories. Each category represents one style of squatting, which is based on the load position and equipment.

The six squat categories are organized from easiest to most difficult. I also include the different equipment and loading options for each category. As a reminder, you can apply the different stances—narrow stance, sumo stance, and B-stance—to all of the variations.

LEARNING TO SQUAT: SQUAT PROGRESSION

On the surface, squatting seems like a simple, everyday movement: squat down and stand back up. But when you try to squat with good form, add weight, and/or start experimenting with variations, it becomes a highly coordinated effort. To make learning how to squat easier, it's helpful to follow a progression. Here's the sequence of squats that I use to help beginners develop the coordination to squat with good form.

I start with a bodyweight box squat and teach them how to sit their hips back while counterbalancing with their arms held out in front of their body. I position the box height to about parallel (knee height) to test their range of motion. Once they can squat with good form, I do one of several things, depending on their technique, mobility, age, and experience. If the parallel bodyweight box squat looks good, I lower the box to rock bottom and see if they can perform a full squat. If they continue to demonstrate good form, the next thing I do is remove the box and have them perform the movement without a depth gauge. It's important to note that you can use a box to gauge distance with all of the squat variations, but at a certain point the box needs to be removed so they know when and how to reverse the movement in midair. From there, assuming everything still looks and feels good, I introduce the goblet squat to test their ability to squat with load. Once they can do that without struggle, I start to experiment with the more complex squat variations, such as the barbell front squat and back squats.

It's important to mention that some people skip right to goblet squats after experimenting with the box squat, while others need to stick with a parallel bodyweight box squat to dial in their mechanics. Put simply, everyone needs to progress at their own pace. Use the squat progression sequence that I've provided here as a learning and teaching template, and move on to the next squat once you can perform the movement safely and effectively.

BOX SQUATS

I've trained thousands of people, and every one of them has been able to squat to some degree. Yet some people say that not everyone is built to squat. The reasons cited usually relate to poor mobility, hip socket orientation and depth, femur length—the list goes on and on. I agree, these characteristics can make squatting problematic, but that's only the case for full-range squats. Unless someone has a medical condition that prevents them from squatting, every healthy individual I've trained could squat to a box positioned at their knees or higher.

Again, squatting with good form and knowing how far to descend creates some challenges. But if you have something to aim for, it's a lot easier. You don't have to think about reversing the movement in midair; you can just sit down as if you were sitting in a chair. In this way, the box squat is a tool to help people gauge distance and overcome their fear of squatting.

Think about it: most lifts have a beginning and an end point. Take the bench press, for example: you lower the bar to your chest and then go back up. Or the deadlift: you start with the bar on the ground and then stand upright. But the squat is different in that the end point is where your form breaks down, which adds another layer of complexity and coordination. The box squat is useful because it provides an end point. You don't have the think about when to reverse the motion because the box tells you. Now you can focus on mechanics while incrementally adjusting the box height lower and lower as you dial in your technique.

This is known as *progressive distance training,* which is another form of progressive overload. But instead of increasing weight over time, you're increasing range of motion over time. When it comes to progressive distance training, it's important to use form as your guide. If you can adhere to the guidelines previously covered and it feels good, then keep progressing. But if your form starts to fall apart—you round forward, you hyperextend through the lower back, or your knees cave inward—then you might need to squat to a taller box. I've worked with elderly clients for whom it took a year just to get to parallel (hip crease and knees in line). And that is perfectly fine. In fact, I work with a lot of advanced lifters who squat only to parallel, and they have the same level of glute development as people who squat below parallel (hip crease below knees).

The point is, we all progress at different rates. With time and consistent practice, you will improve. Once you get to a point where you can squat with control and coordination, you can remove the box and start experimenting with free squats. But that doesn't mean the box squat is obsolete. Even the most advanced lifters incorporate box squats in their training. In fact, there are many different methods of box squatting, each of which offers specific benefits. Let's review all of the box squatting techniques, starting with the most basic variation.

Sit-to-Box Squat

It should come as no surprise that the shape of your pelvis determines how deeply you can squat without butt winking. To put this in more technical terms, the way the head of your femur articulates within your hip socket governs how deep you can squat. For example, say the head of your femur jams into the ridge of your acetabulum (hip socket) as you squat to parallel. In this scenario, it doesn't matter how mobile and flexible you are; there's nowhere for your femur to go. The only way to drop below parallel is to butt wink. That is, your pelvis has to rotate posteriorly to accommodate deeper ranges of hip flexion, causing your lumbar spine to round with it.

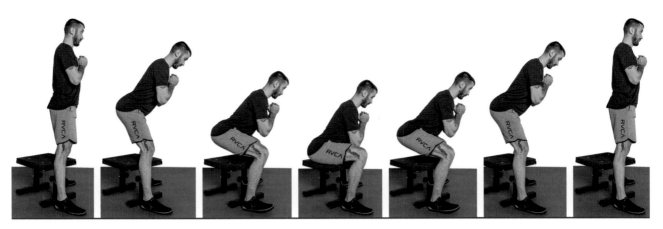

Choose a plyometric box, padded box, or squat box and adjust the height so it's just below your knee line. If you're just starting out, you might want to set the box above knee height. Next, angle the box so the corner is positioned between your feet. Assume your squat stance and back up to the box until your legs make contact with the box, then brace your spine. You can hold your arms at your chest, extend them out in front of you, or raise them as you descend. To execute the squat, lower your butt to the box by hinging from your hips and bending your knees, keeping your back as flat as possible. If you're performing a parallel box squat, sit your hips back and keep your shins vertical. If you're performing a full squat, you sit your hips almost straight down between your thighs (see the low-bar and high-bar back squat variations). With both squats, the key is to lower down with control. Don't just plop onto the box. As soon as your butt makes contact with the box, reverse the position and stand upright by extending your knees, hips, and torso in one fluid motion. Put simply, the moment your butt makes contact with the surface, you stand back up.

BENCH SQUAT

You can use a bench in place of a box, or as a tool to get comfortable squatting. With this variation, you straddle the bench, so you can see it out in front of you, which provides a sense of security as you initiate the squat. But there are a couple of caveats. First, it's harder to adjust the height of the bench. If you are tall, the bench might be a good height for you, but it tends to be too high for most people. You can add padding or bumper plates or even elevate the bench to adjust the height, but I generally don't recommend any of these methods because they're not as safe: if the bench is unstable or you misread the height, your chances of getting injured are much higher. You need to use a stable bench with a wide enough base that it won't tip over or rock from side to side. This creates another potential problem, though, because most sturdy benches also have a wide top, forcing you to take a wide stance. So the bench is a good option, but only in the right circumstances.

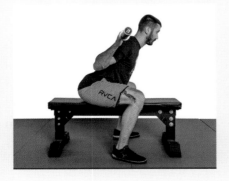

Straddle the center of the bench. With the front of the bench in your line of sight, you can effectively gauge your squat depth. From here, execute the squat exactly as previously described.

Box Pause Squat

With the box pause squat, you sit down, relax the muscles of your legs and hips, pause for one or two seconds, and then stand up. Even though you're actively relaxing your leg muscles, you keep your spine stable and your postural muscles engaged. More specifically, you maintain an arch with your erectors activated and keep your spine braced by maintaining tension in your trunk and upper body. If you're performing the barbell variations, I recommend starting out light, but some people actually become stronger with the box squat compared to the back squat.

To my knowledge, there is no research assigning any particular muscle- or strength-building benefits to this particular variation. In theory, it may improve your ability to drive out of the bottom position because you lose the rebound effect, and research shows superior acceleration off the box compared to back squats. What I can say is that it's another useful tool to practice the squat movement pattern. Remember, performing a variety of exercises is important not only for working the muscle in a unique way but also for developing and honing your technique. By performing the same movement pattern in a slightly different way, you bring a heightened sense of awareness to your movement and force your body to adapt to a novel stimulus, which fosters adaptation, growth, and technique.

Rocking Box Squat

The rocking box squat is similar to the box pause squat, but instead of sitting down and then standing back up, you sit down, lean back into an upright position, and then lean forward and stand back up. It's a rocking motion, and you use the momentum of your forward lean to push out of the bottom position. This is my favorite box squat variation because you can get into a nice rhythm when you do it correctly. However, a lot of trainers don't like it because people have a hard time keeping their spine braced, and the rocking motion is not characteristic of a conventional back squat. Even so, it's another valuable box squat variation that can help develop strength and technique with the squat movement pattern. Like the box pause squat, it's best to keep the load light, and you really have to focus on keeping your spine neutral. Rounding or overemphasizing arching your back with a heavy load while sitting on a box is a recipe for disaster, so you have to be careful and focus on maintaining good form.

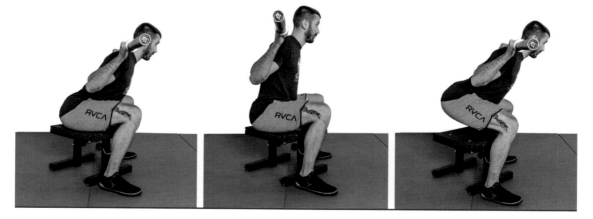

Set up exactly as you would when performing a sit-to-box squat, angling the corner of a box between your legs and backing your legs up to the base. Sit down to the box, but instead of standing back up, rock back by bringing your torso into an upright position, then lean forward and stand up. When you rock back, don't relax all of your muscles—your erectors in particular should stay engaged so that you never round your back. Keep your chest up and your spine braced and rigid (slightly arched or straight) as you sit down and drive out of the bottom position.

BODYWEIGHT SQUATS (FREE SQUATS/AIR SQUATS)

Once you're comfortable squatting down to a box and initiating the squat with your hips, it's time to remove the box and work on reversing the position in midair. If you train with the box enough, your body will remember how far to go down. Most veteran squatters squat to the same height every time, whether there is a box or not. This is the goal. A box can help ingrain that depth, but you will never pattern it by just box squatting. At a certain point, you have to free squat. Beginners use the bodyweight squat (also referred to as the free squat or air squat) to develop strength and coordination. But as you gain proficiency, you should reserve the free squat mainly for warming up, high-repetition burnouts, and conditioning work.

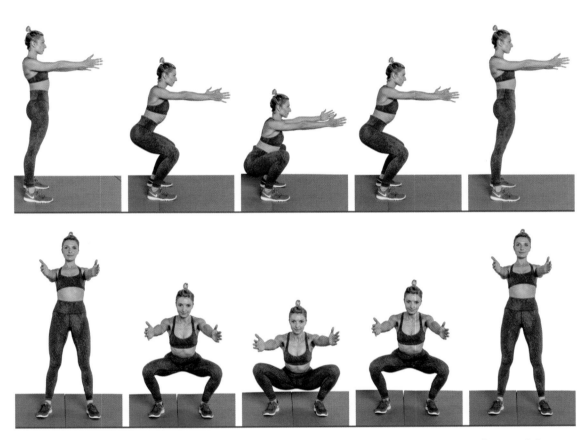

Assume a wide (sumo), medium, or narrow squat stance. Make sure you're standing upright with your back flat and head neutral, looking straight ahead or roughly 10 feet out in front of you. You can start with your arms at your chest, down at your sides, or extended out in front of you like a mummy to counterbalance your weight. If you're performing a parallel squat, initiate the movement by sitting your hips back, tilting your torso forward, and bending your knees, keeping your shins as vertical as possible. If you're performing a full squat (as in the photos above), sit your hips straight down between your thighs and allow your knees to drift forward over your feet as you descend. With both variations, drive your knees out as you lower your hips and bend your knees. If your arms are down at your sides, start to raise your arms as you lower your elevation. When you reach your ideal depth, reverse the movement by driving through your heels, and extending your knees and hips in one fluid motion while continuing to drive your knees out. Squeeze your glutes slightly as you stand upright and return to the start position.

FRONT SQUATS

This category encompasses all of the squats that require you to stabilize a load in front of your body, on either your chest or your shoulders. With the load positioned in front of your body, you have to stay more upright to maintain balance, which places more tension on your quads. However, based on my EMG research, people tend to get the same levels of glute activation with front squats (sometimes more) compared to back squats when the same relative loads are used.

Because each front squat variation has unique characteristics—you might use one for building strength (e.g., the barbell front squat) and another for targeting your glutes (e.g., the goblet squat)—it's important that you learn and practice them all and then select the variation that best suits your goals. *Note:* You can perform the front squat variations from a narrow, medium, or wide (sumo) stance. If you have limited ankle mobility or you struggle to keep your torso upright, I recommend elevating your heels using weight plates or a wedge—see page 422 for a more detailed breakdown of the heel lift variations.

Goblet Squat

The goblet squat, created by world-renowned strength coach Dan John, is my go-to exercise when teaching people how to transition between the bodyweight squat and barbell variations. They're not quite ready for the barbell, but they can perform goblet squats just fine. What I like about the goblet squat variation is that it's a self-limiting exercise in that your elbows go between your knees as you descend into the bottom position, which forces you to drive your knees out and prevents the knee valgus fault.

In addition to being great for beginners, goblet squats are good for advanced front squatters. I still perform goblet squats in my training and use them regularly with my advanced clients in the form of high-rep knee-banded goblet squats at the ends of workouts. Most of the women I train love the goblet squat and see great glute development, especially when performing the knee-banded variations.

It's interesting to note that with some individuals, goblet squats scored the highest of all of the standing squat variations when measuring glute activation, even though the loading was much lighter. According to my EMG research, the farther away the load is from your center, the less glute activation you get out of the exercise. The goblet squat positions the weight close to your body, so you might get better glute activation compared to the other squat variations. I tested this on one of my clients, and she got higher glute activation from a 50-pound goblet squat than a 205-pound back squat.

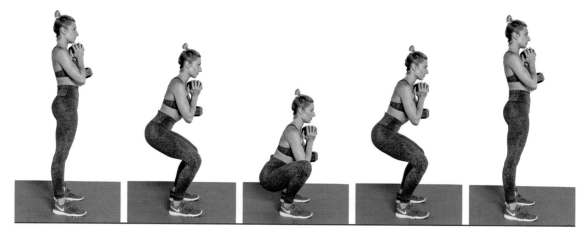

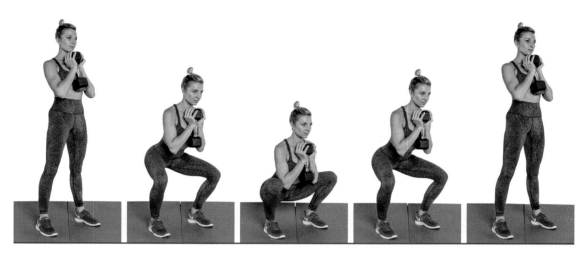

You can perform the goblet squat using either a dumbbell or a kettlebell. Notice the different grip options. Experiment with both types of weights and tinker with your grip, then adopt the variation that feels best. To execute the goblet squat, assume your squat stance, then hoist the weight up to your chest. Keeping your elbows tight to your body and the weight positioned at your chest, drop your hips straight down and drive your knees out as you lower into the squat. To maintain balance, keep your torso upright and the weight tight to your body. As you lower into the squat, allow your elbows to sink between your knees. To reverse the movement, continue driving your knees out and pushing through your heels as you stand upright.

Cable Goblet Squat

You can also perform goblet squats using a cable machine with the V-handle attachment. It's a slightly different feel than the kettlebell or dumbbell goblet squat because you have to lean back slightly to counter the forward pull of the cable. This encourages a more upright position, which many people love. Consider cable goblet squats as another useful variation to include in your arsenal of squat techniques, one that you may choose to employ to break the monotony of your typical squat routine, or simply because you like the way they feel.

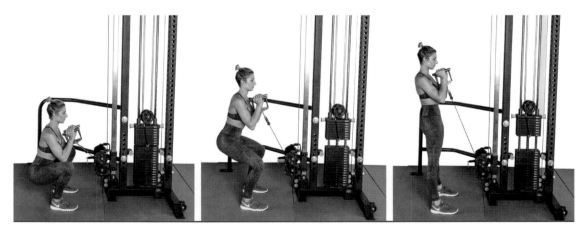

To set up, connect the V-handle to the cable attachment and lower it all to the bottom of the machine. Grip the V-handle with your palms facing upward and lift it into the front rack position. Note: You will probably need to lean back a little bit to counter the forward resistance from the cable. From here, the movement is performed exactly the same as the conventional goblet squat—see previous technique.

Double Dumbbell/Kettlebell Front Squat

In most cases, you can lift more weight with two dumbbells or kettlebells than a traditional goblet squat. For this reason, I sometimes progress people to the double dumbbell front squat before teaching them the barbell variation. The double dumbbell front squat variation is also great in situations where you don't have access to a barbell, like at a hotel gym. One caveat is that the dumbbells are hard to get into position and stabilize, so you might be limited to lighter loads.

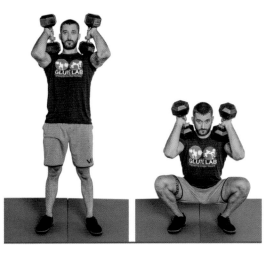

You can rest the dumbbells or kettlebells on your shoulders and keep your elbows high or keep your elbows low as if you were going to press them overhead. The option you choose is a matter of personal preference. To set up for the exercise, curl or clean the dumbbells or kettlebells into the front rack position with the weights resting on your shoulders, and then assume your squat stance. The execution is exactly the same as the goblet squat: keep your torso upright—keeping your back flat—and then lower into the squat by breaking at the knees and hips simultaneously. As you descend into the bottom position, push your knees out, and keep your weight distributed over your heels. It's also important to keep your chest up to prevent from rounding your upper back.

Landmine Front Squat

The landmine front squat is a relatively new variation, and it is another great way to add load to the front squat movement pattern. Although you have to lean forward a bit at the onset of the movement, it feels very similar to a goblet squat out of the hole as you rise upward, which means it's great for beginners and people who get high levels of glute activation with goblet squats.

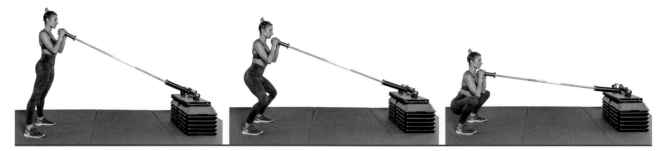

It's best to perform the landmine front squat with the bar elevated off the ground. So you need to either use an adjustable landmine attachment on a power rack or set the landmine unit on a plyometric box, steps, or blocks, making sure that the unit is tightly wedged into a corner and highly stable. If you perform the landmine front squat with the bar positioned on the ground, you'll have to lean forward initially before you lower into the squat so that you end up upright at the bottom, especially if you're tall, which can feel unnatural. Note: If you don't have a landmine unit, you can make do by jamming the barbell in a corner; just know that doing so can beat up the wall. Other than that, you perform the movement in a similar fashion to the goblet squat: keep your elbows in tight to your body, maintain a good arch in your back, allow your elbows to sink between your knees as you lower into the bottom position, and drive your knees out and push through your heels as you stand upright.

Barbell Front Squat

I love barbell front squats. Like all barbell variations, you can add more load compared to the dumbbell and kettlebell counterparts, which is ideal for both strength and muscle development. The barbell front squat is one of my favorite squat variations for both athletes and physique competitors. There is not enough research to determine which squat is best for athleticism or physique training, but a strong case could be made for the deep barbell front squat. To front squat properly, you have to stabilize the load out in front of your body, maintain an upright torso, and stiffen your trunk/core, and you need good hip and ankle mobility. Put simply, it's a true test of leg strength, mobility, and stability, which are crucial in just about every sport.

A certain percentage of people can't comfortably do barbell front squats due to their clavicle and shoulder girdle anatomy. If front squatting with a barbell is too painful for you, then stick with the goblet and double dumbbell variations.

BARBELL FRONT SQUAT LOAD POSITIONS

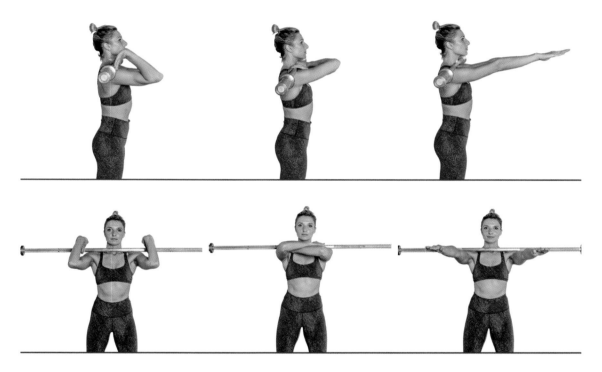

BARBELL FRONT SQUAT

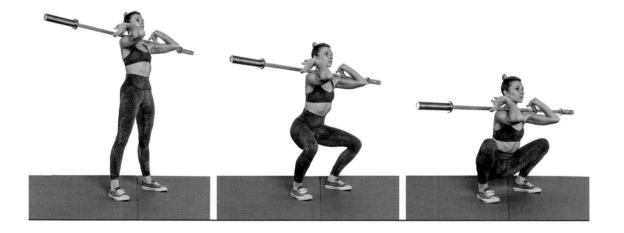

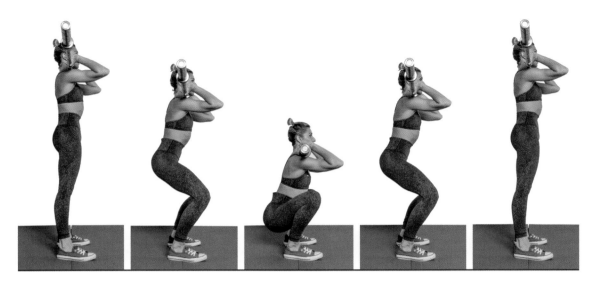

To stabilize the bar on your chest, you can use a traditional front rack, which is what Olympic lifters do, or a cross-arm grip, which is popular among bodybuilders. If you have flexible shoulders, you like Olympic lifting, or you train CrossFit, then the front rack is more sport specific and the variation you should prioritize. If you have inflexible wrists, or relatively long forearms, or tons of upper body muscle mass, then you might like the cross-arm variation. Regardless of the style you choose, there is a sweet spot, a little groove where the bar should sit, which is between the neck and your delt muscles. It is easier to get into this position if you spread your shoulder blades, also known as protracting the scapulae. When it comes to executing the movement, it's exactly the same movement as the other front squat variations: drop your hips between your thighs, keep your back flat and torso upright, drive through your heels, and push your knees out in the bottom position. The key difference with the barbell variations is to keep your elbows up, roughly horizontal with the ground. In other words, you have to counter the forces encouraging you to lean forward or round by maintaining a good arch in your back and keeping your chest up.

BACK SQUATS

Back squats are considered the crème de la crème of the squat variations. With the load positioned on your upper back, you can handle a lot more weight, making it the best squat variation for strength development. The back squat also requires a forward torso lean, which increases tension on some of the posterior chain muscles. And since you can handle more weight, you'll recruit more overall muscle compared to the other squat variations to carry out the task.

The one drawback to back squatting is the same thing that makes them great, which is it's a movement you can load with a lot of weight. This makes the back squat inherently more dangerous. You have to make sure you lift from squat stands or a power rack and, even more important, you have to learn how to safely dump the weight. That is, if you can't complete the lift because it's too heavy, you have to set it down onto the safety pins or jump out (forward) from underneath the barbell, otherwise it will crush you like an accordion. Before you start lifting heavy, make sure to practice with light weight and learn how to bail out so you don't hurt yourself.

There are two back squat variations based on bar position: the low-bar back squat and high-bar back squat.

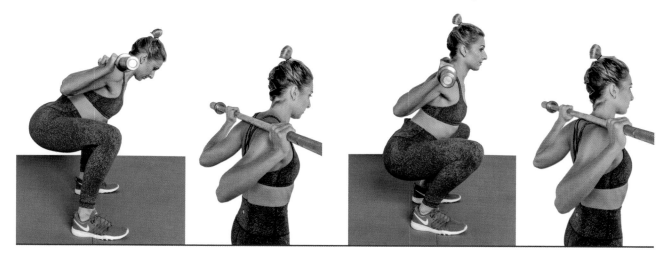

Low-Bar Back Squat

The low-bar back squat is popular among powerlifters because most people can lift more weight—usually around 10 percent more. With the bar positioned lower on your back, you have to lean farther forward to stay balanced (compared to the high-bar variation), which forces you to sit your hips farther back. This combination of actions is thought to place slightly more load on your glutes and hamstrings (hips) instead of your quads (knees). Stated differently, it's considered a hip-dominant squatting movement, meaning that it places more tension on your hips.

However, low bar back squats are not for everyone. It requires more shoulder mobility and a lot of people can't get their wrists into a good position. It's important to point out that wrist pain from low bar back squats typically occurs because there is an excessive bend in your wrists. You can remedy this problem by simply correcting your technique or wearing wrists wraps, which helps support your wrists with load. That said, if low bar back squats hurt your wrists or shoulders or it doesn't feel right on your lower back, then perhaps the high bar back squat is a better option.

If you're new to the low-bar back squat, I recommend using an empty barbell to find the right grip and bar position. The bar should be just on top of your rear delts. Once you find the right placement, experiment with your grip width and elbow flare. Ideally, you want your wrists in a neutral position or slightly bent—meaning there is not an excessive bend—and your elbows positioned underneath or slightly behind the bar. Many people, especially muscular men, lack the shoulder external rotation mobility to remain neutral during low-bar back squats and are therefore forced to bend their wrists. The bar should feel stable, and your upper back should be on tension.

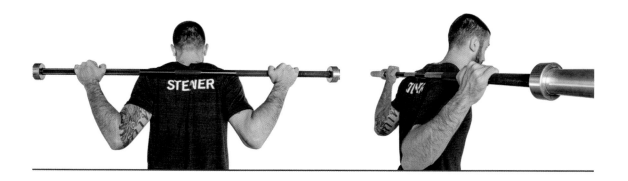

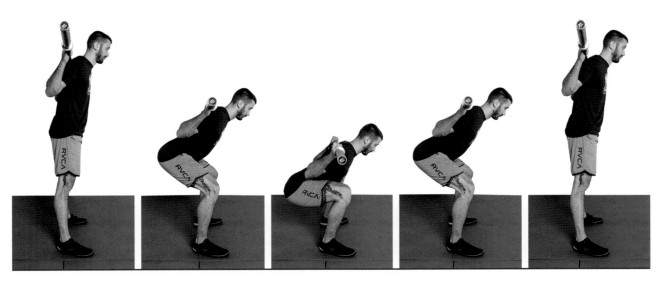

Set the rack a couple of inches below where the bar will rest on your back. With the bar set to the appropriate height, form your grip, dip your head underneath the bar, and slide your back up the bar (bigger people might need to wiggle or squirm a little bit) until it is in the right position. Again, the bar should be roughly positioned on top of your rear deltoids, your wrists neutral or slightly bent, and your elbows positioned slightly behind the bar. Get into your squat stance, lift the bar out of the rack, and take two steps back. From here, brace your spine by taking a big breath and tightening the muscles of your diaphragm, obliques, and abdominals. To execute the squat, sit your hips back, tilt your torso forward, and bend your knees. You don't have to sit way back and keep your shins as vertical as possible, but I like to teach people this form to see if they prefer it. So either sit your hips down and let your knees migrate forward or sit back more and keep your shins more vertical. Once your hips hit parallel (the top surface of your legs at your hip joint is lower than the top of the knees), reverse the motion by driving through your heels, pushing your knees out, and simultaneously extending your hips, raising your torso, and straightening your knees. You can squeeze your glutes slightly as you reach the top position to lock out your hips, but this is not necessary to complete the lift.

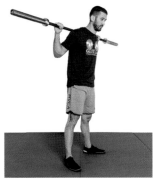

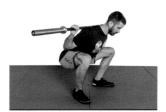

High-Bar Back Squat

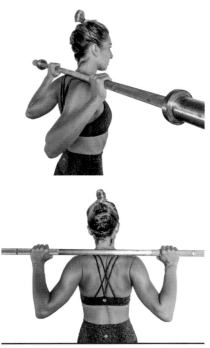

As the name suggests, the high-bar back squat positions the barbell high on your back on your trapezius muscles and shoulders. Now, you probably have an image in your mind of what a perfect high-bar back squat looks like, based on what people have told you and what you've seen from weightlifters. For instance, you might think that you should be perfectly upright. But really you shouldn't. In general, you should be at roughly a 35-degree angle at the bottom; that is the most powerful position. Yes, your torso is more upright compared to the low-bar variation, but there is still a slight lean. Most women I work with prefer the high-bar variation because they can get into a better squat position and it's initially more comfortable on their upper back. It is a more knee-dominant squat, meaning you're staying more upright and letting your knees travel forward over your feet. But even though you may feel it more in your quads, it still works the glutes to roughly the same degree as low-bar back squats. So, like all of the variations outlined in this book, experiment with both and then prioritize the one that feels better.

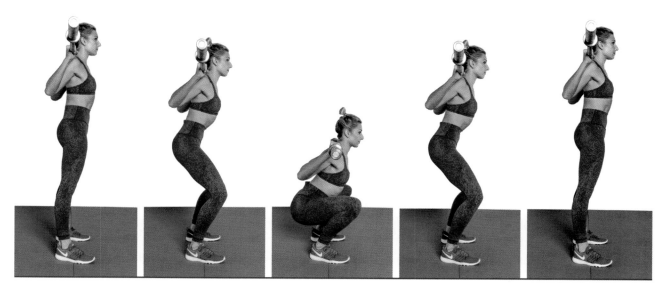

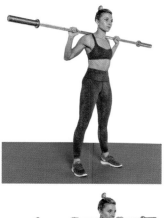

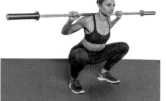

Like the low-bar back squat, set the height of the rack a couple of inches below where the bar will rest on your back. Once the barbell is set to the correct height, form your grip, dip your head underneath the bar, and then slide your back up the bar until it is in the right position. With the high bar back squat, the bar should be resting on your traps, just below the base of your neck. Like the low bar variation, you can align your wrists in a neutral position or keep them slightly bent with your elbows positioned slightly behind the bar. From here, assume your squat stance, brace your spine, lift the bar out of the rack, and take two steps back. Now brace your spine again by taking another big breath and tightening the muscles of your diaphragm, obliques, and abdominals before you initiate the movement. To execute the squat, sit your hips straight down between your thighs while pushing your knees out as you lower your elevation. Once your hips dip below your knee crease (feel free to go rock bottom if you have the mobility), reverse the motion by driving through your heels, pushing your knees out, and simultaneously extending your hips, raising your torso, and straightening your knees.

KNEELING SQUAT

The kneeling squat, interestingly, scored the highest glute activation out of all of the squat variations on an EMG experiment I did on myself. I suspect that this is due to the increased load I used and to the fact that the knees are bent, which—as you know—inhibits the hamstrings, causing the glutes to do more.

The problem with this variation is that there is very little hip range of motion (you don't even get to parallel), which means that you don't lengthen your glutes under tension, which, in the context of glute training, is the primary reason for implementing squats.

Now, does that mean the kneeling squat is useless? Not necessarily. I suppose it could help a lifter retain squat strength while rehabbing an ankle injury. And Louie Simmons of Westside Barbell Club had some of his lifters perform these to develop their hip strength, which might be useful for serious squatters.

But when it comes to glute training, I think a much better option is to prioritize full-range squats—all of the variations previously covered—to work the glutes at longer muscle lengths and stick with glute dominant exercises like the hip thrust and upright hip thrusts (kneeling and standing) to work the glutes at shorter muscle lengths.

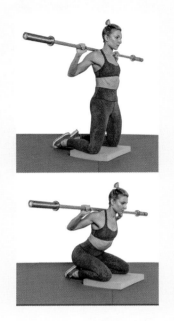

If you happen to like kneeling squats, be sure to perform them inside a power rack with the pins placed at an appropriate height or use a Smith machine so you can safely dump or rack the weight should something go wrong. You can lift heavier loads with this variation due to the decreased range of motion, and it's easy to get carried away and forget about safety. You can't bail out underneath the bar or drop it behind your back on a failed rep, so you need to take this into consideration before loading the bar and getting to work. I also recommend kneeling on a pad to protect your knees.

HANG SQUATS

Hang squats include squat variations where the load is hanging from your body either from your elbows, hands, or hips. In other words, "hang" is a word I assigned to this particular category to help classify the Zercher, hack, and other squat variations in which you hold the weight below your chest. In most powerlifting programs, these squat variations fall into the category of "assistance lifts," meaning they are not main staples, but rather accessory exercises that are injected into the program for variety. However, we perform the double dumbbell hang squat and between-bench squat a lot with our clients and athletes at Glute Lab because they are easy to do, they're easier on the body than traditional squats, and they're less likely to cause injury.

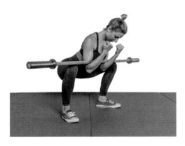

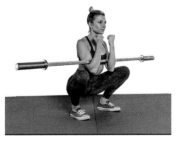

Zercher Squat

The Zercher squat is one of the most underrated and underutilized squats. Some people avoid it because it initially hurts their arms, but you can use padding or just use lighter loads if that's a problem. Eventually—typically after around three weeks of performing them—your arms won't hurt and the pain won't be so bad. Overall, the Zercher squat is well tolerated by most people, and my clients love it because the movement feels very natural and stable.

There are two ways to Zercher squat. The first is to adopt a wide stance and lean forward. This is the more popular variation, as people tend to feel more stable and are less likely to butt wink. They just go to parallel and then reverse the position (parallel Zercher squat). The second option is to adopt a narrow stance, stay more upright, and go deeper (full Zercher squat). Both variations are great, just as in the case of low-bar versus high-bar variation.

FULL ZERCHER SQUAT

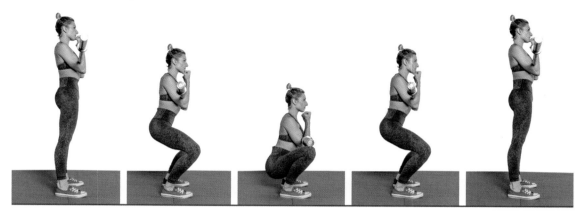

PARALLEL ZERCHER SQUAT

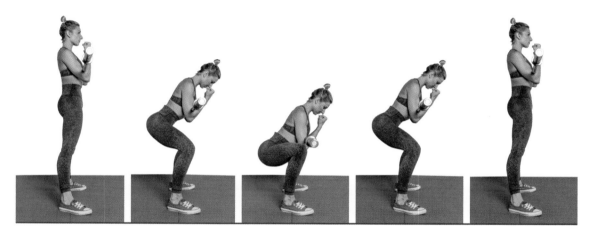

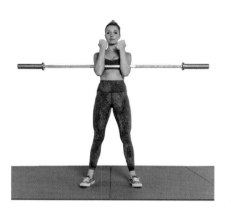

Stand upright with an empty barbell held in the crooks of your arms to determine where you should set the height of the rack, which should be a couple of inches below the bar. With the rack set to the appropriate height, wrap your elbows underneath bar, positioning it in the crooks of your arms. Be sure to use the notches in the barbell to ensure your grip is symmetrical. You can clasp your hands in front of your chest or keep them separated. Choose the option that feels more stable. Keeping the bar against your chest, assume your squat stance, then unrack the weight. Take a couple of steps back, then get braced. If you're performing the full Zercher variation, assume a medium to narrow stance, sit your hips between your thighs, and drive your knees outward as you descend into a full squat. If you're executing the parallel Zercher, assume a wide stance, sit your hips back, and push your knees out as you descend to parallel (hips just below knee crease). Reverse the movement by continuing to push your knees out, driving through your heels, and extending your hips. Focus on keeping your back rigid (straight or slightly arched), your chest up, and the bar close to your body.

Although coaches and trainers have speculated that deeper squats lead to greater glute growth, we never had a study examining actual glute hypertrophy. We did have EMG studies, which show similar glute activation between different squat depths. Despite half squats allowing for heavier weights, full squats still trumped them for glute and adductor growth. Range of motion trumps load for muscle gains (for glutes but not quads in this study).

This paper also showed what several others have—no hamstring and rectus femoris growth from squats, which makes sense biomechanically.

I want to emphasize that you should squat only as deep as your form and mobility will allow. If full squats are not well tolerated or your form degrades, pick a range that you can perform safely and effectively and then progressively increase the range of motion as your form and mobility improve.

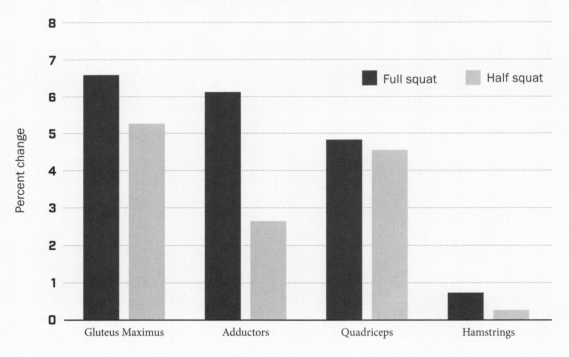

10 WEEKS OF TWICE-WEEKLY SQUATTING IN MALE BEGINNERS WITH DIFFERENT DEPTHS (FULL VERSUS HALF) SHOWED SIMILAR QUAD GROWTH BETWEEN THE TWO GROUPS. HOWEVER, DESPITE USING LESS WEIGHT, THE FULL SQUAT GROUP SAW GREATER GLUTE AND ADDUCTOR GROWTH. THE HAMSTRINGS AND RECTUS FEMORIS DIDN'T GROW IN EITHER GROUP.

Kubo, K., Ikebukuro, T., and Yata, H. (2019). "Effects of squat training with different depths on lower limb muscle volumes." *European Journal of Applied Physiology.* Published ahead of print.

Between-Bench Squat

The between-bench squat is essentially a deficit hang squat. The load position is similar to a dumbbell or kettlebell deadlift because you're holding the weight between your legs, but it's considered a squat because you're in an upright position and expressing full hip and knee range of motion. To prevent the weight from hitting the ground, you stand on two boxes, aerobic steps, blocks, or benches. I use the BC T-Bell (loading pin or plate loading device) to allow for heavier loading options, but you can still do it if you don't have access to a BC T-Bell. Even if you have a moderately heavy kettlebell or dumbbell—which most home and hotel gyms have—you can increase the difficulty by altering the tempo. I generally recommend 3 sets of 20 reps for this exercise, or 3 sets of 10 reps with a 4-second lowering phase (eccentric accentuated).

BC T-BELL BETWEEN-BENCH SQUAT

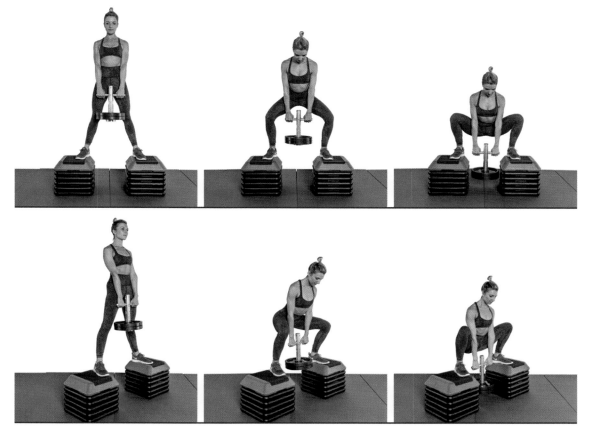

Position two boxes or aerobic steps about your stance width apart. Make sure the stacks are high enough to allow you to lower the weight into a full squat without hitting the ground. You can perform this exercise with a BC T-Bell (plate-loading device), kettlebell, or dumbbell. If you're using a loading pin with a handle characteristic of the BC T-Bell, or a kettlebell, simply grip the handle with a double overhand grip (your palms facing toward your body). If you're using a dumbbell, you can either grip the weight in a vertical position, cupping your hands around the weight portion or head of the dumbbell, or grip it in a horizontal position by wrapping both hands around the handle or interlocking your fingers around the handle. To execute the movement, stand on the boxes or blocks, holding the weight along your center line, and assume your squat stance. Sit your hips between your thighs, keeping your back flat and torso upright as you descend into the squat. Reverse the movement by driving through your heels while simultaneously extending your hips and knees. Keep your arms relaxed, allowing the weight to hang between your legs through the entire range of the exercise.

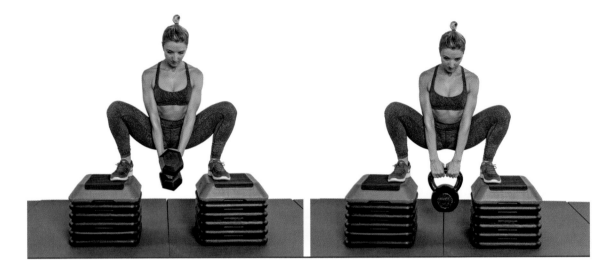

Dumbbell Carry Squat

The dumbbell carry squat is probably one of the most functional squat variations that hardly anyone ever does. You can't go quite as deep as a conventional squat, so it doesn't work your glutes quite as much. But it's a great one to implement, again, if you don't have access to a lot of weight or you want to target your quads. To keep your torso upright and prevent posterior pelvic tilting, I typically tell people to elevate their heels using wedges, weight plates, or weightlifting shoes. This is another variation typically done for high reps, with 3 sets of 20 repetitions being a good baseline.

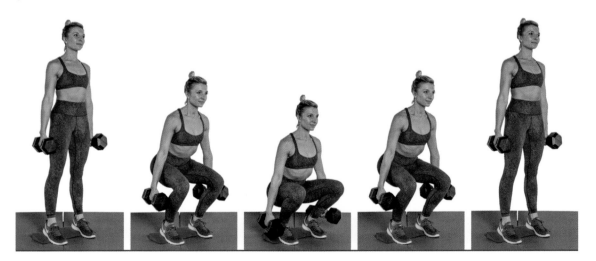

Hold two dumbbells at your sides and assume your squat stance. Keeping your torso upright and your weight on your heels, sit your hips down between your thighs and bend your knees. As you do, actively push your knees outward and keep your spine rigid (straight or slightly arched). Descend as far as you can without butt winking or posterior pelvic tilting. Most people get only to parallel or just above parallel, and that is fine.

Belt Squat

There are several ways to perform the belt squat. My favorite way to belt squat is off of a lever system machine such as the Pit Shark, which is specifically designed for belt squatting. Unfortunately, most commercial gyms don't have this machine.

The best alternative is to stand on two boxes, aerobic steps, or blocks and use a dip belt to hold the weight. You can hook it to weight plates, a heavy kettlebell, or a loading pin. This is the most practical setup for most people. The one drawback is that it can be hard to set up and sometimes the belt is uncomfortable on the hips in that the chain digs into the groin region. Another problem is that the weight tends to swing, so you have to go up and down with rhythm and a coordinated tempo. Like most lifts, however, there is usually a load and cadence that feels right, which will take some tinkering.

Belt squats are particularly great if you have an upper-body injury or you want to take some pressure off your back. Having the weight hang from your hips reduces some of the compressive forces on your spine because the axial load is not positioned on your back and you're not using your erectors as much. This is my go-to squat variation for people who have lower back pain or tend to get lower back pain from barbell squats.

WEIGHT PLATE BELT SQUAT

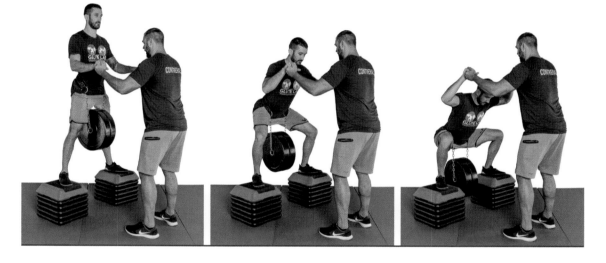

KETTLEBELL BELT SQUAT

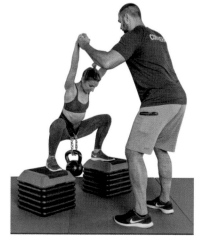

Unless you have a belt squat machine, you will need two boxes, a dip belt, and a weight. Position the boxes close enough to assume your squat stance, but far enough to allow the weight to pass between them. Set the weight on a box to elevate it off the ground, wrap the dip belt around your waist with the chain hanging in front, and attach the weight. Pick the weight up by gripping the chain with both hands, get onto the boxes, and then let the slack out of the chain and let the weight down. Stand back up and make any necessary adjustments to the belt and your stance. From here, you're ready to squat. To reiterate, you want a slow, smooth, and rhythmic tempo to prevent the weight from swinging forward and backward.

LOADING AND EQUIPMENT VARIATIONS

As you learned, there are many ways to create squat variations based on load position and equipment. There will be a few variations that work best for you, and these are the squats you will do most often. However, it's important to switch things up from time to time. Maybe you get injured or bored and want to try something else, or perhaps your progress is stalled. These are good reasons to play around with different squats or experiment with different equipment.

I have already covered the majority of these options, so I'm only going to cover the universal pieces of equipment that you can apply to all of the squat variations—the resistance band (Glute Loop), Smith machine, and leg press.

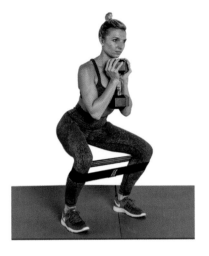

KNEE-BANDED VARIATIONS

Whether you're using a resistance band (Glute Loop) or a mini band, positioning a band around your knees (a L/XL Glute Loop band is ideal for this purpose) is the best way to increase glute activation for the squat movement patterns.

Like the hip thrust and glute bridge, you can position the band above or below the knees. Most people like it above the knees, but I encourage you to experiment. Some people prefer to position the band above their knees when hip thrusting but like it below their knees when squatting. It might depend on the style of squat. You may find that you like the band above your knees when back squatting but below your knees when goblet squatting.

Though I've seen some powerlifters use a band during heavy squats, I never recommend it. The reason I don't like using a band with heavy loads—and it's the same for the hip thrust and glute bridge—is that you're focusing on strength, not necessarily the mind-muscle connection. You're trying to progressively overload the squat, and adding resistance in another plane might compromise your mechanics or reduce the amount of weight you can lift, which is counterproductive to your goal of lifting more weight. In other words, you want your glutes focusing on the hip extension task, not doubling their duty to carry out hip extension and hip abduction against resistance simultaneously.

I like using a band with lighter loads to increase glute activation or to help teach people to drive their knees out. With the band wrapped either below or above your knees, you have to drive outward into the band to maintain a good position, and this outward pressure helps increase upper glute activation. Because squats work mostly the lower subdivision of the glutes, adding a band is a great way to tie in the upper subdivision.

BARBELL VARIATIONS

The vast majority of you will only be able to squat with the bar that's available to you at your commercial gym. However, there are many different types of barbell apparatuses you can use to squat. You can use a standard bar, squat bar, cambered bar, safety squat bar, or Buffalo bar, as well as barbells of varying lengths, thickness, and weight. It's hard to offer specific recommendations because everyone has different preferences. I sometimes use the trainer bar that weighs 35 pounds with women who begin back or front squatting as a transition between dumbbell goblet squats and traditional barbell squats. We have a variety of bars at Glute Lab, and some of my clients prefer the feel of a particular bar over the others. So, once again, I encourage you to find a gym that has different barbells to help you determine the best fit for your body and goals.

When it comes to the barbell you will use most, or if you're looking for one barbell for your home gym, then the standard bar (I like the Texas Power bar) is your best option due to the versatility. You can do everything including squats, deadlifts, lunges, hip thrusts, glute bridges, and the list goes on and on. However, as you progress in your training, it's nice to play around with different barbells, such as the cambered bar and safety squat bar. It's usually my male clients who prefer to use these specialty bars, but there are situations where women prefer to use them too. These specialty bars not only provide a novel stimulus, but also have a specific feel.

For example, a squat bar is great for serious squatters because it has knurling in its center, which helps prevent the bar from sliding down your back. With the cambered bar, the load is positioned farther in front of your midline. In addition to placing more emphasis on your hamstrings, glutes, and lower back, the arch in the bar causes the weights to swing, forcing you to not only stay more upright, but also stabilize your spine to a higher degree compared to the standard barbell. The safety squat bar (also referred to as a yoke bar) has two arms that protrude from the center of the bar with thick padding that wraps around the back of your neck and top of your shoulders and traps. With the weight sitting on your shoulders and traps, the weight distribution falls between a front squat and high bar back squat. This is a great option for people who feel pain during front squats or back squats or lack the shoulder mobility to get into a good position. It's also considered a safer option for lifting maximal loads—the bar balances itself, so you don't need to use your hands to grip the bar—and many people can lift more weight compared to standard barbell back squats.

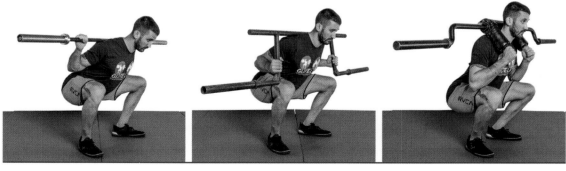

SQUAT BAR   CAMBERED   SAFETY

SMITH MACHINE VARIATIONS

I love the Smith machine and encourage my clients to use it for all of the barbell squat variations. However, not all strength coaches agree. In fact, a lot of trainers contradict themselves by saying that unstable surface training is bad because your muscles don't fire optimally. But those same trainers will say that Smith machines are stupid because they're too stable. So free weight offers just the right stability and therefore is all you should do? It's nonsense.

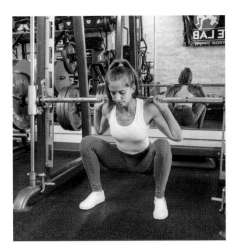

I've said it before and I'll say it again: the more stable the exercise, the safer and easier it is to perform. This is great not only when you're first learning to squat and trying to dial in your coordination, but also to supplement in your training. It's easier on your joints, making it a great tool to use when you're feeling beat up or coming back from an injury. What's more, it doesn't take anything away from your free weight strength. In fact, supplementing or taking some time away from free weights might actually improve your strength, with one big caveat—you perform the squat in the Smith machine just like you do with free weights. This means that you don't position your feet in front of you like you would in a hack squat machine, and you end up leaning forward around 45 degrees at the bottom of the movement. The vast majority of people don't Smith machine squat this way, but you can indeed make your Smith squat feel very similar to your barbell squat.

I did an experiment in which all I did was work out with machines for six weeks, and by the end of it, my free weight squat strength had gone up. I did tons of Smith machine squats but also incorporated machine hack squats and lever squats. Granted, I'm an experienced lifter, so my technique didn't degrade, but it felt good to do something different. Unfortunately, my knees took a beating, mostly due to the machine hack squats, but my quads definitely got stronger.

Most people are training for physique purposes anyway. So what are you going to say to a client who just wants better legs and loves the Smith machine—that they can't use it because it's too stable? No way! I would prefer that client do both free weight and Smith machine squats. I want them to use the Smith machine if they happen to like it because it's more stable, meaning they're less likely to get injured. And they can adjust their stance to be more like a free weight squat or more like a machine hack squat depending on their preference for that session.

The whole functional argument falls flat when it comes to weightlifting because increasing strength indeed improves your functional capacity, but at the end of the day, you'll need to develop some skills outside the weight room. If you want to be the most functional human you can be, you need to do everything from weightlifting, track and field, and gymnastics to mixed martial arts and Parkour. You could theoretically do all of your training on machines and still be strong as hell, and you might even be more functional outside the gym because you're not as beat up. If you don't like machines, then you don't need to use them, but to say that they are never safe or have zero functional carryover is simply not true. It makes sense to utilize all available tools as a lifter. A carpenter uses a hammer or screwdriver more often than a specialty tool, but that doesn't mean the specialty tool isn't important. Throughout the year, there will be times when that specialty tool is vital for the task at hand. As a lifter, you want to have access to a large arsenal of exercise variations to allow for more versatile training.

PIT SHARK

As I said, the Pit Shark machine is what we use at Glute Lab and is my favorite way to perform belt squats. However, many of my powerlifting friends prefer other styles of belt squat units, so do your homework as to whether you want a pendulum style unit that has an arced path of loading or a cable style unit that has the load coming straight up and down. You can add resistance in the form of weight and bands, and the design allows you to squat up and down with great control. You can also adjust your stance by positioning your feet higher or lower on the platform. In general, the higher up you position your feet, the more you will

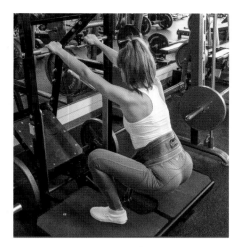

feel the exercise in your quads. There's also a bar you can hold onto for balance, which allows you to accentuate sitting your hips back and putting a deep stretch in your glutes. Like the free weight belt squat variation previously covered, the belt squat machine reduces loading on the spine, making it a great option for people who get lower back pain from conventional squats.

PENDULUM AND LEVER SQUAT MACHINES

The pendulum and lever squat machines produce an arcing motion, which is different than the barbell action, which is straight up and down. There are two primary benefits to these machines. First, there are fewer balance and stabilization requirements, which makes them safer than conventional barbell squats. More specifically, you don't have to worry about the side to side and rotational stability that you have to deal with when squatting with a barbell, allowing you to focus on form and the mind-muscle connection.

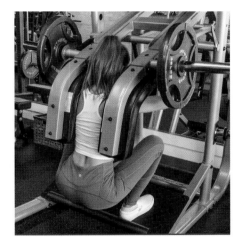

The second benefit is people are not as concerned with how much weight they are lifting. Though chasing PRs with the barbell lifts is great for all of the reasons mentioned throughout this book, you have to be careful not to get carried away. If all you're doing is barbell lifts, there's a tendency to push the envelope and go heavy or go for a PR when you shouldn't. But when you squat on a machine, lifting heavy is not the primary goal. Instead of lifting as much weight as possible, people direct their attention to the muscles they're trying to work. I credit our extremely low rate of injuries at Glute Lab (at the time of this writing, we've had zero injuries) to using more machines.

In short, the lever and pendulum squat machines, though not as common in commercial gyms, are a great substitute for barbell squats, they are safe, and—like the Smith machine—provide a smooth motion. What's more, you can target your glutes by sitting your hips back while remaining stable and balanced, as well as perform loaded reverse lunges.

LEG PRESS

The leg press is a staple in almost every commercial gym and is one of the most popular machines for strengthening the legs and lifting heavy loads. It's stable and relatively safe, assuming you intelligently moderate your working weight and use good form. The one caveat is you can't go super deep. Even if you go as deep as possible, your hips don't move through a full of a range of motion. More specifically, your torso is at an angle, which prevents you from reaching full hip extension. For this reason, it's not the best exercise for working the glutes, but it's a great option for building the legs and for people who tend to get hurt while squatting.

Another advantage of using a leg press machine is it gives you a lot of options. For example, if you want to emphasize your quads, you can position your feet lower on the platform. If you want to emphasize your hamstrings, you can position your feet higher on the platform. And if you want to emphasize your glutes, you can perform knee-banded variations. You can also adjust the width of your stance or target one leg by performing B-stance and single-leg variations. Some of my bikini competitors will even turn onto their side and perform single-leg leg presses to hit the legs from a different angle.

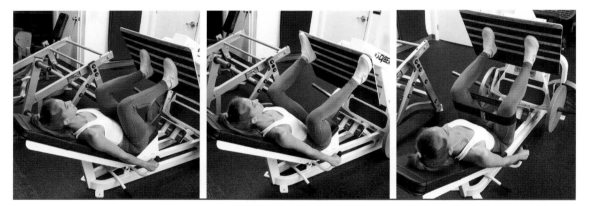

LEG PRESS   WIDE-STANCE LEG PRESS   KNEE-BANDED LEG PRESS

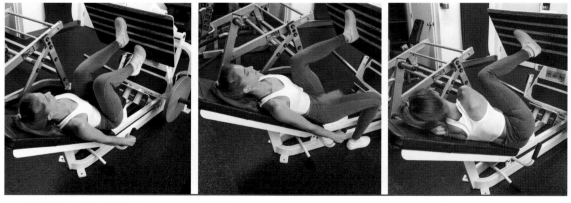

B-STANCE LEG PRESS   SINGLE-LEG PRESS   ANGLED SINGLE-LEG LEG PRESS

2 Split Squats

Split squats encompass staggered-stance squat patterns in which you have one leg out in front of you and one leg behind you, such as lunges and Bulgarian split squats (also known as rear-foot-elevated split squats). What's great about split squats is that just about everyone can do them; they don't favor certain body types like squats do. If someone has long femurs or poor ankle or hip mobility, for example, squatting with proper mechanics is difficult and can pose problems.

But with split squats, nearly everyone can use good form because there is stability from front to back, and you don't have to work around your anatomical restrictions. Sure, you still have to balance your body from side to side in a split squat, but that's not as difficult as balancing your body from front to back, especially if you have an unfavorable skeleton for squatting. And this side-to-side balancing has other advantages in that it builds coordination and stability in a stance that we're in all the time (think walking, running, and stepping). You're working different muscles and developing left-to-right stability, which strengthens the hip muscles responsible for keeping you balanced. What's more, split squats are not as dangerous. Yes, you will wobble a little from side to side when split squatting, but that doesn't carry the same risks as front-to-back wobbling. I've been doing lunges for over 20 years, and a few of my reps on every set are still shaky, especially if I'm lifting a lot of weight or pushing the set close to muscle failure. Yet I can't remember a time that I've ever been injured. I cannot say the same about squats.

In addition to being well tolerated and safe for most people, split squats can be loaded with a lot of weight in a variety of load positions. In fact, some people can lunge with nearly as much weight as they can back squat. So, if squatting is a movement you loathe, you can replace it with a split squat variation as your main quad-dominant lift and still experience substantial strength gains. And it won't take much away from your squat strength, assuming that you're hammering away at single-leg strength and performing other movements that build the squat, such as hip thrusts. In short, people often assume that squatting is a mandatory movement for developing the lower body, but it's not. No exercise is mandatory; what's important is that you find the variations of each movement pattern that work well for your body.

There is one problem with split squats, however: they tend to make your glutes sore. As I outlined in Part 2, muscle damage—which causes muscle soreness—occurs when the muscle is stretched or lengthened under peak tension. The eccentric phase of a movement contributes to muscle soreness because you're contracting the muscle as it is lengthening. With split squats and lunge variations, you lower the weight slowly at the bottom of the movement as you prepare to reverse the weight out of the hole. So you're stretching your glutes maximally as you reach the bottom position, which is why these variations cause a lot of muscle damage and soreness.

As with all of the exercises in this chapter, you have to find a balance between doing enough to get the right stimulus, but not so much that you get overly sore and can't train productively. When I perform single-leg squat patterns, I perform only 2 hard sets per workout, and I do them only twice a week at most. Many people can handle more volume than this, but if you're carrying out your sets close to muscle failure, you won't be able to handle a ton of volume. For this reason, I recommend performing only one single-leg squat pattern per workout. In other words, don't do Bulgarian split squats and high step-ups in the same session.

GUIDELINES AND CUES

Because the squat and the split squat share a similar movement pattern, there is some overlap between their guidelines and cues. But, as you will soon learn, a few nuances are worth noting when you are applying these guidelines to the split squat variations.

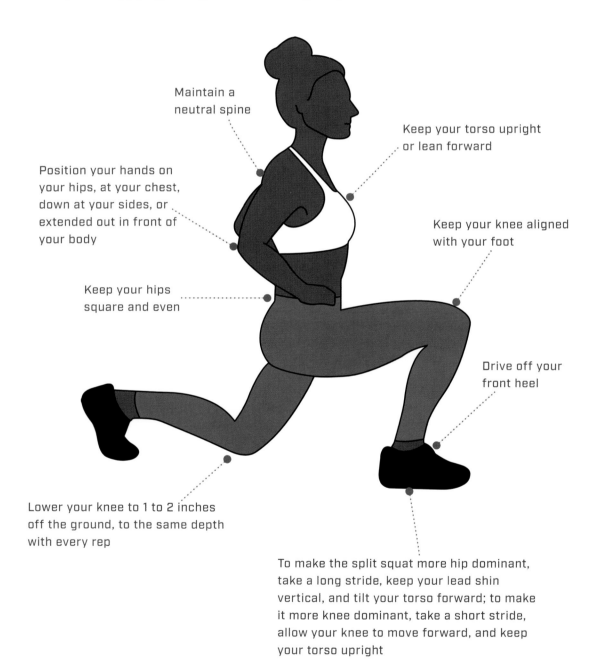

Maintain a neutral spine

Keep your torso upright or lean forward

Position your hands on your hips, at your chest, down at your sides, or extended out in front of your body

Keep your knee aligned with your foot

Keep your hips square and even

Drive off your front heel

Lower your knee to 1 to 2 inches off the ground, to the same depth with every rep

To make the split squat more hip dominant, take a long stride, keep your lead shin vertical, and tilt your torso forward; to make it more knee dominant, take a short stride, allow your knee to move forward, and keep your torso upright

STANCE AND STRIDE: FIND YOUR SWEET SPOT

There are two main considerations when it comes to stance: width and length. To determine your stance width, start by standing with your feet shoulder width apart. Next, take a long, straight step forward. From there, widen or narrow your stance by moving your front foot. There's a sweet spot where you will feel the most stable and balanced, and that is the stance you want to adopt.

Once you feel balanced, drop down to your rear knee. It may take you a few reps with minor adjustments to your stance to get it just right. Keep your front foot straight or slightly turned inward (around 10 degrees). When you drop down to the bottom of the movement, your shin should be angled forward slightly such that the front of your knee lines up with the front of your shoe. You don't want to take such a long stride that your shin slopes downward (we call this a negative shin angle) or such a short stride that your shin angles so far forward that you're forced to come up onto your toes when you sink to the bottom of the movement. It will take some tinkering to find your sweet spot.

In the beginning, adopt the stance that feels best. As you get more comfortable with the movement, you can target different areas of your lower body by taking shorter or longer strides. For example, a shorter step is more knee dominant, meaning that you will feel more tension in your quads, while a longer stride is more hip dominant, meaning that you will feel more tension in your hips and glutes.

NARROW STANCE

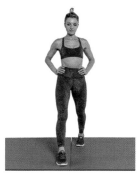

WIDE STANCE

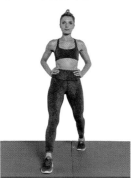

KNEE-DOMINANT SPLIT SQUAT **HIP-DOMINANT SPLIT SQUAT**

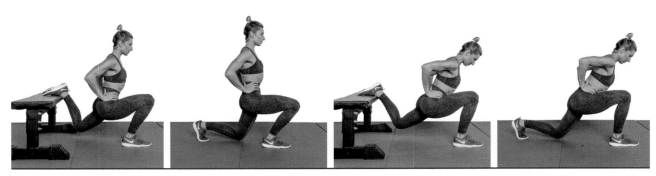

A shorter stride with a more upright torso is more quad/knee dominant, while a longer stride with a forward-leaning torso is more glute/hip dominant.

POSTURE AND TORSO ANGLE: STAY IN THE NEUTRAL ZONE

Like all squat patterns, you want to keep your spine in the neutral zone—that is, keep your back as flat as possible. This is much easier to accomplish with the lunge because you're balanced from front to back, you don't have to lean forward as much, and you don't go as deep unless you're performing a deficit variation. Although many coaches teach an upright torso with split squat variations, I teach them with a slight forward lean. Around 15 to 30 degrees of forward lean is good. This setup shifts a little bit of the emphasis off the quads and places a little more on the hips. However, once you gain proficiency in split squats, you can target your quads by staying more upright or lean substantially forward to shift focus to your glutes and hips.

HIP POSITION: KEEP YOUR HIPS SQUARE AND IN LINE

While you're in the lunge, focus on keeping your pelvis square and even. In other words, don't let it droop to one side or the other. You do this simply by keeping tension in your hips and trunk and focusing on maintaining a good position (more on this in the Faults and Corrections section that follows).

KNEE ACTION: ALIGN YOUR KNEE WITH YOUR FOOT

Just like when you squat, your knee should track over your foot. Allowing your knee to cave inward (knee valgus) puts unnecessary stress on your knee joint, which can eventually manifest as knee pain. A lot of people chalk this habit up to weak glutes, but I disagree. The more likely culprit is ignorance (not knowing it's wrong), poor hip or ankle mobility, or lack of coordination. It also might be due to hip anatomy, in which case there is a slight mechanical advantage to cave inward. In any event, it's best to practice aligning your front knee with your lead foot. It's the safest position for your knees and ensures that all of the right muscles are recruited during the exercise. If you have a tendency to cave inward, think about driving your knee outward as you descend into the lunge.

LUNGE   **BULGARIAN SPLIT SQUAT**

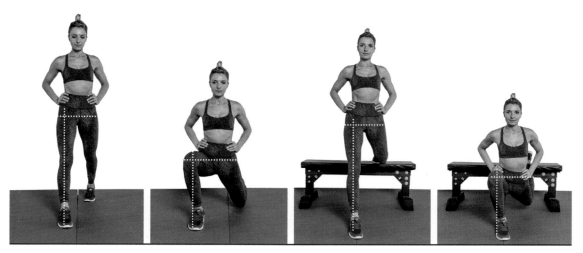

For the lunge and the Bulgarian split squat, make sure to keep your hips square and your front knee aligned over your lead foot.

DRIVE THROUGH YOUR FRONT HEEL

Driving through your lead heel not only helps you maintain balance but also forces you to use the muscles of your hips to carry out the movement. Coming up onto the ball of your lead foot reduces your base of support and places more tension on your calf and quadriceps. If you don't feel balanced pushing through your heel, focus on driving your weight through the center of your foot.

It's worth noting that you will drive off the ball of your rear foot when performing walking lunges, but you want most of the loading to be on your front leg. When you go heavier, you'll naturally rely on your back leg a bit more, but think 80/20 with lunges, meaning that 80 percent of the load should be on your lead leg, with the remaining 20 percent coming from your rear leg.

KNEE DEPTH: MAKE SURE EVERY REP LOOKS THE SAME

There are a couple of things to note here. The first is to pick a consistent knee depth. If you're performing a split squat where you stay in one spot (static lunge, forward lunge, reverse lunge, or Bulgarian split squat), you can tap your knee down to the pad to ensure a consistent depth. If you're performing walking lunges or deficit split squats, then reverse the position roughly an inch off the ground. The keys are to perform the same range of motion with every rep and to control your descent to avoid crashing your knee into the ground.

The second noteworthy point is to raise your hips and torso in one fluid motion. As you drive off your lead foot, raise your hips and torso simultaneously. Put another way, don't shoot your hips up and then raise your torso. Raising your hips and keeping your torso forward shifts tension away from your quads and glutes and onto your hamstrings and back.

FAULTS AND CORRECTIONS

The most common faults associated with the split squat are

- Rounding the back
- Pushing through the ball of the lead foot
- Letting the knee cave inward
- Shooting the hips up
- Not going deep with each rep
- Allowing the pelvis to drop to one side

Rounding the back isn't that common because you have a more upright torso—making it easier to maintain a neutral spine—and your split stance automatically places your weight over the center of your foot, reducing your chances of coming up onto the ball of your foot. You still need to be conscious of your knee position, but the valgus knee fault doesn't occur as often during a split squat compared to a conventional one. Shooting your hips up and not going deep with each rep are also common, but like the other faults, they are easy to correct with a little bit of conscious effort and practice. The pelvic drop fault is a little harder to fix, however, so I am highlighting it here.

FAULT: PELVIC DROP

A lot of people say that pelvic drop is due to weak glutes, but that is hard to determine. More than likely, it's a lack of coordination or an ingrained habit. If you don't put conscious effort into maintaining tension in your hips (contracting your muscles), your body will follow the path of least resistance, which is to sag to one side. More specifically, you're relying on passive tension rather than active tension, causing your pelvis to drop toward your downed knee. Think of it like rounding your back to pick something up; it's much easier because you don't have to activate your muscles to keep your back flat.

CORRECTION:

Simply focus on keeping your hips square and even, as well as maintaining tension in your hips. Like all corrections, this takes some practice and a lot of repetitions to get right. But once you pattern the correct mechanics, you won't have to devote as much conscious effort, and you will naturally move with your hips in line. If you struggle with this, have someone film you from the front and back so that you can see where you are going wrong and make the necessary corrections.

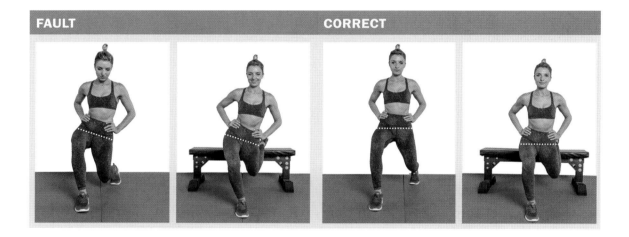

FAULT   CORRECT

SPLIT SQUAT CATEGORIES

The split squat is broken into two main categories: lunges and Bulgarian split squats. Here, I cover only the bodyweight variations and describe what they are good for and how to execute the techniques correctly. In the "Equipment and Loading Variations" section, you will learn all of the ways to load the split squat movement pattern.

LUNGES

There are six lunge variations: static, reverse, walking, forward, side, and curtsy. They all share the same movement pattern and work the glutes in a similar way, but each one provides a slightly different exercise stimulus. At Glute Lab, we lunge in the 8- to 20-rep range most of the time. However, sometimes we go higher with walking lunges and do a set of 50 or even 100 reps.

Static Lunge (Split Squat)

The static lunge is the most basic variation in that you're not moving forward or backward. This version is great for beginners because it's easy to maintain your balance. In fact, with new clients, I sometimes either hold their hands or let them grip a post or brace against a wall for support until they get a feel for the movement. Once they get the movement down, I remove the support and have them practice out in the open. The static lunge is also a good technique for advanced practitioners because you can load the position and increase the range of motion by performing deficit split squats.

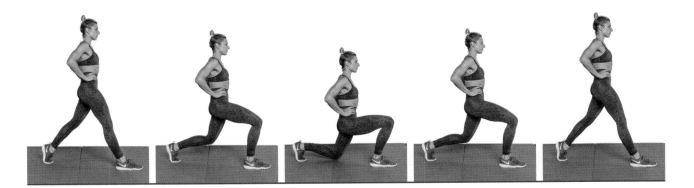

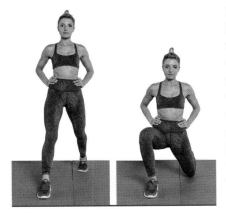

Get into your split stance and drop to your rear knee to check your balance and position. Your lead knee should be roughly aligned with your big toe, and your feet should be roughly shoulder width apart. Once you find your balance, stand upright, coming up onto the ball of your rear foot. To execute the movement, drop straight down slowly, lowering your back knee toward the floor and leaning your torso slightly forward as you descend. Tap your knee to the ground or a couple inches off the ground, then reverse the position by driving off your front heel. The key is to keep your hips square and even and raise your hips and torso at the same time as you stand upright. Rise upward to a full lockout. Note: You can keep your arms down at your sides, on your hips, or at your chest, whichever feels best.

Reverse Lunge

The reverse lunge is great because you don't need a lot of space, you can add load and increase the range of motion by standing on a box, and it's a hip-dominant lunge, meaning that you feel slightly more tension in your glutes. Even though glute activation is similar between the hip- and knee-dominant lunges, some people prefer the feel of the hip-dominant variation because they can feel their glutes working during the exercise.

You can alternate legs from rep to rep or isolate one leg at a time. My preference is to alternate legs, for a couple of reasons:

- It's easier to count. You have to do only one straight set of, say, 20 reps instead of doing 10 reps on the first leg and then 10 reps on the other.
- It works both legs equally. Isolating one leg at a time fatigues your non-squatting or extended leg. By the time you switch, your extended leg is weakened, and you might not get the same quality of reps with the other leg.

REVERSE LUNGE

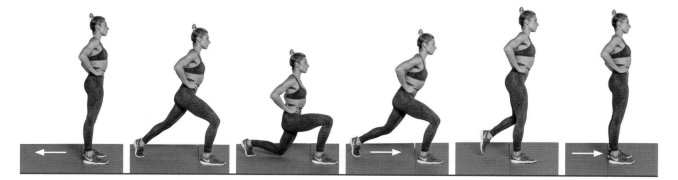

GLIDING REVERSE LUNGE

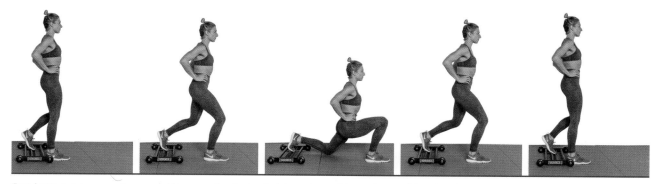

Get into a square stance with your feet straight and positioned roughly shoulder width apart. You can extend your arms out in front of you as you step back to counterbalance or keep them at your sides, on your hips, or at your chest. Keeping your back flat, step one leg straight back, landing on the ball of your rear foot. The goal is to step right into your split stance—see the static lunge on the previous page. As you step back, bend your lead knee slightly and start lowering your elevation the moment your rear foot touches the ground. With roughly 80 percent of your weight on your front leg and the remaining 20 percent on your rear leg, lower your rear knee to the ground while leaning forward slightly, then immediately reverse the position by driving through the heel of your front leg and stand upright. You can also perform the reverse lunge using a glute ham glider.

Forward Lunge

The forward lunge—as the name implies—is a forward-stepping lunge, but you don't keep stepping as you would when performing a walking lunge. In this way, it's similar to the reverse lunge in that you spring back into your stance. But instead of being a hip-dominant lunge, it's knee dominant, meaning that it places more tension on your quads. Interestingly, the forward lunge elicits similar glute EMG activity as the reverse lunge, but you don't feel it as much in your glutes. This could be due to the additional quad activation or because it is performed explosively.

When it comes to glute development, I prefer the reverse lunge and walking lunge because I can feel them working my glutes more. But if I were training someone who plays sports, I would implement the forward lunge because you have to spring backward, which is a similar movement pattern and works the same muscles as decelerating from a sprint or changing directions in sports.

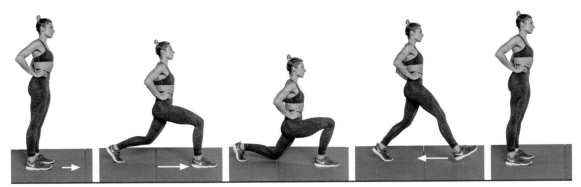

Assume a square stance with your feet positioned roughly shoulder width apart. You can let your arms hang at your sides, place your hands on your hips or chest, or raise your arms as you step. To initiate the lunge, take a straight forward step, landing heel to toe or with your whole foot. As your foot makes contact with the ground, lower your rear knee to the floor, keeping your back flat and your torso upright. Then, in one fluid motion, explosively push off your lead leg and spring back into the start position.

Walking Lunge

The walking lunge is one of my favorite split squat variations. It's challenging, it's easy to load, it gets your heart rate up, and it always makes your glutes sore. But what makes the walking lunge great can also cause problems. You need a lot of space, especially if you're doing barbell walking lunges, and you have to be careful not to be overzealous; otherwise, your glutes will get so sore that you won't be able to train the next day. Walking lunges are a nice blend of hip- and knee-dominant lunges, meaning that you feel the exercise hitting your quads and glutes. They are ballistic just like reverse and forward lunges in that you have to spring off your back leg as you transition between reps. This dynamic action occurs while your glutes are stretched, and you propel yourself upward and forward at the same time, which is perhaps why walking lunges tend to make your glutes more sore than the other lunge variations.

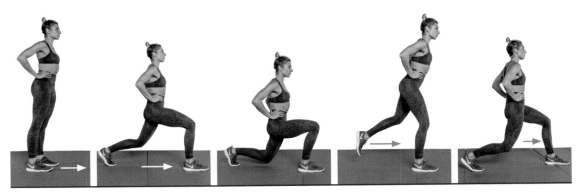

Get into a square stance with your feet straight and positioned roughly shoulder width apart. Take a long step forward—you can step straight forward or slightly to the side. Land with your lead foot straight and come up onto the ball of your rear foot. As your lead foot touches the ground, slowly lower your rear knee to the floor. The moment it touches down, reverse the position by driving off the heel of your front foot. As you stand upright, step your rear leg forward. Note: You can either step into a square stance and then repeat the sequence with your other leg or step forward in one fluid motion into a lunge. Like the other lunge variations, you can keep your arms at your sides or on your hips, whichever feels better.

Side Lunge

The side lunge is technically not a split squat because your stance is square; it's essentially a cross between a single-leg squat and a split squat. But it's classified as a lunge, so I'm placing it here for easy reference. Think of it as another option for injecting variety into your program. Like all lunge movement patterns, you can use the side lunge in the middle of a workout as an accessory exercise (usually with load), toward the end of the workout as a burnout, or at the beginning of the workout as a warm-up. For instance, the side lunge is a great warm-up exercise for the squat because it stretches the glutes and adductor muscles and prepares the quads for more strenuous activity.

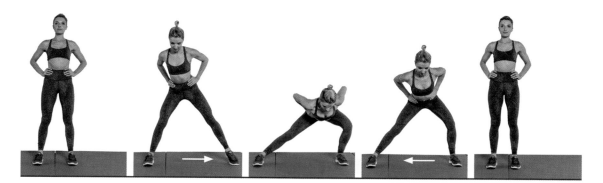

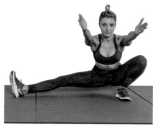

DEEP SIDE LUNGE (COSSACK SQUAT)

Starting from your squat stance, take a lateral step outward as if you were stepping into a sumo stance. You can land with your foot straight or slightly turned out. As your foot makes contact with the ground, shift your weight toward your stepping leg, raise your arms in front of you to counterbalance, and sink your hips back and tilt your torso forward slightly. As you drop into the bottom of the squat, drive your knee out and either come up onto the heel of your opposite foot for a deeper squat or keep your foot flush with the ground and squat to parallel. Return to the starting position and stand upright by driving off the outside of your foot while simultaneously extending your knee, hips, and torso.

Curtsy Lunge

The curtsy lunge is a unique variation in that you're stepping back, behind, and around your lead leg. This not only loads your glutes but also puts them into a deep stretch. In short, you will feel your glutes more with curtsy lunges compared to the other split squat variations.

Because the curtsy lunge is more dynamic and requires a lot of balance, it is often done with only body weight. If you want to make the movement more challenging, you can step off a box and perform deficit curtsy lunges. These are typically placed in the middle of a workout, and the goal is to perform rhythmic repetitions.

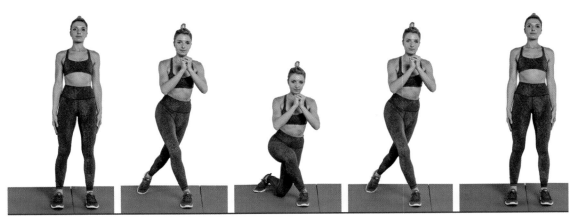

Stand in a square stance with your feet straight. Again, your feet should be roughly shoulder width apart. Keeping your hips even and as square as possible (they will rotate slightly), shift your weight onto one leg and swing your other leg behind your grounded leg. You can elevate your arms as you step back to maintain balance or keep your arms at your sides, whichever you prefer. As you step around your grounded leg, bend your knee slightly and plant the ball of your rear foot on the ground so that your heel is facing away from your body. The moment your foot touches down, lower your knee to the ground. Driving off your lead heel, extend your knee, stand upright, and swing your leg back into the starting position. As you do, keep your back flat and your torso leaned forward slightly, and fight to keep your hips even and as square as possible.

BULGARIAN SPLIT SQUATS (REAR-FOOT-ELEVATED SPLIT SQUATS)

The Bulgarian split squat (BSS) works your quads and, to a lesser degree, your hamstrings and lower glutes. Although it's not the best exercise for glute growth, it's a phenomenal lower-body exercise that builds single-leg strength, stability, and perhaps a little bit of mobility, all of which are essential for functional performance.

There are a few ways to set up the Bulgarian split squat based on equipment availability.

Low Setup Option

Although not as popular, positioning your rear foot on a low step is an effective way to work your lead quad. This setup works especially well when performing rear foot–elevated goblet squats or barbell front squats. With the low setup, it's easier to maintain balance and keep your torso upright, which allows you to lift much heavier weight compared to the conventional Bulgarian split squat.

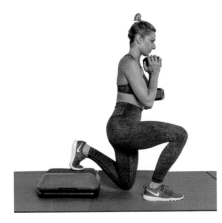

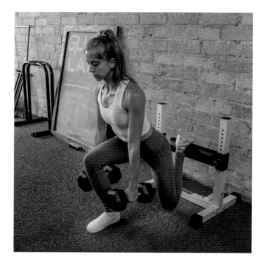

Single-Leg Squat Stand

The best way to perform Bulgarian split squats is to use a single-leg squat stand or single-leg squat pad power rack attachment, which is specifically designed for the BSS. It maximizes stability, which in turn maximizes muscle activation. I don't like the stands with giant rollers or ones that turn. Smaller rollers that stay in place and don't roll are ideal.

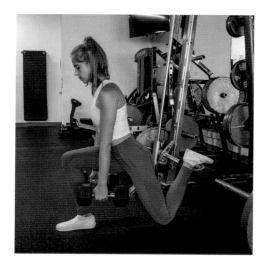

Smith Machine/Power Rack Barbell Squat Stand

Although a single-leg squat stand is best, most commercial gyms don't have one. The good news is that you can create your own single-leg squat stand with a Smith machine or power rack, a couple of long bands (jump stretch bands), and a squat sponge (the Hampton bar pad is ideal because it's thick and has a strap to keep the pad in place), which are common equipment in most commercial gyms. To put together your squat stand, set the height of the barbell to roughly your knee height on the front of the rack. Next, attach a squat sponge around the center of the barbell, and then secure the barbell in place by wrapping a long band around the sleeves of the barbell and the storage pegs of the power rack (this last step is not required if using a Smith machine).

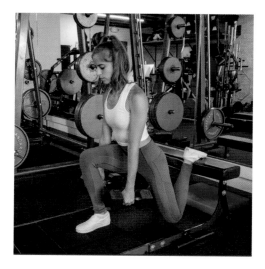

Hip Thruster

You can also perform Bulgarian split squats using a Hip Thruster bench. Even though a flat surface is not ideal, the pad on the Hip Thruster is narrow, so you can still wrap your lower shin and foot around the pad as you would with a single-leg squat stand. Most of my clients prefer the Hip Thruster over a bench (opposite) because the pad is smaller, it's not as high off the ground, and they get an additional 2 inches of range of motion. (The gap between the bench and the mat creates a natural deficit.) As with the bench, you can hook your foot around the pad or flex your toes by posting up onto the ball of your foot.

Bench

You can perform Bulgarian split squats using a standard bench, but it's not ideal. Elevating your rear leg on a bench doesn't feel very natural or comfortable on the lower leg and foot. Nonetheless, in the absence of a single-leg squat stand and power rack, it's the best option.

There are two ways to position your foot on the bench: you can either plantarflex your ankle so that the top of your foot is flush with the flat surface (laces down) or maintain ankle dorsiflexion and flex your toes by posting up onto the ball of your foot (laces forward). The majority of people feel better using the laces-down option, but some, especially those who have great toe and foot mobility, use the latter. Like all variations, experiment with both options to see which works better for you.

LACES DOWN

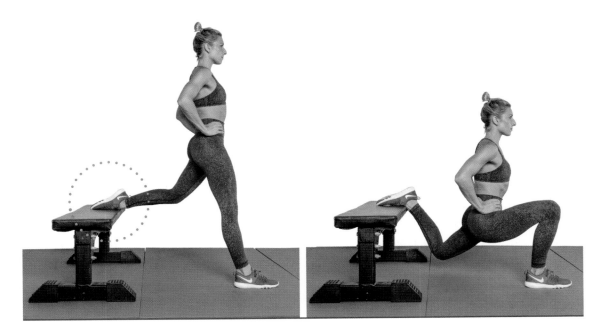

LACES FORWARD

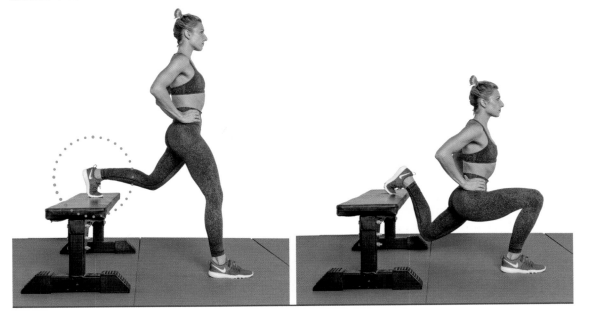

Bulgarian Split Squat Execution

Whether you set up on a squat stand, a Hip Thruster, or a bench, the execution is the same. It's important to rest in the middle of the set. Perform all of your reps with one leg, recover, and then finish the set with your other leg. Unlike reverse, forward, and walking lunges, you can't alternate legs to balance the workload. If you immediately switch legs without resting, you might not be able to match your reps because your extended leg—specifically your rectus femoris—is stretched, which momentarily weakens the muscle. You might get 12 reps with the first leg and 8 with the second. But if you take a minute to recover between legs, you will bounce back quickly and get quality reps with the second leg. Again, you can adopt a shorter stride with a more upright torso to make the exercise more quad/knee dominant or a longer stride with a forward-leaning torso to make it more glute/hip dominant.

FORWARD-LEANING (HIP-DOMINANT) BULGARIAN SPLIT SQUAT

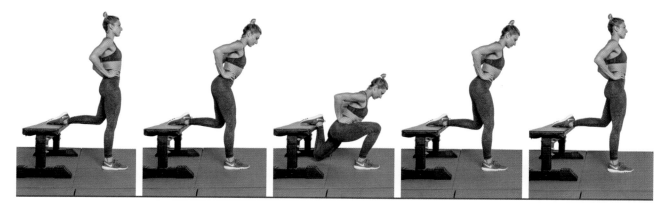

UPRIGHT (KNEE-DOMINANT) BULGARIAN SPLIT SQUAT

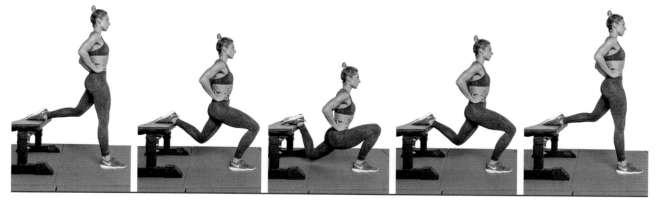

Stand with your back to the pad with your feet roughly shoulder width apart, then step back, hooking your instep around the pad. If you're using a flat bench and you prefer to dorsiflex your foot, position the ball of your foot in the center of the bench. You may need to adjust your lead foot forward, backward, or to the side. Once you find your balance, shift your weight forward with a slight torso lean (about 30 degrees), centering your body over your lead foot. To reiterate, a shorter stride with a more upright torso places more tension on your quads, while a longer stride with an exaggerated forward lean places more tension on your hips. With the majority of your weight (about 85 percent) over your lead foot, descend by bending your lead knee and lower at a diagonal. The moment you reach end range—when your knee taps the ground or pad, or you can't lower any farther without compromising your form—reverse the position by driving off your lead heel and extending your knee. Try to keep your hips square and even as you stand upright.

LOADING AND EQUIPMENT VARIATIONS

The split squat category includes powerful exercises that build strength, stability, muscle, and coordination. Below, I outline the loading and equipment variations for the split squat exercises.

DEFICIT SPLIT SQUAT VARIATIONS

You can increase the range of motion for the split squat, reverse lunge, forward lunge, and rear foot–elevated split squat by standing on a box or an aerobic step. Six inches in height is more than adequate for most people. If you're performing a static split squat, you can stand on one box or two boxes; I prefer two boxes for added range of motion. If you're working a reverse lunge, forward lunge, or Bulgarian split squat, you need only one box. The key to performing these variations correctly is to position your entire foot on the box so that you can drive through your heel. To summarize the benefits of deficit split squats and confirm why you should include them in your program: they accentuate lengthening the glutes under tension, improve mobility and strength at end ranges of motion, and transfer to deep squats.

DEFICIT SPLIT SQUAT   **DEFICIT BULGARIAN SPLIT SQUAT**

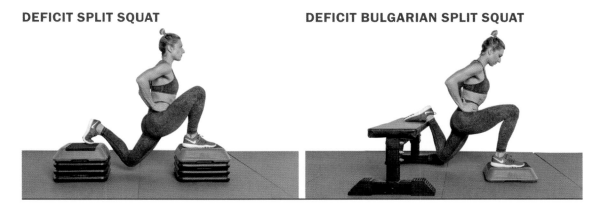

DEFICIT REVERSE LUNGE   **DEFICIT CURTSY LUNGE**

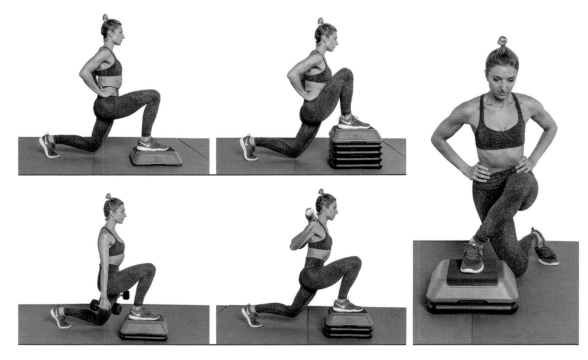

DUMBBELL VARIATIONS

Dumbbells are the best and easiest way to load the split squat exercise. Below I outline several load positions and variations.

Dumbbell Carry

BSS DUMBBELL CARRY   LUNGE CARRY

The most common and perhaps the most effective load position is to hold the dumbbells at your sides. It's a stable position, making it great for both beginners and advanced lifters. You can employ this variation with all of the split squat exercises. The one drawback is that you're limited by your grip strength, meaning that once you get strong with the split squat, you might be able to lift more weight than your grip can handle. In such a situation, use wrist straps or employ the barbell variations instead.

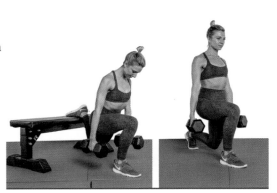

Dumbbell split squats are very simple: all you do is hold the dumbbells at your sides as you execute the movement. However, sometimes this is easier said than done. People tend to lean forward excessively and rock the dumbbells out in front of their bodies slightly as they go heavier or carry their repetitions to failure. They do so to create a counterbalance, which shifts some of the emphasis off the quads and onto the big engine of the hips. But this is sloppy form and is a slippery slope that's best avoided.

Contralateral and Ipsilateral Dumbbell Split Squat

When it comes to training for functional fitness—and to a lesser degree, strength and muscle development—you could argue that all split squat variations should be performed with a wide range of loading because, in addition to working the muscle from a variety of angles, each loading option has slightly different stabilization requirements. For example, in the case of the contralateral and ipsilateral split squat, which requires you to hold a dumbbell or kettlebell on one side of your body (with the opposite-side hand for the contralateral variation, which works more glute medius, and with the same-side hand for the ipsilateral variation), you have to focus on keeping your hips level and your spine braced to counter the opposing load. In short, it's a novel stimulus that might bring more awareness to your spinal mechanics and potentially improve coordination. Or perhaps you have access to only one dumbbell, or you just enjoy doing this type of split squat. In any case, it's one more loading option that you can apply to all of the split squat movement patterns for variety.

If you're training for muscle and strength, I recommend bracing your position by placing your non-weight hand on a wall or pole because your muscles won't fire as hard when balance is a factor. If you're training for function (or you're performing walking lunges), on the other hand, then it might be beneficial to work on your balance, in which case it's better to perform the exercise out in the open.

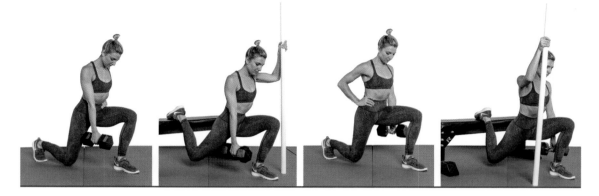

Goblet Split Squat

You can perform goblet split squats with one dumbbell or kettlebell. Again, you can't usually load the position with a lot of weight, so if you're strong, stick to high-rep sets. This loading variation is particularly popular with a lot of my female clients because they feel their glutes working hard during the exercise, and they can keep their torsos upright, which is unique to the goblet loading position. Upright split squats are usually more knee dominant,

GOBLET BSS   GOBLET LUNGE

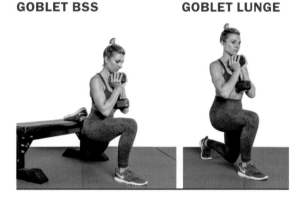

meaning that they increase quad activation, but that is not the case here. With the goblet split squat, you're more upright, but it feels like a hip-dominant movement, so it's easier on your knees and places tension on your glutes.

BARBELL VARIATIONS

Placing a barbell on your back is, in my opinion, the most effective way to load the split squat with significant weight. Unlike the dumbbell loading options, you're not limited by your grip. Furthermore, using a barbell is more stable than trying to balance with two dumbbells, making it a great option for both beginner and advanced lifters.

The only problem with the barbell variations is that you need a lot of space to perform them, especially walking lunges. You can remedy this by using a narrower barbell, such as a preloaded bar or Hip Thruster bar, but getting your hands in closer to your body requires good shoulder flexibility.

Back (Low and High Bar)

Like the barbell back squat, you can place the bar high or lower on your back for the split squat. The high bar position is more knee dominant with an upright torso, and the low bar position is more hip dominant with a more forward-leaning torso. In my experience, most lifters find the high bar position more comfortable because it's easier to position and feels more natural. *Note:* You can perform all of the split squat variations from both the high and the low bar positions.

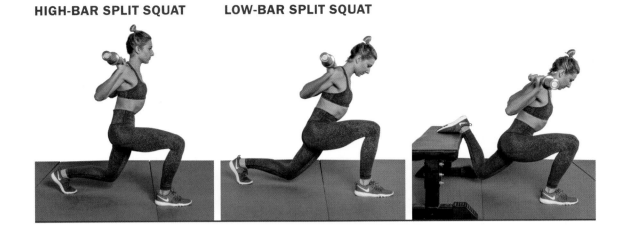

HIGH-BAR SPLIT SQUAT **LOW-BAR SPLIT SQUAT**

Front (Cross-Arm and Front Rack)

Some people prefer the front (cross-arm or front rack) loading position because they can stay more upright and squat a little deeper, while others avoid it because it hurts their shoulders and is harder to get right. If the position is comfortable, you want to lift heavy weight (more than you could in the goblet squat loading position), and you enjoy doing it, then the barbell front split squat is a great loading variation that you can apply to all of the split squat variations.

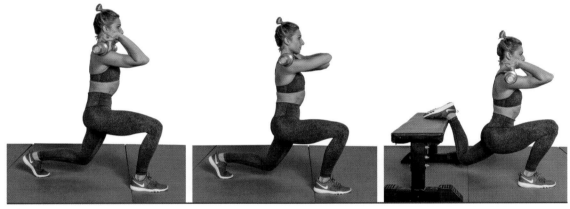

FRONT RACK LUNGE   **CROSS-ARM LUNGE**   **FRONT RACK BSS**

Zercher Split Squat

The Zercher is a hang squat variation in which you cradle the barbell in the crooks of your arms. This is a less common loading position, but whenever I introduce it to clients—especially using lighter loads—they always comment on how stable and good it feels. It becomes problematic, however, when you start to increase the weight. The higher the load, the more uncomfortable it is on your arms. For most of my clients, I keep the weight under their pain threshold, which is typically under 135 pounds for women and under 225 pounds for men, and use a bar pad to reduce pain.

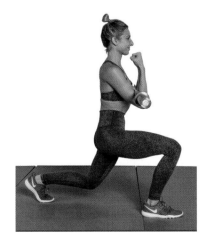

Landmine

The landmine is an effective loading implement for a few reasons. First, you can perform all of the loading positions with every single-leg squat pattern. Second, it's a unique loading pattern in that it's easier in the bottom position, which is where most people struggle. Third, it's a great loading option if you don't have access to heavy dumbbells. My one recommendation is to elevate the landmine unit off the ground at about hip level. If you don't have a power rack attachment, you can place it on a plyometric box. This helps equalize the resistance throughout the range of motion, meaning that it's similar in the bottom and top positions. With the unit on the ground, there is a more pronounced bar path arc, meaning that there is more resistance in the bottom position and less resistance in the top position. But some people prefer that, so experiment with both and choose the option that feels better.

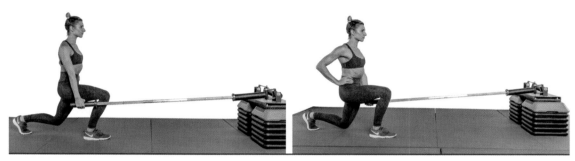

IPSILATERAL SPLIT SQUAT

CONTRALATERAL SPLIT SQUAT

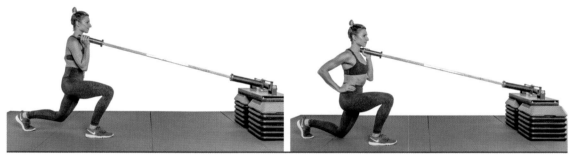

IPSILATERAL FRONT RACK SPLIT SQUAT

CONTRALATERAL FRONT RACK SPLIT SQUAT

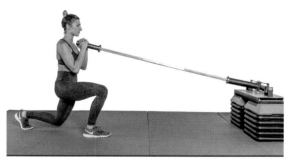

FRONT RACK SPLIT SQUAT

Step-ups

The step-up is one of my favorite squat pattern exercises because it's easy to learn, it transfers to the back squat and other functional movements, and it doesn't beat you up as badly as the split squat. To help you understand why, I'll address each of these benefits in more detail.

Like the split squat, the step-up is a squat pattern that transfers well to the back squat. Obviously, if you're trying to increase your one-rep max back squat, you still have to back squat for specificity. But if you do not tolerate squats well and you're not worried about increasing your barbell back squat 1RM, then you can get away with performing just split-squats and step-ups without losing much strength or compromising your glute gains. In fact, step-ups work the glutes to the same degree as squats in that they lengthen the muscle under tension and primarily work the lower subdivision of the gluteus maximus.

Unlike walking lunges and other single-leg squat patterns, step-ups don't make your glutes as sore, which remains a mystery to me. Remember, it's the eccentric loading that creates the most muscle damage. In the lowering phase of the step-up, you lose tension and fall to the ground. So, in theory, you reduce the amount of eccentric loading with each rep and thereby reduce the amount of muscle damage. Seems legit, but I proved this theory wrong when I started implementing the step-down variation, which accentuates the lowering phase. Now, you would think that this would increase muscle soreness since you're lengthening your glutes under tension, but that is not the case. With no explanation as to why, I've simply accepted it as a key benefit. That is, you can perform more volume without over-damaging your glutes while still reaping the lower glute–building benefits of the exercise.

Step-ups are also great for beginners who need to build functional movement patterns. Think climbing stairs, hiking, or stepping up onto an elevated surface—these are functional tasks that you need to be able to perform in everyday life. The step-up not only helps build this movement pattern but also improves hip flexion mobility, coordination, and lower-body strength.

Whether you're a novice or an advanced lifter, step-ups are a great exercise to program into your training once or twice a week. I typically place the step-up in the middle of the workout as an accessory exercise, but you can treat it as a main lift on squat days if—as I said—back squats are not well tolerated.

What a lot of people fail to realize is that the step-up is an easy movement to progressively overload either by raising the elevation of the step or by adding load in the form of dumbbells. For example, I might start a novice client on a small step and keep them there for 2 weeks or until they can perform 2 sets of 10 reps with good form. As they gain strength and coordination, I incrementally increase the height of the step. Over the course of several months, they'll go from a low step to a high step, which is a clear measure of progress. (This is also a great way to improve squat depth.)

In summary, step-ups are challenging for everyone if the right variation and height are utilized. If I use a high plyometric box, 2 sets of 12 reps at just body weight is very hard for me. The best part is, you probably have a high step or can stack two things to create one—either a box, bench, or some kind of elevated surface—at home, so you can get in a good leg workout without having to go to the gym.

GUIDELINES AND CUES

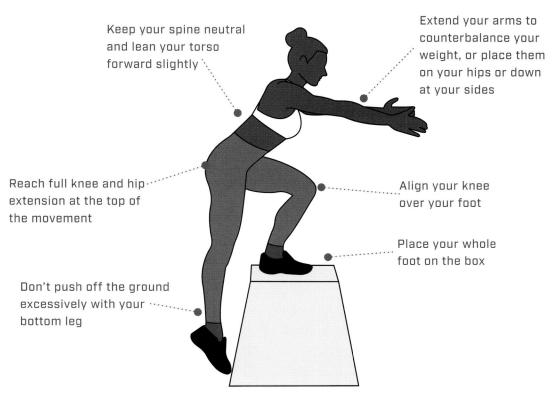

Keep your spine neutral and lean your torso forward slightly

Extend your arms to counterbalance your weight, or place them on your hips or down at your sides

Reach full knee and hip extension at the top of the movement

Align your knee over your foot

Place your whole foot on the box

Don't push off the ground excessively with your bottom leg

The step-up shares a lot of the same guidelines as the squat and split squat in that you want to keep your back in your neutral zone (as flat as possible), avoid excessive inward knee movement, drive through your heel or midfoot, and raise your torso and hips in one fluid motion. However, there are some specific technique cues that will make your step-up experience more fruitful, which I cover in the following pages.

SET THE BOX HEIGHT TO YOUR SQUAT DEPTH

The easiest way to determine step height is to experiment with the free squat and see how far down you can squat with good form. If you can squat only a quarter of the way down, then you should start on a low box that comes up only to your mid-shin. If squatting to parallel feels best, stepping onto a box that is just below knee height is probably best. If you can perform a full-range squat, then stepping onto a high box is ideal. The idea is to test the height of the box by placing your foot on the elevated surface and assessing your balance and pelvic position. If you're falling over backward or butt winking (posterior pelvic tilting), or you have to swing your leg laterally around the box to get your foot up, then it is probably too high.

When it comes to building bigger, stronger glutes with the step-up, I recommend prioritizing range of motion over load. In fact, I would rather you step up onto a high box with just body weight (assuming you have the mobility and coordination to perform the movement with good form) and express you full range of motion than step up to a low box with heavy dumbbells.

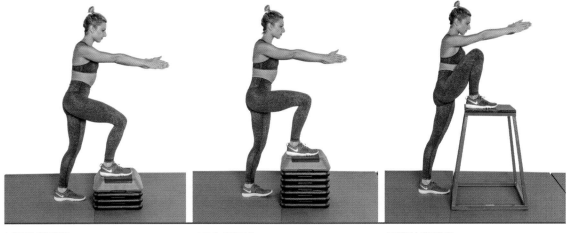

LOW STEP   MID STEP   HIGH STEP

STANCE AND SETUP: ALIGN YOUR KNEE OVER THE FRONT OF YOUR FOOT

Although stance width and foot placement will differ from person to person, positioning your feet directly underneath your hips is a good place to start. When you step your foot on the box, your feet are still roughly hip width apart, with your knee aligned over the front of your foot. Depending on the height of the box and your anthropometry, you might deviate slightly by positioning your foot closer to your center line. But to avoid excessive inward knee movement and swaying from side to side, your knee needs to be slightly forward and aligned over your elevated foot.

The vast majority of individuals prefer a straight foot with the step-up, but a small minority prefer turning their foot slightly inward or outward.

STEPPING MECHANICS: PLACE YOUR ENTIRE FOOT ON THE BOX OR ELEVATED SURFACE

As with the squat, deadlift, and hip thrust movements, you need to push through your heel as you extend your hips. The key, therefore, is to position your entire foot on the box. A lot of people step only half of their foot on the elevated surface, forcing them to drive off the ball of their foot. This shifts tension to the knee and quad and away from the hip and glute. To get the most from this exercise, you need to drive through your heel or midfoot, which is only possible if you step your entire foot onto the box.

HIP MECHANICS: KEEP YOUR HIPS SQUARE

Just like the squat, you want your hips and torso to come up at the same time. If you allow your hips to shoot up, you will shift tension away from your quads and onto your hamstrings. With the step-up, the goal is to use the power of your leg to lift your body upward. But—and this is key—you have to keep your hips square. Let's say you start with your feet positioned underneath your hips. When you step up on the box, you maintain that same stance width, with your knee aligned over your foot. Then, as you tilt your torso forward and step up, you raise your hips and torso in one fluid motion while keeping your hips square. By square, I mean that your hips are on the same horizontal plane and don't tilt or droop to one side or the other. In some cases, you might have to rotate slightly to maintain balance, but the idea is to limit twisting motion and keep your hips square as you step up and down.

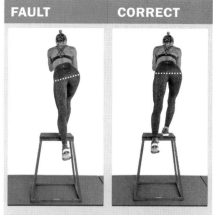

FAULT   CORRECT

PELVIC DROOP   HIPS SQUARE

SPINAL MECHANICS: LEAN YOUR TORSO FORWARD SLIGHTLY

You will have to lean your torso forward slightly in order to step up. Doing so not only is important for balance, but also places tension on your hips and glutes. And as you can see in the photos, the higher the box, the farther forward you have to lean. It's also important to keep your back as flat as possible (or in your neutral zone) as you lean. In other words, don't round your back. Instead, hinge from your hips and think about keeping your back flat as you step up.

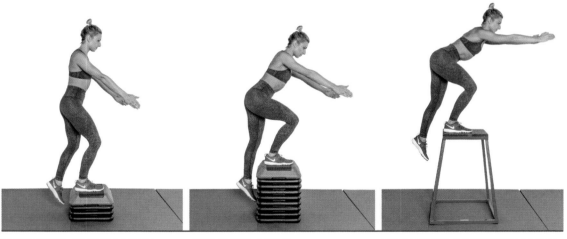

LOW STEP: SLIGHT LEAN   MID STEP: LEAN   HIGH STEP: FORWARD LEAN

BACK LEG MECHANICS: USE YOUR BACK LEG FOR STABILITY AND CONTROL

The initial phase of the step-up is the most challenging part of the movement because you have to propel your body upward using the power of mostly one leg. In this sense, the step-up is a single-leg squat. But, unlike a true single-leg squat, your back leg is there to provide stability and some propulsion. To perform the step-up correctly and get the most from the exercise, you have to get all of your weight over your elevated leg while driving off your heel to stand up. Now, you will need to push off the ground a little to get your weight over your elevated leg and maintain a rhythmic tempo from rep to rep, especially if the step is very high. But you don't want to push so much that you create excessive momentum out of the bottom position.

Your bottom leg also plays a role in the step-down phase. As you lower down, the idea is to control your descent for as long as possible. In other words, you're not just dropping to the ground and then bouncing back up; you're lowering yourself slowly to increase eccentric time under tension. The first third of the movement is easy to control, but there is a "breaking point" where you can no longer support your weight and you drop to the ground. The goal is to control your descent as far as you can. If you're using a plyometric box that has flat sides, you can slide your bottom foot down the box to help maintain balance and control your descent. Otherwise, you will have to step back slightly (away from the step) to keep your balance.

FULL HIP AND KNEE EXTENSION OPTIONS

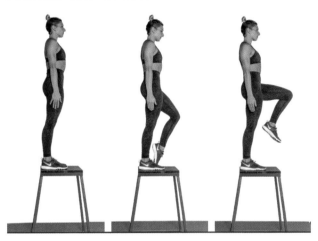

FULL KNEE AND HIP EXTENSION: EXTEND YOUR HIPS IN THE TOP POSITION

As you step up and stand upright, always extend your hips before stepping down. To accomplish this, make sure you fully lock out your knee and hips before stepping down. For example, if you're stepping up with your left leg, you straighten your left knee and fully extend your hips, then gently tap your right foot down onto the elevated surface. You can also raise your right knee to encourage full hip extension (more on this in the Faults and Corrections section below).

COMPLETE REPS ON ONE SIDE BEFORE SWITCHING LEGS; DO NOT ALTERNATE AFTER EACH REP

Let's say you're performing 2 sets of 12 reps. To complete a set, perform 12 reps with your left foot on the step and then 12 reps with your right foot on the step. In other words, choose a side (either your right or your left leg), position your foot on the box, and then keep it there until you have finished 12 reps. Then switch sides and do 12 reps with your other leg. When you perform reverse lunges, switching feet after each rep is fine; it's easier to count reps, the transition feels natural, and you work both legs equally during the set. But that is not the case with step-ups. If you try to step up with one leg and then step down with the other, you not only compromise your rhythm and balance but also lose time under consistent tension. So perform the step-up on one side at a time, and rest between legs as needed.

FAULTS AND CORRECTIONS

Just as the step-up shares many of the same guidelines and cues as the squat and split squat, it shares many of the same faults, all of which can be avoided simply by following the guidelines and cues previously outlined. For example, rounding your back, pushing off the ball of your foot, butt winking, and knee valgus are easy to prevent and correct if you understand the proper mechanics. So, rather than waste your time addressing these faults, I'll focus on the two biggest errors that are common with the step-up.

FAULT: PUSHING OFF YOUR GROUNDED LEG

There is a strong tendency to push off excessively with your grounded leg, especially when stepping onto a high box or platform. Realize that at the bottom of the step-up, or the initial phase of the movement, your glutes are stretched. If the goal is to work your glutes, then you need to drive out of the bottom of the step-up using the power of your elevated leg.

Correction: Reducing the height of the box is the easiest and most practical way to avoid this fault. If you have to push off the ground in order to step up, then the box is too tall or you're not strong enough. In either case, lowering the height of the box is an easy solution.

FAULT: USING YOUR OPPOSITE LEG TO COMPLETE THE MOVEMENT OR EXTEND YOUR HIPS

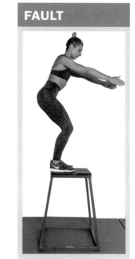

FAULT

One of the most common mistakes is to step halfway up and then touch down prematurely with your opposite leg, catching yourself in a quarter squat, and then stand upright under the power of two legs. Remember, the step-up is a single-leg exercise, and you want to use the power of one leg to complete the movement. You can implement a few tricks to prevent this fault:

CORRECTION 1:
Extend your hips and then tap your other foot on the box once you reach full hip extension. But if you need to touch your opposite foot to the box to catch your balance, do it! Always prioritize your balance and safety over completing a rep.

CORRECTION 2:
Elevate your knee slightly as you extend your hips. So, instead of touching your foot down, you actually lift your knee and raise it to hip height. People see this and wonder, "What's that for—are they trying to work the hip flexor of the opposite leg?" When I first saw people doing it, I thought it was silly, but now I understand; it prevents them from catching themselves in a quarter squat with both legs.

CORRECTION 3:
Perform the side step-up variation. With your leg hanging off the side of the box, there's nowhere to place your opposite foot, making it impossible to catch yourself in a quarter squat.

STEP-UP VARIATIONS

You can create variations for the step-up by changing the height of the box, changing the direction of your step (stepping forward or to the side), or loading the movement with dumbbells, kettlebells, or a barbell. Regardless of the variation you're implementing, it's imperative the step be flat, hard, and stable. Stepping onto a squishy, unstable platform is a recipe for disaster. The best step-up apparatuses are aerobic steps and risers, wide benches with firm padding, regular and adjustable squat boxes, and plyometric boxes, or any step-up platform that is secure and flat, such as a concrete park bench, retaining wall, brick fire pit, or flat boulder.

BODYWEIGHT STEP-UP

As I said, the bodyweight step-up is great for both beginners and advanced athletes. If you're new to glute training, start out with a small or medium step—say, mid-shin to knee height—and progress to a high box once you can perform 2 sets of 10 reps with good form and without pain or discomfort. Generally, 2 or 3 sets of 8 to 12 is challenging for the vast majority of people. Even if you're an advanced athlete, 2 or 3 sets of 12 reps using a high box with body weight will provide a potent leg workout. The best part about bodyweight step-ups is that you can do them just about anywhere. All you need is an elevated, stable platform.

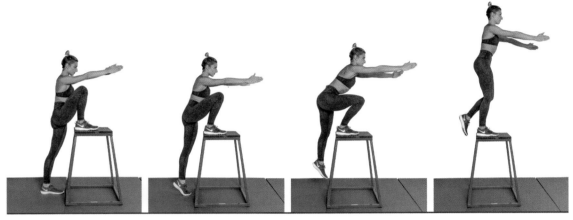

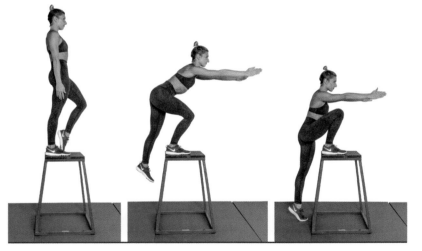

Stand in front of the box with your feet directly underneath your hips (narrow stance). Keeping the same stance width, step onto the box, positioning your entire foot on the box. You can orient your foot straight or turn it slightly inward, whichever feels better. With your foot on the box, lean forward with a neutral spine and get your center of mass balanced over your foot (shift your weight solely onto your lead leg). As you do, allow your knee to translate slightly forward over your toes so that the front of your knee is in line with the front of your foot. Make sure your hips and upper body are square. To execute the step-up, you do several things at once: drive off your lead heel or midfoot, raise your hips and torso in one fluid motion using the power of your leg, and extend your arms out in front of you to counterbalance your weight. Remember, your rear leg is there for balance and stability; don't push off the ground excessively as you initiate the movement. As you stand upright, make sure you fully extend your hips before stepping down. To lower yourself, tilt your torso forward, sit your hips back, and slowly lower your opposite leg to the ground. As you do, keep your front knee aligned over your foot and step your rear leg back slightly (not straight down). Also, try to control your descent as far down as possible. Note: You can push off the ground a little with your bottom foot to help transition to the next rep and maintain a rhythmic tempo as long as you don't rely too much on the momentum to aid in the initial phase of the step-up.

SIDE STEP-UP

You can vary the bodyweight step-up by stepping up and to the side. Instead of positioning the step in front of you, you position it on the same side as your stepping leg. Both variations work your glutes in exactly the same way, so the option you choose is a matter of personal preference.

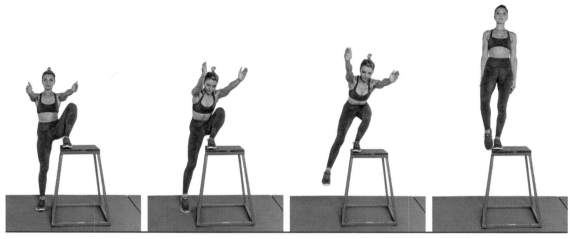

The side step-up shares the same technique and execution as the front step-up. The only difference is that you set up to the side of the box and lean forward at a diagonal over your elevated foot.

DUMBBELL STEP-UPS

In general, the higher the step, the more awkward it is to hold weights because you can't use your arms for balance. I prefer range of motion over loading, so given the option, I will always choose a high step-up with body weight or light weight over a mid-range or low step-up with heavy weight. That said, if you don't have the range of motion to perform a high step-up, or you simply want to target your quads, then holding two heavy dumbbells at your sides or a single dumbbell in a goblet position and performing a low- to mid-range step-up—equivalent to your parallel squat height—is a perfectly viable exercise.

DUMBBELL CARRY STEP-UP

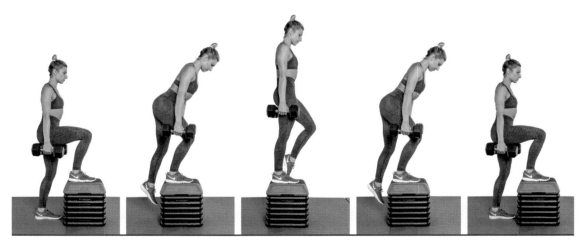

GOBLET STEP-UP

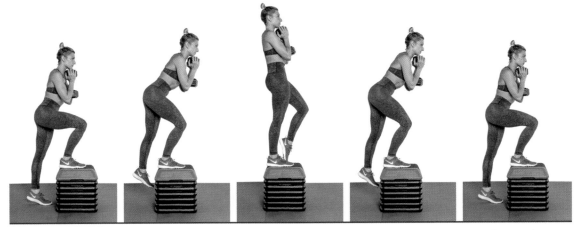

The setup and execution for the dumbbell carry and goblet variations are very similar to the bodyweight step-up. The only difference is that you hold two dumbbells at your sides or one dumbbell at your chest in the goblet position. Focus on keeping your back flat—that is, hinge from your hips as you lean forward, and don't allow the weight of the dumbbells or kettlebell to pull your upper back into flexion.

KETTLEBELL OR DUMBBELL (CONTRALATERAL LOADING) STEP-UP

To perform a high step-up, you need to be able to extend your arms out in front of your body. You do so not only to shift your center of mass over your stepping leg and propel your body upward but also to maintain balance. However, you can hold a kettlebell or dumbbell in a front rack position by resting it on your shoulder while extending your opposite arm for balance and stability. The key is to hold the kettlebell or dumbbell with the arm opposite your stepping leg. So, if you're stepping up with your right leg, you hold the kettlebell or dumbbell on your left shoulder in the front rack position. This variation doesn't work nearly as well with the ipsilateral loading (kettlebell or dumbbell on the same side as your stepping leg). For it to work, you need the arm on the same side of your stepping leg free to counterbalance your body weight, which is why I have included only the contralateral loading option.

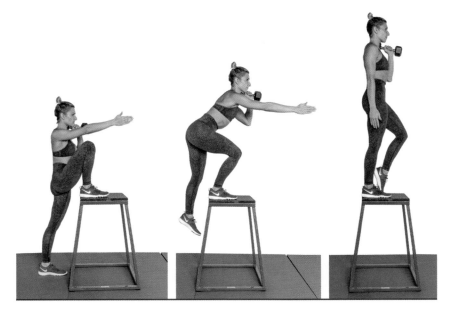

ZERCHER STEP-UP

The Zercher step-up is the best barbell step-up variation because the weight is positioned in front of your body in the crooks of your arms, so if something goes horribly wrong—say, you lose your balance at the top of the step-up—you can dump the weight out in front of you without getting hurt. Unlike the dumbbell variations, you're not limited by your grip. This means you can generally handle more weight, making it a great option for people who want to target their quads with a unique exercise.

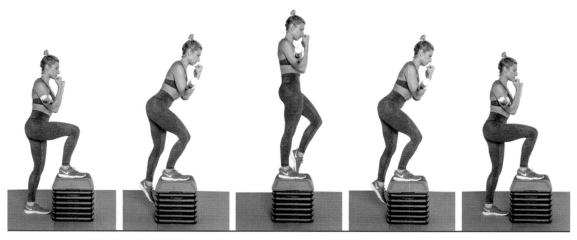

To get the barbell into position, take it out of the rack by hooking the crooks of your arms around the barbell and then walking it over to your box or platform. Once you get the weight in position, you perform the step-up exactly as previously described. Just make sure to keep your back flat (don't round your upper back) and step onto a stable box or platform.

RING/HUMAN-ASSISTED STEP-UPS (ACCENTUATED STEP-DOWN)

I started experimenting with assisted step-ups about 12 years ago to help my clients stay balanced. First, I did them with beginner, elderly, and overweight clients, but then I started doing them with advanced athletes to help the athletes perform faster reps while going very deep. For example, they could bust out 20 reps in 20 seconds and would actually feel their glutes more than when performing conventional bodyweight step-ups because they were able to keep their glutes on tension as they lowered and reversed out of the bottom position. What's more, they were breathing hard, their glutes were on fire, and they felt like they were getting a good workout. One client said, "I love this variation because I feel my glutes and it makes me feel athletic—like how I used to train when I played sports."

Though I still implement assisted step-ups, I've made a couple of modifications over the years. The first is the ring-assisted variation. Holding a client's hands is great if you're coaching one-on-one, but it's impossible when coaching a big class like the Glute Squad. The rings are great because people can do the assisted step-ups on their own. The only caveat is that this variation is challenging to set up; the rings have to be at an appropriate angle, roughly 45 degrees or even more horizontal, when you're holding them in the bottom position. In other words, it won't work if they are straight up and down; they have to be between a diagonal and horizontal. I usually attach them to a pull-up bar on a power rack, and that setup seems to work for most people. Like all step-up variations, the platform needs to be ultra-stable.

The second modification accentuates the step-down portion and keeping the glutes on tension as you lower and come out of the bottom position. This increases eccentric time under tension, which is a good mechanism for muscle growth.

Whether you're performing the human-assisted or the ring-assisted variation, the goal is to use the support to help you keep tension in the bottom position where you would otherwise lose control and fall to the ground. Interestingly, these variations don't make the glutes as sore as lunges (I'm not sure why), making them one of my favorite ways to lengthen the glutes under tension.

HUMAN-ASSISTED STEP-UP

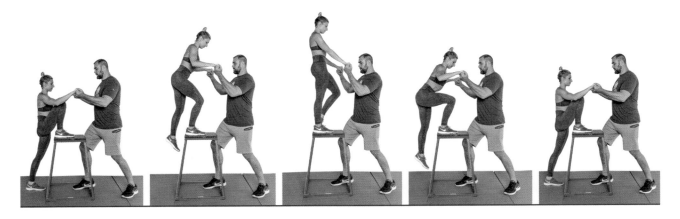

RING-ASSISTED STEP-UP

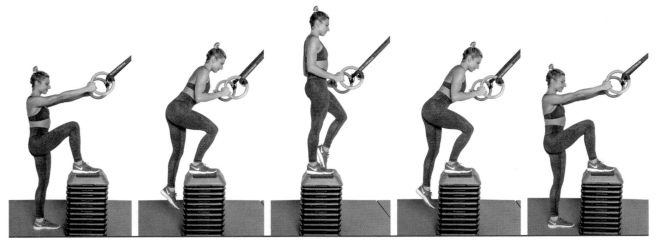

If you're performing the human-assisted step-up, have your training partner stand in front of the box and hold your hands. If you're performing the ring-assisted variation, position the rings at roughly a 45-degree angle with your arms extended diagonally. The execution is the same as for the bodyweight variation: you step your entire foot on the box, align your front knee over your front foot, tilt your torso forward and hinge from your hips with a flat back, and extend your hips and knee simultaneously as you stand upright. Try not to pull excessively on your partner's hands or the rings to assist with the upward motion. Instead, pull just enough to control the latter phase of the movement, keeping as much tension on your glutes as possible. As you lower into the bottom position, pull on the hands/rings just enough to maintain balance and tension (you should feel your glutes stretch while under tension), then reverse the movement when you reach end range.

4 Single-Leg Squats

When it comes to the squat movement pattern, you have a lot of options, all of which work your glutes in a similar way. Choosing the exercise variations you want to perform boils down to your goals and movement preferences.

If you're interested in powerlifting or you have strength-specific goals, prioritizing the back squat makes the most sense. If you're just interested in functional performance, you might prefer the split squat, step-up, and single-leg variations and stick with higher-rep sets that are easier on your body. If your goal revolves around building stronger, higher-performing glutes and quads, you can essentially choose the exercises that you enjoy the most and get results. Again, this is why I chose to include so many exercise variations in this book—to give you options.

Although exercise variety is important, you are sure to love certain exercises and loathe others. The single-leg squat, for example, happens to be an exercise that I loathe because I'm not good at it. It took me 20 years to get my first single-leg squat (also known as a pistol), not because I was weak, but because I didn't practice it. I'm a big, tall guy, and my anthropometry isn't well suited to pistols. They're uncomfortable for me. I much prefer testing my strength with squats.

But that's just my preference. I coach and train a lot of people who prefer the pistol over the back squat, and they are just as strong and functional as people who can back squat double their body weight. Suppose you want to get stronger in the squat pattern and grow your glutes and quads, but back squats hurt your lower back, hips, or knees. Instead of working toward a double bodyweight back squat, which is a common strength goal, a much better option would be to focus on the pistol. In short, doing multiple reps of the single-leg squat or loaded pistol is a true test of leg strength and is just as impressive as doing a double bodyweight back squat.

This is what makes the single-leg squat such a great exercise: not only is it a challenging movement that lengthens the glutes under tension through a full range of motion, but it's also one of the best ways to increase mobility and strength in the squat movement pattern. What's more, single-leg squats (pistol and skater squat variations) are great for addressing differences in leg strength and size. Whether it's an adaptation from your sport or you're recovering from a leg injury, performing single-leg squats or step-ups with your weaker leg is an effective strategy for correcting the imbalance.

Even though single-leg squats are not my favorite exercise and not everyone can do them, they should definitely have a place in your exercise library. In fact, not being able to do a pistol motivated me to work on it and gave me a goal to work toward. I still prioritize the back squat first in my workouts, but now I cyclically employ the pistol as an accessory exercise for the aforementioned reasons. Not only does my squat feel better, but my leg strength, mobility, and coordination have improved markedly.

GUIDELINES AND CUES

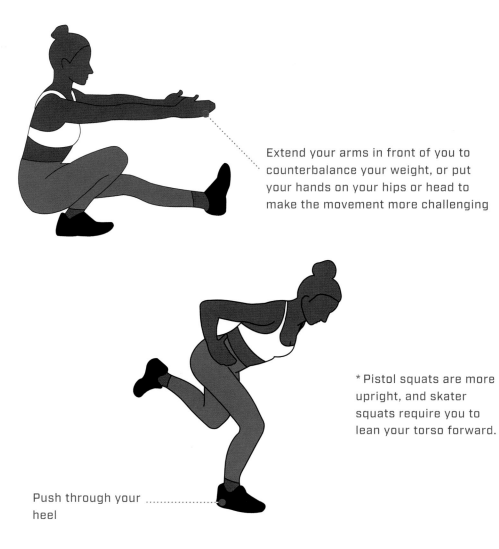

Extend your arms in front of you to counterbalance your weight, or put your hands on your hips or head to make the movement more challenging

* Pistol squats are more upright, and skater squats require you to lean your torso forward.

Push through your heel

Single-leg squats share a lot of the same technique guidelines as the split squat and step-up: you want to drive through your heel or midfoot, align your knee over your foot, keep your hips square, and move your hips and torso in one fluid motion—that is, tilt your torso forward on the way down and keep your torso angle constant during the first half of the rising phase out of the bottom position. However, there is some additional wiggle room when it comes to spinal mechanics, specifically in the bottom position of the pistol. The goal is to stay within your neutral zone throughout as much of the range of motion as possible. But everyone will posterior pelvic tilt if they drop into a low enough squat.

Because the pistol is the lowest you can squat, everyone butt winks to some degree. It's not a bad thing as long as it doesn't cause you discomfort. In fact, most people don't feel any pain and can get away with butt winking when they do pistols because it's an unloaded exercise. More specifically, there is not as much compressive force on your spine, and you don't have the same erector requirements. Like a high step-up, just body weight is challenging.

Later in this section, you will learn a progression or sequence of exercises organized from easiest to most difficult for both the pistol and skater squat movements. Before I delve into those variations, let's review a couple of important technique guidelines.

STANCE AND SETUP: EXPERIMENT WITH YOUR STANCE IN THE BOTTOM POSITION

There are two types of single-leg squats:

- **The pistol requires you to extend your opposite leg out in front of your body.**
- **The skater squat requires you to extend your leg behind your body.**

Setting up in the right stance is the first step to single-leg squatting with good form. The best thing to do is simply to get into the bottom position of each movement. For this drill, allow your leg to rest on the ground while you experiment with the different foot positions.

Some people position their foot directly underneath their hip, some prefer to position it along their center line, while others adopt a stance somewhere in between. To find your optimal foot placement, experiment by getting into the bottom position and feeling it out. Try each stance and tinker with your foot orientation by positioning your foot straight and slightly turned out. Like the other squat variations, the goal is to center your weight over your heel or midfoot and align your knee with your foot. Choose the foot position in which you have the most balance, meaning that you're not falling backward or wobbling from side to side.

Once you've found a comfortable foot position, the next step is to distribute your weight over your grounded foot by lifting your opposite leg off the ground. If you're performing a pistol from the floor, then you hold your leg out in front of you or raise it gradually as you

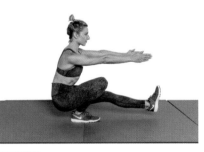

PISTOL

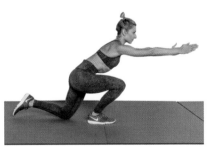

SKATER

descend. If your opposite leg prevents you from lowering all the way into the bottom of the pistol position or it's uncomfortable, try standing on a box and letting your other leg hang off the side of the box. This will allow you to get into the bottom position without having to hold your opposite leg off the ground straight out in front of you. If that still doesn't feel right or you don't have the mobility to get into the right position, start with the box squat variation on page 485.

If you're performing a skater squat, keep your knee on the ground while curling your heel toward your butt. If that's too difficult to manage, you can try resting your knee on a BOSU ball or Airex balance pad.

COUNTERBALANCE: RAISE YOUR ARMS IN THE BOTTOM POSITION

To remain balanced in the bottom position, you need to lean your torso forward and extend your arms to counterbalance your weight. With your arms extended, you will have an easier time leaning forward and staying balanced as you lower and rise out of the bottom position. For example, as you lower into the pistol or skater squat, raise your arms—keeping them straight—and then lower them as you stand upright. If you still have a hard time staying balanced in the bottom position, try the counterbalance dumbbell variation.

SINGLE-LEG SQUAT VARIATIONS

PISTOL SQUATS

Everyone can eventually perform a split squat or step-up, and most people can eventually perform a skater squat to a certain range, but not everyone can do a pistol squat. People have hired me as their online personal trainer with the sole goal of getting a pistol. Like the pull-up, the pistol is a bodyweight strength goal that everyone should work toward. It moves your hip, knee, and ankle through a full range of motion, lengthens the glutes under tension, and is a true test of leg strength and body awareness. The best part is, most people will get it quickly if they stick with it and follow the progression provided here.

If your goal is to get a pistol, prioritize it first in your workout. Remember, what gets done first in the workout gives you the best results. You're fresh, you're focused, and you're recovered. If you can already perform a pistol or it's not your main focus, then you can place it in the middle of your workout.

Ring-Assisted Pistol

The ring-assisted variation is a good place to start. By holding onto rings or TRX handles, you can use your arms to support the weight of your body and stay balanced. This does two things: it allows you to perform the full range of the movement and lower and rise out of the bottom with more stability. To get the most from this variation, however, you need to keep your goal in mind. For example, if you want to progress to a full bodyweight pistol, then you need to perform the movement using the same mechanics as the bodyweight pistol. This is challenging, as you'll naturally lean backward into the rings for support. You should rely on your arms primarily for balance and for some assistance out of the hole so that you develop the leg strength and coordination needed to perform the movement. But don't rely too heavily on your arms to assist with the movement. When you first start out, you might have to lean a lot. The goal is to reduce the degree of your lean as your technique and strength improves. To drill the proper body mechanics, I also recommend performing single-leg box squats. The ring-assisted pistol will move you through a full range of motion, while the single-leg box squat will help you drill proper free pistol mechanics.

Now, if you're only interested in getting a good workout, then these things don't matter as much. Not everyone cares about being able to do a pistol, and some people can do a pistol but just want to get a good leg workout. In such a situation, you can perform ring-assisted pistols for high reps.

RING-ASSISTED LEANING BACK PISTOL

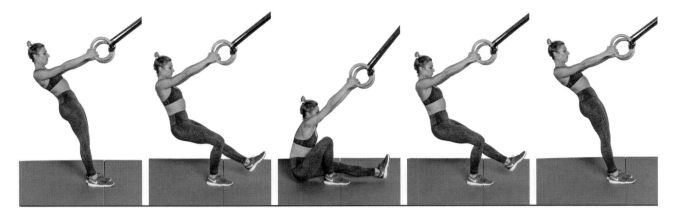

RING-ASSISTED UPRIGHT PISTOL

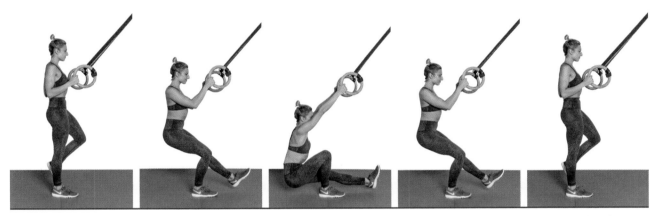

Begin by setting the rings to the correct height. Lower the rings to roughly mid-torso or chest height, then take a few steps back so the rings are at a diagonal. With your arms extended, assume your pistol stance, lean back, and lower into the squat position, keeping your knee aligned over your foot. Don't pull on the rings until absolutely necessary. The goal is to lower into the pistol under the power of your leg, then pull on the rings when you feel like you're going to fall. Even then, you're just using your arms for balance and relying mostly on your leg strength to lower into the bottom position. To reverse the movement, drive through your heel or midfoot, raise your hips and torso in one fluid motion, and pull on the rings just enough to maintain a rhythmic tempo. Note: If your front leg gets in the way or you don't have the hip flexor strength to keep your leg extended in front of you, perform the movement on a box and let your leg hang off the side. (You'll need to adjust the height of the rings if you go this route, of course.)

Single-Leg Box Squat

The single-leg box squat is similar to the double-leg box squat in that you use a box to control your depth and give you a target to aim for. This is another form of progressive distance training where you start with a high box and then incrementally lower the height of the box until you reach a full pistol. You can also use the counterbalance pistol or ring-assisted pistol in conjunction with the box squat variation.

SINGLE-LEG BOX SQUAT

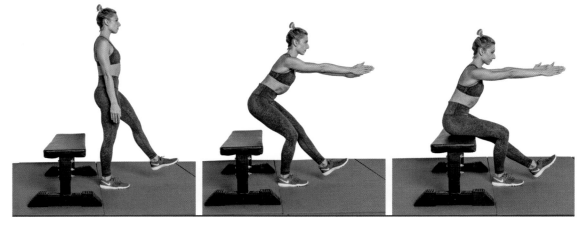

Position a box so that one corner is between your legs or a bench so that it is perpendicular to your body. Stand with your heels positioned just in front of the bench or box in your pistol stance. Next, lift one leg, begin to squat by sitting your hips down and leaning your torso forward, and lower your elevation until your butt touches down to the box or bench. From here, you can immediately reverse the position, or you can sit all of your weight on the box or bench and relax your hip and leg muscles, or you can rock back and then forward before standing back up—see pages 428 to 430 for more detailed descriptions of all of the box squat options.

Counterbalance Dumbbell Pistol

If you're close to getting a pistol but have a hard time keeping your balance in the bottom position, then the counterbalance dumbbell pistol is a great variation to implement. When I teach seminars and am going over pistol squats, I ask the attendees, "Who here is close to being able to do a pistol?" Someone will raise their hand and I'll say, "Okay, let's see it." They'll demonstrate a pistol, and, in most cases, they get close but struggle to maintain their balance in the bottom position. They're almost strong enough to pistol and can lower into the bottom position with control, but they don't yet have the balance and power to reverse the position and stand up. Next, I hand them 5- or 10-pound dumbbells (depending on how big and strong they are) and tell them to raise their arms out in front of their body as they lower into the bottom position. And, like magic, they get it. People are always surprised that they can pistol when holding 10 to 20 extra pounds, but not with body weight. This is the counterbalance mechanism at work.

The hardest part of the pistol is coming out of the bottom position, which requires serious balance and quadriceps strength. If you hold 5- or 10-pound dumbbells out in front of you, you can keep your weight forward and stay balanced long enough to spring out of the bottom position, and the counterbalance mechanism shifts some of the requirements from your knees to your hips. Scientists would say that it shifts your center of mass forward, which increases torque output at the hips and decreases torque output from the knees. Because the hips are capable of being stronger than the knees, it makes sense that you would be stronger this way. So, if you struggle in the bottom position of the pistol, try the counterbalance variation and see what happens.

COUNTERBALANCE DUMBBELL PISTOL

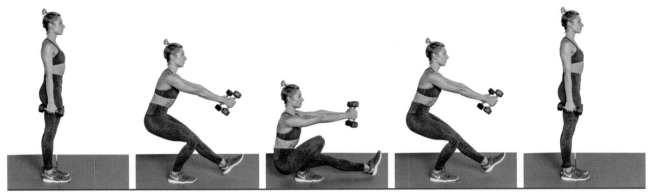

For this variation, you can use dumbbells or a light (10-pound) weight plate. Hold the weights at your sides or out in front of you (if you're gripping a weight plate) and get into your pistol stance. Extend one leg out in front of you and then lower into the bottom position, letting your knee move forward and your hips move backward while leaning your torso forward and keeping your knee aligned over your foot. You can also let your leg dangle and gradually raise it as you descend into the squat. As you do, raise the weights by lifting your arms and keeping them extended. When you reach the bottom position, your arms should be straight out in front of you. Reverse the position by driving through your heel or midfoot and raising your hips and torso in one fluid motion. As you stand upright, lower your arms back into the start position. You can also perform this variation using a box to gauge your depth.

Bodyweight (Free) Pistol

Although the single-leg box squat and counterbalance dumbbell pistol are great for building strength, mobility, and coordination, at a certain point you need to take away the crutches. The bodyweight pistol—as I already covered—is the best single-leg exercise for strengthening the legs and lengthening the glutes under tension through a full range of motion. It's what the pull-up is for the upper body, in that it's the truest expression of bodyweight strength and control. If you can perform a full-range bodyweight pistol with proper form, it demonstrates that you have not only strength and coordination but also good ankle and hip range of motion. In the following sequences, you will learn three bodyweight (free) pistol variations.

BOX PISTOL

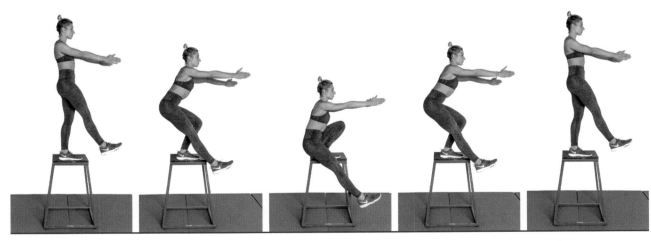

If you have a hard time keeping your opposite foot elevated off the ground in the bottom position, try standing on a box and letting your leg hang off the side.

COUNTERBALANCE PISTOL

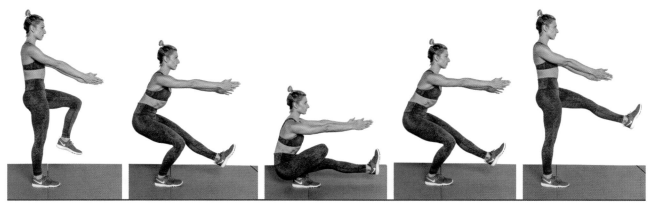

Start by getting into your pistol stance. Extend one leg out in front of you, keeping your foot just above the ground. In one fluid motion, squat down while letting your knee move forward and your hips move back, tilting your torso forward and lowering into the bottom position of the pistol, keeping your knee aligned over your foot. As you lower into the squat, raise your arms out in front of your body to counterbalance your weight. To reverse out of the bottom position, drive through your heel or midfoot and simultaneously extend your hips and knee while raising your torso. If you're using the counterbalance method, lower your hands as you stand upright. Again, if you're unable to keep your opposite leg off the ground, you can perform this variation while standing on a box to give your leg more clearance.

HANDS ON HIPS PISTOL

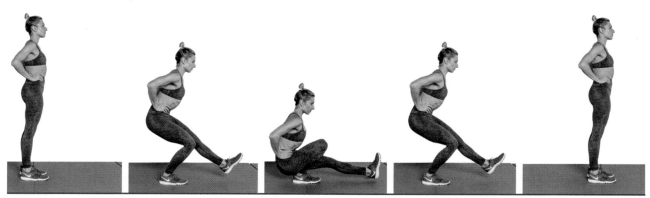

If you're advanced or you want to make the movement more challenging, remove the counterbalance by crossing your arms in front of your chest or placing your hands on your hips or behind your head.

Loaded Pistol (Dumbbell and Weight Vest Variations)

There are a couple of ways to load the pistol. One is to hold a dumbbell in the front rack position (goblet pistol). You will also see people performing double dumbbell front rack pistols, but you don't have as much balance with that variation and there's added risk—say you lose your balance and drop the weights.

A weight vest is another great option. It can restrict your breathing a little when you get really strong, and not everyone has one, but you retain the use of both arms.

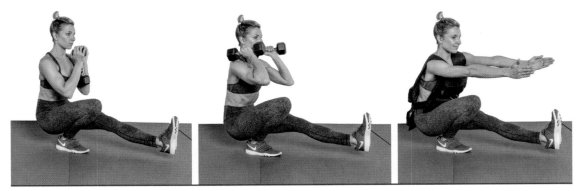

The goblet, double dumbbell, and weight vest pistol variations are performed in exactly the same way as the bodyweight pistol. The only difference is that you're holding a dumbbell (goblet) or dumbbells (front rack) or wearing a weight vest. As with all of the pistol variations, you can stand on a box and let your foot dangle if you can't keep your front leg off the ground.

SKATER SQUATS

If your goal is to hammer your quads, then the skater squat is a great exercise to employ. It shares more similar joint angles to the deadlift, but extending your leg behind your body turns it into a more knee-dominant movement, meaning that it works your quads more than your glutes and hamstrings. It still strengthens the glutes, but not through quite as much range of motion as a pistol, and it transfers well to hip-dominant movements like the deadlift. Like the pistol, the skater squat is a challenging movement that requires a ton of quad strength, balance, and coordination.

To perform the skater squat variations correctly, you extend your leg behind your body and bend your knee. As you lower into the squat, you can touch your knee to a pad or reverse in midair an inch shy of the ground. Most people can't do a skater squat without dropping their shin to the floor. For this reason, I have provided a series of techniques organized from easiest to most difficult.

Half Skater Squat

If you can't perform a full-range skater squat, begin by performing partial skater squats. In the beginning, you may be able to go only halfway down. As you get better, you can use a BOSU ball or thick pad to provide a depth target.

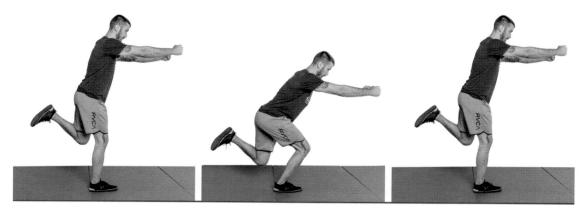

Get into a narrow squat stance with your feet underneath your hips. Now you do several things at once: extend one leg behind your body with your knee bent, tilt your torso forward with a flat back, extend your arms out in front of you for balance, and sit your hips down, keeping your front knee aligned over your front foot. Keeping your arms extended, lower into a squat and touch your knee to the pad, then immediately reverse the movement and stand upright. If you don't have a pad or it is too low, reverse in midair and descend as far as you can without falling to the floor.

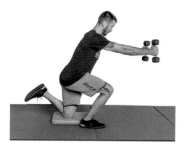

Full Skater Squat

The full-range skater squat is right up there with the pistol as a superior bodyweight exercise for building and strengthening the quads. Like the pistol, doing 2 or 3 sets of 8 to 12 reps of skater squats is challenging for even the most advanced athletes. There are two ways to perform the full skater squat. The first is simply to touch your knee to the ground, which you can do anywhere. The second is to stand on an aerobic step or 3-inch box and come down to a BOSU ball or balance pad. You're still performing a full range of motion, but instead of dropping your knee to the hard floor, you touch down to a padded surface that's level with the ground. In addition to providing a layer of safety, the pad gives you a target, allowing for a more rhythmic and consistent tempo. You can also perform a deficit skater squat by increasing the height of the step, but this variation is tough.

FULL SKATER SQUAT

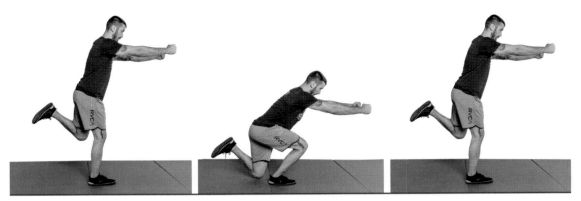

The full skater squat shares the same setup and technique as the half skater: extend one leg behind your body with your knee bent, tilt your torso forward with a flat back, extend your arms out in front of you to counterbalance your weight, and drop your hips, keeping your front knee aligned over your front foot. The only difference is that you're moving through a larger range of motion.

Loaded Skater Squat (Dumbbell Carry and Weight Vest Variations)

The best way to load the skater squat is to wear a weight vest or hold two dumbbells at your sides. You have to lean farther forward for the skater squat, so the kettlebell front rack, counterbalance, and ring-assisted variations are not as effective or advised. Like the loaded pistol, this variation is reserved for advanced athletes who can perform 2 or 3 sets of 8 to 12 reps of full-range bodyweight skater squats without struggling.

WEIGHT VEST SKATER   DUMBBELL CARRY SKATER

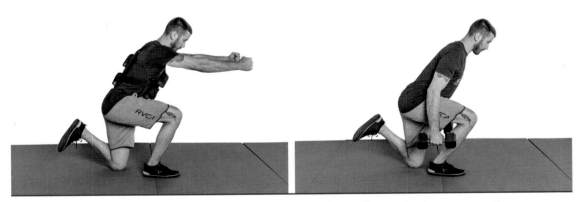

The weight vest and dumbbell carry variations are performed exactly the same as the bodyweight skater squat. Your form should look identical. If adding load causes you to compromise your form—say, round your back—consider increasing the range of motion by performing a deficit variation or increasing the number of reps using just body weight rather than adding load.

Sled Pushes

There are exercises that people can't or shouldn't do. Reasons for avoiding exercises include mobility or anatomical restrictions, susceptibility to injuries, pain or discomfort, or a failure to align with your goals. Simply put, if a particular exercise doesn't feel right or align with your goals, then you shouldn't do it. If it causes you pain or discomfort every time you do it, even when you execute the movement with good form, then it's time to find a variation that feels better or move on to another exercise for the time being.

I have the great fortune of training and interacting with a lot of people—from athletes and physique competitors to people who simply want to look and feel better—and all of them have different exercises that they can't or shouldn't do. For instance, the barbell hip thrust is one of the most well-tolerated glute training exercises, yet probably one in four people aren't huge fans because they feel this exercise working their quads or hamstrings too much for their liking. The squat and deadlift are universally regarded as the most functional strength movements, but in a certain percentage of people, they cause knee and lower back pain, even when done with good form.

This is another reason why it's so important to have a large toolbox of exercises to choose from, especially as a trainer. In most cases, you can find a variation that is well tolerated. But even then, some movement patterns might be off the table. In short, there are very few exercises that everyone can do. The sled push happens to be one of those exercises.

Whether you have a mobility restriction, unique anthropometry, or lower back pain or you're overly sore and beat up, chances are you can still push a sled. It requires very little coordination, you can scale the loading to suit all skill and strength levels, and you don't need a ton of flexibility to perform the exercise correctly. What's more, there is no eccentric activity during the sled push movement. As a quick recap, there's the concentric phase of a lift, during which the muscle shortens, and the eccentric phase of a lift, during which the muscle lengthens. The eccentric phase tends to cause more muscle damage. So pushing a sled won't make you as sore as other exercises because you're not lengthening the muscles under load.

For this reason, I recommend sled pushes when you are feeling beat up, overly sore, or recovering from injury. You can also employ the sled push at the end of a workout as a conditioning and strength-building exercise. You're not quite as likely to grow bigger, stronger glutes with the sled push as you are with full-range dynamic exercises like the squat and hip thrust, but you will maintain muscle mass and build stamina, and those things always have a place in glute training.

SLED PUSH VARIATIONS

The sled push is a hard movement to screw up. As long as you follow the universal principles and technique guidelines—keep your back flat (in your neutral zone), keep your shoulders stable, and don't allow your knees to cave inward excessively—you're good to go. As I said in the abduction section, just because a movement is easy doesn't mean that you can throw technique out the window. Take the movement seriously, think about being athletic while you do it, and be conscious of your form.

There are three different sled push variations based on hand placement and posture:

- High-handle (upright)
- Mid-handle (slight lean)
- Low-handle (leaning)

Each position works different hip ranges of motion and therefore works your glutes in a slightly different way.

In general, the lower you are, the harder the movement is, because you're working your glutes through a larger range of motion and using more muscle to stabilize your body. With regard to distance and tempo, I typically recommend 10 rounds of 20 to 30 meters at a slow pace. Heavy sled pushes are slow and better for building strength, while light sled pushes are fast and better for conditioning.

HIGH-HANDLE (UPRIGHT) SLED PUSH

The upright sled push works the glutes more at end-range hip extension positions. It is the easiest sled push variation because you don't have to use as much overall muscle and you move your hips through a smaller range of motion. It's the best variation for beginners and people who are recovering from injury. The one caveat is that you can't load the sled with as much weight. With your body upright, you don't have a ton of leverage to push the sled forward.

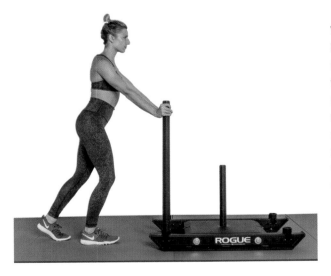

Where you form your grip on the sled handles depends on your height and the height of the bars on the sled. To push with an upright posture, you will probably need to position your arms straight at a downward angle or bend them at roughly a 90-degree angle. The idea is to maintain this arm position—not allowing your arms to come back or reach forward—as you push the sled forward.

MID-HANDLE (SLIGHT LEAN) SLED PUSH

The mid-handle sled push is the most common and universally well-tolerated sled push variation. Tilting your torso forward at roughly a 45-degree angle moves your glutes through a larger range of motion, and you have more leverage to push the sled forward. It is not as hard as the low-range sled push but still provides a potent stimulus.

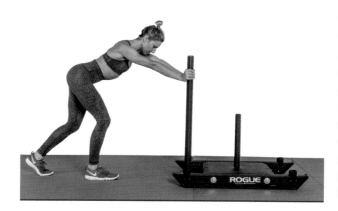

Hinge from your hips, tilt your torso forward—keeping your back flat—and form your grip on the sled handles. As a starting point, form your grip just below or on the same horizontal plane as your shoulders, then adjust up or down based on your preference. You can keep your arms straight or slightly bent, whichever you prefer. The key is to drive off the ball of your foot with each step. Keep your gait straight (step forward in a straight line) and maintain a rhythmic stride.

LOW-HANDLE (LEANING) SLED PUSH

This is the most advanced sled push variation. With your torso nearly parallel with the ground, you are less balanced, and you must rely heavily on the strength of your legs to push the sled forward. More specifically, this variation strengthens your glutes in a flexed position, as you never reach full hip extension during the set. It also works your calves more because you have to stay on your toes throughout the exercise.

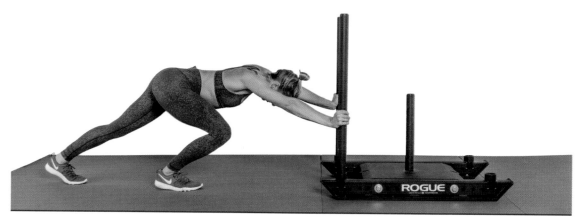

Get into a low sprinter's stance so that your torso is nearly horizontal. Form your grip on the sled handles, positioning your hands just below or on the same horizontal plane as your shoulders. Keep your arms straight and your back flat throughout the entire pushing distance. Again, step forward in a straight line, drive off the ball of your foot with each step and maintain a rhythmic stride.

LOADING AND EQUIPMENT VARIATIONS

There are only a couple of ways to add resistance to the sled push: you can use a resistance band or add weight to the sled.

BANDED SLED PUSH

Using a resistance band (such as a Glute Loop) is the best way to increase glute activation when pushing a sled. This variation is basically a monster walk combined with a sled push. You can perform it only from the upright and mid-handle positions. It's best to use a larger resistance band. You position the band above your knees when pushing the sled so that you can move your legs through a larger range of motion. Lastly, you can walk by keeping your feet in a wide stance or by swinging your leg inward and then outward—stepping outward in a diagonal direction—with every step.

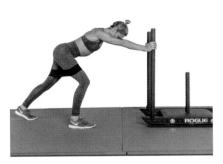

LOADED SLED PUSH

The loading strategy for the sled push depends on your position or posture, the surface and type of sled you're using, and your exercise goals. Some sleds glide better than others and require more loading, and some surfaces provide more friction than others and require less loading. If you want to work on speed, it's best to keep the weight light and push the sled as fast as possible while trying to keep your gait mechanics consistent. If you want to work on conditioning, then any load will do as long as you can utilize it for the desired duration, as you'll naturally push the tempo and move faster with lighter weight. If your main goal is to work your glutes, create enough resistance so that you can maintain a rhythmic stride at a slower pace.

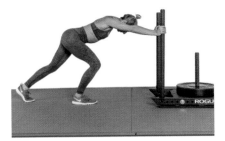

FORWARD SLED DRAG

You can drag the sled instead of pushing it, but this variation requires a harness.

BACKWARD SLED DRAG

The backward sled drag is an amazing quad exercise and is great for rehabilitating knee injuries.

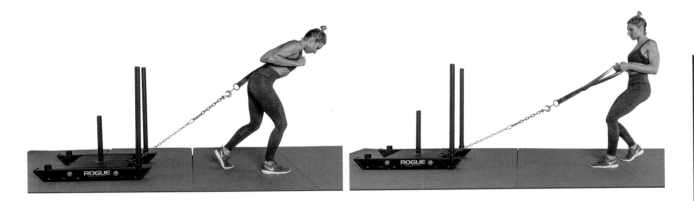

Hamstring-Dominant Exercises

In this chapter, you will learn how to perform hamstring (ham)-dominant exercises, which include the deadlift, good morning, back extension, reverse hyper, swing, straight-leg bridge, and knee flexion exercises. To state the obvious, hamstring-dominant exercises primarily work the hamstrings. But just as quad-dominant exercises also work the glutes and sometimes the hamstrings, ham-dominant exercises also work the glutes and sometimes the quads.

Although you don't always get the same level of glute activation from ham-dominant exercises as you do from glute-dominant exercises, ham-dominant exercises still work your glutes, especially if you perform the exercises the way I teach them. For example, tucking your chin and rounding your upper back during a back extension reduces erector involvement and increases upper glute activation. But even then, you will feel your hamstrings working during these exercises, which is not a bad thing.

Even if you want to grow your glutes without growing your legs, it's important to sprinkle in some quad- and ham-dominant exercises because—as I've covered—these exercises especially work the lower regions of the glutes and lengthen the glutes under tension, which targets different muscle fibers. You still prioritize glute-dominant movements, however, because in this scenario that is the primary goal.

Far too many women I work with say, "I don't want big legs," so they avoid exercises that work the quads and hamstrings. But here's the rub: well-developed hamstrings look good and help shape your legs, and they are responsible for extending your hips, which is a joint action buried in just about every athletic and practical movement we humans perform. In short, your hamstrings are important muscles, and you need to perform lifts that strengthen all ranges of hip extension. This means performing quad- and ham-dominant movements as well as glute-dominant movements.

Remember, glute training is not just a vanity-centric exercise system. Yes, it's a system for developing bigger, stronger glutes, but it's so much more. If you follow the guidelines outlined in this book and train a variety of glute-, quad-, and ham-dominant movements (as well as upper-body exercises), you will also develop functional strength and coordination—that is, the ability to move safely and effectively in a variety of situations—make your body more resilient, improve your mobility, and build a well-balanced frame. What's more, you're training movements that will help you in both life and sport.

Consider all the sports that involve hinging from the hips with a forward-tilted torso: volleyball, baseball, and tennis players getting ready to receive the ball, golfers setting up to swing, and football and rugby linemen in the ready position, to mention a few examples. And think about how often you bend over to pick something up. If your hamstrings are weak and you don't know how to bend and lift with proper form, you might compensate by lifting dynamically with your back, which is how a lot of people get injured and develop lower back pain. The fact is, most people use the hinge pattern more than the squat pattern in everyday life. By implementing the exercises in this chapter, you will learn how to use the power of your hips and posterior chain (erectors, glutes, and hamstrings) to perform this all-important movement, potentially reducing the risk of injury and pain. Equally important, you will develop the muscles needed to carry out those actions, which caters to a wide range of physique goals.

STRUCTURE AND ORGANIZATION

This chapter is divided into seven sections based on the exercise. The seven exercises are all similar in the sense that they work your hamstrings and involve a hip hinge and hip extension movement pattern, but they are unique in that they work your posterior chain in slightly different ways.

- The deadlift is the most popular hip hinge movement and is the best lift for improving functional strength and performance. It's considered a primary lift, so placing it at the beginning of your workouts will give you the best results.
- The good morning shares the same movement pattern as the deadlift, but instead of picking the bar up off the ground, you hinge forward with the load positioned on your back.
- Back extension and reverse hyper exercises elicit higher glute activation than the other ham-dominant exercises, especially if they are performed the way I teach them. They are typically placed in the middle of a workout and done with moderate to lighter loads.
- Swings, such as the kettlebell swing, are used primarily as a conditioning exercise, which I generally program at the end of a training session.
- Straight-leg bridges and knee flexion movements are isolation exercises designed primarily to develop the hamstrings.

Again, if you're mainly interested in developing strength or you love powerlifting, then the deadlift is the best movement for you to perform. But for many hamstring-dominant exercises, the goal isn't always to progressively overload with weight, but rather to focus on the mind-muscle connection.

HAMSTRING-DOMINANT EXERCISES

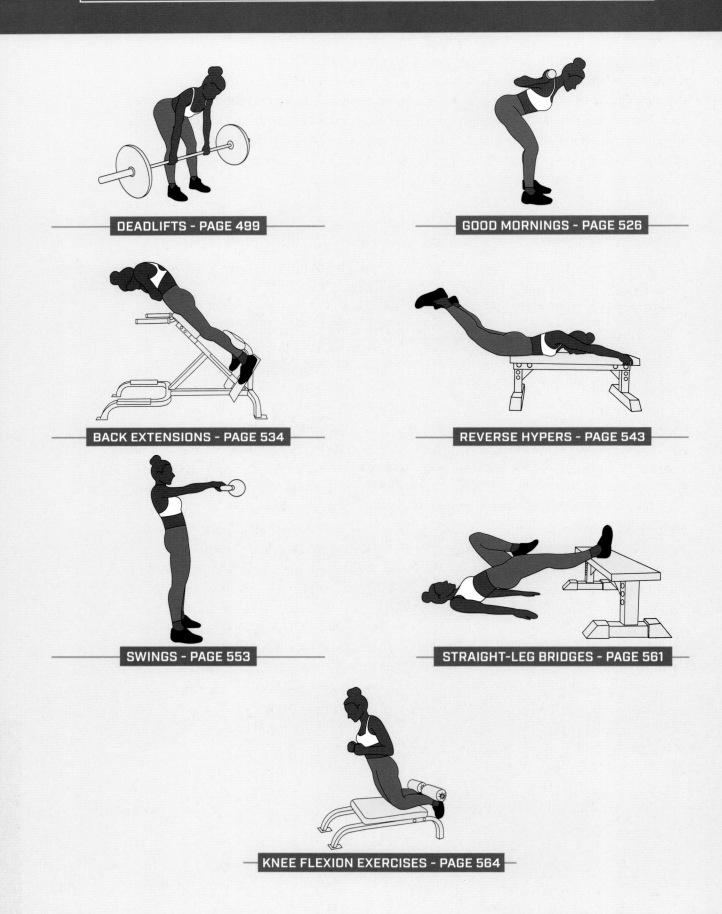

DEADLIFTS - PAGE 499

GOOD MORNINGS - PAGE 526

BACK EXTENSIONS - PAGE 534

REVERSE HYPERS - PAGE 543

SWINGS - PAGE 553

STRAIGHT-LEG BRIDGES - PAGE 561

KNEE FLEXION EXERCISES - PAGE 564

1 Deadlifts

In the gym, the deadlift is quite possibly the ultimate test of strength. Like the squat, it is often referred to as the king of all exercises. Looking in from the outside, the deadlift doesn't seem to require much thinking or technique, but nothing could be further from the truth. When broken down, the deadlift is very technical and quite difficult to master. The movement might appear to be a simple hip hinge, which is present in many activities of daily living. However, it's not that simple, especially under very heavy loading.

The deadlift is a brutal movement and may be the trickiest of all lifts in terms of programming due to its insanely high cost to the central nervous system (CNS). Well, actually, the research doesn't support that the deadlift taxes the CNS, but we iron warriors have a hard time letting go of this notion. It may just be that it's so exhausting due to the microdamage to muscle and connective tissue structures that occurs. Nevertheless, one thing is certain: heavy deadlifting is akin to bringing Everclear to a keg party; things can go really well or end up in utter disaster.

Finding the frequency, effort, and exercise selection that suits you best—which I cover in Chapter 12—is the key to excelling in this lift. Some lifters do best by pulling heavy every week, while others do better when they pull heavy every other week. Some pull hard twice per week, while others prefer to mix in submaximal sessions throughout the week. Then there are those who prefer to avoid the deadlift movement altogether until it's time to max, relying on movements like squats, lunges, good mornings, hip thrusts, and grip work to build their deadlifts. And then there are people who never deadlift heavy and prefer working with lighter loads.

Although most lifters use the deadlift to measure strength, you don't need to lift heavy to get the most from the exercise. In fact, if you're concerned only with building bigger, stronger glutes, then it might be better never to max out or deadlift super heavy due to the risk of injury. Lower back tweaks and random aches and pains go hand in hand with heavy, routine deadlifting. For people who are chasing strength goals, the benefits might be worth the cost, but for people who are primarily interested in building their physique, simply practicing the movement with moderate weight, focusing on form and technique, and pushing sets to failure from time to time will help build and maintain strength while moving them closer to their physique goals.

It's also important to realize that the deadlift is not just a barbell exercise. There are numerous variations based on stance, knee action, range of motion, and equipment. In this section, you will learn all of these variations. But first, let's review some important guidelines for practicing the deadlift movement pattern.

GUIDELINES AND CUES

When it comes to deadlifting with good technique, you need to keep a few things in mind. As with the hip thrust and the squat, the idea is to experiment with different stances, setups, and ranges of motion to dial in your form. In the following pages, I provide some general guidelines to get you moving in the right direction.

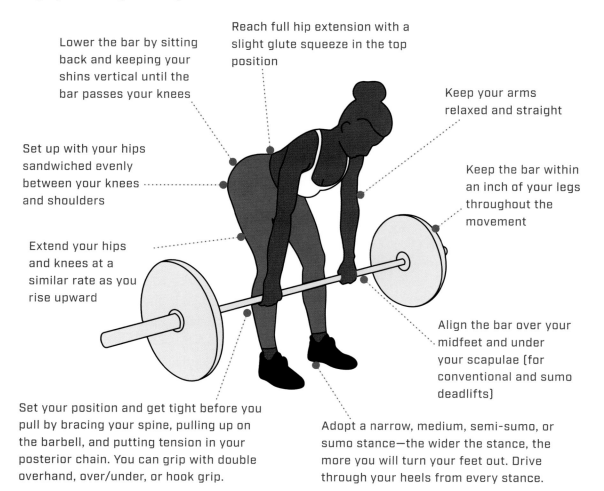

Lower the bar by sitting back and keeping your shins vertical until the bar passes your knees

Reach full hip extension with a slight glute squeeze in the top position

Keep your arms relaxed and straight

Set up with your hips sandwiched evenly between your knees and shoulders

Keep the bar within an inch of your legs throughout the movement

Extend your hips and knees at a similar rate as you rise upward

Align the bar over your midfeet and under your scapulae (for conventional and sumo deadlifts)

Set your position and get tight before you pull by bracing your spine, pulling up on the barbell, and putting tension in your posterior chain. You can grip with double overhand, over/under, or hook grip.

Adopt a narrow, medium, semi-sumo, or sumo stance—the wider the stance, the more you will turn your feet out. Drive through your heels from every stance.

STANCE AND FOOT POSITION

You perform the conventional deadlift with your feet about shoulder width apart (sometimes closer together and sometimes farther apart), with your hands placed just outside your legs. Most lifters prefer to keep their toes pointed straight ahead, while others like to turn their feet out slightly. As with the squat, foot flare is influenced by hip anatomy, so it's important to experiment to find the stance that works best for you.

If you're having trouble finding a comfortable foot position, try this: take the same stance you would if you were performing a vertical jump. This may help get your body into a more advantageous deadlift position. Tinker from there by adopting a slightly wider stance. You can go even wider and have your arms track inside your legs, which is known as the *semi-sumo* position. And you might find that deadlifting with a sumo (wide) stance feels better and works your glutes more.

It's important to mention that if you're used to only one stance, the others will feel strange. This doesn't mean they aren't good stances for you—I recommend performing deadlifts from wide, medium, and narrow stances for variety—you just need to spend some time getting used to them. If, after some experimentation, you still don't like one of the stances—perhaps the sumo stance hurts your hips or the conventional stance irritates your back—then don't do it.

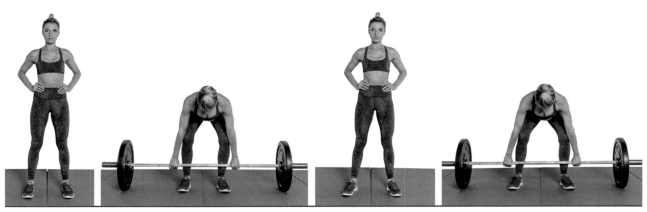

NARROW STANCE   **MEDIUM STANCE**

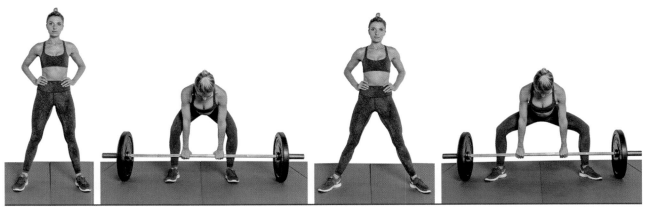

SEMI-SUMO STANCE   **SUMO STANCE**

The wider your stance, the more you have to turn your feet out and the more upright your torso position becomes. This not only positions the bar close to your body, which is necessary to lift the weight with proper form, but also reduces the distance your hips have to travel, which for most people increases the amount of weight they can lift.

EQUIPMENT AND BARBELL SETUP

Once you assume your stance, the next step is to figure out where to position the load in relation to your body. In general, you want the load to be very close to you to reduce the load on your lower back, but the exact distance depends on the width of your stance, your anatomy, and the equipment you're using.

For instance, if you're performing a barbell sumo deadlift, the bar will usually touch your shins or be very close to them. If you're performing a conventional deadlift, on the other hand, you have a little more wiggle room. Some lifters prefer to line up with their shins directly up against the bar, while others like to position the bar about 4 inches away. For most of my clients, I recommend positioning the bar over the midfoot, or along the line that bisects your foot lengthwise.

Another way to determine body placement relative to the bar (or bar placement relative to the body) is to take a photo from the side and make sure that the bar is positioned directly underneath your scapulae and directly above the midfoot. Note that this applies to conventional and sumo deadlifts, not to stiff-leg deadlifts or good mornings. Mark Rippetoe—strength training coach and author of *Starting Strength*—pointed this out years ago, and it's spot on.

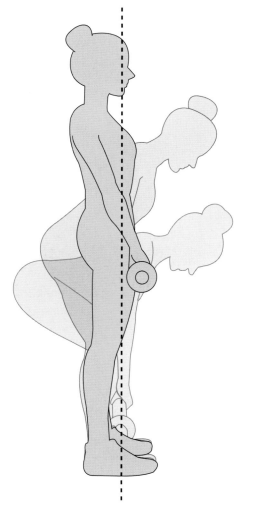

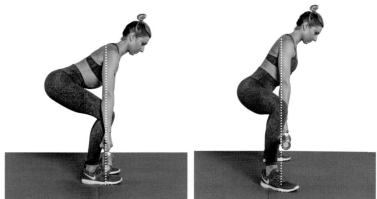

CONVENTIONAL DEADLIFT   SUMO DEADLIFT

STIFF-LEG DEADLIFT

The wider your stance, the more you have to turn your feet out and the more upright your torso position should be. This not only positions the bar close to your body, which is necessary to lift the weight with proper form, but also reduces the distance the hips have to travel, which, for most people, increases the amount of weight they can lift.

Anthropometry also plays a large part in terms of how far away from the bar you should line up. Lining up with the bar too close to your body can interfere with leg drive, while lining up with the bar too far away from your body can impair your balance and generate excessive spinal loading.

With regard to bar path, the bar should skim your legs as it rises and descends. It should not stray more than an inch from your body at any point during the lift. Allowing it to stray makes the lift harder and places more pressure on your lower back.

BARBELL GRIP OPTIONS

There are a few different strategies for gripping the barbell, all of which cater to certain people, lifts, and sports.

Double Overhand Grip

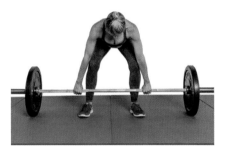

The double overhand grip—in which both palms face the body—is perhaps the most common. I recommend using a double overhand grip as long as possible during your warm-up sets to build grip strength. However, very few lifters can rely on the double overhand grip when the weight approaches maximal loads or the set approaches failure. In short, their grip usually fails before their legs and hips do, meaning that they can't hold onto the bar even though they still have juice in their lower bodies.

Over/Under (Mixed) Grip

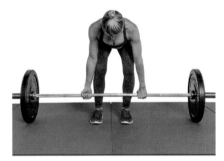

In the over/under, or mixed, grip, one hand is in a pronated position (palm facing the body) and the other is supinated (palm facing away from the body). This grip is well tolerated by most lifters and is the preferred option for powerlifters and when lifting maximal loads. There is a slight risk of experiencing a distal biceps tendon tear in the supinated arm, so be sure to alternate arms from one set to the next. Switching arms between sets also ensures that you don't create muscular imbalances.

Hook Grip

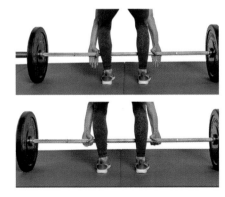

The hook grip is most commonly used in Olympic weightlifting. This strong and secure grip is safer than the over/under grip in that it eliminates the risk of a biceps tear. But it can be quite painful at first. To secure the hook grip, wrap your thumb around the bar, then hook your index and middle fingers around your thumb to secure it in place. After four to six weeks or so, you build up calluses, the pain diminishes, and your body becomes accustomed to it.

Lifting Straps

The last option when it comes to gripping the bar is to use lifting straps. Training with straps diminishes the benefits of forearm and grip strengthening, so I advise using them sparingly. In my first eight years of lifting, I relied on straps, and I could never get in a good workout if I forgot them because I was so weak without them. It's never ideal to be reliant on training aids.

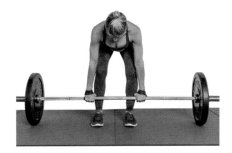

Grip strength can indeed be a limiting factor with regard to maximal deadlifting. If this is the case for you, I highly recommend using chalk, as well as working with a bar with good knurling and performing specialized grip work. To give you an idea of how important these factors are, I can deadlift around 455 pounds with an old, smoother barbell and no chalk. If I use a good knurled barbell, I can deadlift about 545 pounds. And if I add chalk to the mix, I can deadlift up to 620 pounds. In short, I get 165 extra pounds by chalking my hands and using a good bar. If you're concerned only with physique training and grip strength is not something you care about, then using straps fine; just make sure you always have them with you when you train.

SPINAL MECHANICS: KEEP YOUR SPINE IN THE NEUTRAL ZONE

As in squatting, maintaining a neutral spinal position with braced abdominals is ideal. (To learn more about neutral spinal positioning, flip back to page 139; refer to page 140 for more on bracing.) Again, there is some wiggle room when it comes to your spinal and pelvic position. For example, a lot of women I work with prefer to tilt their pelvis forward slightly (anterior pelvic tilt). As long as they stay within the neutral zone and it doesn't cause them any back pain, then a little bit of anterior pelvic tilt is fine.

Some advanced lifters—specifically powerlifters—purposely round their upper backs (thoracic flexion). This enables them to lift more weight, but it comes with added risk. Therefore, it's not something I recommend for beginners; I recommend rounding only for powerlifters who are educated and okay with accepting more risk.

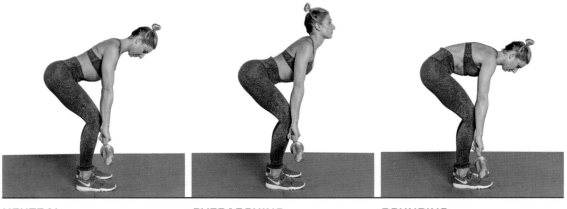

NEUTRAL   OVERARCHING   ROUNDING

According to biomechanical analysis and anecdotal feedback, the safest deadlift posture is neutral. Rounding and overarching through the lower back (lumbar flexion and lumbar hyperextension, respectively) should be avoided, as they can cause damage to ligaments, discs, and other spinal structures.

NECK AND HEAD POSITION

When it comes to neck position, there is some debate as to whether keeping your head neutral, looking slightly up or down, or neck packing (cervical retrusion combined with capital flexion, or making a double chin) is best for performance. Personally, I believe this debate is overblown; clips from the strongest deadlifters in the world portray a variety of neck and head positions. My general recommendation is to avoid any type of excessive overextension or flexion.

HIP HEIGHT AND TORSO ANGLE

Finding the optimal starting position (or hip height) is highly dependent on your body, lever, and limb lengths. In general, from a side view, you want your hips to be sandwiched between your shoulders and knees. Lifters with anatomical proportions such as short femurs, long torsos, or long arms will be more upright, whereas lifters with long femurs, short torsos, and short arms will be more horizontal.

MOVE YOUR HIPS WITH THE BAR

Regardless of your hip height, the key is to move your hips in concert with the bar. In other words, you want to avoid elevating your hips before you pull the bar off the ground. A lot of beginners initiate the pull by lifting their hips first, before the bar leaves the ground. This is an error, and it is commonly committed by lifters who set up with their hips too low or are impatient off the floor. Find the optimal position and stick to it as the bar leaves the ground. Your knees and hips should extend at a similar rate, and your torso should remain at a similar angle during the first half of the concentric (rising) phase.

BRACING MECHANICS: SET YOUR POSITION AND GET TIGHT BEFORE YOU PULL

It's important to build tension in your posterior chain and scapulae before you execute the pull. A lot of lifters accomplish this by forming their grip on the bar and then pumping their hips up and down to create tension in their bodies. So they grip the bar, raise their hips, and then lower their hips while pulling on the barbell, raising their chests, and pulling their shoulders down (scapular depression). These actions not only create tension in the hips, hamstrings, erectors, and lats but also pull the barbell snug with the weights, removing all slack from the system. In short, getting tight helps these lifters maintain a rigid position as they pull the weight from the floor. Now, you don't need to pump your hips up and down as just described (it's one of many strategies), but you should have a pre-deadlift ritual for taking the slack out of your body and getting in a tight position before you lift; otherwise, your hips are likely to shoot up, and the load will pull you into a rounded position the moment you lift it from the floor.

Once you set your position and line up the bar, there's one more important step: to brace your position by taking a deep breath (around 70 percent of your maximum lung capacity) in through your belly and chest and then stiffening the muscles of your trunk. With your spine stabilized and your body tight, you can execute the lift.

DEADLIFT SETUP: PUMPING THE HIPS

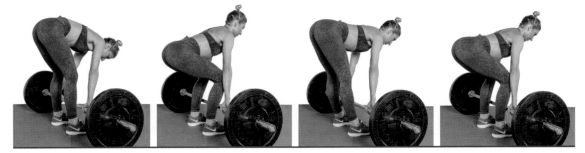

An effective deadlift begins with creating tension in the body in a good position. Grip the bar, then pull it snug to the weight and over the middle of your feet. You can also raise and lower your hips while pulling your shoulders down, which not only creates tension in your back, hips, and hamstrings but also helps you maintain a rigid position as you lift.

FOOT PRESSURE: PUSH THROUGH YOUR HEELS

As with the squat and hip thrust, you want to push through your heels as you initiate and execute the deadlift. When you do, you end up pushing through your whole foot anyway. If you actively strive to push through your whole foot, however, you're more likely to shift forward onto the balls of your feet, which compromises your mechanics and disrupts your balance.

KEEP YOUR ARMS RELAXED AND STRAIGHT

Never pull with your arms or shrug your shoulders when deadlifting. Think of your hands as hooks attached to the barbell and your arms as ropes. That is, keep your arms relaxed and straight and rely on the power of your legs and hips to stand upright with the weight while keeping your back in your neutral zone.

FINISH POSITION: REACH FULL HIP EXTENSION

The finish position is characterized by full hip extension or slight hip hyperextension, with a strong glute contraction. A lot of lifters make the mistake of exaggerating the lockout with lumbar hyperextension (fault: left image). A strong glute squeeze will cause hip hyperextension, but the hyperextension comes from the hips while the lumbar spine remains neutral. In other words, you push your hips forward by squeezing your glutes and stop once your hips run out of range of motion. When people learn how to posterior pelvic tilt with hip thrusts and back extensions, they sometimes transfer this form to the deadlift and take things too far. You see a too-aggressive glute squeeze combined with "soft knees," where you don't lock out your knees with your quads (fault: left image). This can create too much posterior pelvic tilt, which leads to lumbar flexion. This is the fault you want to avoid. To remain safe and prevent injury, make sure to hyperextend at your hips, not your back, and invoke a strong quad contraction to lock out your knees.

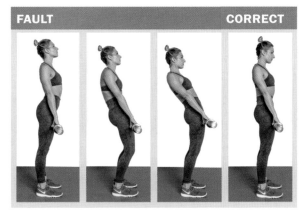

FAULT | CORRECT

Powerlifters need to demonstrate to the judges that they own the deadlift. The only difference in form that I recommend for powerlifters is to pull the shoulders back and stand tall (slight scapular retraction and thoracic extension).

CONTROL THE RANGE OF MOTION

You can change the difficulty of the deadlift by decreasing or increasing the range of motion. For example, you can make it easier by performing block pull deadlifts, which decrease the range of motion, or make it harder by performing deficit deadlifts, which increase the range of motion.

Block Pull Deadlifts

Block pulls are done off a block or mats (usually 2 to 4 inches tall). Rack pulls are done off the pins in a power rack. I prefer the block pull because it's more similar to the deadlift, but if you don't have a way to elevate the plates, the rack pull will suffice.

The block pull is useful in a few situations. For instance, some people just don't have the hamstring or hip flexion flexibility to get into good position when lifting from the floor, so they have to compensate by rounding their backs. For these people, lifting from 3- to 4-inch blocks and then incrementally lowering the blocks as they gain mobility, strength, and coordination is a great option. Block pulls are also less taxing on the body, making them great for both beginners and advanced lifters. Say I'm working with a novice who gets hurt every time they pull from the floor. Rather than avoid the deadlift altogether with that client, I reduce the range of motion and experiment with different variations, such as the Romanian deadlift, until we find a movement and range that doesn't beat them up. If I'm working with an advanced lifter, I might have them pull from blocks as an assistance exercise. Maybe they've stalled in the deadlift or they're getting bored with their training. In either case, performing block pulls for a four- to six-week cycle can inject some variety into the routine and potentially increase deadlift strength. Not only is it less taxing on the body, which gives the lifter more time to recover, but most people are stronger when pulling from blocks, which increases their confidence.

You can also reduce the range of motion by using bigger plates (Hip Thruster plates or wagon wheel plates), but most gyms don't have them. You can make use of other common gym equipment by elevating the plates on steps, mats, blocks, or bumper plates. Note that lifting from blocks (or performing rack pulls) that position the bar higher than your knees will not transfer to the deadlift, and there is diminishing return on glute development the higher you go. So start with a 4-inch lift and then progress accordingly—meaning that you can maintain optimal spinal mechanics from a lower lifting position (a 2-inch block, or the floor).

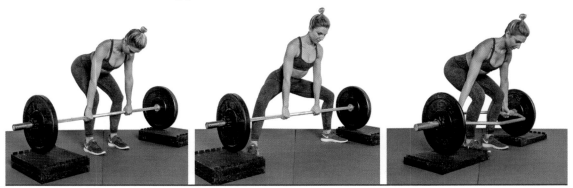

BLOCK PULL DEADLIFT   BLOCK PULL SUMO DEADLIFT   BLOCK PULL TRAP BAR DEADLIFT

Deficit Deadlifts

Just as you can make the deadlift easier by decreasing the range of motion, you can make it harder by increasing the range of motion, which you do by standing on a box(es) or an elevated, stable platform. I don't program deficit deadlifts that often because not a lot of people can do them without rounding their backs, and deficits don't necessarily work the glutes any better than lifting from the floor. However, they are good for variety and for improving strength and mobility, especially for people who have long arms and shorter torsos.

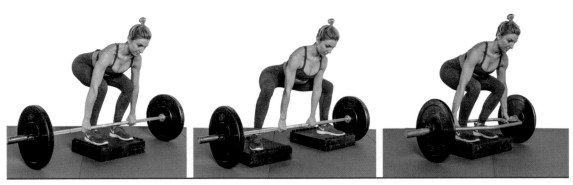

DEFICIT CONVENTIONAL DEADLIFT

DEFICIT SUMO DEADLIFT

DEFICIT TRAP BAR DEADLIFT

FAULTS AND CORRECTIONS

I've already hinted at the most common deadlifting errors and how to avoid them. Here I cover the most prevalent faults in more detail and offer simple corrections, which mirror some of the guidelines and cues already covered.

FAULT: ROUNDED BACK

As I said in the "Guidelines and Cues" section, the safest way to deadlift is to keep your spine as neutral as possible. However, a lot of powerlifters and advanced strength athletes make the choice to round their upper backs. They're willing to risk safety in order to lift a little more weight. Now, if you do opt to round your back, it's important that you round mostly in the thoracic spine (upper back) and keep the lumbar region (lower back) in a neutral position. This requires practice; it's not something beginners can master right off the bat. The reason it's safer to round the thoracic spine is that your ribcage provides stability and protects the region. If you round your entire back, you're asking for trouble.

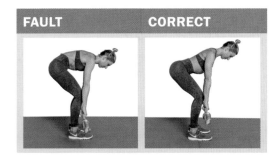

CORRECTION:
Make sure to get tight in the bottom position and brace your spine, then maintain that rigid position as you extend your hips and elevate your torso.

FAULT: LOCKOUT HYPEREXTENSION

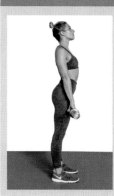

Spinal hyperextension occurs during the lockout phase, or when you're extending your hips in the top or finish position. The spine is very robust and can handle a ton of load in the neutral zone, but moving at the spine under heavy loads can be problematic. You can damage or irritate some of the small structures on the backs of your lumbar vertebrae (referred to as the *posterior elements*), which can cause pain or injury. This occurs when people have weak glutes, they don't understand proper form, or they try to create the illusion of full hip extension without actually locking out their hips.

CORRECTION:

Keep your spine rigid (in your neutral zone) throughout the entire range of the movement and squeeze your glutes to full hip extension. Film yourself from the side to make sure you're doing it right. You can also practice standing glute squeezes and RKC planks (see page 404) to connect the dots between feeling your glutes contract and locking out your hips.

FAULT: SQUATTING THE WEIGHT UP

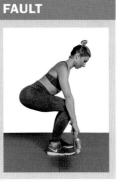

If you position the bar too far forward, you will likely set up in a squat position. This not only places unnecessary stress on your back but also changes the mechanics of the lift, meaning that it works your quads more than your hamstrings and glutes. This is probably the most common fault I see on social media, which suggests that people think they're doing it right when, in fact, they're doing it wrong. However, if you prefer deadlifting (pulling weight from the floor) in a squat position because you like the way it feels, I recommend performing the snatch grip deadlift or the straddle lift, which I cover in the coming pages.

CORRECTION:

As with most corrections, you need to learn the proper setup and execution. Make sure that the bar is positioned at midfoot level and your hips are sandwiched horizontally between your shoulders and knees.

FAULT: STIFF-LEG DEADLIFTING THE WEIGHT UP

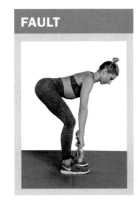

It's common for people to set up in a stiff-leg deadlift position. This typically occurs with people who perform only stiff-leg deadlifts and with beginners who don't understand the proper lifting mechanics and/or have weak quads.

CORRECTION:

This is a form or motor control–related fault, so the solutions revolve around practicing proper mechanics. Revisit the guidelines and cues and keep the load light until you dial in your technique. If weak quads are the culprit, consider incorporating more quad-dominant exercises into your program.

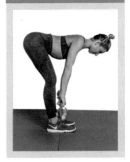

FAULT: LIFTING YOUR HIPS TOO EARLY (NOT GETTING TIGHT)

When you fail to get tight or you are impatient in the bottom position of the deadlift, your hips will typically rise before you lift the weight. This turns it into a stiff-leg deadlift, which places more tension on your back and reduces the amount of weight that you can lift.

CORRECTION:

Again, get tight and stabilize the bottom position by taking all of the slack out of your body, pulling on the barbell, and bracing your spine before you execute the lift.

FAULT: SETTING UP ASYMMETRICALLY

I covered this in Chapter 11, but it's worth repeating here. Far too many people set up with their feet oriented in different directions or grab the barbell off-center. Remember, if you don't set up in a good position, you will not lift in a good position.

CORRECTION:

Make sure your grip is symmetrical in terms of spacing and your feet are in alignment, using the markings on the barbell as a guide.

DEADLIFT VARIATIONS

As I mentioned earlier, there are several different ways to deadlift depending on your stance, depth, grip, knee action, and equipment. As with any lift, the idea is to experiment and find the variation that works best for your body and goals. Some people shouldn't do sumo deadlifts because of their hip anatomy, and others shouldn't perform conventional deadlifts from the ground because they lack hamstring flexibility (block pulls are a good option in this case). At the end of the day, the best deadlift for you is whichever variation you can consistently perform in a progressive manner without compromising form and risking injury.

With all of the deadlift variations, you should have a slight knee bend and torso lean, but the degree of your knee and torso angle depends on the variation. For example, a stiff-leg deadlift requires just a little bit of knee bend and an almost horizontal or 90-degree torso lean relative to vertical. A conventional deadlift requires more knee bend, with a 45- to 60-degree torso lean relative to vertical. The trap bar and kettlebell (or T-bell) deadlifts look almost like a squat, with considerable knee bend and a 30- to 45-degree torso lean relative to vertical. As I've discussed throughout this book, you can make a lift more hip dominant or knee dominant by altering the hip and knee angles. Lifts with a more pronounced knee bend and upright posture work your quads more (knee dominant), while lifts with straighter legs and a hip hinge work your hamstrings more (hip dominant). But even though the upright deadlift variations work your quads, they are still considered hamstring-dominant movements because your knees don't move through a full range of motion as compared to a squat.

All of the deadlift variations are similar in terms of glute activation as well. A lot of people say that they feel the sumo deadlift more in their glutes, but the research shows that glute activation is similar to the other deadlift variations. Everyone will have one variation that feels a little better than the others based on body type, form, experience, and preference. It could be kettlebell, trap bar, sumo, conventional, or Romanian. So, if your primary goal revolves around glute gains, then prioritize the variation that you feel working your glutes the most. It's that simple.

TORSO ANGLES

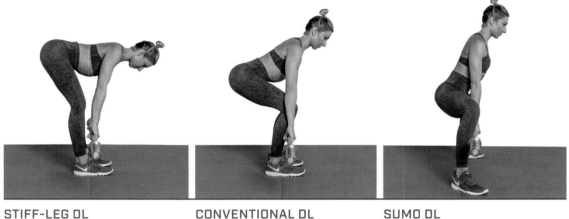

STIFF-LEG DL   CONVENTIONAL DL   SUMO DL

Later in this section, I show you how to create variations using different equipment. But for now, I want to focus on the individual variations, such as the Romanian deadlift, sumo deadlift, and conventional deadlift. Because a barbell is the most common implement, this is what's used to demonstrate the variations.

DEADLIFT CATEGORIZATION

The deadlift is one of the most difficult exercises to categorize due to the overlap in stances, knee actions, grips, ranges of motion (block pull and deficit), and equipment options. For example, if you're lifting with a barbell, you can create seven different variations based on stance, knee action, and grip.

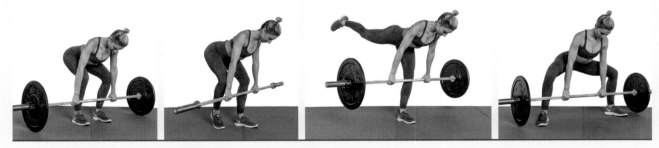

CONVENTIONAL   B-STANCE   SINGLE LEG   SUMO

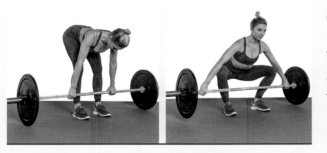

STIFF LEG   SNATCH GRIP

If you're lifting from the ground, you can perform all of these variations from a deficit to increase range of motion or from blocks to decrease range of motion. You can also start the movement from the top position and perform Romanian deadlift variations with all of these stances, knee actions, and grips. And that's just using the barbell! You can create even more variations by using implements such as a trap bar, landmine, loading pin, kettlebells, and dumbbells.

HIP HINGES

The hip hinge is the movement pattern that sets the stage for all of the deadlift variations. However, this technique is more of a teaching tool than an actual exercise. That is, you don't perform the movement to develop your hamstrings, but rather to teach and instill good hip hinging mechanics, such as sitting your hips back and tilting your torso forward with a flat back. Put another way, it's reserved for people who have never learned how to deadlift properly. Once you can hinge from your hips while maintaining a neutral spine, you don't need to do it anymore unless you're using it as a warm-up or as a way to stretch your hamstrings.

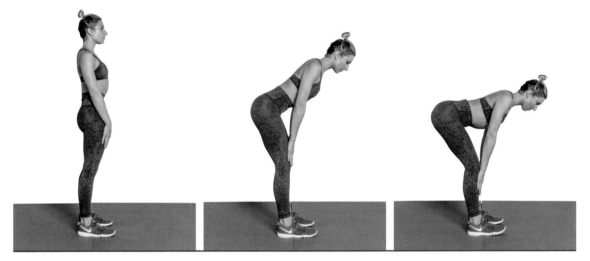

To perform this drill, you can stand in front of a wall and then try to sit your butt back to the wall, or you can do it out in the open. If I'm employing the latter strategy, I tell clients to imagine a rope pulling their hips straight back. In both scenarios, the technique is the same: assume your deadlift stance, brace your spine, and then pull your hips and hamstrings back, keeping your shins vertical and allowing your knees to bend as needed. You can let your arms hang toward the ground or place your hands on your hips. As you reach your hips back, tilt your torso forward while maintaining a neutral spine. Once you reach your end range of motion—meaning that you can't go any farther without rounding your back—drive your hips forward and elevate your torso in one fluid motion.

Single-Leg Hip Hinge

The single-leg hip hinge is surprisingly challenging. It puts a deep stretch on the hamstrings and requires a good deal of balance. To get the most out of the exercise and dial in your mechanics, I recommend posting your hand on a wall or gripping a pole or tall box for support and stability. This will prevent you from rotating, twisting, or swaying as you hinge, which is especially common when performing the bodyweight variation. As you gain proficiency, you can remove the base of support and reach toward a small box or the ground. Once you can single-leg hip hinge with good form, you can add load in the form a barbell, a single kettlebell or dumbbell, two dumbbells or kettlebells, a trap bar, or a landmine. For most of my clients, I encourage bracing onto something for stability—especially when adding load—because I would rather they challenge the muscle than worry about staying perfectly balanced. Like the B-stance variation that follows, you can apply the single-leg hip hinge to most of the deadlift variations, specifically the Romanian, conventional, and stiff-leg deadlifts.

SINGLE-LEG HIP HINGE

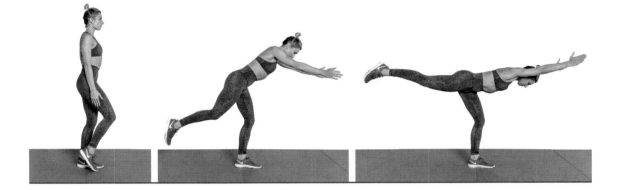

DUMBBELL BRACED SINGLE-LEG HIP HINGE

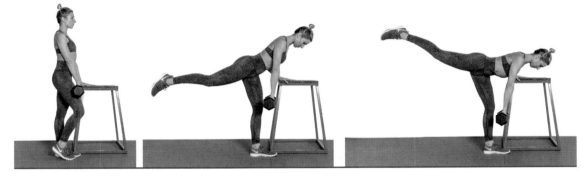

Stand in a narrow stance, with your feet straight and positioned directly under your hips. To initiate the movement, you do several things at once: keeping your weight centered over one leg, hinge from your hip, tilt your torso forward with your spine neutral, and extend your opposite leg directly behind your body. As you do, bend your knee slightly, keeping your shin as vertical as possible and your hips square (on the same horizontal plane). You can place your hand on a wall or grip a pole as an extra base of support, reach toward a target like a bench or box, or let your arms relax and hang toward the ground. To reverse the position, bring your rear leg forward and elevate your torso while extending your hip.

B-Stance Hip Hinge

As with all B-stance variations, the idea is to load about 70 percent of your weight on one leg. Obviously, it's hard to know exactly what percentage of your body weight is on one leg, so as long as the majority of your weight is on one leg and you're using the other leg primarily for support and balance, chances are you're doing it right. As you add load, be sure to stick with moderate weight and rep schemes. People go wrong with B-stance deadlifts when they try to lift too much weight and end up placing more weight on their support leg. This makes it an asymmetrical conventional deadlift and fails to prioritize one leg over the other. When it comes to loading, you can use a barbell, a kettlebell, dumbbells, or a trap bar, all of which I cover in the "Equipment and Loading Variations" section.

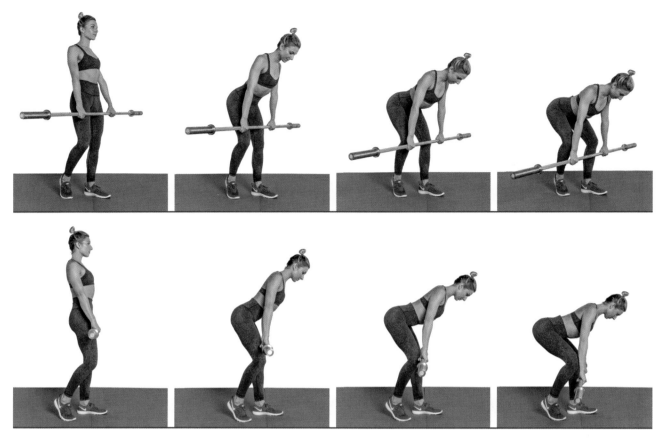

Stand with your feet straight and positioned directly underneath your hips. Shift the majority of your weight (about 70 percent) onto one leg. Slide the foot of your support leg back slightly so that the toes are lined up with the heel of your front foot, turn your back foot out, and elevate your back heel off the floor. From here, the mechanics are the same as the hip hinge: sit your hips back while tilting your torso forward with a flat back. But instead of distributing your weight evenly between both legs, the majority of your weight is centered on one leg. So, as you hinge from your hips, keep your weight over the heel or midfoot of your weight-bearing leg and bend your knee slightly. Allow your arms to relax and hang. Go as far down as you can without rounding your back, then reverse the position by extending your hips and knees in one fluid motion.

Romanian Deadlift (RDL)

The Romanian deadlift is essentially a hip hinge with weight. That is, the movement starts in a standing position, and then you lower the weight just below your knees, meaning that you don't perform a full range of motion. People have an easier time hinging from their hips with a flat back when starting from the top rather than the bottom. However, you still have to deadlift the weight to the top position to begin the movement, so RDLs are typically done with lighter loads and moderate rep ranges. What's great is that you can accentuate the eccentric phase and really focus on hip hinging mechanics and lowering the weight with control. Most people feel a big stretch in their hamstrings, which is a great way to improve flexibility. If you already have flexible hamstrings, however, you may not feel as big of a stretch, and there is a tendency to lower the weight all the way to the ground. But doing so changes the exercise. Hypermobile and flexible athletes should focus on staying rigid and reversing the position while maintaining stability.

You can perform RDLs in a double-leg stance (narrow, medium, or sumo), a B-stance, or a single leg stance with a barbell, a trap bar, a kettlebell, or two dumbbells.

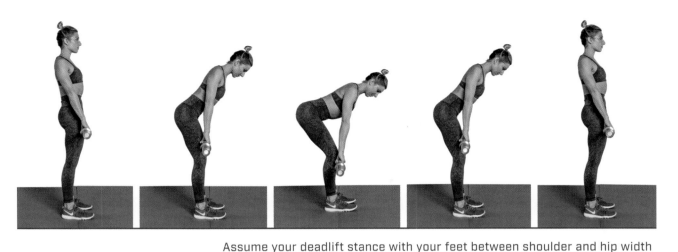

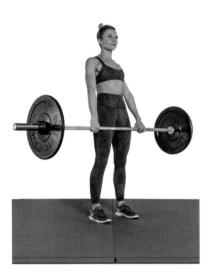

Assume your deadlift stance with your feet between shoulder and hip width apart, positioning the bar over the centers of your feet, then hip hinge with a flat back and form a symmetrical grip on the bar at about your thumbs' distance away from your legs. I recommend a conventional double overhand grip with both palms facing your body. You're not lifting a ton of weight here, so there's no need to use a mixed or hook grip. Deadlift the weight up to the top position, then take a moment to adjust your position if necessary: slight glute squeeze, get your back flat, and pull your shoulders back slightly. The next phase requires you to do several things at once. Keeping your arms relaxed, your shins vertical, and your weight over your heels, sit your hips back and hinge forward from your hips with a flat back. As you sit back and tilt your torso forward, keep the barbell close to your body—it may slide down your thighs—and lower it just past your kneecaps. Then reverse the position by extending your hips, elevating your torso, and straightening your knees. As you stand upright, keep the bar in contact with your legs and think about squeezing your glutes slightly to extend your hips.

American Deadlift

The American deadlift is similar to the Romanian deadlift, but instead of keeping a neutral pelvic position throughout the entire range of the movement, you anterior pelvic tilt in the bottom position and then posterior pelvic tilt in the top position. You're still staying within a neutral zone but titling your pelvis back and forth throughout the range of motion. This accomplishes three things: 1) an anterior pelvic tilt at the bottom provides a greater stretch on the hamstrings; 2) a posterior pelvic tilt at the top elicits greater glute activation; and 3) the exercise teaches you pelvic control and coordination. Obviously, you want to keep the load very light for this variation. If you have a history of lower back pain, you may want to avoid it altogether. This exercise is intended for medium to higher reps and involves a rhythmic action.

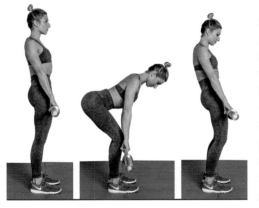

Stand with the barbell in your hands. Descend just as you would in a Romanian deadlift, making sure to sit back as much as possible and keep your shins vertical. As you descend, slide the bar along your thighs and tilt your pelvis anteriorly. Stop when the bar is just below your kneecaps. Reverse the movement and pelvic position as you rise upward, finishing the lockout by pushing your hips forward with a strong posterior pelvic tilt. Unlike the RDL, which involves a purely vertical bar path, there will be some horizontal movement caused by pushing your hips forward. People with very long arms may want to widen their grip on the bar (sort of like a snatch grip) so that the bar is more level with their hips at lockout.

CONVENTIONAL DEADLIFT

The conventional deadlift is what I referred to earlier as the ultimate test of strength and the king of all exercises. When done correctly, it engages more muscles than any other exercise, including the squat. There's something very primal about lifting a heavy load off the ground. For these reasons, the deadlift is the lift that the majority of people care the most about, which creates problems for a serious lifter chasing PRs.

More than any other exercise, you see people—even advanced lifters—deadlift too heavy or push their sets past the point of technical breakdown. I'm a big advocate for progressive overload, but there will be days when you're not feeling your best, you're banged up, you have lower back pain, or your knee is bothering you, and on those days, you need to listen to your body and take it easy. The point I'm trying to make is this: don't be afraid to go lighter and perform higher reps, especially if your goals revolve around sculpting a better physique. Sure, the deadlift is the ultimate test of strength, and, assuming that lifting heavy aligns with your goals, you should utilize progressive overload with this lift. However, don't get obsessed with deadlifting super heavy or going to failure every time you set foot in the gym. It's too taxing on your body, and you will end up hurting yourself. Remember, you can't improve your glutes if you're sidelined with injury.

You can also perform conventional deadlifts in a B-stance to emphasize one leg. To learn how to perform the B-stance variation, see page 513.

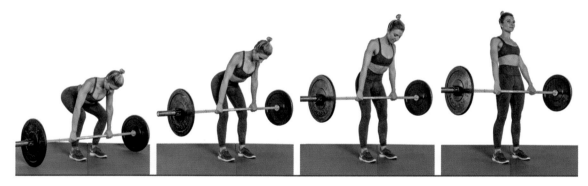

Get into your deadlift stance with the barbell positioned over your midfoot. Hinge from your hips, bend over, and assume your grip on the bar—you can use a double overhand, mixed, or hook grip—at roughly your thumbs' distance from your legs. Use the marks on the barbell to make sure your grip is symmetrical. Next, take all of the slack out of your body and get tight. To accomplish this, pull on the barbell, pull your shoulder blades down, get your back flat, and raise your hips so that your shins are vertical with a slight knee bend. You should feel a ton of tension in your entire posterior chain. Take a big breath, then create core tension by engaging the muscles of your trunk and diaphragm. To execute the lift, you do several things at once: drive through your heels, extend your hips and knees, and raise your torso, keeping the bar close to your body. As the bar passes your knees, slide the barbell up your thighs as you extend your hips and stand upright. Squeeze your glutes to lock out your hips while maintaining neutral alignment. The eccentric, or lowering, phase should look exactly like the concentric, or lifting, phase, but in reverse: sit your hips and hamstrings back as you bend your knees and tilt your torso forward, keeping your shins vertical. As you do, think about painting your thighs with the barbell. Continue to lower the weight with control by hinging from your hips, setting the weight down in the same position as you started. Think leg press off the ground, hip thrust to lockout, then RDL on the way down. (If these cues confuse you, ignore them, but many people find them valuable.)

SUMO DEADLIFT

The sumo deadlift is essentially a wide-stance deadlift, which changes the mechanics of the lift. With your feet spread wide and turned out, you're forced to adopt a more upright torso position. This variation is popular among powerlifters. In fact, most of the strongest deadlifters in the world prefer to lift from a sumo stance, probably due to a combination of 1) a shorter bar distance, 2) more reliance on the quads and adductors, and 3) less taxation on the back, allowing for slightly greater training volumes. If you train for strength, you should train your stronger stance most often. However, I believe you should still train the conventional deadlift even if you're a sumo puller, as it transfers well to sumo. In fact, I've found that a combination of sumo squats and conventional deadlifts seems to build my sumo deadlift better than sumo deadlifts and full squats, which is strange.

When it comes to glute training, most people feel their glutes more with the sumo variation. So, based on anecdotal feedback, the sumo might activate your glutes to a higher degree than the conventional deadlift. However, you get more range of motion from the latter, so it might be a wash for glute hypertrophy. What's more, there's been only one study comparing muscle activity between the sumo and conventional deadlift in powerlifters, and it showed a similar amount of glute EMG activity. My recommendation is to play around with both. When I write programs for clients, I mix in both for variety and to prevent boredom, assuming both lifts are well tolerated.

Some people (myself included) have a hard time getting into a proper sumo stance due to hip anatomy and anthropometry. If you fall into this category, consider reducing the width of your stance, or simply stick with the variations that do feel right.

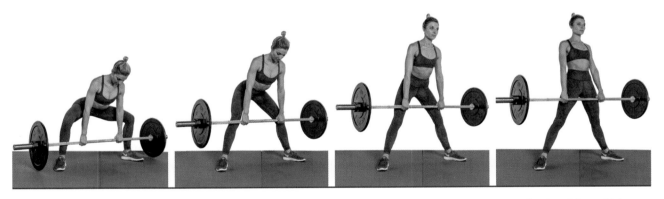

First, figure out your stance width and foot flare. Most people position their feet far outside shoulder width and turn them out more than 45 degrees. If your shins are fairly vertical from both the front and the side and you can reach the bar while maintaining a flat back and an upright torso, then that is probably a good stance width for you. Once you find your ideal stance, set up with the bar touching your shins (or very close to your shins), hinge forward from your hips, externally rotate your hips as you descend (turn your knees outward), and form your grip on the bar. The vast majority of lifters reach their arms straight down and assume a mixed grip. I recommend that smaller lifters take a slightly wider grip so that some of their hands are on the bar knurling, which helps with grip. The next step is to get tight. Lower your hips and raise your torso while pulling your shoulder blades down. Remember, you are more upright in a sumo than in a conventional deadlift. As you set up, keep your arms straight (relaxed) and your back flat. Brace the position by taking a big breath in and engaging your diaphragm and the muscles of your trunk, then execute the pull by driving through your heels and extending your hips and knees in one fluid motion. Due to the angle of your body, the barbell will slide up your legs as you stand upright. Squeeze your glutes to lock out your hips, then lower the weight using the same form in reverse.

STIFF-LEG DEADLIFT (SLDL)

The stiff-leg deadlift is a great exercise for stretching the hamstrings and improving strength at end ranges (the limits of your mobility). Exercises that stretch your muscles to long lengths, as well as eccentric-focused exercises, increase flexibility by increasing actual muscle length. (In science speak, they add sarcomeres in series.) This is in contrast to static stretching, which works mostly by changing the brain's tolerance to the stretch without changing any muscle properties. Although the name of this variation implies that you keep your legs completely stiff, you actually want a slight bend in your knees.

The full-range SLDL is generally reserved for mobile athletes and people who have flexible hamstrings/good hip flexion range of motion. If you can't get set up or bend over with a straight spine and grip the bar, stick with the RDL variation until you develop the hamstring flexibility to get into a good position. You can also perform single-leg SLDLs and sumo-stance SLDLs.

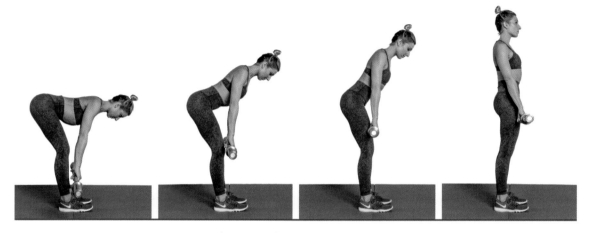

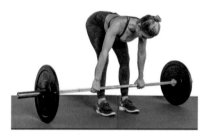

The setup for the stiff-leg deadlift is the same as for the conventional deadlift, but with less of a knee bend. Instead of a 45- to 60-degree lean, your torso is almost parallel to the ground. If you want an even greater stretch in your hamstrings, you can descend deeper by taking a wider grip on the bar. If you are an advanced athlete, you can let the weight drift out in front of you a little bit as you lower into the bottom position. This increases the load on your hamstrings and provides a more aggressive stretch. As you come up and the bar passes your knees, pull the bar toward you so it slides up your thighs. Squeeze your glutes to lock out your hips. Again, you can stand on a plate, a block, or mats to create a deficit as long as you are able to maintain a fairly neutral spine. In other words, don't go so deep that you round your back excessively.

SNATCH GRIP DEADLIFT

The snatch grip deadlift is really just a deadlift done with very wide grip. But, as in the case with widening the stance for the sumo deadlift, widening the grip for the snatch grip deadlift changes the overall mechanics. It's popular among Olympic weightlifters for sport specificity reasons, but for people interested in glute training, it's just another variation to throw in for variety. What's great about this variation is that it increases your hip and knee range of motion and utilizes a more upright position. In this sense, it's a hybrid deadlift and squat.

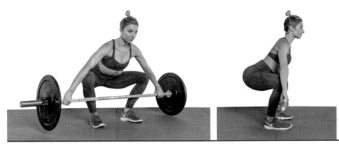

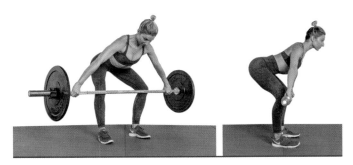

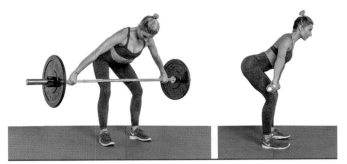

Approach the bar and get into your deadlift stance, just as you would when setting up for a conventional deadlift. If you're an Olympic weightlifter, form your grip on the bar as if you were performing a snatch lift. If you're just glute training, you need to find your ideal grip. Stand up with the bar and position your hands so that the bar is right in your hip crease. For taller people like me, it's all the way out to the ends of the bar. You'll likely need to use wrist straps with this variation, as it's hard to hold onto ample weight. When you drop down to set up for the lift, you'll notice that the wide grip requires you to descend much deeper, almost as if you're squatting. In other words, your knees have to travel forward a bit to get into good position. From here, the mechanics are the same as a deadlift: leg press the weight off the ground, keeping the bar close to your body as you extend your hips and knees, and squeeze your glutes to lock out your hips as you stand upright. Reverse the movement by sitting back and then dropping straight down after the bar passes your knees.

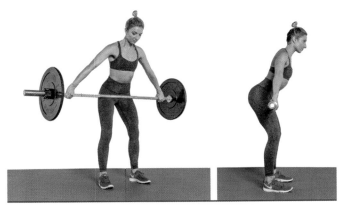

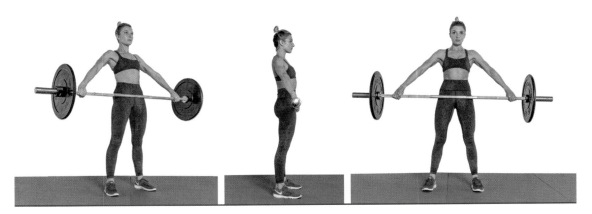

LOADING AND EQUIPMENT VARIATIONS

To demonstrate the deadlift variations, I used a barbell because it's the most common deadlifting implement. However, you can perform most deadlift variations using other equipment, including kettlebells, dumbbells, a trap bar, a BC T-Bell (loading pin), and a landmine.

BANDED BARBELL VARIATIONS

The best thing about barbell deadlifts is their versatility. Not only can you perform all of the deadlift variations, but you can also moderate the weight, meaning you can lift light, heavy, or anything in between. You can also perform a banded barbell variation by looping mini bands next to the weight sleeves. If you have access to a Hip Thruster or deadlift platform, you can use the band attachments; otherwise, you can set it up by crisscrossing two dumbbells on top of each other or using two heavy dumbbells. What's great about the banded barbell variation is that it challenges the lockout phase of the lift without adding load to the lift-off portion.

BANDED DEADLIFT USING DUMBBELLS

BANDED DEADLIFT USING HIP THRUSTER

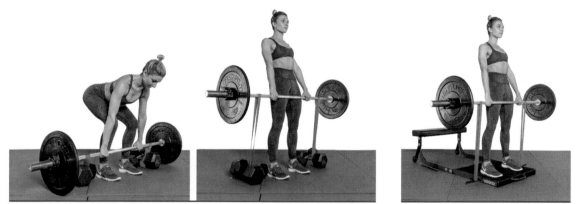

Though a barbell is great for most people, not everyone is well suited for it. Moreover, most hotels and home gyms don't have barbells. So, if you're someone who hates the barbell deadlift variations, you get hurt every time you deadlift with a barbell, or you don't have access to one, then you have plenty of other good variations to choose from.

TRAP BAR VARIATIONS

A trap bar positions the weight at your sides with your body in the middle of the implement, which allows for a more natural movement pattern. You don't have to worry about moving the weight around your knees, and you can adopt a more upright torso and forward knee position, similar to a squat (but not quite as deep). This not only makes the movement easier but also reduces loading on your spine. So, if you have a history of lower back pain or if barbell deadlifts aggravate your back, then the trap bar variation might be a good fit. But it's not for everyone. A lot of women I work with don't like the trap bar because the handles are too wide and it feels awkward on their shoulders. You can use a trap bar for most of the deadlift variations: RDLs, single-leg variations (if the bar has an opening), conventional deadlifts, and stiff-leg deadlifts.

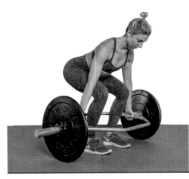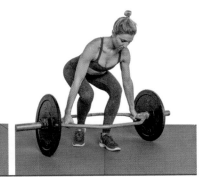

CONVENTIONAL TRAP BAR
DEADLIFT

STIFF-LEG TRAP BAR
DEADLIFT

B-STANCE TRAP BAR
DEADLIFT

KETTLEBELL VARIATIONS

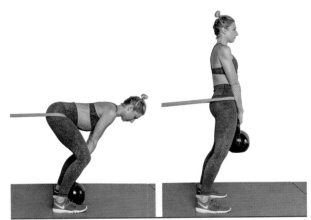

The kettlebell deadlift is one of my favorite ways to teach a beginner how to deadlift. In fact, a lot of people prefer the kettlebell over the barbell because the bell is right underneath you, the movement pattern is more natural, your grip is centered, and the weight is easier to manage. In this sense, it's similar to a trap bar deadlift but with the weight positioned between your legs. Not only that, but kettlebell DLs are extremely versatile: you can perform every deadlift variation from every stance, including contralateral (holding the weight on the opposite side of your grounded leg) and ipsilateral (holding the weight on the same side as your grounded leg) single-leg variations. You can also perform a standing banded upright hip thrust combined with a kettlebell deadlift to accentuate hip extension and place greater emphasis on your glutes.

To get the most from the kettlebell deadlift, it's important to lift heavy weight. The problem is, most gyms don't have heavy kettlebells. If you're strong and you don't have access to heavy kettlebells, then you're better off using a trap bar or barbell.

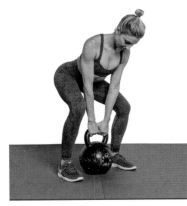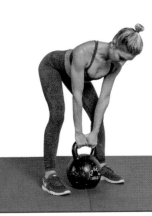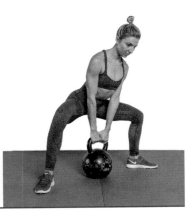

CONVENTIONAL
KETTLEBELL DEADLIFT

STIFF-LEG
KETTLEBELL DEADLIFT

SUMO KETTLEBELL
DEADLIFT

DOUBLE DUMBBELL VARIATIONS

The dumbbell carry (double dumbbell deadlift) is another way to load the deadlift movement pattern. Most people use dumbbells only for stiff-leg deadlifts and RDLs, but they are an equally effective loading tool for conventional deadlifts and single-leg RDLs. What's especially great about the dumbbell variations is that you can do them just about anywhere—most people have dumbbells lying around the house, and nearly every hotel gym has them—and you can substitute dumbbells for a barbell in nearly every deadlift variation.

For dumbbell stiff-leg deadlifts, I like to hold the weights at my sides at a 45-degree angle relative to my body, but for dumbbell deadlifts, I like to hold the weights at my sides with a neutral grip so that the handle grips are pointing forward and backward. The main differences between the two variations are the knee bend and the torso angle. With the SLDL, you have less knee bend and a more horizontal torso, whereas with the dumbbell deadlift, you have more knee bend and a more upright torso. The dumbbell deadlift movement pattern is exactly the same as the trap bar deadlift. The main difference is that you may need to take a slightly narrower stance, and you want to reverse the movement before the dumbbells touch the ground (descend to lower shin level and then stand back up).

DOUBLE-LEG VARIATIONS

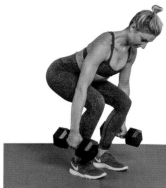
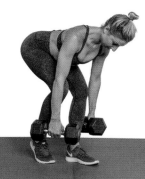
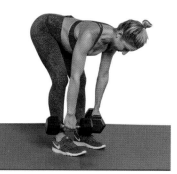

DUMBBELL DEADLIFT

B-STANCE DUMBBELL DEADLIFT

DUMBBELL STIFF-LEG DEADLIFT

SINGLE-LEG VARIATIONS

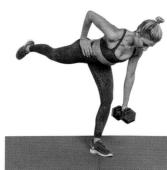
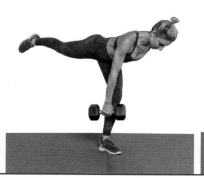
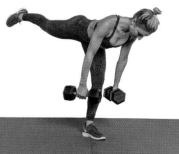

IPSILATERAL DUMBBELL SINGLE-LEG RDL

CONTRALATERAL DUMBBELL SINGLE-LEG RDL

DOUBLE DUMBBELL SINGLE-LEG RDL

Some time ago, people started implementing an RDL variation with the rear foot elevated—like a Bulgarian split squat (see page 464), but instead of actively bending your knee to hinge, you sit back and keep your shin vertical. In theory, this is a great idea. Elevating one leg places the majority of your weight on your grounded leg, creating a unique single-leg variation. However, elevating your leg behind your body and then hinging forward doesn't feel right. It's unstable, and you end up wobbling from side to side. That's why I didn't include the Bulgarian single-leg RDL in this book. The single-leg abducted stiff-leg deadlift fixes this problem. By posting your leg out to the side on an elevated surface, you have additional side-to-side stability, which you might find easier than the other single-leg variations. Like the B-stance variation, think about distributing 70 percent of your weight on your grounded leg and the remaining 30 percent of your weight on your abducted leg. You can load the movement with a dumbbell or kettlebell—holding it in either hand—or with two dumbbells.

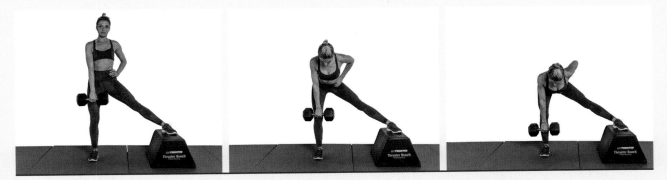

Position one foot on a small box or bench. Drive your hips back, keeping your grounded shin as vertical as possible. Bend your knee slightly as you tilt your torso forward.

LOADING PIN VARIATIONS

A loading pin is used for between-bench squats, stiff-leg deadlifts, and straddle lifts, which are essentially a mix between a squat and deadlift. Your knee angle is similar to a squat, but you're leaning forward more and pulling the weight from the floor as you would when deadlifting. In this way, the movement closely resembles a snatch grip deadlift. But instead of taking a wide grip on a barbell, you form a narrow grip on a V- or T-handle. You also stand on boxes, which allows you to sink deeper and express a larger hip and knee range of motion. This subtle grip difference, body position, and increased range of motion are what make the straddle lift unique. It combines the best qualities of the squat and deadlift into one exercise and may even be a safer alternative. In other words, if squatting and deadlifting are problematic for you—say the barbell hurts your shoulders when back squatting and the deadlift aggravates your lower back—the straddle lift might be a great alternative. In fact, I've been performing and prescribing straddle lifts for over two decades, and I have never been injured by them. What's more, we perform straddle lifts all the time in Glute Lab, and they are well tolerated by the majority of our clients.

Although you can perform the straddle lift using a dumbbell or kettlebell, neither is ideal. The dumbbell is awkward to grip, the kettlebell handle is usually too thick, and neither one allows you to adjust the weight in small increments or effectively lift heavy loads (above 100 to 200 pounds).

This is why I recommend using a loading pin. However, most loading pins are not adjustable and are too long. This is why I developed the BC T-Bell, which is essentially a loading pin with the aforementioned features.

Whether you use a loading pin, a dumbbell, or a kettlebell to perform straddle lifts, I recommend medium to high reps (8 to 20). I typically place them in the middle of a workout.

LOADING PIN DEADLIFT

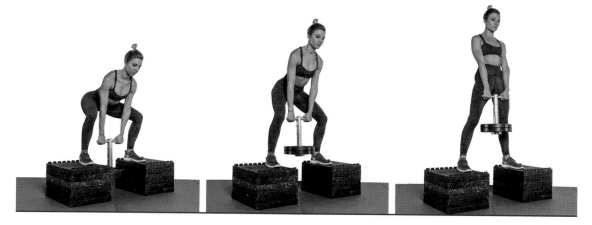

TORSO AND HIP POSITIONS

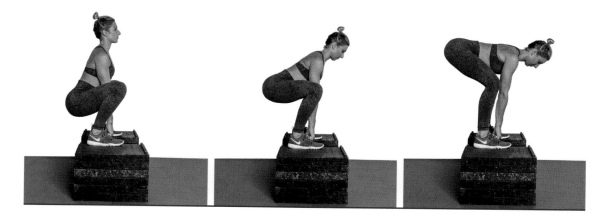

LANDMINE VARIATIONS

The landmine is a barbell variation that you can apply to all of the deadlift movement patterns. Admittedly, the landmine is not my favorite implement because the pivot point is low, creating a strength curve that is hard at the bottom and easy at the top. It also changes your mechanics because you have to lean forward to maintain your balance. However, this problem is easily solved by elevating the unit using a landmine rack attachment or by setting the landmine unit on a plyometric box. But solving one problem creates another. When you elevate the bar, you can't load the landmine with a ton of weight, so you either have to get creative by elevating the weighted end of the bar on a box or lift with lighter loads. Despite these challenges, a lot of my colleagues and clients like to use the landmine, and it caters to a wide range of deadlift variations, which is why I'm including it as an option.

LANDMINE DEADLIFT

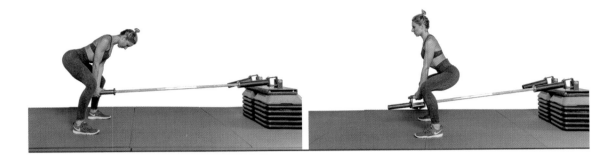

STIFF-LEG LANDMINE DEADLIFT

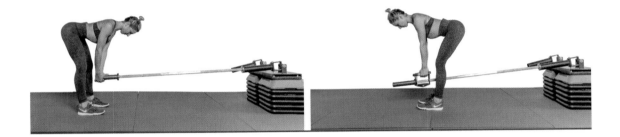

CONTRALATERAL SINGLE-LEG LANDMINE DEADLIFT

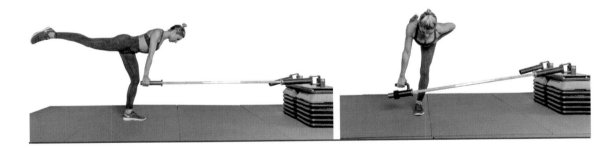

IPSILATERAL SINGLE-LEG LANDMINE DEADLIFT

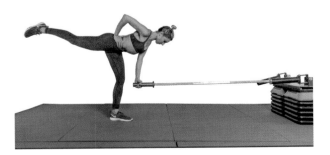

Good Mornings

The good morning exercise is similar to the deadlift in that it is a hip hinge movement pattern that primarily works the hamstrings, glutes, and erectors, but instead of hinging from your hips with the load in your hands, you hinge from your hips with the load on your back.

Good mornings get a bad rap in the fitness industry because they are dangerous when done incorrectly or with heavy weight. The same can be said about most exercises, but it's particularly true with good mornings.

The reason might have something to do with how powerlifters have traditionally used good mornings in their training. Louie Simmons—a legendary powerlifter and the founder of the Westside Barbell Club—popularized this exercise as a substitute for deadlifts. I remember reading about his methods 20 years ago, and his reason for implementing good mornings still holds up today. He implemented good mornings as a substitute for deadlifts because—as I covered—heavy deadlifts are extremely taxing on the body. As it turns out, good mornings don't beat you up quite as badly. This provides a couple of key benefits for serious powerlifters.

First, the good morning strengthens the muscles used in deadlifting without compromising total training volume. In other words, you can train more often and still get stronger in the deadlift without having to deadlift heavy throughout the week.

Second, the good morning helps reduce the risk of injury in a squat-gone-wrong situation when the hips shoot up out of the bottom position, which is a common occurrence when squatting with maximal loads. Because the good morning mimics this exact movement pattern, the rationale is that the lifter strengthens the muscles used to carry out the movement, which might help prevent injuries if or when the fault occurs.

The problem is, the powerlifters who perform good mornings are generally lifting a ton of weight and, in some cases, are rounding their backs. And this is exactly how people get injured: they get overconfident and try to lift too much weight, perform the movement with questionable form, or load up the bar without warming up. This is how martial artist Bruce Lee famously injured his back while performing the exercise. He loaded too much weight—135 pounds, which was his body weight—without taking adequate time to warm up. The outcome was catastrophic. He injured one of his sacral nerves (a nerve in the lumbar spine) and spent the next six months bedridden and in extreme pain. Even worse, he never fully recovered. He reportedly suffered lower back pain for the rest of his tragically short life.

But we shouldn't assume that good mornings will automatically cause injuries. As long as you apply the right technique and don't get overzealous with loading, good mornings are perfectly safe. Not only that, in a number of situations, good mornings are a great option. Say you hurt your knee and can't squat, or you hurt your wrist and can't deadlift. In such situations, good mornings are a good substitute. And there are many benefits to performing this exercise that people fail to consider. In addition to transferring to the squat and deadlift, good mornings, when done correctly, strengthen the back muscles, which might help prevent lower back injuries instead of causing them. The exercise lengthens the glutes under tension, making it a great accessory hip hinge exercise for people interested solely in glute training. And lastly, it stretches and strengthens the hamstrings at end ranges, which improves hip flexion mobility.

GUIDELINES AND CUES

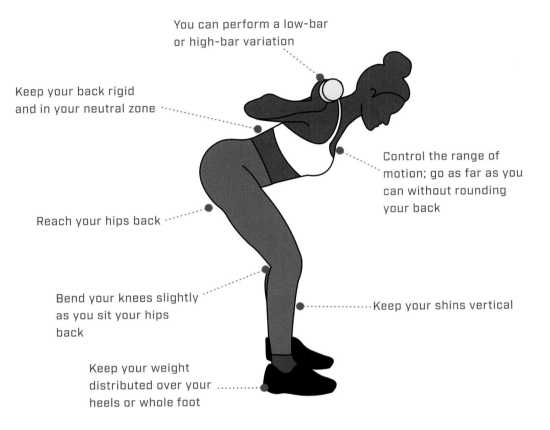

You can perform a low-bar or high-bar variation

Keep your back rigid and in your neutral zone

Control the range of motion; go as far as you can without rounding your back

Reach your hips back

Bend your knees slightly as you sit your hips back

Keep your shins vertical

Keep your weight distributed over your heels or whole foot

Because good mornings share a similar movement pattern to the low-bar back squat and deadlift, many of the technique guidelines and cues are the same. However, redundant as they may be, it's important to address, especially given the perceived risk and reputation that doing good mornings will lead to lower back injuries. In short, the following guidelines are overtly obvious, and they apply to all exercises, but I feel they are necessary to include given that some people are irrationally fearful of this exercise.

STANCE AND SETUP

When it comes to stance and setup, it's exactly the same as the deadlift and squat: you can adopt a narrow stance (feet positioned underneath your hips), medium stance (feet positioned shoulder width or more apart), or a wide/sumo stance (feet turned out and positioned far outside your shoulders). Moreover, you can position your feet straight, turn them out slightly, or turn them out a lot—whichever you prefer. As I've repeated throughout the book, experiment to find the stance that feels best, and as long as they are well tolerated, try to mix in different stances from one training session or training cycle to the next for variety.

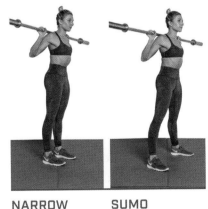

NARROW   SUMO

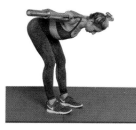

NARROW

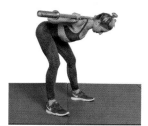

SUMO

HIP AND SPINAL MECHANICS

Whether you're in a narrow, medium, or wide stance, always hinge from your hips while maintaining a neutral spine. The key is to brace your spine by taking a big breath in and then tightening the muscles of your diaphragm and trunk to stabilize your position before you initiate the hinge. As you sit your hips back, you can also arch your back a little bit; just be sure you don't hyperextend too much through your lumbar spine. You should feel tension in your glutes, hamstrings, and back. From there, it's all about keeping your spine in a neutral zone as you continue to sit your hips back and tilt your torso forward. Your shins will remain almost perfectly vertical on this exercise if you do it correctly. To encourage hinging from the hips and not the back, I often tell my clients to imagine there is a rope tied around their hips, pulling them rearward. You can also think chest up, which is another way of saying don't round, and keeping your gaze at a spot on the floor ten feet in front of you.

WARM UP BEFORE ADDING LOAD AND PROGRESS SLOWLY

Let's all learn from Bruce Lee's mistake. Never jump into this exercise without warming up thoroughly. In fact, many people use light—barbell only or banded—good mornings as a warm-up for deadlifts. You should take the same approach when adding load to good mornings. It's also important to realize that good mornings can make your hamstrings excessively sore. That is a hint to progress slowly and keep your set and rep ranges low (2 or 3 sets of 8 to 12 reps is a good starting point) until you know how your body is going to react.

DON'T GO TOO HEAVY

If you're just interested in glute training, there is no good reason to ever go super heavy with this exercise. Keep the weight light and focus on the mind-muscle connection. If you're chasing deadlift PRs, then that is a different story. Even then, I caution you to exercise perfect form, never max out or go quite to failure, and keep the rep ranges and loading moderate.

CONTROL THE RANGE OF MOTION

The goal with good mornings is to eventually get your torso parallel with the ground. But that is only if you have adequate hamstring flexibility and hip flexion range of motion. The downward movement stops when you can no longer hinge from your hips with a flat back. If you feel the arch in your back start to break or you round forward, you've gone too far. You will feel when your hamstrings run out of flexibility—that's when you reverse the movement and go back up.

FAULTS AND CORRECTIONS

I've already provided the most essential guidelines to avoid injury and get the most from the good morning exercise. Put simply, follow the guidelines and cues, and your chance of committing an injurious error is slim. However, there are two faults that you must avoid at all costs: rounding forward and overarching.

FAULT: ROUNDED BACK

When you bend forward from your spine while performing a good morning, you use your back as a prime mover rather than a stabilizer. Instead of rotating purely through your hips, you're moving partially through your hips and partially through your spine. This not only puts added pressure on your spinal discs and some of the ligaments in your lumbar spine but also increases the risk of straining an erector muscle. This tends to happen either right off the bat, as a result of poor coordination and knowledge of proper form, or at the bottom of the movement when the hamstrings run out of flexibility and the only way to go deeper is to round the back.

CORRECTION:

The best defense is master the bodyweight good morning prior to adding load, which I cover shortly. Brace your spine and keep it rigid (flat or slightly arched), keep the weight light, warm up thoroughly, and don't move past the limits of your range of motion. It might also be helpful to keep your gaze forward, focusing your eyes about 10 feet out in front of you.

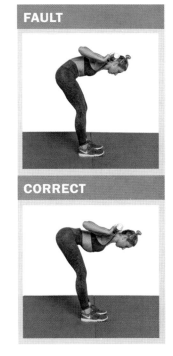

FAULT: OVERARCHING FAULT

Another fault associated with the good morning is spinal hyperextension. I see this occur more often with women than men, probably because more women have higher levels of spinal hyperextension mobility than men. Whatever the case may be, it is important to set up with a fairly neutral spine and keep this position constant throughout the range of motion. Many people set up with an excessive arch and this exposes the vertebrae and ligaments to greater risk of injury in both the top and bottom positions.

CORRECTION:

Start with just the bar and add load and volume incrementally as you gain and demonstrate proficiency. Again, maintain a neutral spine, move within your workable ranges of motion, and don't get overconfident when selecting your load. If you're lifting with a barbell, make sure it is centered and symmetrical on your back. Stop your lockout once your torso is erect and your glutes push your hips forward; don't keep bending backward with your spine.

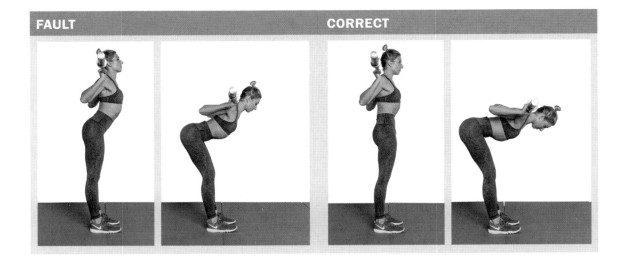

GOOD MORNING VARIATIONS

When I start working with clients, I throw a lot of exercises at them in the first few training sessions and pay close attention to their feedback. This is how I determine which exercises they like and, equally important, which exercises are well tolerated. If a client is new to lifting weights, I generally start them out with body weight, introduce the different stances, and then layer on more advanced variations as they gain experience. The good morning is an exercise I introduce only when the client feels comfortable and expresses competency with the deadlift.

Let's say I have an experienced client who wants to strengthen their hamstrings, glutes, and erectors and improve their squat and deadlift. First, I take them through the basic technique and introduce the different stances with an unloaded barbell. If they can perform the movement with good form and enjoy doing it, I'll experiment with B-stance good mornings or modify the tempo in the form of an eccentric-accentuated or pause variation. Conversely, if they don't like it, it doesn't align with their physique goals, or they have a history of lower back pain, then we won't do them.

There are a few different ways to perform good mornings. You can do them with body weight using a dowel, PVC pipe, or broomstick; with a barbell on your back; or with a band, all of which can be done from a narrow, medium, or wide stance. In the following pages, I break down each good morning variation, explaining what it is good for and how to perform it correctly.

BODYWEIGHT (BROOMSTICK/DOWEL/PVC PIPE) GOOD MORNINGS

The best way to teach or learn the good morning is to start out using a dowel or light rod of some kind, such as a PVC pipe or broomstick. With the dowel positioned along the long axis of your back, you can maintain three points of contact: one at the back of your head, one at your thoracic spine, and one at your sacrum. This teaches you to keep a neutral spine as you bend at your hips. If you lose contact with the dowel, you know you're no longer in neutral and you either rounded or overarched your spine. This is also where you can dial in your workable ranges of motion. For beginners, performing 2 or 3 sets of 8 to 12 reps is a good starting point; you might be surprised to feel a little soreness the following day from the active stretch. In addition to a great teaching tool, you can use bodyweight good mornings as a warm-up for more strenuous hamstring and hip hinge work or as a way to improve hamstring flexibility.

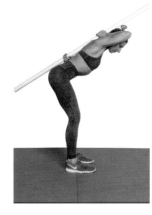

Place the dowel along your back and form a comfortable over/under grip so that one arm is positioned behind your lower back and the other is behind your neck. Assume your good morning stance, then brace your spine. To initiate the movement, you do several things at once: with your spine rigid (straight or slightly arched), sit your hips back, lean your torso forward, and bend your knees slightly, keeping your shins as vertical as possible. The idea is to go down as far as you can without rounding your back. Again, your depth is determined by your hamstring flexibility. Some people can descend only 45 degrees, while others can go down to 90 degrees and get their torsos parallel with the ground. As you tilt your torso forward, try to keep your weight evenly distributed over your feet (don't elevate your heels off the floor). To reverse the movement, think about squeezing your glutes to extend your hips while simultaneously elevating your torso and straightening your knees.

BANDED GOOD MORNINGS

By hooking a long (41-inch) resistance band around your feet and the back of your neck, you can effectively add resistance to the good morning movement pattern. You can use this as a warm-up or use a thicker band (multiple bands are also an option) to increase resistance and make it more challenging. In most cases, the banded variation is performed with higher reps, such as 2 or 3 sets of 12 to 20. What's more, there is less resistance the farther you hinge, putting less stress on your spine. People generally tweak their back in the bottom position as they reverse the movement, so less resistance in this range is great if you're worried about injury.

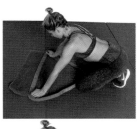
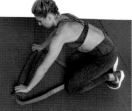

I also recommend placing a towel between the band and your neck. This not only reduces friction but also prevents you from smelling like rubber after your training session. I had an ex-girlfriend who would tease me, saying I smelled like a condom after I did these. The towel solved this problem.

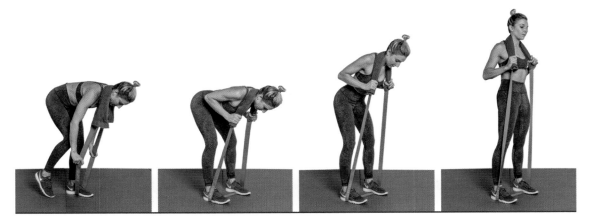

Wrap a towel around the band, and then place that section around the back of your neck, positioning as low on your neck as possible. Hook the band around the arches of your feet and assume a narrow stance to keep slack in the band. You will probably have to hinge forward and dip your head through the loop while pulling it upward with both hands. Stand upright and then make any necessary adjustments, such as widening your stance. With the band positioned around the base of your neck, form a grip on the band (you can pull up slightly to reduce tension on your neck if it's uncomfortable), brace your spine, and then initiate the movement by sitting your hips back, bending your knees slightly—keeping your shins as vertical as possible—and lowering your torso. Once you reach your end range, extend your hips and knees, and think about squeezing your glutes as you stand upright.

BARBELL GOOD MORNINGS

If you have a history of lower back pain or you feel your back light up when performing bodyweight or banded good morning variations, then perhaps this is an exercise you shouldn't do. If it feels good, on the other hand, then the barbell variation is a great option, especially if you're interested in building squat and deadlift strength.

Newcomers to the exercise should start out with just the barbell, then add weight incrementally. Most important, I recommend performing heavy good mornings in a power rack with the safety pins set a couple of inches below your end range. That way, if you accidentally round your back or your form is compromised, you can drop your hips, bend your knees, and set the barbell down instead of powering through the movement with questionable form.

When it comes to barbell placement, you can perform high-bar and low-bar variations, just as you would when back squatting. Most people prefer the high bar position because they feel their hamstrings more during the exercise, but the low bar position allows you to use more load. Like all exercise variations, experiment with both to see which you like better. Although you can use similar technique for both the high-bar and low-bar good mornings, I prefer to perform the high-bar variations with straighter legs and the low-bar variations with more knee bend. My low-bar technique almost looks like a squat gone wrong when the hips shoot up from the bottom position.

If you're using the good morning to improve your deadlift, I recommend the high-bar variation because it transfers better to that movement pattern. If you're using it to improve your squat, the low-bar variation with a greater knee bend more closely mimics the squat movement pattern. If you're performing good mornings with the goal of building your glutes, play around with the different bar placements and stances and prioritize the one where you feel the most tension in your glutes.

HIGH-BAR GOOD MORNING

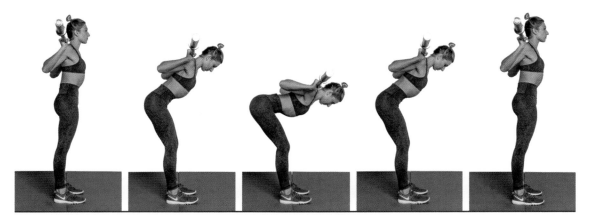

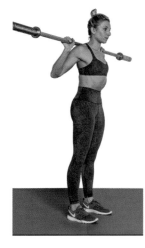

With the bar in the rack, step underneath and position the barbell on your traps below the base of your neck. Form your grip so that your wrists are neutral and your elbows are behind the bar, creating tension in your upper back. Get into a stable stance, then unrack the bar by standing upright. Take a couple of steps back, get into your good morning stance (narrow or sumo), and then brace your spine by taking a big breath in and tightening the muscles of your diaphragm and trunk. To initiate the movement, sit your hips back and tilt your torso forward, keeping your spine rigid (slightly arched or straight) and your gaze forward. As you do, bend your knees slightly, keeping your shins as vertical as possible and your weight distributed evenly over both feet. Once you reach end range or get to parallel, drive through your heels, extend your hips and knees in one fluid motion, and raise your torso. Squeeze your glutes as you extend your hips and stand upright.

LOW-BAR GOOD MORNING

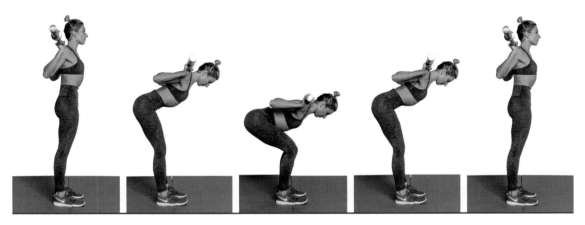

You can also bend your knees to increase the range of motion, sort of mimicking a low-bar back squat but with a little less knee bend and a little more trunk lean. The setup for the low-bar variation is the same as for the high-bar version, but instead of positioning the bar just under the base of your neck, you position it 2 to 3 inches lower on your traps, just above your rear shoulder muscles (posterior deltoids). After you unrack the bar, assume your good morning stance, brace your spine, and then sit your hips back and tilt your torso forward, keeping your spine rigid (slightly arched or straight) and your gaze forward. Depending on your anthropometry and hamstring flexibility, your torso angle at the bottom might be between 60 and 90 degrees relative to vertical. To reverse the movement, drive through your heels and extend your hips and knees in one fluid motion. As you stand upright, squeeze your glutes and return to a neutral upright position.

B-STANCE GOOD MORNINGS

You can perform good mornings with a staggered stance or B-stance (also known as a "kickstand"). With any B-stance variation, the goal is to get about 70 percent of the loading on your front (working) leg and 30 percent on your back (supporting) leg. Many people who don't like bilateral good mornings find that they tolerate the B-stance well.

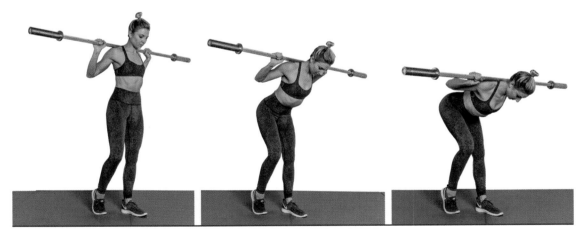

Unrack the bar and take a couple of steps backward. Get most of your weight on one leg and place the foot of your other leg at the heel of your front foot. In other words, slide your support leg backward at roughly the length of your lead foot. Angle your back foot outward about 45 degrees. Keeping a neutral spine, sit back and bend at your hips, allowing your torso to lean forward and your knees to bend slightly. Sit back as far as possible while keeping a vertical shin on your front leg until your hamstring runs out of flexibility. Then reverse the motion by extending your hips and knees and erecting your torso.

Back Extensions

Traditionally, back extension exercises are used to strengthen your back, which they do. But they also work your hamstrings and glutes to a very high degree. In fact, if you examine the mechanics, the title of the exercise is not exactly accurate because you're extending your hips using the power of your glutes and hamstrings, not your back. They should therefore be called "hip extensions," but that name is a bit generic, so I'll stick with the traditional term.

To perform back extensions, you need a hyperextension bench—either a 45-degree hyper, a horizontal back extension, or a glute ham developer (GHD). With your feet anchored and your legs straight, you hinge and extend from your hips just as you would when performing a good morning or stiff-leg deadlift. But instead of standing, your body is angled—horizontal or at a 45-degree angle—which creates a different torque angle curve. Put simply, good mornings are more challenging in the bottom position and get easier as you extend your hips. Back extensions are the opposite in that they are easier in the bottom position and get more challenging in the top position, which is the zone where you get maximal glute activation. In other words, good mornings elicit peak glute activation at longer muscle lengths, while back extensions elicit peak glute activation at shorter muscle lengths. In fact, based on my EMG experiments and research, back extensions get the second highest glute activity behind hip thrusts.

The 45-degree hyper is unique in that the hardest part is when you're straight out horizontally. The load on the hips gets easier as you rise up from parallel or descend deeper than parallel (since your center of mass gets closer to your fulcrum). It therefore creates an inverted U-shaped hip extension torque-angle curve. What's unique about the 45-degree hyper is that there's more consistent tension on the hips throughout the movement, since there's always high torque requirements.

For this reason, back extensions are my favorite non-glute-dominant glute-building exercise. They are still considered ham dominant because your legs are straight and you're working a hip hinge pattern. And like the other exercises in this section, they work your entire posterior chain. So, not only are they great for glute development, but also for strengthening your lower back and hamstrings, making back extensions an excellent accessory and supplemental exercise to the deadlift. However, we never place back extensions first in the training session because you generally don't load the movement with a lot of weight. In most cases, it falls in the middle or end of the training session with medium to high reps (2 or 3 sets of 10 to 30 reps is the ideal range). And we typically prescribe this movement once or twice a week in the program.

In this section, I teach you how to perform conventional back extensions, which work your entire posterior chain, as well as how to modify the exercise to make it more of a glute-dominant exercise. But before we delve into the individual exercise variations, let's review some all-encompassing guidelines and cues to get you moving in the right direction.

GUIDELINES AND CUES

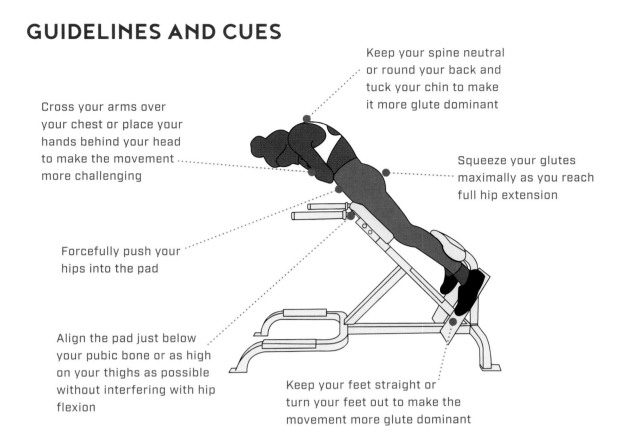

Keep your spine neutral or round your back and tuck your chin to make it more glute dominant

Cross your arms over your chest or place your hands behind your head to make the movement more challenging

Squeeze your glutes maximally as you reach full hip extension

Forcefully push your hips into the pad

Align the pad just below your pubic bone or as high on your thighs as possible without interfering with hip flexion

Keep your feet straight or turn your feet out to make the movement more glute dominant

There are two apparatuses you can use to perform back extensions. You can do them on a 45-degree hyper with your body positioned at a diagonal or on a horizontal back extension or GHD with your body positioned at a horizontal angle. (I break down each movement later in the section.) Angled and horizontal are equally effective, and there's not a big difference between the two. In short, the guidelines covered here apply to both variations.

SETUP: ALIGN THE PAD WITH YOUR PUBIC BONE

Adjusting the pad to the appropriate position is crucial for executing back extensions correctly. In general, you want the pad positioned just below your pubic bone, or as high as possible on your thighs without interfering with hip flexion. You should be able to hinge from your hips with your back flat and stretch your hamstrings maximally without the pad getting in the way. If the pad is too high on your hips, it will cause you to round your lower back as you hinge forward, which reduces the stretch on your hamstrings and glutes and potentially places unnecessary stress on your lower back. If it is too low and there is a big gap between your hips and the pad, you won't feel your glutes fire nearly as much, and your hamstrings will take over the exercise.

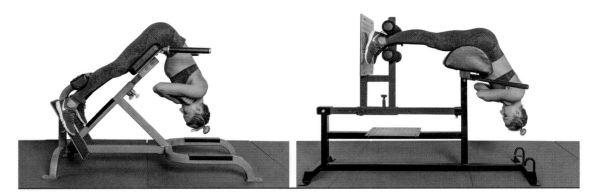

45-DEGREE HYPER PAD POSITION **HORIZONTAL BACK EXTENSION PAD POSITION**

Position the pad just below your pubic bone, or as high as possible on your thighs without interfering with hip flexion.

FOOT POSITION: TURN YOUR FEET OUT TO EMPHASIZE THE GLUTES

Your foot position depends on which muscles you want to target. If you want to work your entire posterior chain (glutes, hamstrings, and erectors), keep your feet straight or neutral. If you want to emphasize your glutes, turn your feet out. Externally rotating your hips by turning your feet out has been shown to increase glute activation by up to 30 percent. However, turning your feet out will cause you to hit your lateral hamstrings more than your medial hamstrings. This isn't a big deal as long as you're still performing hip extension exercises with a more neutral foot alignment, such as with deadlifts and good mornings. I turn my feet out roughly 45 degrees, while others like to turn them out even more. Play around with your foot flare and stance width and adopt the position that feels best for your body.

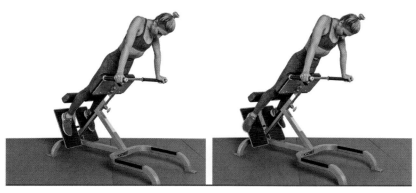

FEET STRAIGHT **FEET TURNED OUT**

SPINAL MECHANICS: ROUND YOUR BACK TO EMPHASIZE THE GLUTES

Just as altering your foot position changes the emphasis of the working muscles, your spinal movement determines which muscles you target with the exercise. There are three spinal strategies you can implement for back extensions, each of which targets your posterior chain in a unique way.

The first strategy is to maintain a neutral spine throughout the entire range of motion. This is a great strategy for people who want to target the entire posterior chain. It's safe and effective, and it works your glutes, hamstrings, and erectors.

NEUTRAL SPINE

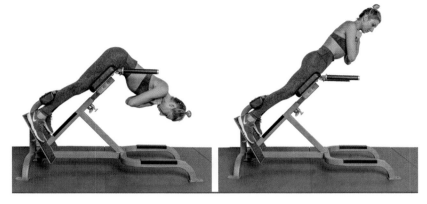

ROUNDED (BOTTOM) NEUTRAL (TOP)

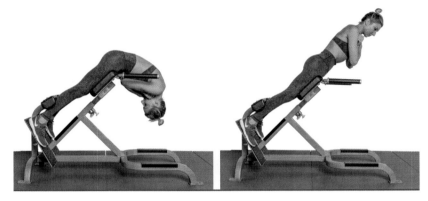

The second strategy is to round your back in the bottom position and then straighten and arch your spine as you reach the top position. This is more of a back-dominant strategy because it places greater emphasis on your erectors. Some people prefer to position the pad at belly button level when aiming to target their erectors, as this prevents the hips from flexing, forcing all of the movement onto the spine.

The third strategy is to posterior pelvic tilt slightly and keep your back rounded throughout the entire range of motion. Keeping your back rounded decreases tension in your erectors and might place greater emphasis on your glutes, making it more of a glute-dominant variation. The job of the erectors is to erect the spine, so not erecting the torso will shut down the erector muscles. This is the recommended strategy for people who primarily want to target their glutes. Rather than ending the set because your erectors are fatigued, you'll end the set when your glutes and hamstrings can't do any more work.

To perform this variation, get into the bottom position, relax your upper body, and then tuck your chin and round your entire back. Holding this position, drive your hips into the pad and squeeze your glutes. Do not unravel your spine; keep it flexed. The key is to think about driving your hips forward and keeping your upper back rounded and chin tucked as you raise your torso.

GLUTE-DOMINANT BACK EXTENSION

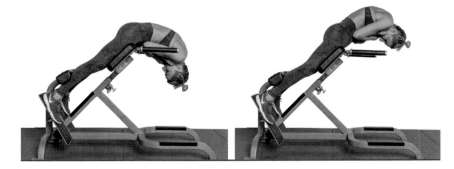

FAULTS AND CORRECTIONS

There are only two faults you need to be aware of when performing back extensions. The first is not setting up correctly, which I already addressed. The second is not achieving the proper spinal mechanics for the intended variation. If you're striving to target your erectors, then you can dynamically move your spine as long as you don't feel any pain. But if you're performing traditional back extensions, you need to move almost exclusively at your hips with very little spinal motion. If you're striving to target your glutes, then you need to keep your spine flexed and not unravel it as you rise upward, which a lot people struggle with. They think they're not reaching full hip extension, so they unravel their back and straighten their spine. This is fine if you're trying to build your erectors, but it's an error if you're executing the glute-dominant variation. To correct this error, focus on three things: keep your chin tucked, keep your ribcage down (back rounded), and squeeze your glutes maximally as you reach full hip extension.

WHEN IT IS AND IS NOT SAFE TO ROUND YOUR BACK

You may be wondering at this point why I caution against rounding your back with squats, deadlifts, and good mornings but advise it with back extensions. The short answer is experience. Having spent a ton of time in the gym in the last 28 years, I know which exercises and what type of form tends to hurt people. Lower-load exercises that involve spinal flexion (rounding), like crunches, hanging leg raises, sit-ups, hollow-body holds, RKC planks, and glute-dominant back extensions, are well tolerated even when exceeding the neutral zone. But heavy barbell exercises from a standing position, such as squats, deadlifts, and good mornings, are not considered safe, especially if you round your back excessively (outside your neutral zone).

The long answer is that the spine is well suited to handle a lot of flexion with a little load or a lot of load with a little flexion, but not a lot of flexion combined with a lot of load. What's interesting is that it's not the barbell itself that generates the high spinal loads; it's the spinal stabilization requirements. The erectors have to work hard to stabilize the spine during heavy lifts, and this creates a lot of compression on the discs of your spine. (Picture the erectors contracting hard and generating tension between the ribcage and pelvis.) To put this another way, when your erectors contract to stabilize your spine, your discs compress. And when you add spinal flexion, the front side of each disc gets pinched by the bending vertebrae, which squeeze the nucleus rearward out of the disc until a herniation emerges. Put simply, rounding your back when performing an exercise with high spinal stabilization requirements makes you more susceptible to spinal damage and injury.

So keep your spine in your neutral zone with standing barbell exercises, but know that you have more freedom with back extension variations.

BACK EXTENSION VARIATIONS

The best way to perform back extensions is on a 45-degree hyper, horizontal back extension, or glute ham developer (GHD). The former positions your body at a 45-degree angle, while the latter two variations position your body at a horizontal angle. As I've said, there isn't a big difference between the two in terms of how they work your glutes, and you can perform the same techniques on both pieces of equipment. In other words, anything you can do off a 45-degree hyper, you can do from a horizontal position. So the variation you choose boils down to accessibility and personal preference. If you don't have access to a hyperextension bench, you can still perform the movement on a flat bench, which I demonstrate on page 541.

45-DEGREE HYPER

The 45-degree hyper is the most common and most popular back extension variation. With your body at a diagonal angle, you don't get as dizzy when performing the movement, and many people report feeling a slightly better glute pump compared to its horizontal counterpart. What's more, the 45-degree hyper is a common piece of equipment and is a staple in most commercial gyms. In fact, you can purchase one for a reasonable price, and it doesn't take up nearly as much space as a GHD, making it a better option for home gyms. For bodyweight back extensions, I generally prescribe 3 sets of 20 to 30 reps with a 1-minute rest between sets.

GLUTE-DOMINANT BACK EXTENSION   **NEUTRAL BACK EXTENSION (PRISONER POSITION)**

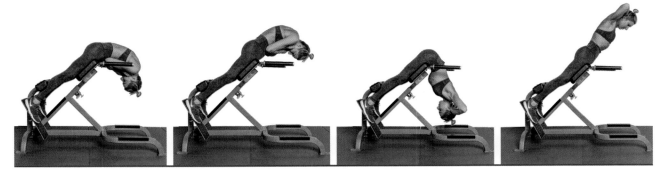

To set up, adjust the pad so that it is aligned with your pubic bone—as high up on your thighs as it can be without interfering with hip flexion—and slip your feet into position. You should be able to hinge from your hips without rounding your lower back. If you want to target your glutes, turn your feet out roughly 45 degrees, purposely round your back, fold your arms over your chest, and tuck your chin (see glute-dominant back extension). Now drive your hips into the pad and squeeze your glutes as you elevate your torso. Make sure to keep your back rounded; don't unravel. In other words, the distance between your ribcage and pelvis should not change throughout the set. Once you reach full hip extension, stop the movement and hold for a slight pause, squeezing your glutes maximally. If you want to target your entire posterior chain, keep your feet and back straight (see neutral back extension). To reiterate, keep your lower back flat and avoid overarching. If you want to make the bodyweight movement more challenging, you can position your hands behind your head in the prisoner position instead of on your chest.

You can also perform single-leg variations for all of the 45-degree hyper and horizontal back extension exercises. However, they primarily work your hamstrings and do not work your glutes nearly as well as the double-leg variations.

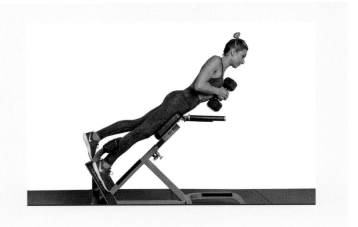

HORIZONTAL BACK EXTENSION

Horizontal back extensions share the same glute-building benefits as the 45-degree hyper variations. However, some people just prefer the feel of the glute ham developer (GHD) machine and get slightly higher peak glute tension with the horizontal variations. The main drawback is that the horizontal position makes some people dizzy, and the equipment is not nearly as common in commercial gyms. Moreover, it's a lot more expensive and takes up more space than a 45-degree hyper. Though it does give you more exercise options, such as glute ham raises and straight-leg sit-ups, it's not as practical for most home gyms. As with the 45-degree hyper, 3 sets of 20 to 30 reps is a good bodyweight goal to shoot for.

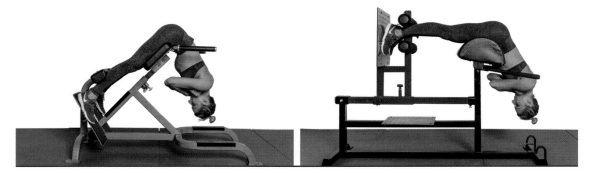

The setup and execution for the horizontal back extension are exactly the same as the 45-degree hyper. The only difference is your body position. So, again, get into position with your feet turned out, allow your torso to drop, round your back, tuck your chin, and then drive your hips into the pad while squeezing your glutes to elevate your torso. You can position your hands across your chest or over the back of your head for added load. Momentarily hold the top position while squeezing your glutes and avoid arching or hyperextending through your lumbar spine.

A lot of people wonder how to perform back extensions without a hyperextension bench from their home gym. Here's how:

To perform horizontal back extensions, you need a flat bench and a heavy dumbbell, which most home gyms and all commercial gyms have. If you have access to a balance pad you can place that under your hips for extra cushion. To set up the bench, place a heavy dumbbell on one side, line your pelvis up on the end of the bench, and then hook your feet underneath (you can also have someone sit on the bench and hold your feet). Hooking your feet underneath the bench mimics a frog stance, which is characterized by hip abduction and external rotation. This works more glutes and lateral (as opposed to medial) hamstrings. From here, you're ready to execute the movement.

It's important to point out that if the bench is flat on the ground, you won't be able to use a full range of motion. To remedy this problem, you can either elevate both ends off the ground by stacking the bench on plyometric boxes or elevate just one end and perform the 45-degree hyper variation, with the latter being the preferred method. Also, you can perform the bent-leg variation by placing the arches of your feet against a loaded barbell.

You can also perform back extensions in a power rack, which works just as well as performing them in a 45-degree hyper apparatus. You need a rack, two barbells, and two thick bar pads (trust me, you need them to protect your ankles and hips). As you can see in the photos, you need to add significant weight to the barbell on the ground and wedge it between two bumper plates so that it doesn't move. The elevated barbell is positioned on the outside of the rack. When you set up, make sure your body is pushing the barbell into the steel uprights and not into the opening of the pins. You have to tinker with the height and distance, but once you get it just right, it feels no different than most 45-degree hyper machines.

While these variations are not as good as the real thing (having an apparatus), they are still worthwhile, assuming it feels right for your body.

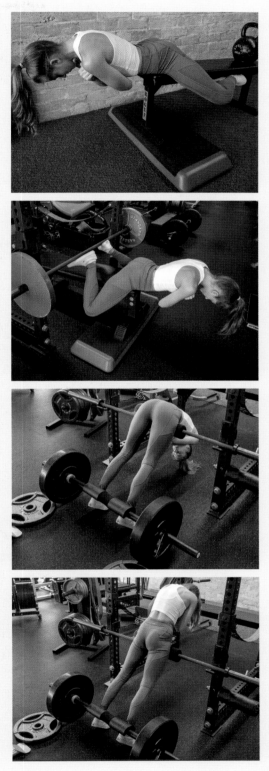

LOADING AND EQUIPMENT VARIATIONS

You can load back extension variations by using a band or by holding a dumbbell or barbell.

DUMBBELL VARIATIONS

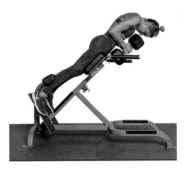

The dumbbell is perhaps the easiest and most common way to load back extension exercises. Though you can still do high reps with lighter dumbbells, I generally recommend choosing a weight that is challenging for 3 sets of 12 reps. To perform the variation, position the dumbbell underneath or just in front of the pad, then get into the machine. Once in position, get into the bottom position, grip the handle with both hands, and pull it to the center of your chest, positioning it vertically and holding it underneath your chin.

BANDED VARIATIONS

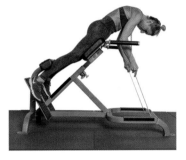

To execute the banded back extension variations, you need a 41-inch resistance band. What's great about the band is that it enhances the lockout, which is the zone in which you get the highest glute activation. The only problem is setting it up. Some back extension machines have band attachments, but many do not. In this case, setting up might require some ingenuity. You can hook the band around the feet of the machine, or if that doesn't work, you can use heavy dumbbells to anchor the band.

BARBELL VARIATIONS

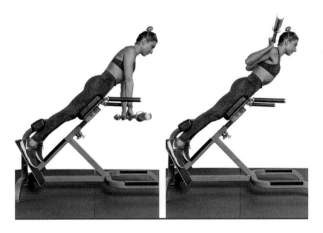

The barbell variation is used primarily for improving strength. For example, if your main goal is to improve your deadlift, then performing 3 sets of 6 to 10 heavy barbell 45-degree hypers is great. Simply place a loaded barbell in front of the apparatus, form a wide grip on the barbell (consider wearing wrist straps for these), and raise your upper body in the same manner described previously. Alternatively, you can place the bar on your upper back like a back squat.

If you're mostly interested in glute training, on the other hand, you can stick with the bodyweight, dumbbell, and banded variations.

4 Reverse Hypers

The reverse hyper exercise is like a back extension but in reverse. Instead of anchoring your legs, hinging from your hips, and moving your upper body, you stabilize your torso on a flat bench, hinge from your hips, and move your lower body. As with back extensions, the reverse hyper variations work your entire posterior chain—hamstrings, glutes, and lower back—when done as traditionally taught. But the variations I teach are more glute dominant. This creates a unique classification conundrum, where the line between hamstring dominant and glute dominant is blurred and the categorization system based on the dominant muscle isn't perfectly accurate.

With the reverse hyper, you hinge from your hips, which is characteristic of hamstring-dominant movements, but you can modify the exercise to home in on your glutes. For instance, the conventional reverse hyper is done with your feet together and legs straight, making it a hamstring-dominant exercise. But doing it with bent legs takes your hamstrings out of the equation, making it a glute-dominant exercise. And there are other ways to make the reverse hyper more glute dominant, such as by performing the knee-banded spread eagle variation.

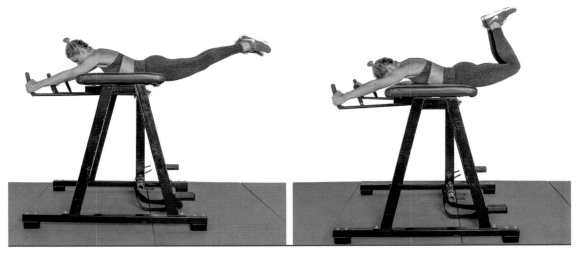

HAMSTRING-DOMINANT REVERSE HYPER
(LEGS STRAIGHT)

GLUTE-DOMINANT REVERSE HYPER
(LEGS BENT)

In short, you can make the reverse hyper more glute or ham dominant based on the knee action, loading, and exercise strategy (tempo), all of which I cover in the following pages. But whether you perform glute- or ham-dominant variations, all reverse hyper exercises work your lower back muscles. In fact, strengthening the lower back is one of the primary benefits of the reverse hyper.

Like many great lower-body exercises, the reverse hyper was made popular by the iconic powerlifter and coach Louie Simmons. Although he didn't invent the exercise, he developed and popularized the reverse hyper machine and brought the straight-leg reverse hyper to the forefront of the powerlifting and athletic training communities. Most notably, he made the connection between reverse hyper exercises and improved back health, which I also found in my practice. That is, people who have or are susceptible to lower back pain tend to feel better and have less frequent flare-ups when they routinely employ the reverse hyper exercise in their training. If I have a client who hurts their back deadlifting, for example, I sometimes use the reverse hyper (both the bent-leg and straight-leg variations) to strengthen and rehabilitate their lower back.

However, to reap the lower back and glute-building benefits, you must apply careful consideration to technique. Doing the movement incorrectly can increase your susceptibility to back pain or make an existing condition worse. What's more, to make the reverse hyper a more glute-dominant exercise, you need to make certain modifications that are not conventionally taught. In this section, you will learn how to execute the movement in a way that will further strengthen your hamstrings and potentially reduce occurrences of lower back pain, as well as strategies to make the exercise more glute dominant.

GUIDELINES AND CUES

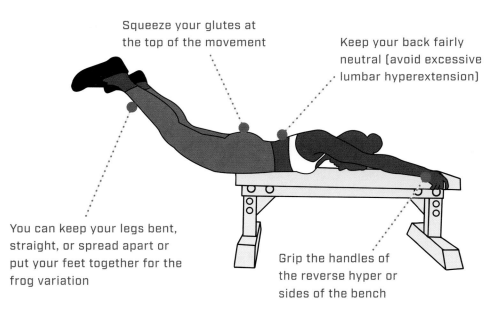

Squeeze your glutes at the top of the movement

Keep your back fairly neutral (avoid excessive lumbar hyperextension)

You can keep your legs bent, straight, or spread apart or put your feet together for the frog variation

Grip the handles of the reverse hyper or sides of the bench

The best way to perform reverse hyper exercises is on a reverse hyper machine. The problem is, most commercial gyms don't have this specialized piece of equipment. You can make do by performing them on anything that is stable, is raised, and has a flat surface, such as a countertop or table. You can also use a bench (ideally elevated on mats or plyometric boxes), which most home gyms and all commercial gyms have.

SETUP: ALIGN THE EDGE OF THE BENCH/PAD WITH THE TOP OF YOUR PUBIC BONE

Whether you're using a reverse hyper machine, a bench, or a tabletop, the setup is the same: lie on your belly and position the edge of the apparatus as low on your abdomen as possible without interfering with hip flexion. Usually, this is just above your pubic bone.

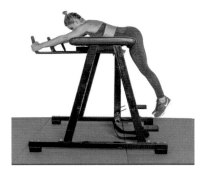

FORM A STABLE GRIP

Gripping the handles of the reverse hyper machine or the edges of the bench not only provides stability and prevents you from sliding up and down the surface but also engages your upper body musculature. Your forearms, lats, and core stiffen maximally, especially when performing the pendulum variation, making it a full-body exercise.

SPINAL MECHANICS: KEEP YOUR SPINE NEUTRAL AND MINIMIZE SPINAL MOTION

Reverse hyper exercises are great for building your lower back muscles and can even be used to treat and prevent lower back pain. However, if you're not mindful of your spinal mechanics, they can have the opposite effect. To get the most out of the exercise and avoid lower back pain, you need to stay in your neutral zone. Lower your legs as much as you can without rounding your back and raise your legs as high as you can without overarching your back. Put simply, move mostly from your hips, not from your spine and pelvis.

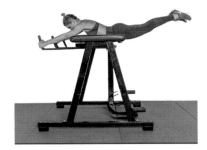

SQUEEZE YOUR GLUTES IN THE TOP POSITION AND CONTROL YOUR DESCENT

To get the most muscle-building benefits from the reverse hyper variations, squeeze your glutes and momentarily pause in the top position and then control your legs down into the bottom position. The only exception is if you're performing the pendulum variation on a reverse hyper machine, which I cover on page 548. With the pendulum variation, you don't pause at the top.

FAULTS AND CORRECTIONS

I've already outlined the essential guidelines for preventing injury and getting the most from the reverse hyper exercises. Put simply, if you follow the guidelines and cues, your chance of committing an injurious error is slim. However, there are two faults that you must avoid: hyperextending and rounding the lower back.

FAULT: HYPEREXTENDING AND ROUNDING THE LOWER BACK

Many coaches and powerlifters teach the straight-leg reverse hyper in a unique way. Instead of performing slow, grinding reps, you explode out of the bottom position during the concentric phase and relax during the eccentric phase. When you do the exercise this way, the lower back typically rounds in the bottom position and hyperextends in the top position. Although this stretches and strengthens the lower back, flexing and hyperextending through the spine can cause problems for some people. Granted, not everyone gets back pain as a result of this technique, and I'm sure you can develop a tolerance over time. However, in my experience, whether you're rapidly swinging your legs or grinding out slow reps, it's best to minimize spinal motion.

CORRECTION:

If you're susceptible to lower back pain, control the eccentric and concentric phases of the movement and stay in your neutral zone.

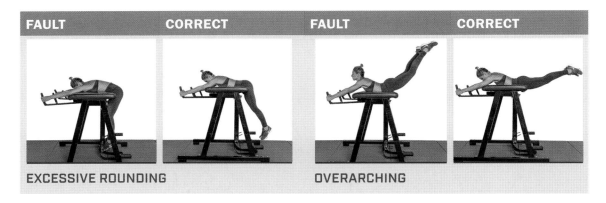

| FAULT | CORRECT | FAULT | CORRECT |
| EXCESSIVE ROUNDING | | OVERARCHING | |

REVERSE HYPER VARIATIONS

There are two ways to perform the reverse hyper: one is to keep your legs straight, and the other is to bend your knees. You can further divide these variations into subcategories based on the resistance and knee action. For example, the straight-leg reverse hyper variations with your feet together are more hamstring dominant, while the knee-banded spread eagle and all bent-leg variations are more glute dominant.

Most people need to perform a ton of reps to get a muscle-building stimulus, so if you can perform 2 or 3 sets of 20 to 30 reps at body weight without struggle, I recommend performing one of the loaded variations, such as the knee-banded spread eagle, or ankle weight variations. Or you can stick with body weight and work on the mind-muscle connection by maximally squeezing your glutes in the top position and controlling the tempo.

STRAIGHT-LEG REVERSE HYPER

Keeping your legs fairly straight and your feet close together is how the reverse hyper is traditionally taught. When done with body weight, it is mostly a glute and erector exercise. To make it more of a hamstring-dominant movement, you need to add resistance by performing the pendulum variation on a reverse hyper machine. You can perform both double-leg and single-leg variations. To execute these techniques, however, you need to be high enough off the ground that your legs don't touch the floor in the bottom position. If you don't have access to a reverse hyper machine, you can place a bench on two plyometric boxes of equal size or do the exercise on a high countertop or table.

BODYWEIGHT STRAIGHT-LEG REVERSE HYPER (DOUBLE LEG)

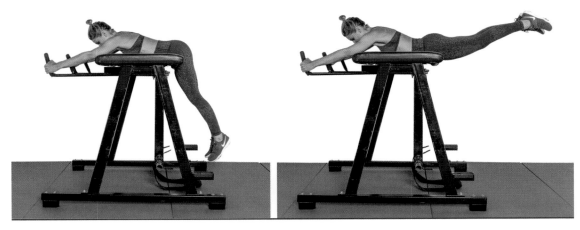

The bilateral bodyweight straight-leg reverse hyper is performed with a slow, deliberate tempo characterized by raising the legs, squeezing for a brief moment at the top of the movement, and then controlling the eccentric phase. To set up, align the top of your pelvis or lower abdomen at the edge of the apparatus, allow your legs to hang off the end with your feet together, and grip the handles of the reverse hyper machine or the edges of the bench. With your torso flat on the bench, raise your legs—keeping your legs straight or your knees slightly bent—and squeeze your glutes as you reach full hip extension. Make sure not to hyperextend your back in the top position or excessively round in the bottom position. Put simply, go as far down as you can without rounding and as high as you can without hyperextending. You want a fairly neutral spine with nearly all of the motion occurring at your hips.

ANKLE WEIGHT STRAIGHT-LEG REVERSE HYPER (SINGLE AND DOUBLE LEG)

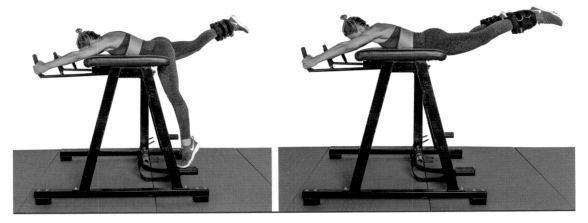

You can also perform single-leg straight-leg reverse hypers. The technique is essentially the same as the bilateral reverse hyper; the only difference is that you raise both legs for the bilateral variation and one leg for the unilateral variation. If possible, try to rest your non-working leg on a box or bench. The single-leg variations can be performed in the middle of a workout for medium reps as a strength exercise or before a workout during the warm-up or as a way to minimize posterior chain imbalances. You can add load to both the unilateral and bilateral straight-leg variations by using ankle weights. You still want to perform these in a slow, controlled style. Don't rely too much on momentum and keep your spine fairly neutral while moving mostly at the hips.

PENDULUM REVERSE HYPER

There are two ways to perform the pendulum reverse hyper: concentric only and concentric/eccentric reps. *Note:* You will need access to a reverse hyper machine for these variations.

Concentric Only

Concentric only means that you activate your muscles during the concentric phase and relax during the eccentric phase. This technique is performed with slight spinal extension on the way up and spinal flexion on the way down, which is usually considered an error. But in this case, it's not as dangerous because you relax your muscles during the lowering or eccentric phase and allow gravity to pull your legs into a stretch, then use the momentum of the pendulum to swing your legs back up. Harnessing the momentum of the swing means that your back is not under a lot of tension when you enter spinal flexion and extension, thereby reducing your risk of injury. In fact, it has the opposite effect. Many powerlifters and athletes use this technique as a rehab tool to prevent and treat lower back pain. In addition to stretching the spine, omitting the eccentric phase doesn't make you as sore or damage your back muscles. What's more, the dynamic and explosive action builds speed and explosive power, which is essential for powerlifters and athletes. So it's a great conditioning exercise for power athletes, but not as good for muscle building.

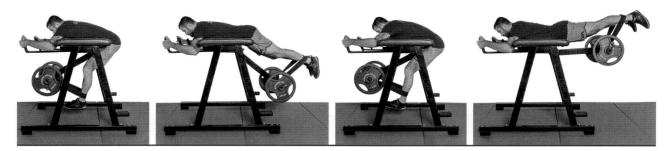

To execute the concentric-only technique, you explode during the concentric phase (raising your legs with great acceleration), then relax during the eccentric phase (lowering your legs and letting gravity do the work). In other words, you're not performing slow reps, but rather swinging your legs dynamically. To start, you need to generate momentum by pulling your legs back and then relaxing into the bottom position. Without pausing, harness the momentum by explosively swinging your legs back. Continue this process—exploding your legs upward and then controlling the descent—until you reach the top position. For example, on the first attempt, you might raise your legs a quarter of the way up, let them fall, and then explode halfway up on your second attempt, and then let them fall, and then again to reach the top position, at which point the set starts. From there, you repeat this action—activating your posterior chain to raise your legs until you hit neutral, then relaxing and letting the momentum and gravity do the rest of the work.

Concentric/Eccentric

You can also perform slower, more deliberate reps by squeezing for a moment at the top of the movement and then controlling the eccentric phase, which is better for building muscle. These are concentric/eccentric reps. With the concentric/eccentric method, you do not hyperextend your back in the top position or excessively round in the bottom position. Put simply, you go down as far as you can without rounding and as high as you can without hyperextending.

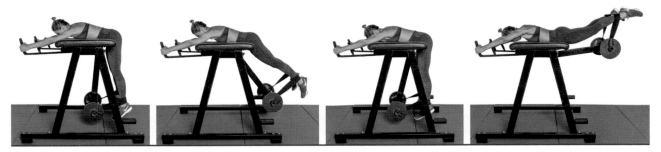

Whether you perform explosive or slow reps, the setup and knee action are the same. Align the top of your pelvis or lower abdomen at the edge of the apparatus, allow your legs to hang off the end with your feet together, put your legs through the strap, and grip the handles of the reverse hyper machine. With your torso flat on the bench, keeping your legs straight or your knees slightly bent, take two "swings" before performing a full repetition. This means you move the pendulum about a quarter of the way up on the first swing and about halfway up on the second swing, and then you move into your working reps with full-range movement. Squeeze your glutes as you reach full hip extension, then control your legs back down into the start position. Keep your spine in your neutral zone and move only from your hips.

SPREAD EAGLE REVERSE HYPER

The spread eagle reverse hyper is a straight-leg variation that is more glute dominant. With your hips abducted, you get higher levels of glute activation than you do when you keep your feet together. What's particularly great about this exercise is that there are many ways to add resistance. For example, the knee-banded variation forces you to drive your legs outward into the band, thereby increasing glute activation throughout the entire range of motion. You can also perform this variation with ankle weights, manual resistance, or any combination of the three.

BODYWEIGHT SPREAD EAGLE

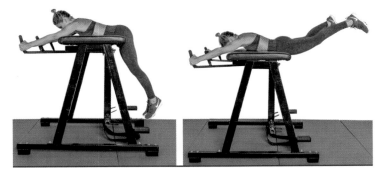

There are two ways to perform the spread eagle reverse hyper. The first is to keep your legs spread throughout the entire range of the movement. The second is to keep your legs together in the bottom position and then spread them as you raise your legs into the top position. Regardless of the method you choose, the setup is the same. Align the top of your pelvis or lower abdomen at the edge of the apparatus, allow your legs to hang off the end with your feet together or spread slightly apart, and grip the handles of the reverse hyper machine or the edges of the bench. From there, raise your legs—keeping your legs straight or your knees slightly bent—squeeze your glutes as you reach full hip extension, and then lower your legs with control. Try not to hyperextend your back in the top position or excessively round in the bottom position. Go down as far as you can without rounding your back and as high as you can without hyperextending your back.

KNEE-BANDED SPREAD EAGLE

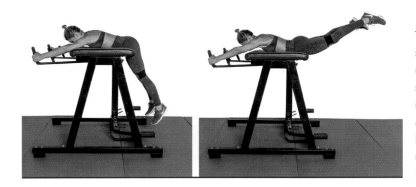

The knee-banded variation shares the same setup and execution as the bodyweight spread eagle. The only difference is that you wrap a band above or below your knees and drive your legs outward into the band as you lower and raise your legs.

ANKLE WEIGHT SPREAD EAGLE

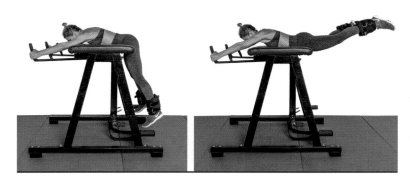

You can use ankle weights to increase the load. Again, the setup and execution are the same as for the bodyweight and knee-banded reverse hyper variations. The key with this variation is to control the eccentric phase so that you don't excessively round your lower back in the bottom position.

ENHANCED-ECCENTRIC MANUAL RESISTANCE SPREAD EAGLE

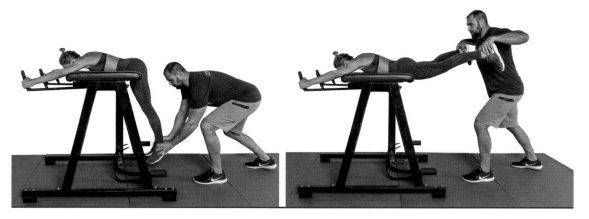

Have a training partner or coach stand between your legs and press down on the backs of your heels during the eccentric phase (lowering your legs). But here's the trick: your partner has to push down and in so that you're forced to resist hip extension and abduction. Getting the rhythm and feel just right takes some practice. You raise your legs just as you would a normal spread eagle reverse hyper. At the top, your hips are extended and abducted (parallel to the ground and legs spread apart), at which point your partner pushes down and inward on your legs. So you're using your glutes and hamstrings to resist the downward push and your upper glutes to resist the inward push.

FROG REVERSE HYPER

This variation is essentially an open-chain frog pump (the frog pump is a closed-chain, supine exercise shown on page 348) performed on a reverse hyper or bench. What's particularly great about the bent-leg variation is that you can perform it on a bench without having to raise it off the ground (see the next page) and add ankle weights to increase the load. People who typically don't feel frog pumps from the ground working their glutes tend to feel frog reverse hypers in their glutes big-time, which is strange because the movement patterns are similar.

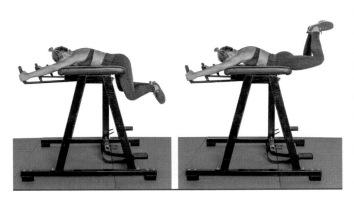

Set up on a bench with your lower abdomen aligned over the edge. With your torso flat against the pad, grip the outsides of the bench and position the bottoms or insides of your feet together. Squeeze your glutes and raise your legs, keeping the heels of your feet together the entire time. Like all reverse hyper techniques, momentarily pause in the top position and control the descent.

BENT-LEG REVERSE HYPER

There are several ways to perform the bent-leg reverse hyper. You can keep your legs bent throughout the entire movement or straighten them as you raise your legs, turning it into more of a kickback movement. You can use a knee band, ankle weights, or a combination of the two to increase resistance, as well as perform both single- and double-leg variations. As with the frog variation, all you need is a bench, so you can do it almost anywhere.

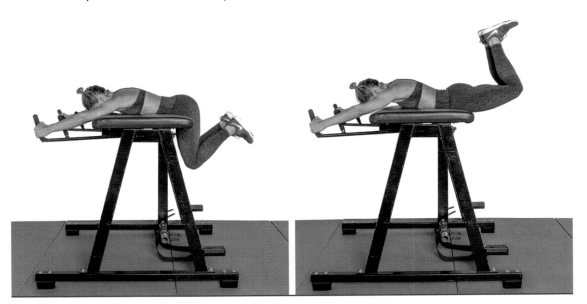

Set up on a bench with your lower abdomen aligned over the edge. Grip the outsides of the bench and curl your legs at roughly a 90-degree angle. Keeping your legs bent and your torso flat with the bench, squeeze your glutes and lift your legs until your thighs are parallel to the ground. If you're performing the knee-banded variation, actively drive your knees outward into the band throughout the entire range of motion. As with all variations, momentarily pause in the top position with a maximal glute squeeze.

BENT TO STRAIGHT LEG

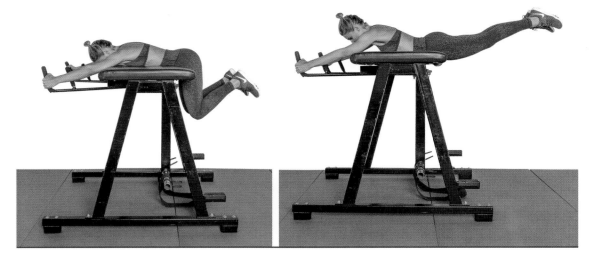

The bent-to-straight-leg variation is similar to the bent-leg variation above, but instead of keeping your legs bent, you straighten your legs as you reach the top position.

BENT TO SPREAD EAGLE

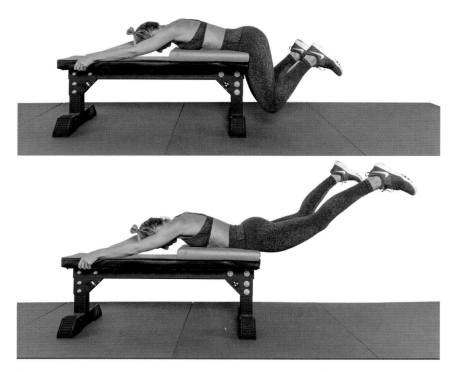

Perform the bent-to-spread-eagle variation by extending and moving your legs outward on the way up and then flexing or bending on the way down.

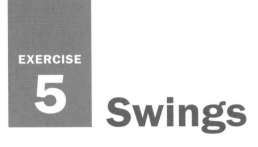

The kettlebell swing is one of the most popular and widely used exercises in the fitness industry. From military operators, fighters, Olympic weightlifters, powerlifters, athletes, and CrossFitters to generalist fitness enthusiasts, nearly everyone uses kettlebell swings in their training.

This popularity is due in part to Pavel Tsatsouline—world-renowned kettlebell master, fitness instructor, and author—who is largely responsible for bringing kettlebell training to the West from Russia and catapulting it into the mainstream. Once reserved for Russian soldiers and athletes, it is now used in all training modalities at all fitness levels as a way to improve conditioning, strength, and physique.

If you've browsed through other sections of this book or frequented my blog and social media platforms, you already know that I use kettlebells a lot in my training, mostly as a tool for loading the squat and deadlift movement patterns. In this section, I cover the kettlebell swing movement pattern, which has something unique to offer to glute training.

Unlike the other movement patterns featured in this book, which are generally stable and performed at slow speeds, the swing is explosive. What is particularly great about the swing is that it's not as challenging to teach or to learn compared to other explosive exercises, like power cleans and snatches. For instance, say I have only a short time to work with an athlete or I want to program a conditioning exercise with an explosive element with beginners or a large group of athletes. In such a situation, the swing offers the most versatility and benefits because it is safe and effective and—equally important—it translates to other movement patterns, like the squat, deadlift, and hip thrust.

In fact, if I'm working with someone who has dabbled in kettlebell training, then my job as a coach is a lot easier because the swing instills essential skills like keeping the spine rigid and neutral while hinging from the hips (as you would when squatting and deadlifting), as well as squeezing the glutes through hip extension without hyperextending through the lumbar spine (as you would when hip thrusting). Put another way, learning how to swing builds solid movement mechanics that translate to the three primary lifts in glute training, meaning that it sets you up to squat, deadlift, and hip thrust with better technique because elements of each of those movements are built into this exercise.

In addition to building explosive power and shortening the learning curve for essential movement patterns, the kettlebell swing is a great conditioning exercise with some muscle- and strength-building qualities. Though not as effective for glute building as the hip thrust, or even the squat and deadlift, it still works the glutes in a unique way and injects some fun and variety into a training program. It's like always eating the same foods: most of the time you have the same meals to stay on track with your goals, but every once in a while, it's nice to eat something different.

Although I work mostly with people who are interested in physique training, I realize that nearly everyone enjoys training like an athlete. People like moving explosively and feeling like they're getting a good workout, and the swing is a perfect exercise for doing just that. For example, when I design programs for my Booty by Bret members, I provide three full-body glute-emphasis workouts per week, as well as two optional workouts. This is when I would program kettlebell swings. So one of the optional workouts might include 3 to 4 sets of 20 to 30 swings on the off-day. This not only provides options and variety but also reinforces good technique, with the added benefit of building stronger, higher-performing glutes.

GUIDELINES AND CUES

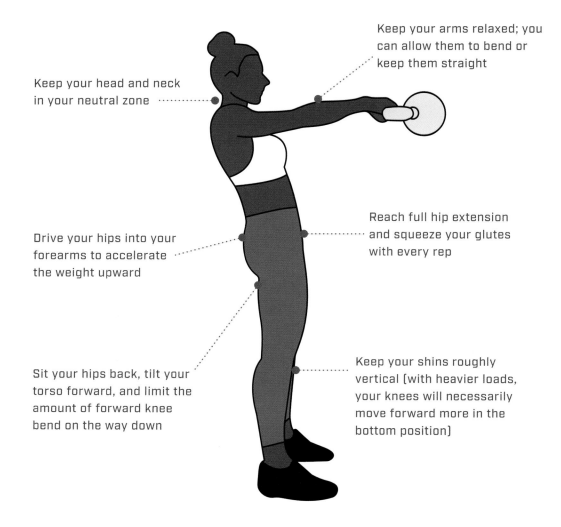

Keep your head and neck in your neutral zone

Keep your arms relaxed; you can allow them to bend or keep them straight

Drive your hips into your forearms to accelerate the weight upward

Reach full hip extension and squeeze your glutes with every rep

Sit your hips back, tilt your torso forward, and limit the amount of forward knee bend on the way down

Keep your shins roughly vertical (with heavier loads, your knees will necessarily move forward more in the bottom position)

The kettlebell swing is a great exercise because it has elements of other lifts built into the movement with an explosive component. Follow the guidelines and cues provided to shorten your learning curve and achieve optimal swing technique.

SETUP AND STANCE

When it comes to the kettlebell swing stance, most people prefer to orient their feet straight and position them just outside shoulder width. This gives you a large base of support with enough space to swing the kettlebell between your legs.

To set up for the swing, position the kettlebell a few feet in front of you along your center line. Bend over by hinging from the hips and grip the kettlebell, holding it at a 45-degree angle. As you can see in the photos, you want your lats and arms stretched, back flat, and shins roughly vertical. From here, generate momentum for the swing by hiking the kettlebell between your legs. Next, harness the momentum by simultaneously raising your torso and extending your hips.

BOTTOM-UP SETUP

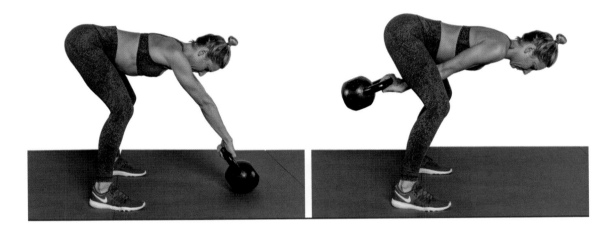

Though common, the hike method just discussed is challenging for some beginners. If you're new to kettlebell swings, you can learn the movement by starting in a standing position and then dropping down into a swing. Like the pendulum reverse hyper, you don't have to worry about performing the full range of motion on your first attempt. In general, I tell people to shoot for a full-range swing on the third rep, so rep 1 is to get momentum, rep 2 is to get a rhythm, and rep 3 is the start of the set. Keep practicing the hike (literally just the hike; don't even swing the bell) as a separate method and strategy, and as you gain proficiency with the swing, you can switch from the top-down to the hike method. Or you might find that you prefer one method for heavy swings and the other for high-rep, lighter swings.

TOP-DOWN SETUP

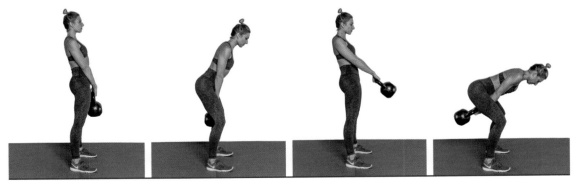

HIP AND ARM MECHANICS: USE THE POWER OF YOUR HIPS AND KEEP YOUR ARMS RELAXED

As the kettlebell passes between your legs, keep your arms straight and move your hips back. To reverse the motion, drive your hips into your forearms, extending your hips, torso, and knees in one fluid motion. The idea is to use the power of your hips to propel the kettlebell upward while keeping your arms relaxed.

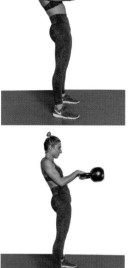

Now, it's fine to raise your arms and have the kettlebell rise up to head height with your arms outstretched, but this form naturally lends itself to using the arms to carry out the lift (doing a front raise and using the delts). If you struggle with this tendency, think about holding pencils in your armpits. This will cause you to keep your arms in line with your torso and bend your elbows. The kettlebell won't rise as high simply because you're relying solely on your hips and not using any arm power. It doesn't look as pretty, but it's a better method, in my opinion.

At the top of the movement, you can let gravity do the work by allowing the kettlebell to drop or accelerate the swing by pulling down on the kettlebell. As it drops, stay vertical until the bell descends halfway down, then shoot your hips back and allow your torso to descend forward. To stay balanced, lean your body forward slightly on the way down (during the eccentric phase) and lean back slightly on the way up (during the concentric phase), allowing the kettlebell to pass between your legs.

SQUEEZE YOUR GLUTES AS YOU REACH FULL HIP EXTENSION

In the bottom position, you should feel tension in your hips and glutes. To reverse the motion, rapidly extend your hips into your forearms and squeeze your glutes to reach full hip extension. Hold this glute squeeze in full hip extension with a slight posterior pelvic tilt while the bell rises upward, while the bell starts to drop, and until it approaches your thighs. A lot of beginners prematurely shoot their hips back before the kettlebell gets close to their body, which compromises rhythm and balance. To avoid this fault, think of it like holding a plank position as the kettlebell floats upward and descends. In short, you're squeezing your glutes with your spine neutral for the duration of the upward swing and halfway through the lowering phase.

SPINAL MECHANICS: KEEP YOUR HEAD AND SPINE IN THE NEUTRAL ZONE

Just as it's important to keep your spine neutral when squatting and deadlifting, so too with the swing. To avoid craning your neck in the bottom position and breaking your rigid spinal position, keep your eyes focused about 10 feet out in front of you. In short, keep your head and neck in your neutral zone throughout the entire range of motion. The heavier you go, the more you will lean forward in the bottom position and lean back in the top position. However, you still need to keep your spine in the neutral zone.

FAULTS AND CORRECTIONS

The swing shares a lot of the same faults with the deadlift and squat because it involves a similar movement pattern. More specifically, you want to avoid hyperextending your back in the top position and rounding in the bottom position. For example, a common mistake is to bend over so the kettlebell passes between the knees. To correct this fault, coaches often cue athletes to "attack the zipper," which is another way of saying that your wrists should be aligned with your groin and that you should allow the kettlebell to pass between your upper thighs.

Another common fault is to hyperextend through the lumbar spine, stopping short of full hip extension and trying to muscle the weight using the power of the arms, which usually looks like a front raise. And the front raise begins before full hip extension is reached, making it obvious that the lifter is trying to compensate with the upper body to make up for a lack of power and coordination in the lower body. To avoid these errors, follow the guidelines and cues previously outlined—that is, relax your arms, use the power of your hips to guide and control the weight, and squeeze your glutes to lock out your hips.

SWING VARIATIONS

There are numerous ways to swing a kettlebell: you can swing it with two arms, one arm, up to your chest, or over your head. There are also different ways to move your body during the swing. For example, you can perform the swing with a pronounced hip hinge or adopt a more upright squat style. On the following pages, I describe two swing categories, both of which are double-arm swings that emphasize a hip hinge movement pattern. It's important to point out that the other swings (such as the one-arm swing) are not wrong, but are more challenging to teach and learn and don't work the glutes or transfer to the deadlift quite as well as the double-arm hip hinge swings. In short, the two swing variations that follow are the easiest to perform and are more effective for conditioning, muscle building, and developing hip hinge mechanics and explosive power.

HIP-DOMINANT SWING

In my opinion, the hip-dominant swing (also referred to as the RKC or Russian swing) is the swing pattern that most people should use because it relies solely on the power of the hips to guide the kettlebell upward. This means you can lift heavy or light and focus on muscle building, explosive power, and conditioning. It's important to realize that the height of the swing is determined by your explosive hip drive and the weight of the kettlebell. For instance, if you're swinging a heavy kettlebell, your arms will bend on the upward motion, and the kettlebell may go only as high as your belly button, which is fine. If you're swinging a lighter kettlebell, on the other hand, your arms may stay straight or bend slightly, drift farther out in front of your body, and go as high as your chest. The drawback of the hip-dominant swing is that it's not very conducive to endurance since you're exploding on each rep. To build explosive power by swinging a heavy kettlebell, 3 or 4 sets of 8 reps is a good starting point. For conditioning, 3 or 4 sets of 20 to 30 reps is what we do at Glute Lab.

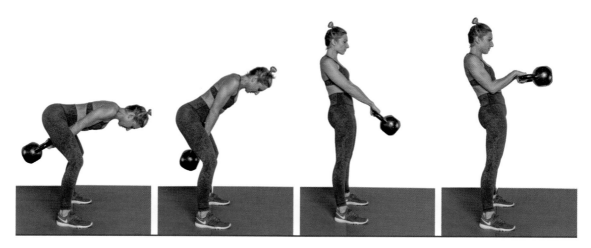

Assume your kettlebell swing stance with the weight positioned along your center line a few feet out in front of you. Hinge from your hips and bend your knees slightly, keeping your back flat and your shins vertical. Form your grip on the kettlebell, tilt it toward you at a 45-degree angle, and then hike it between your legs. As it passes between your legs and your forearms make contact with your groin, rapidly drive your hips forward by extending them as forcefully as possible. Squeeze your glutes, keep your arms relaxed, and maintain a neutral spine as you extend your hips. If you start from the top down, take a few swings to get the bell moving through its full arc of motion. Remember, you're not pulling up with your arms; you're relying on the power of your hips to propel the kettlebell upward. It's also important to keep your weight distributed over the centers of your feet. Avoid rocking back and forth from the balls of your feet to your heels and keep your feet flush with the floor throughout the entire range of the movement.

B-STANCE HIP-DOMINANT SWING

The B-stance hip-dominant swing is great for variety and is an effective strategy for increasing the difficulty of the swing when you only have access to lighter kettlebells or dumbbells. Like all B-stance variations, you place the majority of emphasis (roughly 70 percent of your body weight) on one leg at a time. Because your stance is staggered, swinging one kettlebell between your legs is not optimal. For this reason, it's better to perform B-stance swings with two kettlebells or dumbbells at your sides.

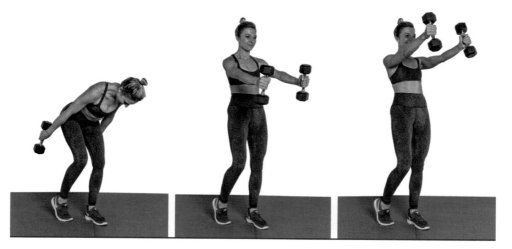

Position your feet roughly hip width apart and keep them straight. Next, slide one foot backward so that your toes line up with your opposite heel. Distributing the majority of your weight on your front leg, lean forward while sitting your hips back, swing the dumbbells back, and then drive your hips forward as you elevate your torso. Keep your arms relaxed, allowing the dumbbells to swing forward.

BANDED HIP-DOMINANT SWING

The banded variation overloads the eccentric phase of the swing, which encourages a more explosive hip drive. Stated differently, the tension in the band accelerates the downward motion of the kettlebell, forcing you to counter the momentum with a rapid hip extension motion. You can mimic this variation with manual resistance by having someone push down on the kettlebell at the top of the movement.

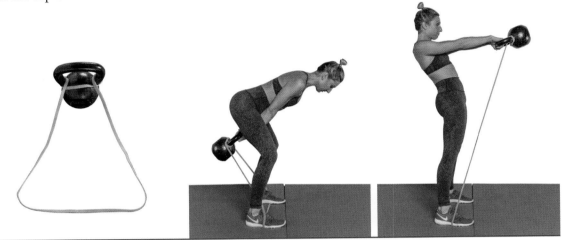

Wrap a thin 41-inch band around the kettlebell where the handle meets the bell, then pull it through the opening. Step on the band, then execute the hip-dominant swing movement as previously described.

HIP-BANDED HIP-DOMINANT SWING

You can also wrap a band around your hips to enhance the hip extension phase of the exercise.

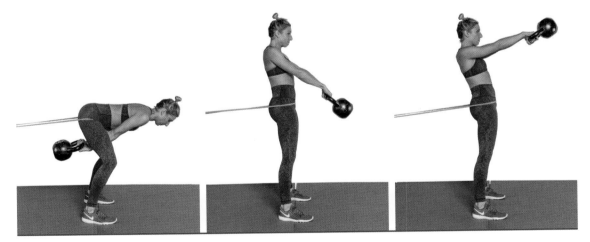

Connect a 41-inch band to a pole or power rack and position the band around your hips. Stand up with the kettlebell and walk forward to put tension in the band. From there, execute the hip-dominant swing movement as previously described.

AMERICAN SWING

The American swing, popularized by CrossFit, is different from the hip-dominant swing in that you increase the range of motion by raising the kettlebell over your head. At the top of the movement, the kettlebell is directly above you. This involves more upper body and overall muscle, turning it into a full-body exercise that is used primarily for conditioning. You won't be able to go quite as heavy with the American swing because you're accelerating it over a longer period and displacing it by a greater magnitude.

You naturally squat the kettlebell up a bit more with the American swing and keep the bell a bit closer to your body. If you have stiff shoulders or you're interested only in getting a good glute workout, stick with the hip-dominant swing.

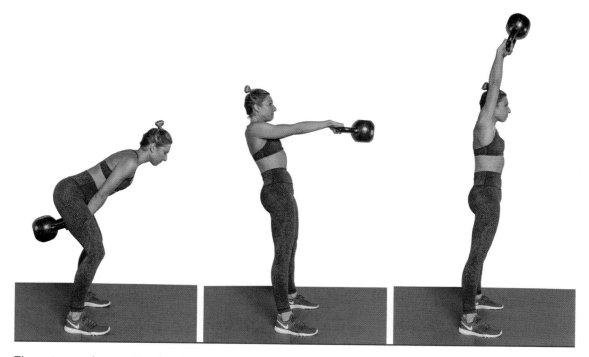

The setup and execution for the American swing are similar to the hip-dominant swing in that you want to harness the power of your hips to power the motion of the kettlebell. However, you raise the bell overhead, remain slightly more upright, and bend your knees a little more than you would for the hip-dominant swing.

6 Straight-Leg Bridges

The straight-leg bridge techniques are among my favorite bodyweight exercises for getting a good hamstring workout when I don't have access to a gym.

If you have access to equipment, you have a lot of great options for building your hamstrings, but there will be times when you don't have anything but your body weight to work with. Maybe you want to train at home, or perhaps you're traveling and the hotel gym—despite being advertised as fully equipped—has nothing but a couple of broken-down cardio machines. In these situations, the straight-leg bridge variations are useful.

GUIDELINES AND CUES

What's great about straight-leg bridges is that there isn't much to the technique, which is to say that they are very easy to perform. All you need to do is set up correctly and keep your spine and knees straight.

SETUP AND STANCE

To perform a straight-leg bridge, you elevate your feet roughly 16 inches off the floor. Most standard benches will work, but you can also use an ottoman, the edge of a chair, a plyometric box, or whatever you have on hand. If the platform is too high, the exercise is easier to carry out and won't work your hamstrings as much. If your feet are too low, then you won't get enough range of motion. The sweet spot is around 16 inches, give or take a couple of inches depending on your height.

The setup is straightforward. Lie on the ground with your back flat and prop your heels on the edge of the bench (or whatever platform you're using) with your feet roughly shoulder width apart.

To work your entire hamstrings, keep your feet pointed straight up. If you want to emphasize your outer or lateral hamstrings, turn your feet outward.

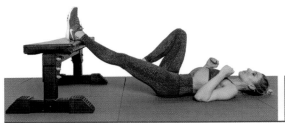

SINGLE-LEG STRAIGHT-LEG BRIDGE

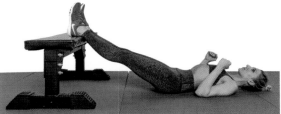

DOUBLE-LEG STRAIGHT-LEG BRIDGE

SPINAL AND KNEE MECHANICS

The straight-leg bridge is similar to the glute bridge, but instead of driving through the bottoms of your heels and keeping your legs bent, you drive through the backs of your heels and keep your legs straight. The key is to keep your back flat and focus on activating your hamstrings as you extend your hips. At the top of the bridge, your body should form a straight line from your shoulders to your feet.

STRAIGHT-LEG BRIDGE VARIATIONS

There are only two ways to perform the straight-leg bridge: double leg and single leg. People often ask me if they can do shoulder- and feet-elevated straight-leg bridges. You can, but when bridging upward, your body straightens out, and therefore the pivot points need to change. The only way to make this happen is to hold onto rings or put the backs of your ankles on rollers that are elevated. I've tried it both ways and both work well, but they're not as good as back extensions and stiff-leg deadlifts, in my opinion. The point of straight-leg bridges is to give you an option for training your hamstrings when you don't have access to equipment, so I'm only going to cover the basic variations.

DOUBLE-LEG STRAIGHT-LEG BRIDGE

This is a great exercise for beginners because it is stable and easier to perform than the single-leg variation. Position your feet on a stable surface, such as a bench or box. A good set and rep scheme is 3 sets of 12 reps. You can place a dumbbell in your lap to increase the difficulty; just make sure it doesn't roll down your torso as you raise your hips.

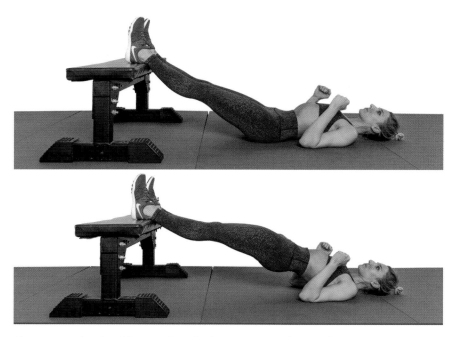

Lie on your back with your feet facing a 16-inch bench (or box, chair, ottoman, etc.). Prop your heels on the bench a few inches from the edge with your feet spaced roughly hip width apart. Drive your heels into the bench and raise your hips—keeping your back and knees straight. Squeeze your glutes to fully extend your hips and momentarily pause in the top position.

SINGLE-LEG STRAIGHT-LEG BRIDGE

As you know, single-leg variations are more challenging and therefore are best utilized when the double-leg variations are too easy. My EMG research showed that the single-leg straight-leg bridge activates the inner hamstrings very well. So, if you want to work the backs of your inner thighs, this is a good exercise to employ. Most fit people can get a good workout by performing 3 sets of 10 to 12 reps.

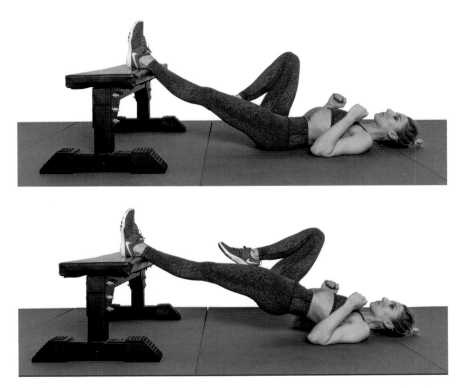

Lie on your back in front of a bench (or any stable 16-inch platform) and prop one heel a few inches from the edge. You can elevate your opposite leg by bending your knee or extending it straight up. The execution is the same as the double-leg variation, but you do it with one leg: drive through your heel while raising your hips.

Knee Flexion

One of my favorite days of the week is the day I coach my Glute Squad, a group of physique competitors who love nothing more than to crush their glutes with hard workouts. Because it's a large group, I structure the session differently than I would if I were training them individually. Instead of having everyone perform the same exercise, I set up each member at an exercise station and have them rotate through each station after a set time or for a predetermined set and rep scheme.

Before each session, I take them through every station and make sure they know what they need to do. Though the majority of the stations are exercises that are considered glute dominant, I also program quad- and hamstring-dominant exercises.

Now, you would think that the squat, lunge, deadlift, or hip thrust movement pattern would be the most popular. But, over the course of many classes, I learned that this is not the case. To my surprise, of all the exercises we implement, the Nordic ham curl (NHC) station is the favorite of several of the Glute Squad members. Every time I introduce the exercise, they get excited and jockey for position to be first at that station. Their interest brought Nordic ham curls to the forefront of my attention.

Though I've always loved Nordic ham curls myself, I used them sparingly with my physique competitors for a couple of reasons. First, if I added isolation exercises that target the quads and hamstrings, such as leg extensions, or knee flexion exercises like leg curls, Nordic ham curls, or glute ham raises, or if I prioritized these movements in their training, then over time, some of them would develop legs that were too big for their liking (and not enough glute prominence). Though this didn't happen with everyone, it did with some, especially after a few years of progressive training. Second, the quads and hamstrings tended to develop just fine alongside the glutes since I always implemented a healthy balance of quad- and hamstring-dominant glute exercises like lunges and back extensions, so there was no need to isolate the quads or hamstrings with single-joint movements.

Now, it's important to point out that knee flexion exercises—which include leg curls, Nordic ham curls, and glute ham raises—are the most hamstring dominant of all of the hamstring-dominant exercises. Unlike deadlifts, back extensions, swings, and reverse hypers, which work the entire posterior chain, knee flexion exercises isolate the hamstrings and don't work other muscles nearly as much as the other movements covered in this section—which is why I never prioritized them with my clients.

But coaching the Glute Squad opened my eyes and helped me realize the importance of knee flexion exercises. This is partly because we have a Nordic ham curl machine set up in our gym, so I get feedback from members based on how often it is used and the results they attain. Not only do they love them, but after only a few months of doing more knee flexion exercises—specifically Nordic ham curls—my competitors had much better hamstring development than ever before. They were being rewarded by judges for their glute-ham tie-in, and their performance in the gym also improved. In fact, Nordic ham curls and other knee flexion variations have been shown in the research to reduce hamstring strain injuries and improve running speed, making them popular exercises in sport training. So, in addition to boosting hamstring hypertrophy and strength, they decrease susceptibility to injury and improve athleticism.

I still consider Nordic ham curls accessory exercises and place them in the middle of workouts after the primary lifts (unless, of course, someone's main goal is to be able to perform unassisted NHCs, in which case I place them first in the workout), but I use them a lot more in my training now than I did in years prior. Whether you're a physique competitor, an athlete, or simply someone who wants to build bigger, stronger hamstrings, knee flexion exercises should have a place in your program.

In this section, you will learn different ways to set up and perform Nordic ham curls and other knee flexion exercises, such as gliding leg curls and glute ham raises, which are great not only for developing the hamstrings but also for progressing to the more challenging Nordic ham curl variations.

GLUTE-HAM TIE-IN

In the world of bodybuilding, the "glute-ham tie-in" receives a lot of attention. Judges examine this region and make sure that there's a smooth transition from the glutes to the hamstrings. It is therefore of great interest for physique athletes to optimize the appearance of this region.

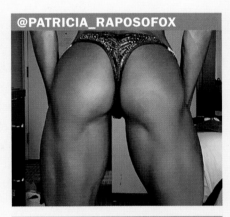
@PATRICIA_RAPOSOFOX

If you're a bodybuilder who wants to improve your glute-ham tie-in, I recommend that you do three things:

1. Strengthen your glutes
2. Strengthen your hamstrings
3. Get lean

As you can see from these recommendations, there is no "glute-ham tie-in" muscle. You have the gluteus maximus and the hamstrings. So please don't ever say, "This exercise really works the glute-ham tie-in." Sure, lunges, Bulgarian split squats, and squats work the lower glutes, and deadlifts, good mornings, and back extensions do a great job of working the glutes and hamstrings together. But the various hip extensors are separate muscles, and you're going to need to do a variety of exercises to maximize gluteal and hamstring shape.

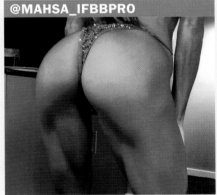
@MAHSA_IFBBPRO

For the glutes, make sure to incorporate plenty of glute-dominant exercises like barbell hip thrusts and hip abduction work, as well as quad-dominant exercises like squats and lunges. For the hamstrings, employ the knee flexion exercises covered in this section as well as the other hamstring-dominant exercises covered in this chapter. Finally, make sure you lean out through proper nutrition. Doing these things will improve your glute-ham tie-in via bodybuilding standards.

I also want to point out that attaining an aesthetically pleasing glute-ham tie-in has a lot to do with personal preference. Most of the women I work with are more concerned with their glutes protruding from their legs and don't care as much about the glute-ham tie-in. In short, the glute-ham tie-in is more specific to bodybuilders; regular folks tend to prefer more separation between their glutes and hamstrings.

GUIDELINES AND CUES

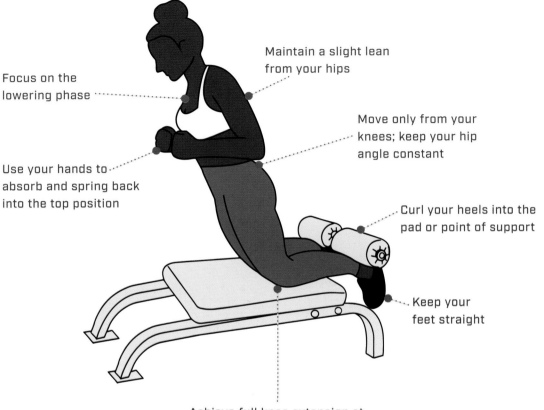

Focus on the lowering phase

Maintain a slight lean from your hips

Use your hands to absorb and spring back into the top position

Move only from your knees; keep your hip angle constant

Curl your heels into the pad or point of support

Keep your feet straight

Achieve full knee extension at the bottom of the movement

As you've learned, knee flexion exercises isolate the hamstrings—and, to a lesser degree, the calf (gastrocnemius) muscles—and involve a leg curl action. Though the variations range from easy to extremely difficult, there isn't much to the technique. The two guidelines covered here apply to all of the variations and are the most important to keep in mind when learning the knee flexion exercise variations. The only other universal guidelines worth mentioning are to focus on the mind-muscle connection and to treat the exercises as athletic movements, meaning that you need to take your form seriously. Like abduction exercises, just because the movement is not overtly complex doesn't mean that you should approach it without consideration for technique.

MOVE ONLY FROM YOUR KNEES (KEEP YOUR HIP ANGLE THE SAME)

Whether you're performing knee flexion exercises (also referred to as leg curls) on your knees, as in a Nordic ham curl, or in a prone position, as in a glute ham raise, always move from your knees and keep your hip angle the same. Note that some knee flexion variations, such as stability ball and gliding leg curls, require you to change your hip angle, so this guideline applies only to kneeling and prone knee flexion exercises.

Even if you start with a slight hip bend, the idea is to keep that hip angle constant throughout the entire range of motion. Most coaches will tell you that it's a good Nordic ham curl only if your hips are neutral in full hip extension and you remain in that position for the entire range of motion. But when people try to perform Nordics in a neutral pelvic position, they never hold that position throughout the set. They always anterior pelvic tilt, which forces them into lumbar hyperextension. Leaning forward slightly lengthens your hamstrings a little, which increases their strength and makes for a more productive repetition. It also decreases the chances of anterior pelvic tilting and lumbar hyperextension, which increases the compressive forces on your spine and places unnecessary stress on your lower back. The caveat is that you don't change that hip angle. So lean forward 30 degrees, then maintain that angle throughout the entire range of motion. This will extend your breaking point, give you more control of the lowering phase, and increase time under tension.

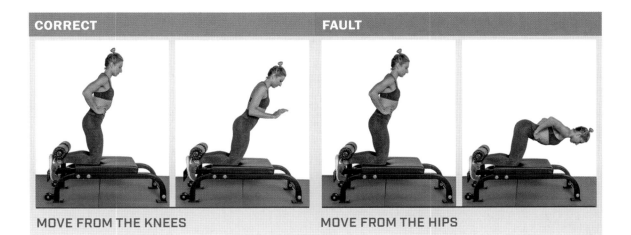

CORRECT   FAULT

MOVE FROM THE KNEES   MOVE FROM THE HIPS

COMPLETE A FULL RANGE OF MOTION

A common error is to prematurely reverse the motion before your hamstrings are fully stretched or to stop short of full knee extension range of motion. To get the most out of the knee flexion exercises, make sure that you achieve full knee flexion and extension. For example, if you're performing supine knee flexion exercises like stability ball leg curls, fully extend your knees as you straighten your legs and pull your heels as close to your butt as possible. If you're performing Nordic ham curls or glute ham raises, allow your thighs to touch the pad or your knees to fully extend at the bottom of the movement. Don't reverse the motion by pulling yourself back up or pushing yourself upright before your thighs touch the pad. You can still use your hands to lower with control; just keep tension in your hamstrings and try to maintain a consistent tempo.

FULL-RANGE-OF-MOTION LEG CURL   **FULL-RANGE-OF-MOTION NORDIC**

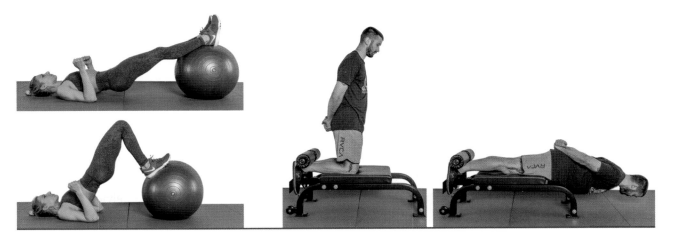

EXERCISES

5

KEEP YOUR FEET STRAIGHT

To strengthen your lateral and medial hamstrings, keep your feet straight when doing knee flexion exercises. Targeting both sides of your hamstrings is optimal when performing these exercises, so I generally don't advise turning your feet out.

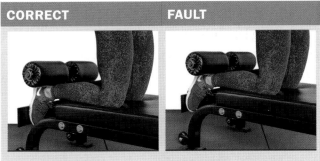

FAULTS AND CORRECTIONS

Following the guidelines and cues is the best way to prevent the most common knee flexion errors. The one fault I want to highlight is excessive lumbar hyperextension and anterior pelvic tilt. Some is acceptable, but too much is problematic—it can produce lower back discomfort and pain. Mind your lumbopelvic posture and stay within your neutral zone.

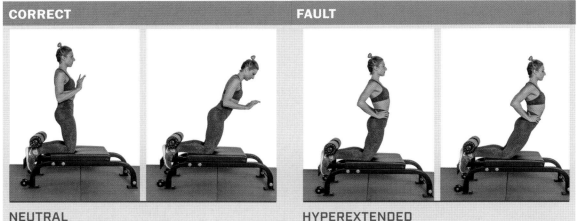

KNEE FLEXION CATEGORIES AND VARIATIONS

In this section, you will learn what each knee flexion exercise is good for, how to regress or progress each exercise to suit your strength and abilities, and how to perform all of the variations with optimal technique.

SUPINE KNEE FLEXION EXERCISES

Supine knee flexion exercises encompass all leg curl variations performed from your back, which include stability ball leg curls, sliding leg curls, and gliding/hanging leg curls. These variations are great for strengthening the hamstrings and serve as a regression for the more challenging Nordic ham curls. So, if Nordic ham curls are too difficult or you don't feel comfortable performing them, supine knee flexion exercises are a good place to start. A common set and rep scheme for these exercises is 3 sets of 10 to 12 reps.

Stability Ball Leg Curl Variations

Performing leg curls on a stability ball is an easy, low-cost option that is great for both beginners and advanced practitioners. I recommend using a 55-cm or 65-cm ball. If you're new to leg curls, start with the double-leg variation. As you get stronger, combine the double- and single-leg variations by pulling with two legs and then lowering with one. Once you can do that without struggling, try isolating the single-leg variation.

DOUBLE-LEG STABILITY BALL LEG CURL

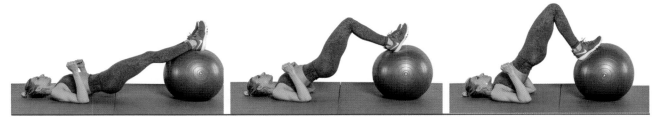

Lie on your back and place your feet on top of the ball with your legs straight. Drive your hips upward while curling your legs and pulling your heels toward your butt. Think of doing a feet-elevated glute bridge combined with a leg curl. You can do it with complete or partial hip extension; both ways are great. To ensure that the ball glides back and forth in a straight line, center your feet on the ball, keep your feet together, apply equal pressure into the ball with both legs, and perform the movement slowly in a controlled fashion. You can also spread your arms and keep them flush with the ground for additional side-to-side stability. Rise upward until the bottoms of your feet are in full contact or flush with the ball.

TWO UP/ONE DOWN STABILITY BALL LEG CURL

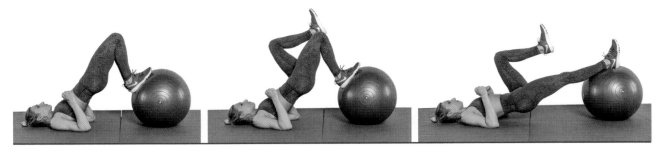

SINGLE-LEG STABILITY BALL LEG CURL

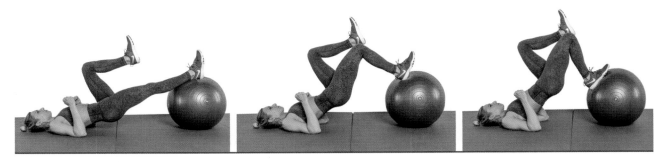

The unilateral variation shares the same technique, but instead of pulling with both legs, you pull with only one. This requires a lot more control, and you may have to adjust your foot and spread your arms across the floor to widen your base and prevent the ball from rolling from side to side. You can keep your opposite leg extended or bent, whichever you prefer. If performing the pulling phase is too difficult, you can combine the variations by pulling with both legs and then lowering with one leg (two up/one down).

Sliding Leg Curl Variations

The sliding leg curl is similar to the stability ball leg curl, but it's slightly more challenging because your feet are on the ground, requiring you to lift a higher percentage of your body weight. There are several ways to perform this variation. If you're on a slick surface such as hardwood, linoleum, or laminate, you can place your feet on a towel or paper plates or even wear thick socks (this option is best performed on a slide board). If you're on a carpeted floor, you can use Valslides—which also work well on slick surfaces—or furniture sliders. Like the stability ball variations, you can perform this technique using both legs, two legs up and one leg down, or one leg.

DOUBLE-LEG SLIDING LEG CURL

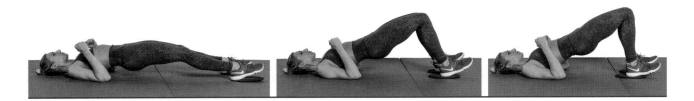

TWO UP/ONE DOWN SLIDING LEG CURL

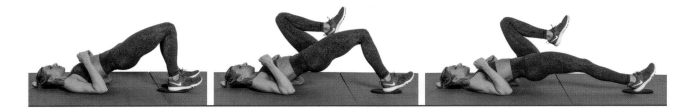

SINGLE-LEG SLIDING LEG CURL

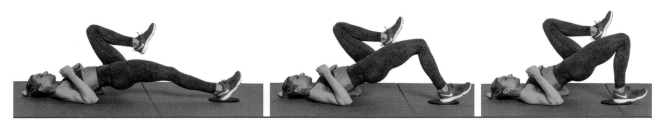

Start with your legs extended, positioning your heels on something that will slide across the floor. You can put your arms at your sides, spread them out to widen your base, or keep them bent, as shown. To execute the movement, pull your heels toward your butt while bridging your hips off the ground. You can get full or partial hip extension on each rep, whichever you prefer; just be consistent. As you do, you will transition from your heels to your feet. Bring your heels as close to your butt as possible. If you're performing the single-leg variation, you can extend your elevated leg or bend it. You can also perform the two up/one down variation by pulling with both legs, then lowering with one leg.

Rolling Leg Curl Variations

The rolling leg curl variations share the same benefits and technique as the sliding leg curl, but instead of sliding your feet across the ground, you use an apparatus with wheels, such as a power wheel or glute ham roller. At Glute Lab, we use the Sorinex glute ham roller, but you can find a lot of other options online. The benefit of using a glute ham roller over a power wheel or similar apparatus is twofold: it is more stable, which creates a smoother glide, and it offers more loading options (single-leg variations and band resistance).

DOUBLE-LEG ROLLING LEG CURL

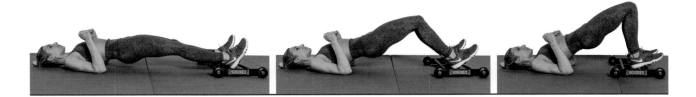

TWO UP/ONE DOWN ROLLING LEG CURL

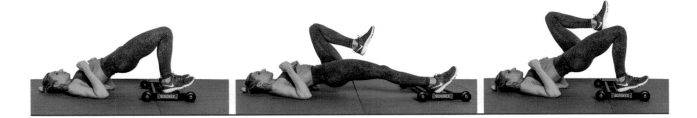

SINGLE-LEG ROLLING LEG CURL

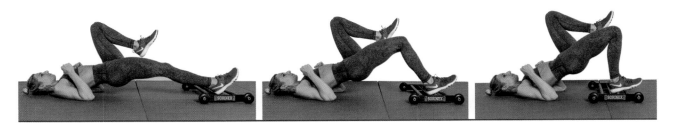

Lie on your back, keeping your arms bent or spread outward. Place your heels in the grooves of the glute ham roller and straighten your legs. Don't put your arms at your sides; the wheels could roll over your fingers—a painful experience. To execute the movement, you do several things at once: elevate your hips, drive your heels down, and curl your feet toward your butt. Like the other sliding variations, you want to pull your heels as close to your butt as possible. To make this exercise more challenging, you can place a dumbbell on your hips to provide hip extension resistance, attach a band to the roller to increase knee flexion resistance, or perform single-leg or two up/one down variations.

Gliding/Hanging Leg Curl Variations

I thought up the gliding leg curl exercise (also referred to as a hanging leg curl) in my garage gym back in 2009. I was doing stiff-leg deadlifts, glute ham raises, good mornings, reverse hypers, and back extensions—all great hamstring developers—but I wanted a high-rep pump-and-burn option. I didn't have access to a leg curl machine, and I sought something a little more challenging than the stability ball and sliding/rolling leg curl options but less challenging than Nordic ham curls and glute ham raises, which work the heck out of your hamstrings but don't produce a pump or burn. So I started experimenting, and eventually I came up with the gliding leg curl.

I programmed these at the ends of my workouts for high reps (around 20), and they had the desired effect. They're more challenging than the stability ball and sliding/rolling leg curl options because you're lifting a higher percentage of your body weight and pulling your body upward as opposed to rolling the ball with your leg, but they're not nearly as difficult as Nordic ham curls and glute ham raises due to the orientation of your body. They're easier in the stretch position and harder in the shortened/contracted position compared to NHCs, making them the perfect hamstring pump-and-burn exercise. Like the other supine knee flexion exercises, you can perform double-leg, two up/one down, or single-leg variations.

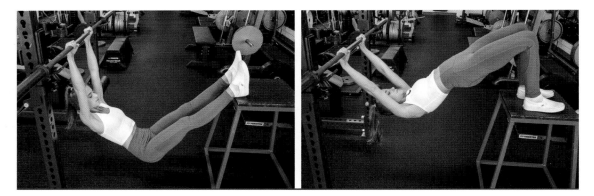

You need a tall plyometric box. If you're using a lightweight box with no sides, place a dumbbell over the base to prevent it from tipping. If you have a medium-sized box, you can stack weights to the appropriate height. I don't recommend using a bench because it's not tall enough and is likely to tip over. To suspend your body, you can hang from a barbell inside a power rack or from rings. If hanging from a barbell, face away from the rack so that your grip is facing the steel uprights (poles) of the power rack, not the opening of the pins. This locks the barbell in place, making it stable and safe. With regard to barbell height, position it so that your shoulders are on roughly the same horizontal plane as the box, then adjust up or down based on strength—a lower box is easier and a higher box is harder. Position the box far enough away that there is roughly a 135-degree bend in your hips. To execute the movement, hang from the bar as if you were doing a pull-up and place your heels on the box. Keep your arms and legs straight in the bottom position with your hips flexed. Next, pull your body upward using the power of your legs by driving your heels into the box while flexing your knees and extending your hips. As you flex and extend, allow your body to swing forward as if you were pulling yourself uphill using your legs. Think of your arms as hooks; don't bend them or try to pull yourself up. As you reach full hip extension, allow your feet to land flush on the platform. Control your descent by slowly lowering into the bottom position.

KNEELING KNEE FLEXION EXERCISES

Kneeling knee flexion exercises encompass Nordic ham curl variations (also known as Russian leans, Russian ham curls, poor man's glute ham raises, natural glute ham raises, bodyweight leg curls, Nordic lowers, and Nordics—yeah, they have a lot of names), which are great for hamstring hypertrophy and strength development. However, you will never feel the burn or pump like you do when performing high-rep supine leg curls. In this way, they're similar to lunges. Your glutes never get a pump or burn from lunges, but lunges make your glutes sore and contribute to muscle hypertrophy. It's the same thing with Nordic ham curls—that is, you won't feel a burn or pump, they can make your hamstrings sore, and they build and develop your hamstrings like nothing else. For this reason, Nordics are programmed either first in a workout if you're trying to progress to a full Nordic, or, more commonly, in the middle of the workout if glute development is your primary goal. I generally prescribe 3 sets of 3 to 5 reps of this exercise, regardless of when in the training session it is performed. It's better to do lower reps on these and fight like crazy during the lowering phase than do high reps with no tension in your muscles.

There are many ways to set up and execute Nordics. First, I will demonstrate all of the ways to set up using different equipment and apparatuses. Then I will show you how to perform Nordics correctly, from the easiest to the most difficult variation.

TRY TO SET PRS WITH BODYWEIGHT EXERCISES WHEN DIETING

What's great about Nordic ham curls and other challenging bodyweight exercises like pull-ups and dips is that they get easier as you diet down and lose weight. Plenty of my bikini competitors have gotten their first Nordic the week of a competition. In fact, last year three of my Glute Squad members hit their first concentric Nordic (they lowered all the way down and rose all the way up without any push-up assistance) on the same day, which happened to be the Monday before their show.

Most bodybuilding coaches don't program much training in the week before a competition. They're checked out and think, "You can't build any muscle, you're dieted down, and the training is done." But I don't like this way of thinking. I prefer to push my competitors to set PRs with bodyweight exercises because they're lighter and stronger from all of their hard training. Absolute strength on barbell lifts might diminish, but strength endurance on bodyweight exercises increases. So they probably won't set PRs on hip thrusts or deadlifts, but they will with bodyweight movements. And setting PRs—say, by getting more pull-ups or a full Nordic—makes their confidence soar, and they carry that confidence over to the stage, where it plays a big role in performance and outcome.

Focusing on Nordics, pull-ups, inverted rows, dips, push-ups, pistols, and other challenging bodyweight exercises is also great for people losing weight through diet. You may not be getting ready for a show, but it will have the same impact. That is, you will get stronger at Nordics as you diet down, thereby increasing your confidence and giving you a sense of accomplishment.

NORDIC HAM CURL SETUP

There are several ways to set up for the Nordic ham curl. The option you choose depends on the equipment available to you and your personal preference.

Nordic Ham Curl Machine

The best way to perform Nordics is on a machine designed for the exercise. At Glute Lab, we have a Sorinex Poor Man's Glute Ham Raise, and it's one of our most popular pieces of equipment. (Rogue and other companies make similar products.) No setup is required—just get in and go. Though a Nordic ham curl machine is the best equipment option, these machines are rare, even in large commercial gyms. The next best options are the partner-assisted, bench and strap, and barbell setups.

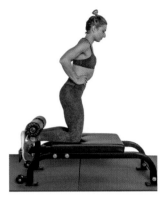

Partner Assisted

The partner-assisted setup is a great option when working with a training partner or coach. All you need is a pad for your knees. To set up, position your knees on the pad with your feet dorsiflexed and your toes extended so that they are bent and pressed into the ground. If your toes are not flexible or it hurts when your partner pushes down, position your insteps over a foam roller or just do the exercise in plantarflexion (this makes it harder, though). Have your partner kneel behind you—positioning their knees behind the soles of your feet—and anchor your legs to the ground by placing pressure on the backs of your heels and ankles. As you extend your knees and fall forward, your partner should apply downward pressure and lean forward to get more weight over your ankles. Your partner needs to weigh close to what you weigh or be heavier, or they won't be able to hold you down as you reach the bottom of the movement. Do not underestimate the importance of this setup; the better your partner stabilizes you, the better your hamstring workout will be.

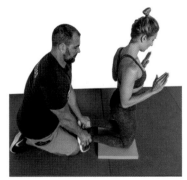

Ideally, you would use a thick pad like an Airex balance pad, which provides plenty of cushioning for your knees, and elevate it about 8 inches off the ground (you can use steps, a block, or a few pads stacked on top of each other). This "deficit" feels better on your feet, allows you to maintain a 30-degree lean, and helps you achieve greater range at the bottom of the movement, and you can actively dorsiflex your ankles to reduce calf contribution, all of which translates to a better training stimulus for your hamstrings.

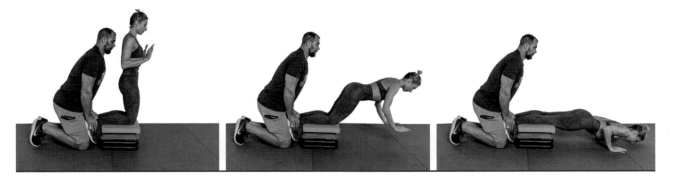

Bench and Strap

This setup is a great low-budget hack for Nordics. Spud, Inc. sells a glute/ham strap that wraps around a bench and keeps your feet locked in place. You can even wrap it around a bench press station and perform band-assisted variations.

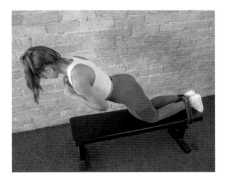

Barbell

If you don't have access to a Nordic ham curl apparatus or a glute/ham strap and bench, you can use a barbell, weights, squat sponge, and pad. To begin, load a lot of weight (more than your body weight) onto the barbell to prevent it from lifting or rolling, wrap a thick squat sponge around the bar to protect your ankles, and position your knees on a thick pad. It's also important to place weights or wedges on both sides of the barbell to keep it from moving backward or forward.

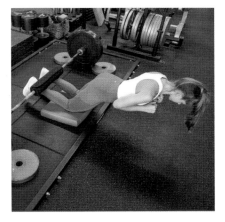

Smith Machine

You can also use a Smith machine instead of a power rack. The setup is exactly the same as the power rack and barbell setup; the only difference might be the barbell height. Many Smith machines don't have a low enough setting, so you might have to set the barbell height higher and perform the movement on a bench or off blocks or steps.

Lat Pull-Down Machine

Another common commercial gym hack is to perform Nordics using a lat pull-down machine. This is not what the machine is designed for, so it's not ideal. For most men, the pad is too narrow, and you have to position a bench or aerobic steps in front of you and set it to just the right height so that you can absorb the weight of your upper body. But if you have nothing else, and assuming your knees fit on the pad, it is a viable option.

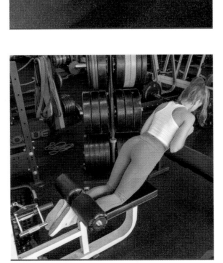

NORDIC HAM CURL REGRESSIONS AND PROGRESSIONS

When you start doing Nordic ham curls, you begin in the top position and then, as you lower into the bottom position, you sink like a ship. It's difficult to control the eccentric, or lowering, phase because the strength demands are so high. As your knees extend, it gets harder and harder to control the weight of your upper body, and there's a "breaking point" at which you go from controlling the descent to just falling. At first, your breaking point occurs early, so the goal is to extend your breaking point as you get stronger and better at performing the exercise.

For this reason, people typically refer to the Nordic ham curl as the "Nordic lowering exercise" or "Nordic drop." In fact, it's better to think of Nordics as a primarily eccentric exercise, especially in the beginning. Instead of trying to perform the full movement, focus on lowering into the bottom position as slowly as possible and extending your breaking point by performing assisted variations. When it comes to the concentric phase, you want to push off with your hands just enough to pull yourself back into the top position. As you get stronger, you will rely more and more on your hamstrings to pull your body upright. Although the end goal is not to use your hands at all, it is extremely difficult; very few athletes I've worked with can do it. So don't get discouraged if you're stuck performing just the eccentric phase or assisted variations. I do Nordics a couple of times per week, and I still can't do a concentric rep without assistance.

To help you progress through the Nordic variations, I've organized the techniques into three categories from easiest to most difficult: assisted, bodyweight, and resisted.

ASSISTED NORDICS

Assisted Nordics encompass techniques that utilize a band, a training partner, or some form of support. If you've never performed Nordics, you can't lower yourself under control when doing bodyweight Nordics, or you simply want to dial in your technique and then progress to the more challenging variations, performing assisted Nordics is a good place to start. Don't make the mistake of performing high-rep Nordic variations; you usually want to stick with 5 or fewer reps per set. To progress to a full Nordic, I recommend sticking with the assisted variations until you are strong enough to lower at least halfway on your own with just body weight. With this base level of strength and technique, the variations offered over the coming pages will put you one step closer to getting a full Nordic.

Manually Assisted Nordic

Having a training partner or coach kneel in front of you and holding their hands is a great way to learn how to lower with control and perform the technique correctly. With your partner's hands for support, you can focus on curling your legs into whatever apparatus you're using—whether it's a bar, foot pads, or someone else's hands—and lower yourself using the power of your hamstrings. With practice, the spotter and lifter establish a rhythm, and the spotter can figure out just the right amount of assistance to provide at just the right time for the most productive set.

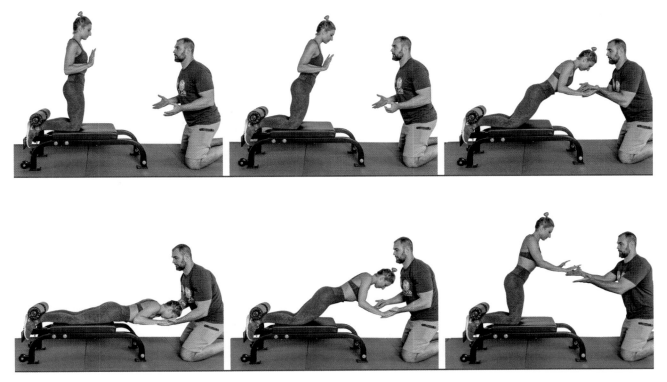

With a training partner kneeling in front of you, slowly lower your body by curling your legs and extending your knees. Your partner should adjust the amount of support being provided based on your ability and strength. The idea is to provide assistance by pulling up on your hands and absorbing the weight of your upper body as you fall forward. The farther you fall, the more support your partner will need to provide. When you get to the bottom position, your partner should help push you back into the top position.

Band-Assisted Nordic

A band is a great tool for progressing Nordics because it helps support your body weight as you descend into the bottom position. More accurately, it provides less assistance during the first phase of the movement, which is easier, and more assistance during the second phase, which is harder. So the band helps distribute the resistance more equally throughout the entire range of motion by providing assistance where you need it most, which is in the bottom position. This means you can perform the entire movement without breaking or having to push off as hard to complete a full rep.

You can adjust the amount of assistance provided by choosing a thicker or thinner band or by adjusting the trajectory. The higher you anchor the band, the more assistance it will give you in the bottom position.

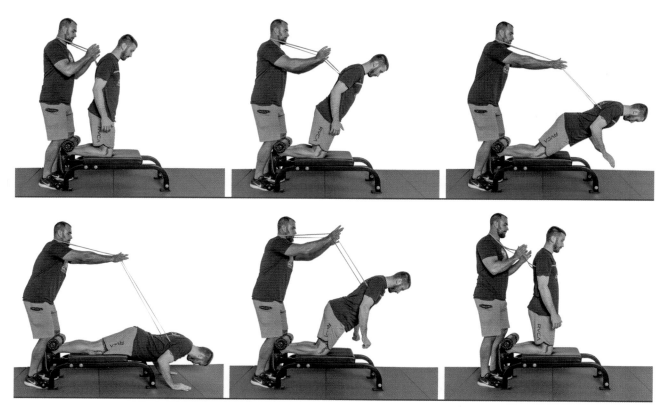

There are a couple of ways to perform the band-assisted Nordic variation. You can have a training partner stand above you or attach the band to a power rack, bench press, or pull-up structure. Regardless of the setup, you should always position the band around your chest and under your armpits. If you're holding the band for your partner, wrap it around the back of your neck and push up and out on the band as they descend. This makes it a more perpendicular and effective support vector when they get to the bottom of the movement.

Pole-Assisted Nordic

This regression is unique in that you can control the degree of assistance through the entire range of the movement by using a pole, such as a dowel or PVC pipe, to support your weight. A large medicine ball can also be used for this purpose (you roll it outward as you descend), but a dowel is better. Although you can perform this variation from the ground, it is better to do it on an apparatus that is elevated off the ground, such as a GHD, Nordic ham curl unit, bench, or lat pull-down station.

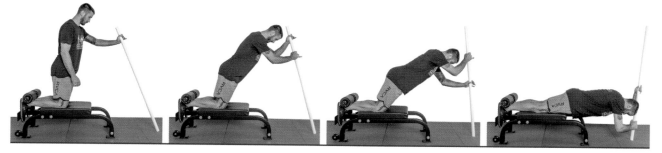

Position the pole out in front of your body, then walk your way down and up the pole. The idea is to use the pole only for support and balance. In other words, try to lower yourself down by keeping as much tension in your hamstrings as possible.

BODYWEIGHT NORDICS

As a strength coach, I'm surrounded by incredibly strong and talented athletes, most of whom can lift more than their body weight in all of the main lifts. However, of all of the coaches and athletes I interact with, only a few can perform a full bodyweight Nordic. For this reason, I've included several bodyweight variations that can be used not only to progress to a full Nordic but also to strengthen and develop your hamstrings.

Remember, you don't need to pursue a full Nordic to get the most from this exercise. The variations included are just as good for developing your hamstrings as they are for improving your strength.

Eccentric-Accentuated Nordic

When it comes to bodyweight Nordics, your primary focus in the beginning is to control the eccentric, or lowering, phase of the movement. As you get better and stronger, the goal is to increase your breaking point, or the point at which you can no longer control your descent and you fall toward the bench or the ground. In short, you will progress faster and develop your hamstrings more by emphasizing the eccentric phase, not the concentric (or rising) phase. Let's say that when you first start performing NHCs, you can control your fall only 50 percent of the way down, and each rep lasts three seconds. In a month, if you can lower yourself with control 65 percent of the way down and make each rep last five seconds (making sure that you're not just spending more time in the top position, which is easy), you've achieved progressive overload, and your hamstrings should be slightly more muscular.

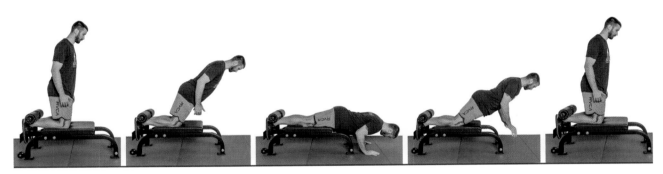

There are a couple of ways to position your body based on your preference: you can keep your upper body and hips neutral or lean forward slightly, no more than 30 degrees—anything past that point and you're performing a different technique (see the flexed-hip variation on page 581). To execute the movement, curl your feet into the apparatus or your training partner's hands and slowly lower your body as a single unit. The key is not to break at your hips; you should see movement only at your knees. As you fall to the floor, use your arms to absorb the weight of your upper body while maintaining tension on your hamstrings. So, when you reach your breaking point, don't just fall; use your arms just enough to continue lowering with control. You should feel tension in your hamstrings during the entire eccentric phase of the movement. Once your thighs touch the pad, floor, or bench, you can either push yourself back into the starting position with the assistance of your hamstrings or crawl or walk your hands back into the top position.

Pause Rep

Executing a pause rep means that you stop near your breaking point for two seconds before using your hands to assist with the eccentric and concentric portions of the movement. Over time, the goal is to increase your breaking point and pause lower and lower to the ground. Put simply, this is another way to progress the Nordic and increase time under tension when performing the eccentric-accentuated variation.

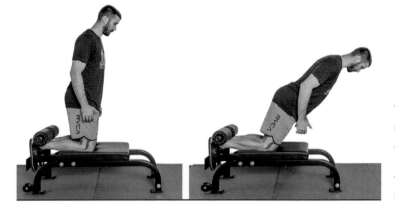

The pause rep Nordic variation shares the same technique as the eccentric-accentuated Nordic. The only difference is that you pause for two seconds right above your breaking point.

Pulse Method

The pulse method requires you to pulse up and down in the bottom position for 3 reps. This increases time under tension in the bottom position, which, as you know, is the hardest phase of the movement.

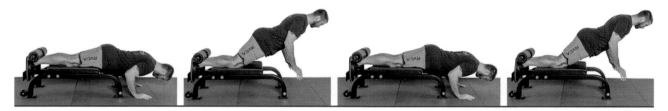

Lower yourself with control until your knees are nearly fully extended. From there, pulse up and down for 3 repetitions, using your arms just enough to maintain maximal tension in your hamstrings. In other words, pulse using the power of your hamstrings and use your arms only for assistance.

Flexed-Hip Nordic

The flexed-hip Nordic variation requires you to bend your hips 90 degrees and keep them locked at that angle for the full range of motion. This makes it slightly easier to perform bodyweight variations due to the lengthening of the hamstrings. As you can see, it's best to set up on a bench or other elevated surface so that you can keep your hips at a 90-degree angle and perform the full range of the movement.

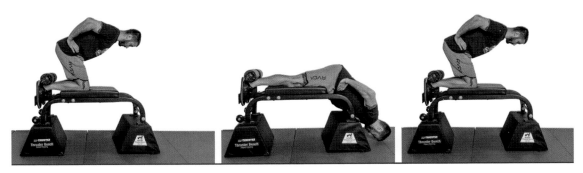

Hinge from your hips until you're at a 90-degree angle, then slowly lower by extending your knees. If you can't perform the full bodyweight variation, use your hands to assist past your breaking point as described for the eccentric-accentuated Nordic.

Razor Nordic

The razor Nordic is a cross between a regular Nordic and a flexed-hip Nordic. With this variation, your hamstrings don't change much in length (they shorten at the hips with extension but lengthen at the knees with flexion), which makes it a quasi-isometric hamstring exercise.

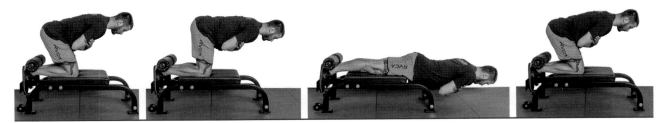

Bend your hips at a 90-degree angle. As you descend, extend your hips and keep your torso parallel to the ground throughout the entire set. The bottom position will look just like a traditional Nordic, but as you rise up, you shoot your butt back and bend at your hips.

Full Nordic

The eventual goal is to perform a full bodyweight Nordic without assistance. I've trained only about a dozen people who can actually do it, so don't get discouraged if you never achieve this level of strength. However, if you stick with the progressions, focus on technique, and stay consistent, you will get there eventually.

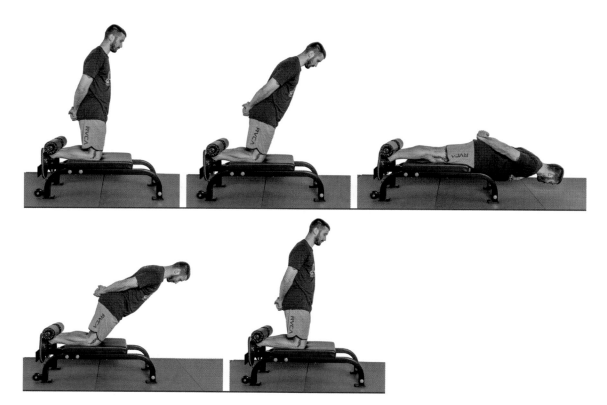

Use one of the Nordic setups previously described. With your feet anchored, bend your hips slightly, then slowly lower yourself toward the ground by extending your knees. As you do, pull your feet into the supports (your partner's hands, the foot pads, a barbell, etc.), and slowly lower your upper body until your thighs touch the pad or ground. Without touching your hands to the ground, pull yourself back into the top position by curling your legs, keeping your torso and hip angle the same throughout the entire range of motion. Even with this variation, you can progress from having your hands at your sides to having your arms crossed, which increases the lever arm of the system of mass above your knee joint, making the exercise harder.

RESISTED NORDICS

Because most of us can't perform full bodyweight Nordics, full-range weighted or resisted variations are not accessible. However, you can modify these variations to work different ranges of the exercise, turning them into valuable progressions.

Slow Manually Resisted Nordic

To create resistance in the top position, which is the easiest part of the movement, have your training partner push on your back and resist in the top position and during the first phase of the range of motion. Creating resistance from the start increases time under tension through the first half of the lowering phase and builds hamstring strength in deep knee flexion.

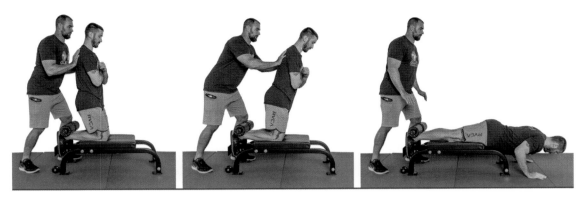

Have a training partner apply slow and steady pressure to your upper back in the top position. Resist the pressure to create tension in your hamstrings. You are quite strong in that range, but as you slowly lower past 45 degrees (the first half of the movement), your partner should stop pushing and let the weight of your body take over to level out the resistance.

Fast Manually Resisted Nordic

This variation is similar to the slow manually resisted Nordic in that your training partner pushes on your back in the top position. But instead of pushing slow and steady, they push faster and more explosively, creating an accelerated eccentric phase. This variation might have better crossover to sport due to the explosive nature of the exercise. (Sports are fast, so it's more specific.)

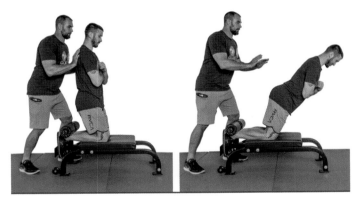

Set up in the top position and brace for an explosive push. Have your training partner push explosively on your upper back. Resist the moment you feel the push to slow your descent. The idea is to slow down as much as possible and control the lowering phase before pushing off the floor and returning to the top position.

Manually Resisted and Assisted Nordic

This is my favorite Nordic variation because there is steady and consistent tension in the hamstrings throughout the entire range of motion. However, this variation shouldn't entirely replace the bodyweight Nordic. One of the main benefits of the bodyweight Nordic is that it gets harder and harder on the way down. This is a great variation to throw in from time to time to level out the strength curve.

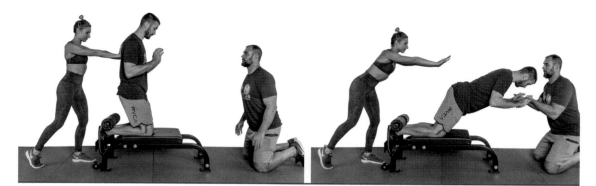

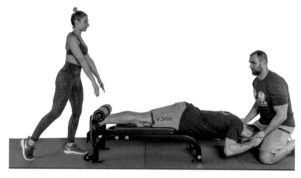

Have your training partner apply slow, steady pressure to your upper back in the top position. The moment you approach your breaking point, your partner should come around to the front and provide counter-resistance by pushing up on your hands so that you can lower into the bottom position with control (as in the partner-assisted Nordic). Next, your partner should assist you back into the top position. Then do 2 more reps.

Band-Resisted Nordic

What's great about this variation is that the band provides the most resistance in the top position, where it's easiest. You also have your hands free to catch your fall as you lower past your breaking point. In short, this variation primarily works the first half of the lowering phase.

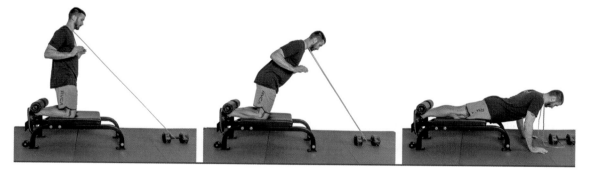

Set up with the band anchored to the ground (using heavy dumbbells or a power rack). Wrap the other end around the back of your neck. With the band fully stretched in the top position, slowly lower and control your descent through the first half of the range of motion. Once you reach your breaking point, use your hands to assist—keeping as much tension in your hamstrings as possible—and complete the lowering phase. Crawl or push yourself back into the top position.

Dumbbell-Resisted Nordic

If can lower yourself with control using your body weight and you feel comfortable with Nordics, you can hold a dumbbell to add resistance. However, you can't use your hands to catch your fall, so it's important that you can lower yourself most of the way down with control.

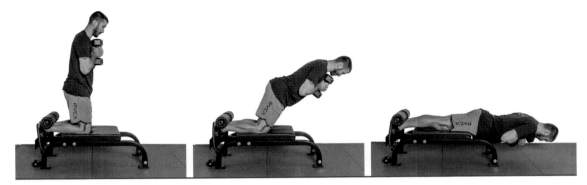

Hold a dumbbell vertically in the center of your chest, gripping the handle with both hands. As you lower into the bottom position, drop the dumbbell and come back up. If you can't get the concentric phase, use your hands to assist for the rest of the range of motion. Have a training partner hand you the dumbbell in the top position to perform another rep. When performed in this manner, it's an enhanced-eccentric variation. You can also perform full reps with a dumbbell (or weighted vest).

PRONE KNEE FLEXION EXERCISES

The category of prone knee flexion exercises encompasses primarily the glute ham raise (GHR), which is performed on a glute ham developer (GHD).

If you don't have access to a GHD apparatus, you can build your hamstrings just as effectively by performing Nordic ham curl variations. In fact, once I took a couple of months off glute ham raises to focus on Nordics, and my GHR strength increased. I realized that Nordics build glute ham raise strength just as effectively as doing glute ham raises. So don't feel like you need to buy a GHD just to work your hamstrings; the other variations covered in this section are just as effective. That said, the curved path of the GHD makes the Nordic motion easier, allowing you to work in higher rep ranges. For example, I might do 3 sets of 3 NHCs but 3 sets of 15 GHRs. Both sets are challenging, but the NHCs might be better for strength and the GHRs might be better for hypertrophy.

In the following pages, I provide a comprehensive progression of exercises for the GHR. Before I delve into the techniques, realize that the settings on your GHD influence how hard the movement is and how many reps you can perform.

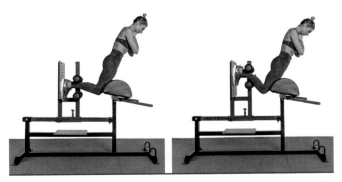

LOW AND FAR [EASY]   HIGH AND CLOSE [HARD]

To make the GHR easier, position the footplate lower and/or farther from the hip pad. To make it harder, position the footplate higher and/or closer to the hip pad. Be aware of the settings and keep them consistent when going for rep PRs. Remember, you have progressive overload only if you use the same form with the same range of motion under the same conditions.

Inverse Curl

The inverse curl is one of my favorite hamstring exercises that hardly anyone does. It's a rhythmic two-part exercise characterized by hip extension followed by knee flexion, making it a perfect mix between a glute ham raise and a horizontal back extension. Shoot for 2 or 3 sets of 20 reps and your hamstrings will scream for mercy.

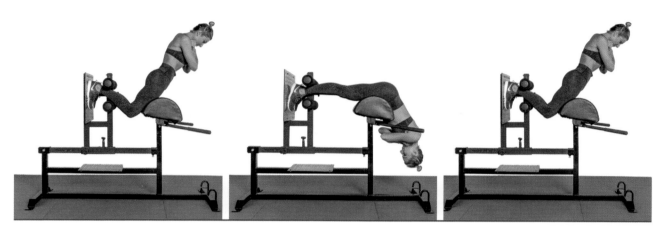

Position the footplate about halfway between your GHR and back extension footplate positions. (The GHR footplate position is closer, and the back extension footplate position is farther out.) Set up in the unit, then lower your torso into deep hip flexion. From there, elevate your torso by extending your hips. Once you reach full hip extension, continue rising upward via knee flexion. You can hold a dumbbell if you like, but I prefer high reps with body weight. You won't be able to rise as high as you would in a normal GHR because the knee pad is positioned farther away.

Flexed-Hip GHR

This variation is like the flexed-hip Nordic, except it's a little easier to perform.

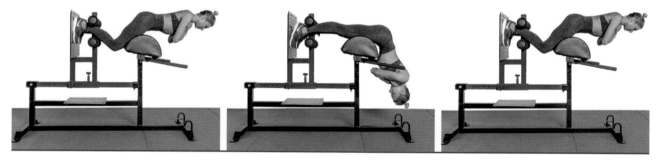

Set up in the GHD, then position your torso so that it is parallel to the ground. Descend by straightening your knees and allowing your torso to drop. At the bottom, your body will form an L shape. Maintaining the same hip angle, reverse the motion by curling your legs and flexing your knees.

Razor Curl

The razor curl is a cross between a regular GHR and a flexed-hip GHR. With this variation, your hamstrings don't change much in length (they shorten at your hips with extension but lengthen at your knees with flexion), which makes the razor curl a quasi-isometric hamstring exercise.

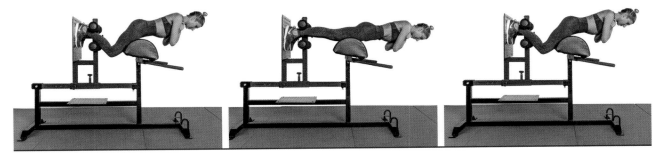

Flex your hips so that your torso is parallel to the ground. Maintaining the same torso position, extend your hips and knees. The moment you reach full hip and knee extension, reverse the motion by curling your legs, shooting your butt back, and bending your hips. The key is to keep your torso parallel to the ground throughout the entire range of motion.

Neutral-Hip GHR

The neutral-hip GHR is much harder than it may seem. It's natural to lean at your hips or anteriorly tilt your pelvis. Your body tends to do that during knee flexion exercises to increase the length of your hamstrings, which increases their strength.

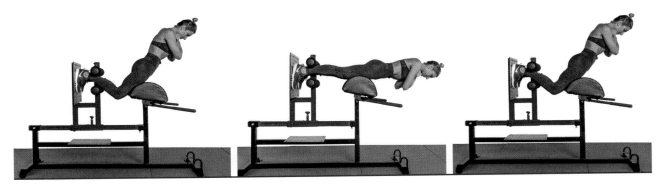

Set up in neutral hip extension and carry out the eccentric and concentric phases while holding this neutral hip and pelvic position.

Prisoner GHR

Raising your arms during exercises like the GHR and the back extension makes them harder because it shifts your center of mass higher up on the body, creating a longer resistance lever.

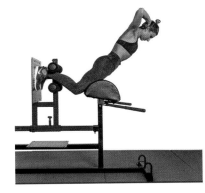

Place your hands behind your head in the prisoner position and perform the GHR movement as previously described.

Dumbbell GHR

You can also make the GHR more difficult by holding onto a dumbbell or weight plate.

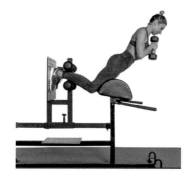

Hold the dumbbell or weight plate just below your chin and execute the GHR movement as previously described.

Banded GHR

Wearing a long band around your neck makes the GHR more difficult. But unlike a dumbbell, which is a constant load, a band provides increasing resistance as it's stretched. This means that down low, where the band isn't stretched as much, there is less tension on your hamstrings, and up high, there is a ton of tension on your hamstrings.

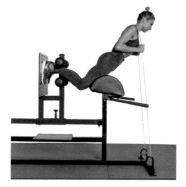

Wrap a long band around the GHD unit and around the back of your neck and perform GHRs as previously described.

Rear-Elevated GHR

A final way to progress the GHR is to elevate the back end of the GHD apparatus. This shifts the strength curve to make the exercise harder at the top and easier at the bottom. In fact, I can get 20 total reps with regular GHRs, but when I perform rear-elevated GHRs, I can get only around 5 reps before my hamstrings are fatigued.

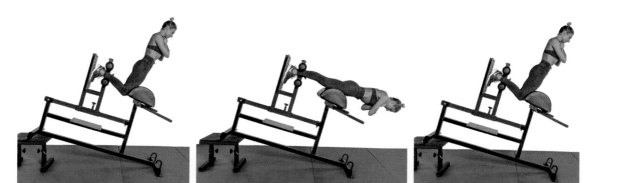

Prop the back end of a GHD on a box or some blocks or steps, then perform the GHR movement as previously described. This variation is very difficult because peak contraction is required of the hamstrings at the top of every rep.

CONCLUSION

Thank you for taking the time to read *Glute Lab*. I hope you have gained valuable insight that will elevate your training to the next level. This edition represents what I know (as of August 2019) to be true. My practical methods and scientific understanding will continue to evolve as I gain more experience and as more research is published. That's how science works. Glen and I intend to update the book every couple of years to keep it up-to-date and comprehensive.

I want to express my unwavering gratitude for every individual out there who has implemented my methods and shared my work. You have helped me popularize the hip thrust and other glute training methods, and I could have never gotten this far without you. Your trust and willingness to try new things have helped advance the fitness industry, and I hope that my methods have added value to your everyday life.

If you enjoyed the book and found some benefit in reading it, I'd love to hear from you. Please share your progress and feel free to ask me questions on Instagram (@bretcontreras1). You can also help the success of the book by taking the time to leave an honest review on amazon.com or barnesandnoble.com. Your feedback and support let me know what you like about the book and what Glen and I can do to make it better, and will provide proof that the principles and methods work, which may inspire others to buy it. So, in addition to helping me out in a big way, you're helping fellow lifters and fitness enthusiasts find the book and advance them toward their glute training goals.

Whether you share the book with your friends on your social media page or leave a review, I want you, the reader, to know how much I appreciate your support.

One of my goals is to create convenient and affordable solutions to improve your glute training. Throughout this book, I've provided pictures of and references to numerous products and services I offer. You can find out more about them at the links below.

To join my Booty by Bret program, visit bootybybret.com

For online training, personalized programming, and other products and services, visit bretcontreras.store

For my range of glute training products, including the Glute Loop, T-Bell, Hip Thruster, Thruster Bar, and Thruster Plates, visit bcstrength.com

For video references demonstrating the exercises included in this book, visit glutelabbook.com

Coming soon—I'm pleased to announce that we'll soon offer Glute Lab certifications and affiliate franchises.

REFERENCES

The references provided refer to the citations numbered in the Science Speak boxes. For a full list of references pertaining to the information covered in this book—more specifically, the studies cited in the main narrative—please go to glutelabbook.com.

Chapter 1: Glute Training for Aesthetics: Science Speak: Improved Aesthetics

1. Kanehisa, H., Nagareda, H., Kawakami, Y., Akima, H., Masani, K., Kouzaki, M., & Fukunaga, T. (2002). "Effects of equivolume isometric training programs comprising medium or high resistance on muscle size and strength." *European Journal of Applied Physiology* 87(2): 112–119.
2. Tracy, B. L., Ivey, F. M., Hurlbut, D., Martel, G. F., Lemmer, J. T., Siegel, E. L. & Hurley, B. F. (1999). "Muscle quality. II. Effects of strength training in 65- to 75-yr-old men and women." *Journal of Applied Physiology* 86(1): 195–201.
3. Seynnes, O. R., de Boer, M., & Narici, M. V. (2007). "Early skeletal muscle hypertrophy and architectural changes in response to high-intensity resistance training." *Journal of Applied Physiology* 102(1): 368–373.
4. Wakahara, T., Fukutani, A., Kawakami, Y., & Yanai, T. (2013). "Nonuniform muscle hypertrophy: its relation to muscle activation in training session." *Medicine & Science in Sports & Exercise* 45(11): 2158–65.
5. Børsheim, E., & Bahr, R. (2003). "Effect of exercise intensity, duration and mode on post-exercise oxygen consumption." *Sports Medicine* 33(14): 1037–60.
6. Heden, T., Lox, C., Rose, P., Reid, S., & Kirk, E. P. (2011). "One-set resistance training elevates energy expenditure for 72 h similar to three sets." *European Journal of Applied Physiology* 111(3): 477–484.
7. Farinatti, P., Castinheiras Neto, A. G., & da Silva, N. L. (2012). "Influence of resistance training variables on excess post-exercise oxygen consumption: a systematic review." International Scholarly Research Notices, 2013.
8. Paoli, A., Moro, T., Marcolin, G., Neri, M., Bianco, A., Palma, A., & Grimaldi, K. (2012). "High-intensity interval resistance training (HIRT) influences resting energy expenditure and respiratory ratio in non-dieting individuals." *Journal of Translational Medicine* 10: 237.

Chapter 2: Glute Training for Health: Science Speak: Reducing Risk of Injury and Pain

1. Alkjær, T., Wieland, M. R., Andersen, M. S., Simonsen, E. B., & Rasmussen, J. (2012). "Computational modeling of a forward lunge: towards a better understanding of the function of the cruciate ligaments." *Journal of Anatomy* 221(6): 590–597.
2. Stecco, A., Gilliar, W., Hill, R., Fullerton, B., & Stecco, C. (2013). "The anatomical and functional relation between gluteus maximus and fascia lata." *Journal of Bodywork and Movement Therapies* 17(4): 512.
3. Bryanton, M. A., Carey, J. P., Kennedy, M. D., & Chiu, L. Z. (2015). "Quadriceps effort during squat exercise depends on hip extensor muscle strategy." *Sports Biomechanics* 14(1): 122–138.
4. Lewis, C. L., Sahrmann, S. A., & Moran, D. W. (2009). "Effect of position and alteration in synergist muscle force contribution on hip forces when performing hip strengthening exercises." *Clinical Biomechanics* 24(1): 35–42.
5. See note 3 above.
6. Vigotsky, A. D., & Bryanton, M. A. (2016). "Relative muscle contributions to net joint moments in the barbell back squat." American Society of Biomechanics 40th Annual Meeting, North Carolina State University, Raleigh, NC.
7. Liu, H., Garrett, W. E., Moorman, C. T., & Yu, B. (2012). "Injury rate, mechanism, and risk factors of hamstring strain injuries in sports: a review of the literature." *Journal of Sport and Health Science* 1(2): 92–101.
8. Mendiguchia, J., Alentorn-Geli, E., Idoate, F., & Myer, G. D. (2013). "Rectus femoris muscle injuries in football: a clinically relevant review of mechanisms of injury, risk factors and preventive strategies." *British Journal of Sports Medicine* 47(6): 359–366.
9. Ryan, J., DeBurca, N., & McCreesh, K. (2014). "Risk factors for groin/hip injuries in field-based sports: a systematic review." *British Journal of Sports Medicine* 48(14): 1089–96.
10. Wiemann, K., & Tidow, G. (1995). "Relative activity of hip and knee extensors in sprinting-implications for training." *New Studies in Athletics* 10: 29–49.
11. Khayambashi, K., Ghoddosi, N., Straub, R. K., & Powers, C. M. (2016). "Hip muscle strength predicts noncontact anterior cruciate ligament injury in male and female athletes: a prospective study." *The American Journal of Sports Medicine* 44(2): 355–361.
12. Hollman, J. H., Ginos, B. E., Kozuchowski, J., Vaughn, A. S., Krause, D. A., & Youdas, J. W. (2009). "Relationships between knee valgus, hip-muscle strength, and hip-muscle recruitment during a single-limb step-down." *Journal of Sport Rehabilitation* 18(1): 104.
13. Hollman, J. H., Hohl, J. M., Kraft, J. L., Strauss, J. D., & Traver, K. J. (2013). "Modulation of frontal-plane knee kinematics by hip-extensor strength and gluteus maximus recruitment during a jump-landing task in healthy women." *Journal of Sport Rehabilitation* 22(3): 184–90.
14. Padua, D. A., Bell, D. R., & Clark, M. A. (2012). "Neuromuscular characteristics of individuals displaying

excessive medial knee displacement." *Journal of Athletic Training* 47(5): 525.

15. Nyman, E., & Armstrong, C. W. (2015). "Real-time feedback during drop landing training improves subsequent frontal and sagittal plane knee kinematics." *Clinical Biomechanics* 30(9): 988–994.

16. Thomson, C., Krouwel, O., Kuisma, R., & Hebron, C. (2016). "The outcome of hip exercise in patellofemoral pain: a systematic review." *Manual Therapy* 26: 1–30.

17. Zalawadia, A., Ruparelia, S. Shah, S., Parekh, D., Patel, S., Rathod, S. P., and Patel, S. V. (2010). "Study of femoral neck anteversion of adult dry femora in Gujarat region." *National Journal of Integrated Research in Medicine* 1(3): 7–11.

18. Beck, M., Kalhor, M., Leunig, M., & Ganz, R. (2005). "Hip morphology influences the pattern of damage to the acetabular cartilage femoroacetabular impingement as a cause of early osteoarthritis of the hip." *Journal of Bone & Joint Surgery,* British Volume 87(7): 1012–18.

19. Lewis, C. L., Sahrmann, S. A., & Moran, D. W. (2007). "Anterior hip joint force increases with hip extension, decreased gluteal force, or decreased iliopsoas force." *Journal of Biomechanics* 40(16): 3725–31.

20. Interview with Stuart McGill by Bret Contreras, retrieved from https://bretcontreras.com/transcribed-interview-with-stu-mcgill/

21. Neumann, D. A. (2010). "Kinesiology of the hip: a focus on muscular actions." *Journal of Orthopaedic & Sports Physical Therapy* 40(2): 82–94.

22. McGill, S. M., & Karpowicz, A. (2009). "Exercises for spine stabilization: motion/motor patterns, stability progressions, and clinical technique." *Archives of Physical Medicine and Rehabilitation* 90(1): 118–126.

23. Gibbons, S. G. T., & Mottram, S. L. (2004). "The anatomy of the deep sacral part of the gluteus maximus and the psoas muscle: a clinical perspective." Proceedings of the 5th Interdisciplinary World Congress on Low Back Pain. November 7–11, Melbourne, Australia.

24. Barker, P. J., Hapuarachchi, K. S., Ross, J. A., Sambaiew, E., Ranger, T. A., & Briggs, C. A. (2014). "Anatomy and biomechanics of gluteus maximus and the thoracolumbar fascia at the sacroiliac joint." *Clinical Anatomy* 27(2): 234–240.

25. Vleeming, A., Van Wingerden, J. P., Snijders, C. J., Stoeckart, R., & Stijnen, T. (1989). "Load application to the sacrotuberous ligament: influences on sacroiliac joint mechanics." *Clinical Biomechanics* 4(4): 204–209.

26. Snijders, C. J., Vleeming, A., & Stoeckart, R. (1993). "Transfer of lumbosacral load to iliac bones and legs: part 1: biomechanics of self-bracing of the sacroiliac joints and its significance for treatment and exercise." *Clinical Biomechanics* 8(6): 285–294.

27. Lafond, D., Normand, M. C., & Gosselin, G. (1998). "Rapport force/déplacement du sacrum et efficacité du mécanisme de verrouillage de l'articulation sacro-iliaque; Étude en conditions expérimentales in vivo." *The Journal of the Canadian Chiropractic Association* 42(2): 90.

28. Cohen, S. P. (2005). "Sacroiliac joint pain: a comprehensive review of anatomy, diagnosis, and treatment." *Anesthesia & Analgesia* 101(5): 1440–53.

Chapter 3: Glute Training for Strength: Science Speak: Hip Thrust Strength

1. Contreras, B. (2015, August 4). "Squats versus hip thrusts part II: the twin experiment." [Blog post]. Retrieved from https://bretcontreras.com/squats-versus-hip-thrusts-part-ii-the-twin-experiment/.

2. Contreras, B., Vigotsky, A. D., Schoenfeld, B. J., Beardsley, C., McMaster, D. T., Reyneke, J. H., & Cronin, J. B. (2017). "Effects of a six-week hip thrust vs. front squat resistance training program on performance in adolescent males: a randomized controlled trial." *The Journal of Strength & Conditioning Research* 31(4): 999–1008.

3. Lin, K. H., Wu, C. M., Huang, Y. M., & Cai, Z. Y. (2017). "Effects of hip thrust training on the strength and power performance in collegiate baseball players." *Journal of Sports Science* 5: 178–184.

4. Hammond, A., Perrin, C., Steele, J., Giessing, J., Gentil, P., & Fisher, J. P. (2019). "The effects of a 4-week mesocycle of barbell back squat or barbell hip thrust strength training upon isolated lumbar extension strength." *PeerJ,* published ahead of print.

Chapter 4: Glute Training for Performance: Science Speak: Function and Performance

1. Shin, S. J., Kim, T. Y., & Yoo, W. G. (2013). "Effects of various gait speeds on the latissimus dorsi and gluteus maximus muscles associated with the posterior oblique sling system." *Journal of Physical Therapy Science* 25(11): 1391.

2. Kim, T. Y., Yoo, W. G., An, D. H., Oh, J. S., & Shin, S. J. (2013b). "The effects of different gait speeds and lower arm weight on the activities of the latissimus dorsi, gluteus medius, and gluteus maximus muscles." *Journal of Physical Therapy Science* 25(11): 1483.

3. Lewis, J., Freisinger, G., Pan, X., Siston, R., Schmitt, L., & Chaudhari, A. (2015). "Changes in lower extremity peak angles, moments and muscle activations during stair climbing at different speeds." *Journal of Electromyography and Kinesiology* 25(6): 982–989.

4. Savelberg, H. H. C. M., Fastenau, A., Willems, P. J. B., & Meijer, K. (2007). "The load/capacity ratio affects the sit-to-stand movement strategy." *Clinical Biomechanics* 22(7): 805–812.

5. McGill, S. M., & Marshall, L. W. (2012). "Kettlebell swing, snatch, and bottoms-up carry: back and hip muscle activation, motion, and low back loads." *The Journal of Strength & Conditioning Research* 26(1): 16.

6. McGill, S. M., McDermott, A., & Fenwick, C. M. (2009b). "Comparison of different strongman events: trunk muscle activation and lumbar spine motion, load, and stiffness." *The Journal of Strength & Conditioning Research* 23(4): 1148–61.

7. Winwood, P. W., Keogh, J. W., & Harris, N. K. (2012). "Interrelationships between strength, anthropometrics, and strongman performance in novice strongman athletes." *The Journal of Strength & Conditioning Research* 26(2): 513–522.

8. See note 6 above.

9. Beardsley, C., & Contreras, B. (2014). "The increasing role of the hip extensor musculature with heavier compound

lower-body movements and more explosive sport actions." *Strength & Conditioning Journal* 36(2): 49–55.

10. Bryanton, M. A., & Chiu, L. Z. (2014). "Hip- versus knee-dominant task categorization oversimplifies multijoint dynamics." *Strength & Conditioning Journal* 36(4): 98–99.

11. Beardsley, C., & Contreras, B. (2014). "Increasing role of hips supported by electromyography and musculoskeletal modeling." *Strength & Conditioning Journal* 36(4): 100–101.

12. Dorn, T. W., Schache, A. G., & Pandy, M. G. (2012). "Muscular strategy shift in human running: dependence of running speed on hip and ankle muscle performance." *The Journal of Experimental Biology* 215(11): 1944–56.

13. Kyröläinen, H., Komi, P. V., & Belli, A. (1999). "Changes in muscle activity patterns and kinetics with increasing running speed." *The Journal of Strength & Conditioning Research* 13(4): 400–406.

14. Kyröläinen, H. K., Belli, A., & Komi, P. V. (2001). "Biomechanical factors affecting running economy." Medicine & Science Sports & Exercise 33(8): 1330–7.

15. Kyröläinen, H., Avela, J., & Komi, P. V. (2005). "Changes in muscle activity with increasing running speed." *Journal of Sports Sciences* 23(10): 1101–9.

16. Willson, J. D., Kernozek, T. W., Arndt, R. L., Reznichek, D. A., & Straker, J. S. (2011). "Gluteal muscle activation during running in females with and without patellofemoral pain syndrome." *Clinical Biomechanics* 26(7): 735–740.

17. Inaba, Y., Yoshioka, S., Iida, Y., Hay, D. C., & Fukashiro, S. (2013). "A biomechanical study of side steps at different distances." *Journal of Applied Biomechanics* 29(3): 336–345.

18. Shimokochi, Y., Ide, D., Kokubu, M., & Nakaoji, T. (2013). "Relationships among performance of lateral cutting maneuver from lateral sliding and hip extension and abduction motions, ground reaction force, and body center of mass height." *The Journal of Strength & Conditioning Research* 27(7): 1851–60.

19. Roach, N. T., & Lieberman, D. E. (2014). "Upper body contributions to power generation during rapid, overhand throwing in humans." *Journal of Experimental Biology* 217 (Pt 12): 2139–49.

20. Campbell, B. M., Stodden, D. F., & Nixon, M. K. (2010). "Lower extremity muscle activation during baseball pitching." *The Journal of Strength & Conditioning Research* 24(4): 964–971.

21. Oliver, G. D., & Keeley, D. W. (2010). "Gluteal muscle group activation and its relationship with pelvis and torso kinematics in high-school baseball pitchers." *The Journal of Strength & Conditioning Research* 24(11): 3015–22.

Chapter 5: Anatomy of the Glutes

Science Speak: Differences Between Male and Female Hip Anatomy

1. Wang, S. C., Brede, C., Lange, D., Poster, C. S., Lange, A. W., Kohoyda-Inglis, C., Sochor, M. R., Ipaktchi, K., & Rowe, S. A. (2004). "Gender differences in hip anatomy: possible implications for injury tolerance in frontal collisions." *Annals of Advances in Automotive Medicine* 48: 287–301.

2. Musielak, B., Rychlik, M., & Jozwiak, M. (2016). "Sexual dimorphism of acetabular anatomy based on three-dimensional computed tomography image of pelvises." *Journal of Orthopedics, Traumatology and Rehabilitation* 18(5): 451–459.

3. Seike, K., Koda, K., Oda, K., Kosugi, C., Shimizu, K., & Miyazaki, M. (2009). "Gender differences in pelvic anatomy and effects on rectal cancer surgery." *Hepatogastroenterology* 56(89): 111–5.

4. Bailey, J. F., Sparrey, C. J., Been, E., & Kramer, P. A. (2016). "Morphological and postural sexual dimorphism of the lumbar spine facilitates greater lordosis in females." *Journal of Anatomy* 229(1): 82–91.

5. Czuppon, S., Prather, H., Hunt, D. M., Steger-May, K., Bloom, N. J., Clohisy, J. C., Larsen, R., & Harris-Hayes, M. (2017). "Gender-dependent differences in hip range of motion and impingement testing in asymptomatic college freshman athletes." *Journal of Injury Function and Rehabilitation* 9(7): 660–667.

6. Hogg, J. A., Schmitz, R. J., Nguyen, A. D., & Shultz, S. J. (2018). "Passive hip range-of-motion values across sex and sport." *Journal of Athletic Training* 53(6): 560–567.

7. Grelsamer, R. P., Dubey, A., & Weinstein, C. H. (2005). "Men and women have similar Q angles: a clinical and trigonometric evaluation." *Journal of Bone and Joint Surgery* 87(11): 1498–1501.

8. Russell, K. A., Palmieri, R. M., Zinder, S. M., & Ingersoll, C. D. (2006). "Sex differences in valgus knee angle during a single-leg drop jump." *Journal of Athletic Training* 41(2): 166–171.

9. Norton, B. J., Sahrmann, S. A., & Van Dillen, L. R. (2004). "Differences in measurements of lumbar curvature related to gender and low back pain." *Journal of Orthopaedic & Sports Physical Therapy* 34(9): 524–534.

10. Preininger, B., Schmorl, K., von Roth, P., Winkler, T., Matziolis, G., Perka, C., & Tohtz, S. (2012). "The sex specificity of hip-joint muscles offers an explanation for better results in men after total hip arthroplasty." *International Orthopaedics* 36(6): 1143–8.

Science Speak: Muscle Size

11. Ito, J. (1996). "Morphological analysis of the human lower extremity based on the relative muscle weight." *Okajimas Folia Anatomica Japonica* 73(5): 247–251.

12. Ito, J., Moriyama, H., Inokuchi, S., & Goto, N. (2003). "Human lower limb muscles: an evaluation of weight and fiber size." *Okajimas Folia Anatomica Japonica* 80(2–3): 47–55.

13. Pohtilla, J. F. (1969). "Kinesiology of hip extension at selected angles of pelvifemoral extension." Archives of *Physical Medicine and Rehabilitation* 50(5): 241–250.

14. Arokoski, M. H., Arokoski, J. P., Haara, M., Kankaanpää, M., Vesterinen, M., Niemitukia, L. H., & Helminen, H. J. (2002). "Hip muscle strength and muscle cross sectional area in men with and without hip osteoarthritis." *The Journal of Rheumatology* 29(10): 2185–95.

15. Kamaz, M., Kiresi, D., Oguz, H., Emlik, D., & Levendoglu, F. (2007). "CT measurement of trunk muscle areas in patients with chronic low back pain." *Diagnostic and Interventional Radiology* 13(3): 144–148.

16. Wu, G. A., & Bogie, K. (2009). "Assessment of gluteus maximus muscle area with different image analysis programs." *Archives of Physical Medicine and Rehabilitation* 90(6): 1048–54.

17. Ahedi, H., Aitken, D., Scott, D., Blizzard, L., Cicuttini, F., & Jones, G. (2014). "The association between hip muscle cross-sectional area, muscle strength, and bone mineral density." *Calcified Tissue International* 95(1): 64–72.

18. Yasuda, T., Fukumura, K., Fukuda, T., Uchida, Y., Iida, H., Meguro, M., & Nakajima, T. (2014). "Muscle size and arterial stiffness after blood flow–restricted low-intensity resistance training in older adults." *Scandinavian Journal of Medicine & Science in Sports* 24(5): 799–806.

19. Niinimäki, S., Härkönen, L., Nikander, R., Abe, S., Knüsel, C., & Sievänen, H. (2016). "The cross-sectional area of the gluteus maximus muscle varies according to habitual exercise loading: Implications for activity-related and evolutionary studies." *HOMO–Journal of Comparative Human Biology* 67(2): 125–137.

20. Uemura, K., Takao, M., Sakai, T., Nishii, T., & Sugano, N. (2016). "Volume increases of the gluteus maximus, gluteus medius, and thigh muscles after hip arthroplasty." *The Journal of Arthroplasty* 31(4): 906–912.

21. See note 10 above.

22. See note 19 above.

Science Speak: Muscle Architecture

23. Lieber, R. L., & Fridén, J. (2000). "Functional and clinical significance of skeletal muscle architecture." *Muscle & Nerve* 23(11): 1647–66.

24. Ward, S. R., Eng, C. M., Smallwood, L. H., & Lieber, R. L. (2009). "Are current measurements of lower extremity muscle architecture accurate?" *Clinical Orthopaedics and Related Research* 467(4): 1074–82.

25. Barker, P. J., Hapuarachchi, K. S., Ross, J. A., Sambaiew, E., Ranger, T. A., & Briggs, C. A. (2014). "Anatomy and biomechanics of gluteus maximus and the thoracolumbar fascia at the sacroiliac joint." *Clinical Anatomy* 27(2): 234–240.

26. Friederich, J. A., & Brand, R. A. (1990). "Muscle fiber architecture in the human lower limb." *Journal of Biomechanics* 23(1): 91–95.

27. Horsman, M. K., Koopman, H. F. J. M., Van der Helm, F. C. T., Prosé, L. P., & Veeger, H. E. J. (2007). "Morphological muscle and joint parameters for musculoskeletal modelling of the lower extremity." *Clinical Biomechanics* 22(2): 239–247.

Chapter 6: Function of the Glutes

Joint Actions

1. Neumann, D. A. (2010). "Kinesiology of the hip: a focus on muscular actions." *Journal of Orthopaedic & Sports Physical Therapy* 40(2): 82–94.

2. Wilson, J., Ferris, E., Heckler, A., Maitland, L., & Taylor, C. (2005). "A structured review of the role of gluteus maximus in rehabilitation." *New Zealand Journal of Physiotherapy* 33(3).

Science Speak: Hip Extension

3. Gibbons, S. G. T., & Mottram, S. L. (2004). "The anatomy of the deep sacral part of the gluteus maximus and the psoas muscle: a clinical perspective." Proceedings of the 5th Interdisciplinary World Congress on Low Back Pain. November 7–11, Melbourne, Australia.

4. Dostal, W. F., Soderberg, G. L., & Andrews, J. G. (1986). "Actions of hip muscles." *Physical Therapy* 66(3): 351.

5. Blemker, S. S., & Delp, S. L. (2005). "Three-dimensional representation of complex muscle architectures and geometries." *Annals of Biomedical Engineering* 33(5): 661–673.

6. Németh, G., & Ohlsén, H. (1985). "In vivo moment arm lengths for hip extensor muscles at different angles of hip flexion." *Journal of Biomechanics* 18(2): 129–140.

7. Contreras, B., Vigotsky, A. D., Schoenfeld, B. J., Beardsley, C., & Cronin, J. (2015). "A comparison of two gluteus maximus EMG maximum voluntary isometric contraction positions." *PeerJ* 3: e1261.

8. Anders, M. (2006). *Glutes to the Max.* ACE, 7.

9. Yamashita, N. (1988). "EMG activities in mono- and bi-articular thigh muscles in combined hip and knee extension." *European Journal of Applied Physiology and Occupational Physiology* 58(3): 274–277.

10. Fischer, F. J., & Houtz, S. J. (1968). "Evaluation of the function of the gluteus maximus muscle: an electromyographic study." *American Journal of Physical Medicine & Rehabilitation* 47(4): 182.

11. Worrell, T. W., Karst, G., Adamczyk, D., Moore, R., Stanley, C., Steimel, B., & Steimel, S. (2001). "Influence of joint position on electromyographic and torque generation during maximal voluntary isometric contractions of the hamstrings and gluteus maximus muscles." *The Journal of Orthopaedic and Sports Physical Therapy* 31(12): 730.

12. Kang, S. Y., Jeon, H. S., Kwon, O., Cynn, H. S., & Choi, B. (2013). "Activation of the gluteus maximus and hamstring muscles during prone hip extension with knee flexion in three hip abduction positions." *Manual Therapy* 18(4): 303–307.

13. Suehiro, T., Mizutani, M., Okamoto, M., Ishida, H., Kobara, K., Fujita, D., & Watanabe, S. (2014). "Influence of hip joint position on muscle activity during prone hip extension with knee flexion." *Journal of Physical Therapy Science* 26(12): 1895.

14. Queiroz, B. C., Cagliari, M. F., Amorim, C. F., & Sacco, I. C. (2010). "Muscle activation during four Pilates core stability exercises in quadruped position." *Archives of Physical Medicine and Rehabilitation* 91(1): 86–92.

15. Sakamoto, A. C. L., Teixeira-Salmela, L. F., de Paula-Goulart, F. R., de Morais Faria, C. D. C., & Guimarães, C. Q. (2009). "Muscular activation patterns during active prone hip extension exercises." *Journal of Electromyography and Kinesiology* 19(1): 105–112.

16. Park, S. Y., & Yoo, W. G. (2014). "Effects of hand and knee positions on muscular activity during trunk extension exercise with the Roman chair." *Journal of Electrophysiology and Kinesiology* 24(6): 972–976.

17. Kim, S. M., & Yoo, W. G. (2015). "Comparison of trunk and hip muscle activity during different degrees of lumbar and

hip extension." *Journal of Physical Therapy Science* 27(9): 2717.

18. See note 15 above.

Science Speak: Hip External Rotation

19. See note 1 above.
20. See note 3 above.
21. Stecco, A., Gilliar, W., Hill, R., Fullerton, B., & Stecco, C. (2013). "The anatomical and functional relation between gluteus maximus and fascia lata." *Journal of Bodywork and Movement Therapies* 17(4): 512.
22. See note 4 above.
23. Delp, S. L., Hess, W. E., Hungerford, D. S., & Jones, L. C. (1999). "Variation of rotation moment arms with hip flexion." *Journal of Biomechanics* 32(5): 493–501.
24. Macadam, P., Cronin, J., & Contreras, B. (2015). "An examination of the gluteal muscle activity associated with dynamic hip abduction and hip external rotation exercise: a systematic review." *International Journal of Sports Physical Therapy* 10(5): 573.

Chapter 7: The Role of Genetics: Science Speak: Mechanisms of Genetic Impact on Hypertrophy

1. Petrella, J. K., Kim, J. S., Mayhew, D. L., Cross, J. M., & Bamman, M. M. (2008). "Potent myofiber hypertrophy during resistance training in humans is associated with satellite cell-mediated myonuclear addition: a cluster analysis." *Journal of Applied Physiology* 104: 1736–42.
2. Bamman, M. M., Petrella, J. K., Kim, J. S., Mayhew, D. L., & Cross, J. M. (2007). "Cluster analysis tests the importance of myogenic gene expression during myofiber hypertrophy in humans." *Journal of Applied Physiology* 102: 2232–9.
3. Puthucheary, Z., Skipworth, J. R., Rawal, J., Loosemore, M., Van Someren, K., & Montgomery, H. E. (2011). "Genetic influences in sport and physical performance." *Sports Medicine* 41(10): 845–859.
4. Seeman, E., Hopper, J. L., Young, N. R., Formica, C., Goss, P., & Tsalamandris, C. (1996). "Do genetic factors explain associations between muscle strength, lean mass, and bone density? A twin study." *The American Journal of Physiology* 270(2 Pt 1): E320.
5. Arden, N. K., & Spector, T. D. (1997). "Genetic influences on muscle strength, lean body mass, and bone mineral density: a twin study." *Journal of Bone and Mineral Research* 12(12): 2076–81.
6. Nguyen, T. V., Howard, G. M., Kelly, P. J., & Eisman, J. A. (1998). "Bone mass, lean mass, and fat mass: same genes or same environments?" *American Journal of Epidemiology* 147(1): 3–16.
7. Bray, M. S., Hagberg, J. M., Pérusse, L., Rankinen, T., Roth, S. M., Wolfarth, B., & Bouchard, C. (2009). "The human gene map for performance and health-related fitness phenotypes: the 2006–2007 update." *Medicine & Science in Sports & Exercise* 41(1): 35.
8. Pescatello, L. S., Devaney, J. M., Hubal, M. J., Thompson, P. D., & Hoffman, E. P. (2013). "Highlights from the functional single nucleotide polymorphisms associated with human muscle size and strength or FAMuSS Study." *BioMed Research International*, 2013.

Chapter 8: How Muscle Grows: Science Speak: Muscle Fibers

1. Scott, W., Stevens, J., & Binder–Macleod, S. A. (2001). "Human skeletal muscle fiber type classifications." *Physical Therapy* 81(11): 1810–16.
2. Ogborn, D., & Schoenfeld, B. J. (2014). "The role of fiber types in muscle hypertrophy: implications for loading strategies." *Strength & Conditioning Journal* 36(2): 20–25.
3. Mitchell, C. J., Churchward-Venne, T. A., West, D. W., Burd, N. A., Breen, L., Baker, S. K., & Phillips, S. M. (2012). "Resistance exercise load does not determine training-mediated hypertrophic gains in young men." *Journal of Applied Physiology* 113(1): 71–77.
4. Campos, G. E., Luecke, T. J., Wendeln, H. K., Toma, K., Hagerman, F. C., Murray, T. F., & Staron, R. S. (2002). "Muscular adaptations in response to three different resistance-training regimens: specificity of repetition maximum training zones." *European Journal of Applied Physiology* 88(1–2): 50–60.
5. Johnson, M., Polgar, J., Weightman, D., & Appleton, D. (1973). "Data on the distribution of fibre types in thirty-six human muscles: an autopsy study." *Journal of the Neurological Sciences* 18(1): 111–129.
6. Širca, A., & Sušec-Michieli, M. (1980). "Selective type II fibre muscular atrophy in patients with osteoarthritis of the hip." *Journal of the Neurological Sciences* 44(2): 149–159.

Chapter 10: Exercise Categorization

Science Speak: Exercise Categorization

1. Loturco, I., Tricoli, V., Roschel, H., Nakamura, F. Y., Abad, C. C. C., Kobal, R., & González-Badillo, J. J. (2014). "Transference of traditional versus complex strength and power training to sprint performance." *Journal of Human Kinetics* 41(1): 265–273.
2. Siff, Mel. *Supertraining*. 5th Ed. Supertraining Institute, 2003: 201.
3. Siff, 240.

Science Speak: Moment Arms and Planes of Motion

4. Dostal, W. F., Soderberg, G. L., & Andrews, J. G. (1986). "Actions of hip muscles." *Physical Therapy* 66(3): 351.

Science Speak: Knee Action

5. Sakamoto, A. C. L., Teixeira-Salmela, L. F., de Paula-Goulart, F. R., de Morais Faria, C. D. C., & Guimarães, C. Q. (2009). "Muscular activation patterns during active prone hip extension exercises." *Journal of Electromyography and Kinesiology* 19(1): 105–112.
6. Kwon, Y. J., & Lee, H. O. (2013). "How different knee flexion angles influence the hip extensor in the prone position." *Journal of Physical Therapy Science* 25(10): 1295.

INDEX